Mastering Competencies in Family Therapy

A PRACTICAL APPROACH TO THEORIES AND CLINICAL CASE DOCUMENTATION

Third Edition

DIANE R. GEHART

California State University, Northridge

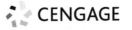 CENGAGE

Australia • Brazil • Canada • Mexico • Singapore • United Kingdom • United States

CENGAGE

Mastering Competencies in Family Therapy:
A Practical Approach to Theories and Clinical
Case Documentation, **Third Edition**
Diane R. Gehart

Product Director: Marta Lee-Perriard

Product Manager: Julie Martinez

Content Developer: Trudy Brown

Product Assistant: Megan Nauer

Digital Content Specialist: Jaclyn Hermesmeyer

Marketing Manager: Zina Craft

Manufacturing Planner: Karen Hunt

Photo Researcher: Lumina Datamatics

Art and Cover Direction, Production
    Management, and Composition: MPS Ltd.

Text and Cover Designer: MPS Ltd.

Cover Image Credit: iStockPhoto.com/BraunS

For product information and technology assistance, contact us at
Cengage Customer & Sales Support, 1-800-354-9706.

For permission to use material from this text or product,
submit all requests online at **www.cengage.com/permissions**.
Further permissions questions can be e-mailed to
permissionrequest@cengage.com.

Library of Congress Control Number: 2017933382

Student Edition:
ISBN: 978-1-305-943278

Loose-leaf Edition:
ISBN: 978-1-337-117739

Cengage
200 Pier 4 Boulevard
Boston, MA 02210
USA

Cengage is a leading provider of customized learning solutions with employees
residing in nearly 40 different countries and sales in more than 125 countries
around the world. Find your local representative at **www.cengage.com**.

To learn more about Cengage platforms and services, register or access
your online learning solution, or purchase materials for your course, visit
www.cengage.com.

Printed at CLDPC, USA, 06-21

In the past few years, the field of family therapy has lost many whose contributions are our mainstay. This book is dedicated to those who have paved the way for the next generation. We are forever in their debt.

Gianfranco Cecchin
Whose laughter, humility, and acceptance transformed me

Tom Andersen
Whose presence was angelic: the most "gentle" man I have ever met

Paul Watzlawick
Whose courage and kind words I shall never forget

Steve de Shazer
Whose brilliance dazzled me

Insoo Kim Berg
Whose energy and enthusiasm inspired the best in me

Michael White
Whose ideas opened new worlds for me

Jay Haley
Who taught me the logic of paradox

Ivan Boszormenyi-Nagy
Who reminded me to focus on what really matters

Peggy Penn
Who taught me how putting pen to paper can transform the world

Brief Table of Contents

Detailed Table of Contents

Becoming Competent with Competencies, or What I Have Learned About Learning

Even though I have been teaching in one form or another since 1978, I was never formally schooled in educational concepts like student learning outcomes, rubrics, and competencies. I, like many of my colleagues, followed a tried-and-true method of teaching—how I remembered being taught by those teachers I admired the most and not teaching how I recalled being instructed by those teachers I dreaded the most. (With this steadfast educational philosophy intact, I, along with my fellow teachers in the elementary, middle, and high schools and community colleges and universities, would approach the latest, greatest new educational theory, model, or fad rolled out by well-meaning, earnest administrators and instructional specialists with the same disinterest as some of our students would embrace our own zealous pronouncements of the importance of mastering algebra, knowing who Charlemagne was, and differentiating between first- and second-order change.) Funny as it seems, we as teachers and students appeared to share the same lament—what does all this learning stuff have to do with being successful in the real world? Now looking back 30 years later, I have come to the realization that learning has everything to do with being successful, and that learning is not the same thing as teaching.

Learning about Learning

I have always loved learning, although I was not always crazy about school. I was one of those students who lived by the proverb to never let my schooling get in the way of my education. Today I live by another proverb when it comes to working—to never let my job get in the way of my career, but that is a preface for another book.

It was this apparent paradox of loving learning but not loving school that led me to think about what made the two processes so different in my mind and life. For me, the main difference between learning and schooling seemed to be predicated on who decided what needed to be learned and who directed the learning process. When I was able to explore what interested me, acquire information I felt I needed to master, and access mentors who could help facilitate my learning, I was always more successful in achieving my goals and objectives.

With this new revelation filling my head, I started to think how I could share this way of learning with my students. The first step in this epiphany was to see that my students were not that different from me. They too liked to learn what they liked to learn, so I made this insight the centerpiece of my learning-centric approach. The second step was to see learning not as an epic dyadic struggle between me as the omniscient and omnipotent teacher who possessed all knowledge and wisdom and the students as reluctant, empty opponents needing to be directed and taught, but rather as a triadic arrangement involving three interrelated parts: the student, a body of knowledge or group of skills, and me. In this configuration, I find I am no longer in conflict with students, forcing them to learn what I deem to be privileged knowledge; instead, I now try to learn what students aspire to become; help them define this aspiration as goals, objectives, and competencies; and work with them to support and facilitate their learning journeys.

Taking this approach was liberating for me and startling for many of my students. In their formal schooling, many of them had never been asked to be proactive with their learning; however, like me, they all found they could learn well when they could be in charge of their own learning. Having confidence that students were really like me and could learn very well on their own was an insight I wanted to put into practice in my work with marriage and family therapy (MFT) graduate students.

Being Competent with Competencies

Most students who choose to matriculate in therapy programs like counseling, clinical psychology, social work, or family therapy really want to be therapists or counselors. The challenge is that students usually do not know all the things they will want to know before they know them. We always wish we knew *then* what we know now. Students who want to become competent marriage and family therapists are no different.

We now seem to be in the world of competencies for marriage and family therapists. The American Association for Marriage and Family Therapy (AAMFT) initiated a dialogue in which marriage and family therapists reflected on what they knew about being effective therapists and shared these insights with one another. Through this ongoing, collaborative process, the AAMFT Core Competencies were born (Nelson et al., 2007), with the result that therapists can now clearly define what competent marriage and family therapists should be able to accomplish in their work with clients.

The effort to create this set of competencies originated within a number of critical contexts. Health care policymakers in Washington wanted practitioners to be clearer about what they did and did not do with their patients and clients. Consumers also wanted clarity in what they could expect licensed professionals to deliver. Higher education accreditation professionals and policymakers wanted educators to take an outcomes-based approach to learning and to become more accountable to students and employers so that all interested parties could know what could be expected from graduates of specific degree and training programs.

The good news was that the competencies were here. We as MFT educators could work from a system that was specific enough to communicate learning objectives and outcomes so that we, along with our students, could have reasonable expectations of what becoming competent family therapists would entail, while being generic enough for us to be creative in facilitating and supporting our students as they began the journey to become therapists.

Of course, the bad news was also that the competencies were here. Most of us had not been educated in this style of learning when we were training to become therapists. We also had not been trained as faculty members and supervisors to educate our students in this manner. The challenge before us was how to become competent with the competencies. And that is where Diane Gehart's delightful new book comes in.

To meet this challenge, Diane, like many of us, has had to learn about learning to become competent with the competencies! She has taken the best of the learning-centered approaches and has woven in the latest clinical innovations and scholarship from the world of marriage and family therapy to create a clear and concise set of learning outcomes that can become that third partner with students and faculty to form a triadic learning model.

In the first part of the book, Diane introduces her readers to this wonderful world of learning in which teachers and students work together to learn new knowledge and

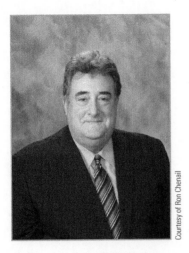

Courtesy of Ron Chenail

skills in the pursuit of transparent and mutually beneficial goals. She then deconstructs the Core Competencies into the basics of case conceptualization, clinical assessment, treatment planning, evaluation, and documentation, making them more readily apparent to the beginning marital and family therapist. Finally, she reconstructs MFT learning by bringing modern and postmodern approaches into this world of learning outcomes and competencies so that we can skillfully conceptualize, assess, treat, evaluate, and document our work, regardless of the clinical approach we embrace.

In this new edition, Diane has taken great care to make the learning more experiential by inviting her readers to try things for themselves via practice prompts for building clinical skills and through reflective questions to consider mindfully what they have learned and how they can apply these ideas to their clinical work in a practical way. These learning practices will help readers to become more active and responsible in their own learning process as they are asked to translate theory and research into clinical practice in a very personal way.

I encourage you to learn how Diane has learned how to learn marriage and family therapy in a loving way so that you too can become proficient with the MFT competencies, common factors, and evidence-based practice. If you do, I think you will come away from this book with a new appreciation and affection for learning and be positioned well to become a more mindful, ethical, and competent therapist.

Ronald J. Chenail, Ph.D.
Ft. Lauderdale, Florida

REFERENCE

Nelson, T. S., Chenail, R. J., Alexander, J. F., Crane, D. R., Johnson, S. M., & Schwallie, L. (2007). The development of core competencies for the practice of marriage and family therapy. *Journal of Marital and Family Therapy, 33*(4), 417–438. doi:10.1111/j.1752-0606.2007.00042.x

Preface

The Purpose of This Book

Mastering Competencies in Family Therapy is designed to be an efficient and highly effective means of teaching new therapists to master the essential competencies necessary to succeed in doing couples and family therapy in the 21st century. As an instructor in an accredited program and university that is required to measure student learning, I needed something that would enable me to effectively measure student learning. Although I created comprehensive assessment systems for measuring student mastery of competencies (Gehart, 2007, 2009), I realized that in order to do so, the students needed resources that meaningfully provided them with the detailed knowledge they need to actually develop real-world skills. In short, I needed something more than a text that simply offered solid but old school "book knowledge"; I needed a resource that eloquently responded to my students' everyday training experiences and needs. This book was written to be the missing link between theory and practice that my students needed.

Text Overview

Using state-of-the-art pedagogical methods, this text is part of a new generation of textbooks, ones that are correlated with national standards for measuring student learning in the mental health professions, including counseling, family therapy, psychology, and social work. Using a learning-centered, outcome-based pedagogy, the text engages students in an *active learning process* rather than delivering content in a traditional narrative style. More specifically, the text introduces family therapy theories using: (a) theory-informed case conceptualization, (b) clinical assessment, (c) treatment planning, and (d) progress notes. These assignments empower students to apply theoretical concepts and develop real-world skills as early as possible in their training, resulting in greater mastery of the material. In addition, the text includes extensive discussions about how diversity issues and research inform the contemporary practice of family therapy.

Furthermore, I use a down-to-earth style to explain concepts in clear and practical language that contemporary students appreciate. Instructors will enjoy the simplicity of having the text and assignments work seamlessly together, thus requiring less time spent in class preparation and grading. The extensive set of instructor materials—which include syllabi templates, detailed PowerPoint slides, test banks, online lectures, and scoring rubrics designed for accreditation assessment—further reduce educators' workloads. In summary, the book employs the most efficient and effective pedagogical methods available to family therapy theories, resulting in a win–win for instructors and students.

What's New in the Third Edition

Students and instructors familiar with the second version of the text will notice a similar style and format and also appreciate numerous enhancements:

- **Video series:** A series of videos designed to accompany the text will be released with this edition. Ranging from 30 to 60 minutes, these videos are designed to teach a single intervention—such as enactment in structural therapy or sculpting in Satir's approach—and provides viewers with very specific instructions from leading experts. In addition, during the interview, significant therapeutic moments are identified and explained on the bottom of the screen to enable new clinicians to understand the thinking of the therapist during the session. Finally, the videos include a debriefing session with clients in which they share their personal experience during the session and their reflections; in virtually every video, the client debriefing provides some of the most useful instructions to viewers. Instructors who adopt the book will have free access to these videos to stream in class via Cengage's www.cengagebrain.com. Students and professionals can access the videos individually for a nominal fee on www.cengagebrain.com. The video topics include:
  - **Systemic–strategic therapy:** Ordeals
  - **Structural therapy:** Enactments
  - **Satir Human Growth Model:** Sculpting
  - **Emotionally focused couples/family therapy:** Tracking the negative interaction cycle
  - **Bowen Intergenerational:** Constructing a genogram in session with clients
  - **Cognitive–behavioral family therapy:** Teaching families with a child diagnosed with ADHD to practice mindfulness
  - **Solution-based:** Solution-focused scaling to designed homework assignments
  - **Narrative therapy:** Preferred narrative
  - **Collaborative therapy with reflecting teams:** Mutual puzzling and reflecting team.
- **MindTap version of text:** The third edition of this text will be available on MindTap, a state-of-the-art learning platform that maximizes and significantly expands the learning experience by integrating video, role-plays, connection with peers and instructors, external journal articles, flash cards, assignments, etc.
- **Theory-specific case conceptualization forms:** In response to instructor requests, theory-specific case conceptualization forms have been added for each theory. New clinicians can use these forms to develop a theory-specific case conceptualization. Still included, the former "Systemic Case Conceptualization" has been renamed "Cross-Theoretical Systemic Case Conceptualization." This form is ideal for programs that want to measure student learning related to all couples and family therapy theories.
- **Cross-theoretical comparison:** Couples and family therapy theories are now compared in each chapter using Karl Tomm's approach to conceptualizing interpersonal patterns. Tomm's approach includes conceptualizing not only pathologizing interpersonal patterns but also healing, wellness, transformation (therapeutic), deteriorating, and sociocultural interpersonal patterns (Tomm et al., 2014). This flexible yet comprehensive approach to conceptualizing systemic patterns provides an unparalleled method for comparing theories and has significantly improved my students' ability to understand the theories presented in this book. The foundations of Tomm's approach is introduced in Chapter 3, and then each chapter on a specific theory includes a section that translates the theory into Tomm's interpersonal patterns.
- **Cross-theoretical comparison table:** Chapter 3, "Philosophical Foundations of Family Therapy Theories," includes a table that compares how each approach: (a) conceptualizes interpersonal patterns, (b) defines wellness interpersonal patterns, and (c) intervenes to transform interpersonal patterns, allowing new practitioners to more quickly grasp similarities and differences between theories.

- Revised treatment plan form: The treatment plan has been streamlined to include more meaningful explorations of diversity and the evidence base. Enthusiastically received by students, the new shorter form is organized as follows:
  - Goals with interventions and option to set measurable targets
  - Treatment tasks, including developing a therapeutic relationship, developing a case conceptualization and assessment, and managing crises/referrals
  - Diversity considerations, which prompts clinicians to discuss how a wide range of diversity factors and contexts were addressed in the plan
  - Evidence-based practice section, which prompts students to identify relevant research to support their plan; the resources for this section are covered both in the general review of the couple and family therapy evidence in Chapter 2 and in the "Research and Evidence Base" section in each theoretical chapter.
- DSM-5 clinical assessment: The clinical assessment form has been updated to include *Diagnostic and Statistical Manual of Mental Disorders* (DSM-5) diagnosis and Cross-Cutting Symptom assessment. The clinical assessment chapter includes an expanded section that introduces readers to the purpose, structure, and technical issues related to the DSM-5.
- New theories: Two new theories have been added: integrative behavioral couples theory (a leading evidence-based couples therapy treatment) and intensive structural therapy.
- Gender and power in couples therapy: Socioemotional relational therapy was introduced to the philosophical foundations section (see Chapter 3) to provide a contemporary approach to address issues of gender, culture, and power that can be used in conjunction with other approaches (Knudson-Martin & Huenergardt, 2015).
- Expanded diversity sections: The diversity sections in each theory chapter were updated and expanded to include specific, practical applications of the theory with specific populations. Each chapter contains a discussion of ethnic/racial diversity as well as sexual and gender identity diversity. Expanded sections on specific populations provide students with detailed suggestions, adaptations, and cautions for using a given theory with a specific population, including African Americans, Hispanics/Latinos, Asian Americans, Native Americans/First Nation/Aboriginals, biracial/ multiethnic individuals, gay men, lesbians, and transgendered youth.
- Expanded section on research and the evidence base: The review of research in Chapter 2 has been expanded to include: (a) a unified treatment protocol for couples therapy, the first in the field of couples and family therapy, and (b) an expanded review of outcome and process findings for couples and family therapy.
- Try It Yourself: Each chapter contains prompts for the reader to practice applying the concept or intervention in the chapter to promote building of practical skills for working with couples and families.
- Questions for Personal Reflection and Class Discussion: Each chapter now contains a set of questions to encourage readers to personally reflect and think critically and practically about the concepts in each chapter.
- Chapter reorganization: The theory chapters in Part II were reorganized to even the length across sections and to include evidence-based treatments in chapters with similar approaches to facilitate more effective learning.

Appropriate Courses

A versatile book that serves as a reference across the curriculum, this text is specifically designed for use as a primary or secondary textbook in the following courses:

- Introductory or advanced family therapy theories courses
- Prepracticum skills classes
- Practicum or fieldwork classes
- Treatment planning and case documentation courses

Assessing Student Learning and Competence

The learning assignments in the text are designed to simplify the process of measuring student learning for regional and national accreditation. The case conceptualization and treatment plans in the book come with scoring rubrics, which are available on the student and instructor websites for the book at www.cengage.com. Scoring rubrics are available for all major mental health disciplines using the following sets of competencies:

- *Counseling:* 2016 Council on the Accreditation of Counseling and Related Educational Programs (CACREP) standards
- *Marriage and family therapy:* MFT core competencies
- *Psychology:* Psychology competency benchmarks
- *Social work:* Council for Social Work Education accreditation standards

Rubrics are provided correlating competencies for each profession to the skills demonstrated on the four learning assignments: case conceptualization, clinical assessment, treatment planning, and progress notes.

Organization

This book is organized into three parts:

Part I: Theoretical Foundations provides an introduction to competencies, research, ethics, and the philosophical foundations of the field.

Part II: Couple and Family Therapy Theories covers the major schools of family therapy

- Systemic–strategic theories: MRI, Milan, and strategic
- Structural family therapies: Structural and functional family therapies
- Experiential family therapies: Satir's human growth model and emotionally focused therapy with a clinical spotlight on Whitaker's symbolic–experiential family therapy
- Intergenerational and psychodynamic theories
- Cognitive–behavioral and mindfulness-based family therapies, including multicouple and multifamily groups
- Solution-based therapies
- Postmodern therapies: collaborative and narrative

Part III: Clinical Case Documentation details the five steps to competent therapy described at the beginning of this chapter:

- Case conceptualization
- Clinical assessment
- Treatment planning
- Evaluating progress
- Progress notes

The theory chapters in Part II are organized in a user-friendly way to maximize students' ability to use the book when developing case conceptualizations, writing treatment plans, and designing interventions with clients. The theory chapters follow this outline consistently throughout the book:

- In a Nutshell: The Least You Need to Know
- The Juice: Significant Contributions to the Field: If there is one thing to remember from this chapter it should be. . . .
- Rumor Has It: The People and Their Stories
- The Big Picture: Overview of the Therapy Process
- Making a Connection: The Therapy Relationship

- The Viewing: Case Conceptualization
- Targeting Change: Goal Setting
- The Doing: Interventions
- Scope It Out: Cross-theoretical comparison using Tomm's interpersonal patterns
- Putting It All Together: Treatment Plan Template
    - Theory-Specific Case Conceptualization Template
    - Treatment Plan Template for Individuals with Depression/Anxiety Symptoms
    - Treatment Plan Template for Distressed Couples/Families
- Tapestry Weaving: Working with Diverse Populations
    - Ethnic, Racial, Gender, and Cultural Diversity
    - Sexual and Gender Identity Diversity
- Research and Evidence Base
- Online Resources
- Reference List
- Case Example: Vignette with a complete set of clinical paperwork described in Part III, including a theory-specific case conceptualization, clinical assessment, treatment plan, and a progress note.

MindTap for Mastering Competencies

MindTap®, a digital teaching and learning solution, helps students be more successful and confident in the course—and in their work with clients. MindTap guides students through the course by combining the complete textbook with interactive multimedia, activities, assessments, and learning tools. Readings and activities engage students in learning core concepts, practicing needed skills, reflecting on their attitudes and opinions, and applying what they learn. Videos of client sessions illustrate skills and concepts in action, while case studies ask students to make decisions and think critically about the types of situations they'll encounter on the job. Helper Studio activities put students in the role of the helper, allowing them to build and practice skills in a non-threatening environment by responding via video to a virtual client. Instructors can rearrange and add content to personalize their MindTap course, and easily track students' progress with real-time analytics. And, Mind-Tap integrates seamlessly with any learning management system.

Instructor and Student Resources

MindTap for Mastering Competencies includes digital study tools and resources that complement this text and help your students be more successful in your course and their careers. There's an interactive eBook plus videos of client sessions, skill-building activities, quizzes to help students prepare for tests, digital forms for all assignments, apps, and more—all in one place.

Instructors will find numerous teaching resources to accompany the book on the Instructor Companion Site (login.cengage.com). These include:

- Online lectures by the author
- Sample syllabi for how to use this book in a theory class, prepracticum skills class, or practicum class
- PowerPoint slides for all chapters
- Scoring rubrics for each assignment correlated to each profession's competencies: counseling, family therapy, psychology, and social work
- An Instructor's Manual
- A Test bank with questions to accompany each chapter

Students can find digital forms, online lectures, and numerous other useful resources on the author's websites: dianegehart.com or masteringcompetencies.com

REFERENCES

Gehart, D. (2007). *The complete marriage and family therapy core competency assessment system: Eight outcome-based instruments for measuring student learning.* Thousand Oaks, CA: Author. Available at www.mftcompetencies.com.

Gehart, D. (2009). *The complete counseling assessment system: Eight outcome-based instruments for measuring student learning.* Marriage, Couple, and Family Counseling Edition. Thousand Oaks, CA: Author. Available at www.counselingcompetencies.com

Knudson-Martin, C., & Huenergardt, D. (2015). Bridging emotion, societal discourse, and couple interaction in clinical practice. In C. Knudson-Martin, M. A. Wells, & S. K. Samman (Eds.), *Socio-emotional relationship therapy: Bridging emotion, societal context, and couple interaction* (pp. 1–13). New York: Springer Science + Business Media. doi:10.1007/978-3-319-13398-0_1

Tomm, K., St. George, S., Wulff, D., & Strong, T. (2014). *Patterns in interpersonal interactions: Inviting relational understandings for therapeutic change.* New York: Routledge.

Acknowledgments

I would like to thank the following content experts who gave their time and energy to ensure that the information in this textbook was accurate and current:

Interpersonal patterns: Karl Tomm, Sally St. George, Dan Wulff, and Tom Strong

Socioemotional relational therapy: Carmen Knudson-Martin

Systemic–strategic therapies: Angela Kahn, Wendel Ray, Todd Gunter, and Allison Lux

Structural therapies: Charles Fishman, Marion Lindblad-Goldberg, Angela Kahn

Satir Model: Kathlyne Banmen-Maki, Lynne M. Azpeitia, Angela Kahn

Symbolic–experiential therapy: Michael Chafin

Bowen Intergenerational Therapy: Michael Kerr, Cynthia Larkby, Jose Luis Flores, Angela Kahn

Psychodynamic: Martha Carr, Dan Alonzo

Cognitive-Behavioral Family Therapy: Norm Epstein, Bill Northey

Integrated behavioral couples therapy: Andy Christensen and Dorothy O'Neil

Gottman's Marriage Clinic approach: Naomi Knoble

Solution-based therapies: Bill O'Hanlon, Terry Trepper, Thorana Nelson

Narrative therapy: Gerald Monk

Collaborative therapy: Harlene Anderson

Emotionally focused therapy: Scott Woolley, Ben Caldwell

Functional family therapy: Thomas Sexton

Emotionally focused therapy case study: Jonathan Vicksburg

Multifamily group therapy: Eric McCollum

Outcome and session rating scales: Scott Miller

Outcome questionnaire: Michael Lambert

Competencies and learning assessment: Ron Chenail, Thorana Nelson, William Northey

Clinical forms: Julie Diaz, Angela Kahn

The following reviewers provided invaluable feedback on making this book work for faculty:

William F. Northey, Jr. (Bill Northey): Former AAMFT staff member

John K. Miller: University of Oregon

Joshua M. Gold: University of South Carolina

Brent Taylor: San Diego State

Randall Lyle: St. Mary's University

Cynthia T. Walley: Old Dominion University
Graduate student research team for the third edition:

- Christopher Abounayan
- Deborah Brown
- Jessica Erker
- Sara Klausner
- Matt Kloeris
- Courtney Markowitz
- Matt Stephan
- Anna Schaerf

The following students and former students assisted in the development of the instructors' manual for the first edition:

Brandy Lucus: Syllabi, test bank, and video lists
Tricia Lethcoe: PowerPoint slides and test bank
Karen Graber: Reference checks and CACREP rubrics
Julie Woodworth: Test bank
Alina Whitmore: Test bank

Instructor and student materials for the second edition were developed by:

Dana Stone: Test bank and web quizzes
Jessica Lopez: PowerPoint slides and glossary
Brooke Clarke: Rubrics and syllabi and test bank
Corie Loiselle: PowerPoint slides, test bank, and glossary

The following students and colleagues assisted in researching and proofing the second edition:

- Hiroko Okuishi
- Alejandra Trujillo

I would also like to thank the following people for their generous assistance:

Bill O'Hanlon: Whose Writing Bootcamp made this book happen much more easily and quickly and whose encouragement kept me going

Michael Bowers: Who provided permission to reprint the AAMFT Core Competencies

Marquita Flemming: The book's initial editor at Cengage, who helped develop its vision and focus

Seth Dobrin: The book's second editor at Cengage, who helped bring it to its final form

Guenther and Anna Gehart: My parents, whose proofreading and editing kept the drafts clean

Michael and Alexander McNicholas: For teaching me about what family is all about.

About the Author

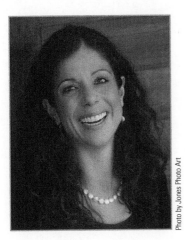

DR. DIANE R. GEHART is Professor in the Marriage and Family Therapy and Counseling Programs at California State University, Northridge. Having practiced, taught, and supervised for over 20 years, she has authored/edited:

Theory and Treatment Planning in Counseling and Psychotherapy
Case Documentation in Counseling and Psychotherapy
Mindfulness and Acceptance in Couple and Family Therapy
Collaborative Therapy: Relationships and Conversations that Make a Difference (coedited)
The Complete MFT Core Competency Assessment System
The Complete Counseling Assessment System
Theory-Based Treatment Planning for Marriage and Family Therapists (coauthored)

She has also written extensively on postmodern therapies, mindfulness, mental health recovery, sexual abuse treatment, gender issues, children and adolescents, client advocacy, qualitative research, and counselor and MFT education. She speaks internationally, having given workshops to professional and general audiences in the United States, Canada, Europe, and Mexico. Her work has been featured in newspapers, radio shows, and television worldwide, including the BBC, National Public Radio, Oprah's *O Magazine*, and *Ladies Home Journal*. She is an associate faculty member at three international postgraduate training institutes: the Houston Galveston Institute, Taos Institute, and the Marburg Institute for Collaborative Studies in Germany. In addition, she is an active leader in state and national professional organizations. She maintains a private practice in Agoura Hills, California, specializing in couples, families, women's issues, trauma, life transitions, and difficult-to-treat cases. For fun, she enjoys spending time with her family, hiking, swimming, yoga, salsa dancing, meditating, and savoring all forms of dark chocolate. You can learn more about her work on www.dianegehart.com.

Author's Introduction: On Saying "Yes" and Falling in Love

I never envisioned myself writing a book such as this. Up to this point, I have focused my career less on the science and more on the heart and soul of therapy, choosing to train as a collaborative therapist who works side by side with clients to create new understandings (see Chapter 10; Anderson & Gehart, 2007), to conduct postmodern qualitative research that introduces the voices of clients into professional literature (Gehart & Lyle, 1999), and to incorporate Buddhist psychology, mindfulness, and spiritual principles and practices into my work (Gehart & McCollum, 2007). Except for my earlier book on treatment planning (Gehart & Tuttle, 2003), nothing in my background points in the direction of writing a book on the competencies or the science-based aspects of family therapy. So, how did I get here? Ironically, what led me here were the very things that one would assume would have prevented it: namely, my postmodern and Buddhist training. More specifically, their practices of saying "yes."

One of the hallmark principles of collaborative therapy, and most family therapies for that matter, is to honor the perspectives of all participants, saying "Yes, I hear you and take your concerns to heart." The Buddhist practice of "saying yes" is the practice of softening and moving toward "what is," even if it is uncomfortable, undesirable, or painful. As a professional, saying "yes" involves taking seriously the perspectives of our colleagues, our clients, third-party payers, state and federal legislatures, licensing boards, professional organizations, and the general public. How do they see us? What questions and concerns do they have about what we do?

Over the years, voices from outside our profession have increasingly demanded clarity on and evidence for what we do. Answering these demands while maintaining integrity with my training is often challenging because the working assumptions of what "counts" as evidence in human relations are not as simple or straightforward as one might think. What an insurance company considers as evidence of successful therapy (i.e., a particular score on an assessment form) is quite different from what a therapist might emphasize (i.e., observing the client move with the ceaseless stream-of-life stressors more gracefully).

As part of our profession's response to the demand for greater accountability, family therapists generated a list of Core Competencies that detail the knowledge and skills that define the practice of family therapy (see Appendix A). For faculty members such as myself, this is essentially a to-do list of what we need to teach our students. As a member of this community, I recognized that I needed to find a positive, respectful way to work with these external priorities and balance them with my own. This book is my answer, my "yes," to these concerns.

My Other Purpose: Falling in Love

I must confess that I had another intention for writing this book: to help you to fall in love. And, preferably to do so again and again—making even Casanova envious. I want you to fall in love with not one but all of the family therapy theories in this book, enthusiastically embracing each while seeing both its beauty and its limitations, much in the same way we help our clients to love each other. I hope you cultivate a profound respect for the brilliant minds that have paved the way for us to help clients with their most complex and intimate problems—their couple and family relationships—or, more essentially, to teach them how to love. I hope you find yourself passionate about the insight each approach offers in understanding human relationships as well as about helping people create the relationships they desire. As family therapists, we inherit a stunning and profound body of knowledge that is difficult to fully appreciate in the beginning. I personally believe that some of the greatest wisdom in the Western world is captured in the philosophical foundations of family therapy. Although these ideas sometimes seem surprising or even objectionable at first, if you sincerely try to put them into practice, I believe you will find that each touches upon a useful truth and reality. Should you choose to seriously study it, the field of family therapy offers an ever-widening exploration of the human experience that cannot help but transform you both personally and professionally. I hope this book inspires you to start on a passionate journey of discovery that lasts a lifetime.

What You Will Find

This book is divided into three sections: the first introduces you to foundational concepts in the field, including competence, the evidence base, professional ethics, and the philosophical foundations. In the second part of the book, you will learn about the major family therapy theories, both the traditional theories and the newer evidence-based therapies. The chapters describe the theory using a highly practical approach that will provide specific instructions on how to use the concepts in session. In addition, each chapter includes a case study with a complete set of clinical documentations: case conceptualization, clinical assessment, treatment plan, and progress note. The final section provides you with detailed instructions for completing this form as well as options for measuring clinical progress.

The Invitation

I invite you to passionately and enthusiastically embrace each perspective, concept, and theory that follows. Savor the big-picture view of case conceptualization while also taking time to examine the intricate matters of clinical assessment. Appreciate the unique wisdom of each theory while also recognizing the *common factors* (see Chapter 2) that they share. Get excited about research and the evidence base of our work (see Chapter 2), while honoring the philosophical foundations (see Chapter 3). Be open to theories that rely on technique and content to promote change as well as to those that rely on process and relationship, knowing that each has its place when working with diverse clients. Say "yes" to all that comes your way, and take pleasure in the incredible journey of becoming a family therapist.

Enjoy the adventure.

Diane R. Gehart, Ph.D.
Westlake Village, California
July 2016

REFERENCES

Anderson, H., & Gehart, D. (2007). *Collaborative therapy: Relationships and conversations that make a difference.* New York: Brunner/Routledge.

Gehart, D. R., & Lyle, R. R. (1999). Client and therapist perspectives of change in collaborative language systems: An interpretive ethnography. *Journal of Systemic Therapy, 18*(4), 78–97.

Gehart, D., & McCollum, E. (2007). Engaging suffering: Towards a mindful re-visioning of marriage and family therapy practice. *Journal of Marital and Family Therapy, 33,* 214–226.

Gehart, D. R., & Tuttle, A. R. (2003). *Theory-based treatment planning for marriage and family therapists: Integrating theory and practice.* Pacific Grove, CA: Brooks/Cole.

Anderson, H., & Gehart, D. (2007). Collaborative therapy: Relationships and conversations that make a difference. New York: Brunner/Routledge.

Gehart, D. R., & Lyle, R. R. (1999). Client and therapist perspectives of change in collaborative language systems: An interpretive ethnography. Journal of Systemic Therapy, 18(4), 78–97.

Gehart, D., & McCollum, E. (2007). Engaging suffering: Towards a mindful revisioning of marriage and family therapy practice. Journal of Marital and Family Therapy, 33, 214–226.

Gehart, D. R., & Tuttle, A. R. (2003). Theory-based treatment planning for marriage and family therapists: Integrating theory and practice. Pacific Grove, CA: Brooks/Cole.

PART I

Theoretical Foundations

CHAPTER

1

Competency and Theory in Family Therapy

Learning Objectives

After reading this chapter and a few hours of focused studying, you should be able to:

- Describe a broad-strokes overview of the elements of competent therapy.

- Outline the reasons why mental health practitioners are focused on competency-based learning methods.

- Identify four key aspects of competency in mental health.

The Secret to Competent Therapy

There is a secret to providing competent family therapy. The secret applies whether you are trained as a psychologist, counselor, or social worker or as a family therapist specifically. Fortunately, it is an open secret, and the goal of this chapter is to sketch a map showing where and, more importantly, how to look for it. You are probably familiar with the basic landscape. You may recognize therapy's more promising pathways and some of the dead-end routes. But like everyone setting out on a journey, your choice between the high road and the low road would be easier if you knew what was in store for you beforehand.

Since I know you will race ahead if I make you wait too much longer, let's lay our map on the table right now and get a better sense of this secret on the first page. Mapping a successful therapeutic journey involves five steps.

THE FIVE STEPS TO COMPETENT THERAPY

Step 1. Map the Territory: Conceptualize the situation with the help of theory (Chapter 11).

Step 2. Identify Oases and Obstacles: Assess the client's mental status and provide case management (Chapter 12).

Step 3. Select a Path: Develop a treatment plan with therapeutic tasks—including how to build a working therapeutic relationship—and measurable client goals (Chapter 13).

Step 4. Track Progress: Evaluate the client's response to treatment (Chapter 14).

Step 5. Leave a Trail: Document what happens (Chapter 15).

Mapping a Successful Therapeutic Journey

These five steps follow a classic method used by all explorers in uncharted territory. And that's what each new therapeutic relationship is: uncharted territory, an unknown region, *terra incognita*. Although it may seem that clients can be easily lumped into groups—depressed clients, distressed couples, children with attention-deficit/hyperactivity disorder (ADHD), for example—any experienced therapist can tell you that each client's journey is unique. The excitement—and secret—to competent therapy is mapping the distinctive terrain of each client's life and charting a one-of-a-kind journey through it.

The first step is to delineate as much of the terrain as possible: to get the big picture. What are the contours of the relationships? Where are the comfort zones? Where is the page marked "Here Be Dragons?" As with all maps, the bigger and more detailed the record, the easier it is to move through the territory. In family therapy, our maps are our *case conceptualizations,* assessments of the client using family therapy theories. Once you have a map of the big picture, you identify the landmarks, the oases and obstacles. You notice where the rest stops are and identify what dangers lie ahead. In therapy, the oases are client resources: anything that can be used to strengthen and support the client. The obstacles are potential or existing hindrances to creating change in the client's life: Are there really dragons there, or is the region just unfamiliar?

Like a cartographer surveying the landscape, therapists carefully assess potential hindrances, ruling out possible medical issues in consultation with physicians, identifying psychiatric issues by conducting a *mental status exam,* and considering basic life needs, such as financial or social resources, through *case management.* When actual or probable impediments are addressed early in the therapeutic process through *clinical assessment,* the therapeutic journey is likely to proceed more easily and smoothly.

Once you have your map with oases and obstacles clearly identified, you can confidently select a realistic path toward the client's chosen destination or *goal.* If you have done a good job mapping, you will be able to choose from among several different paths, depending on what works best for those on the journey: namely, you and the client. This translates to being able to choose a therapeutic theory and style that suit all involved. Seasoned clinicians distinguish themselves from newer therapists in their ability to identify and successfully navigate through numerous terrains: forests, seas, deserts, plains, paradises, and wastelands. The greater a therapist's repertoire of skills, the more able the therapist is to move through each terrain. Once a preferred path is chosen, the therapist generates a *treatment plan,* a general set of directions for how to address client concerns. Like any set of travel plans, treatment plans are subject to change because of weather, natural disaster, human error, and other unforeseeable events, otherwise known as "real life." Therapists can rest assured that unexpected detours, delays, and shortcuts (yes, unexpected good stuff happens also) will be part of any therapeutic journey.

Once you select a course of action, you need to check frequently to make sure that: (a) the plan is working and (b) you are sticking with the plan. In therapy, this translates to *assessing client progress* along the way. If the client is not making progress, the therapist needs to go back and reassess: (a) the accuracy of the map and (b) the wisdom of the plan. It is almost always easy to make improvements in both areas that will get things back on course. The key to assessing client progress is often just to notice when you are off course as soon as possible.

Finally, you need to leave a trail to track where you have been. Leaving a trail always helps you find your way back if you get lost: others (as well as you) can see why and how you proceeded. Therapists leave a trace of their path by generating thorough *clinical documentation,* which helps in two highly prized aspects of therapy: getting paid by third-party payers (i.e., insurance) and avoiding lawsuits (i.e., the state lets you practice). By making it clear where you are going, you can help everyone concerned better understand your specific route of treatment. So, competent therapy is that simple: five basic steps that this book will walk you through, step-by-step.

Try It Yourself

Either by yourself or with a partner, describe what elements of this map of the therapeutic journey make sense to you. What do you find surprising?

From Trainee to Seasoned Therapist

The difference between trainees and seasoned therapists can be found in the quality of the map, the effectiveness of the path of treatment, and the speed it takes to move through the steps. A seasoned therapist may move through the five steps of competent therapy in the first few minutes of a session, whereas a trainee may take more time, collecting information and trying various options. How long it takes is less important than the quality of the journey. This book is designed to help you move through these steps more effectively, whether you are just starting out or have been doing therapy for years.

Competency and Theory: Why Theory Matters

Although much has changed in the past decade in mental health—better research to guide us, new knowledge about the brain, more details about mental health disorders, increased use of psychotropic medication—the primary tool that therapists use to help people, *theory,* has not. Therapeutic theories provide a means for quickly sifting through the tremendous amount of information clients bring; then targeting specific thoughts, behaviors, or emotional processes for change; and finally helping clients effectively make these changes to resolve their initial concerns. Even with fancy fMRI (functional magnetic resonance imaging), neurofeedback machines, and hundreds of available medications, no other technology has taken the place of theory. However, the changing landscape of mental health care has altered how therapy theories are understood and used. Specifically, theory and how it is being used and understood has been recontextualized by two major movements in recent years: (a) the **competency** movement, which includes multicultural competency; and (b) the research- or evidence-based movement, which is discussed in detail in Chapter 2. These movements have not ended the need for theory, but have instead changed how we conceptualize, adapt, and apply theory.

Arguably, working with couples and families often requires greater use of theory. Regardless of professional identity—family therapist, professional counselor, social worker, psychologists or psychiatric nurse—competent therapy with families involves learning to conceptualize not only the psychology of the individual but also the complex web of relationships that constitutes a person's social world *and* the interaction between the two. There are a lot of moving pieces. The theories in this text will help you learn what to focus on to better understand this complex web of interpersonal dynamics. Some readers may be quietly thinking, "I don't want to do couple or family therapy" and may conclude they don't need to worry too much about these theories. The problem is that even if you have only one client in the room, the client's web of relationships is still affecting his or her behavior and mood, often in ways that are difficult to imagine or accurately assess without using couple and family theoretical concepts. In general, the more severe the client problem, the more people you need in the room to effect change (Lebow, 2006).

Why All the Talk about Competency?

All health professions, including mental health, have been abuzz in recent years with talk of *competencies*, detailed lists of the knowledge and skill professionals need to effectively do their job. The main source of this movement has been external to the field and has come from stakeholders who believe that professionals should not only be taught a consistent set of skills but that their learning should be measured on real-world tasks (for a detailed discussion, see Gehart, 2011). Thus, this movement is asking educators to shift their focus from conveying content to ensuring that students know how to meaningfully apply the knowledge and skills of their given profession.

Each major mental health profession—including counseling, marriage and family therapy, psychology, psychiatry, psychiatric nursing, and chemical dependency counseling—has developed a unique set of competencies. Thankfully, there are many similarities across

MFT Core Competencies Task Force Members and Facilitator: Ron Chenail, Thorana Nelson, James Alexander, Russ Crane, Linda Schwalie, and Bill Northey

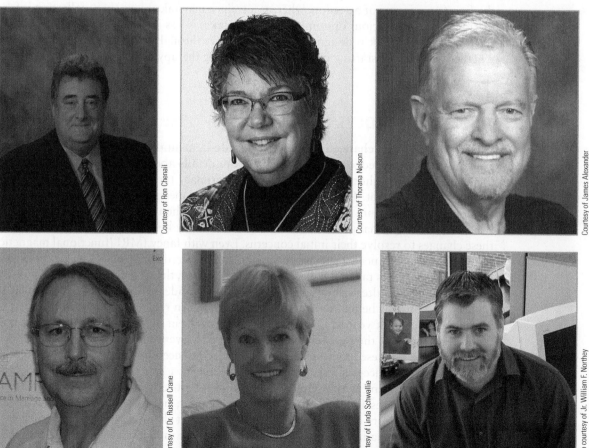

Courtesy of Ron Chenail

Courtesy of Thorana Nelson

Courtesy of James Alexander

Courtesy of Dr. Russell Crane

Courtesy of Linda Schwallie

Photo courtesy of Jr. William F. Northey

them. For working with couples and families specifically, most professionals refer to the Marriage and Family Therapy Core Competencies, which was developed by a task force commissioned by the American Association for Marriage and Family Therapy (Nelson et al., 2007). On nights when you have insomnia, you may find it helpful and interesting to read through what are considered essential skills for working with couples and families, regardless of the title on your license.

These competencies are being used to more clearly define what mental health professionals must know and do in order to be competent. If you are new to the field, this will actually make the task of learning to work with couples and families far easier: the goals are now clearly defined. This book is designed to help you develop these competencies as quickly and directly as possible.

Competency and (Not) You

Although at first it may seem insensitive, the vernacular expression commonly used by my teen clients sums up the mind-set of competency best: *"It's not about you."* It's not about *your* theoretical preference, what worked for *you* in your personal therapy, what *you* are good at, what *you* find interesting, or even what *you* believe will be most helpful. Competent therapy requires that *you* get outside of your comfort zone, stretch, and learn how to interact with clients in a way that works for *them*. In short, you need to be competent in a wide range of theories and techniques to be helpful to all of the clients with whom you work. As you read on, you might even begin to see how this makes some sense and might even be in your best interest.

Perhaps it is best to explain with an example. You will likely either have a natural propensity for generating a broad-view case conceptualization using therapy theories or have a disposition that favors a detail-focused mental health assessment and diagnosis; humans tend to be good with either the big picture or with the details. However, to be competent, a therapist needs to get good at both even if one is easier, preferred, and philosophically favored. Similarly, you may prefer theories that promote insight and personal reflection; after all, that may be what works for *you* in *your* life. However, that may not work for your client, and/or research may indicate that such an approach is not the most effective approach for your client's situation or cultural background. Thus, you will need to master theories of therapy that may not particularly interest you or even fit with your theory of therapy. Even though you may not like this idea at first, I think that by the time you are done with this book, you might just warm up to it.

I first learned this competency lesson when working with families in which the parents had difficulty managing the behaviors of their young children. I was never a huge fan of behaviorism, but it did not take too many hysterically screaming, clawing, and biting two-year-olds before I was preaching the value of reinforcement schedules and consistency. Given my strong—admittedly zealous—attachment to my postmodern approach at the time, I have faith that you will be driven either by principle (ideally) or desperation (more likely) to move beyond your comfort zone to become a well-rounded, competent therapist.

Common Threads of Competencies

Whether you are training to be a counselor, family therapist, psychologist, or social worker, you will notice that are common themes across the various sets of competencies. You will want to take particular note of these:

- Diversity and multicultural competence: The use of therapeutic theory is always contextualized by diversity issues, which means that the application and applicability vary—sometimes dramatically—based on diversity issues, such as age, ethnicity, sexual orientation, ability, socioeconomic status, immigration status, etc.
- Research and the evidence base: To be competent, therapists must be aware of the research and the evidence base related to their theory, client populations, and presenting problem.

- Ethics: Perhaps the most obvious commonality across sets of competencies is law and ethics; without a firm grasp of the laws and ethical standards that relate to professional mental health practice . . . well, let's just say you won't be practicing very long. A solid understanding of ethical principles, such as confidentiality, is a prerequisite for applying theory well.
- Person-of-the-therapist: Finally, unlike most other professions, specific personal qualities are identified as competencies for mental health professionals. These will be discussed in more depth below.

Diversity and Competency

Over the past couple of decades, therapists have begun to take seriously the role of diversity in the therapy process, including factors such as age, gender, ethnicity, race, socioeconomic status, immigration status, sexual orientation, gender identity, ability, language, and religion. These factors inform the selection of theory, development of the therapy relationship, assessment and diagnosis process, and choice of interventions (Monk, Winslade, & Sinclair, 2008). In short, everything you think, do, or say as a professional is contextualized and should be informed by diversity issues. If you think effectively responding to diversity is easy or can be easily learned or that perhaps your instructors, supervisors, or some famous author has magic answers to make it easy, you are going to be in for an unpleasant surprise. Rather than a black-and-white still life, dealing with diversity issues is more like finger painting: there are few lines to follow, it is messy for everyone involved, and it requires enthusiasm and openheartedness to make it fun.

I have often heard new and experienced therapists alike claim that because they are from a diverse or marginalized group, they don't need to worry about diversity issues. Conversely, I have heard therapists from majority groups say things such as, "I don't have any culture." Both parties have much to learn on the diversity front. First of all, we are all part of numerous sociological groups that exert cultural norms on us, with the more common and powerful ones stemming from gender, ethnicity, socioeconomic class, religion, and age. Many, if not most, people belong to some groups that align more with dominant culture and to some that are marginalized. However, it is important to realize that some groups experience far more traumatic and painful forms of marginalization than others, and to further complicate matters, each individual responds to these pressures differently.

To illustrate, some people experienced the process of coming out as gay as highly traumatic and want therapists to address these experiences with extreme sensitivity and care; others find it insulting when therapists *assume* there has been trauma and tiptoe around the issue, because they live in communities that are largely supportive. Furthermore, many Americans seem unaware that there is a very strong and distinct "American culture" of which they are a part; in fact, the various geographic regions of America have very unique characteristics of which therapists need to be aware. As another example, Midwestern men typically express their emotions far differently than do men in California; therapists who expect the two types of men to handle emotions in a similar way are going to unfairly pathologize one or the other.

Suffice it to say, competently handling diversity issues requires great attention to the unique needs of each person; it is a career-long struggle and journey that adds great depth and humanity to the person-of-the-therapist. In this book, you examine issues of diversity in virtually every chapter. In Chapter 2, you will read about diversity relates to research and ethical issues, and in Chapter 3, I review contemporary approaches for conceptualizing sociocultural influences in families, including how cultured gender roles affect power dynamics in couple relationships. In Part II of the book, you will find discussions of diversity related to each theory, including descriptions of how these issues relate to specific theoretical concepts, and an extended section at the end of each chapter covers racial, ethnic, gender, and sexual identity diversity related to the implementation of the specific theory. Finally, in Part III, you will find that diversity issues are prominent in case documentation forms, including the case conceptualization, assessment, and treatment plan.

Research and Competency

Another common thread found in mental health competencies is understanding and, more importantly, *using* research to inform treatment and to measure one's effectiveness and client progress. In recent years, there has been a powerful movement within the field of mental health to become more evidence-based. This involves two key practices: (a) using existing research to inform clinical decisions and treatment planning and (b) learning to use evidence-based treatments, which are specific and structured approaches for working with distinct populations and issues (Sprenkle, 2002). These movements are discussed in detail in Chapter 2 (in perhaps too much detail for some); issues related to the evidence base for each therapeutic theory are also discussed at the end of each theory chapter, with the related evidence-based treatment highlighted. In addition, Chapters 5, 6, and 8 cover leading evidence-based treatments in the field of couple and family therapy. If you were hoping to escape a discussion of research in your theory text, you will initially be disappointed; however, I hope that by the end you find the integration an invigorating addition.

Law, Ethics, and Competency

I often quip with students entering the field that if they think therapists can cut corners with legal or ethical issues, they should transfer to a business program so that they can make some money without worrying about such details and avoid a felony prison sentence after working as an underpaid intern for four-plus years. That might be a bit of an exaggeration, but not much. Therapists who fail to develop competence in legal and ethical issues will not last long. These issues are so central to the profession that even before you begin reading about theories and treatment planning, you need a brief introduction so you don't run off and start applying the concepts in this book to identify the underlying causes of problems in your clients, friends, family, neighbors, pets, and yourself. All mental health professional organization—the American Association for Marriage and Family Therapy, the American Counseling Association, the American Psychological Association, and the National Association of Social Workers—have codes of ethics that their members must follow. Thankfully, there is significant agreement between the various organizations, which results in general agreement on most key issues; federal and state laws also generally agree on the key principles. These issues are covered in depth in Chapter 2.

Person-of-the-Therapist and Competency

Finally, being a competent therapist requires particular personal characteristics that are often difficult to define. Some qualities are basically assumed to be prerequisites for a professional—integrity, honesty, and diligence—and take the form of following through on instructions the first time asked, raising concerns before they spiral into problems, staying true to one's word, etc. It is hard to establish competency in anything without these basic life skills.

The more subtle issues of the person-of-the-therapist come out in building relationships with clients. To begin with, the research is clear that clients need to feel heard, understood, and accepted by therapists, which often takes the form of offering empathy and avoiding advice giving (Miller, Duncan, & Hubble, 1997). Furthermore, therapists need to identify and work through their personal issues to avoid bias and to avoid inappropriately pathologizing a client—what psychodynamic therapists call *countertransference* (see Chapter 7). Although more difficult to quantify, these issues often become quickly apparent by the appearance of strong emotions or unusual interactions in relationships with clients, supervisors, instructors, and peers. Managing these well is part of being a competent therapist.

Finally, a more difficult aspect to define is *therapeutic presence*, a quality of self considered to have intrapersonal, interpersonal, and transpersonal elements, including elements of empathy, compassion, charisma, spirituality, transpersonal communication, patient responsiveness, optimism, and expectancies—making it elusive and difficult to operationalize (McDonough-Means, Kreitzer, & Bell, 2004). Clients—rather than a professional—are the best judges of this subtle quality because in the end, it comes down to how the client experiences the therapist as a human being in the room. Although these competencies are more difficult to measure, they are nonetheless some of the more important to develop.

> ### Try It Yourself
>
> **Either by yourself or with a partner, describe what elements of competency make most sense to you. What surprises you?**

How This Book Is Different and What It Means to You

Mastering Competencies in Family Therapy is a different kind of textbook. Based on a new pedagogical model, learning-centered teaching (Killen, 2004; Weimer, 2002), this book is designed to help you *actively learn* the content and develop real-world competencies rather than simply deliver the content and hope that you will memorize it. Thus, learning activities are a central part of the text so that you have opportunities to apply and use the information in ways that facilitate learning. The specific learning activities in this book are: (a) case conceptualization, (b) clinical assessment, (c) treatment planning, and (d) progress notes; these translate the theory learned in the chapter to practical client situations. This book teaches real-world skills that you can immediately use to better serve your clients.

This book is different in another way: it is organized by key concepts rather than by general headings with long narrative sections. This organization—which evolved from my personal study notes for my doctoral and licensing exams back before I had e-mail (and, no, dinosaurs were not roaming the planet then)—facilitates the retention of vocabulary and terms because of the visual layout. Each year I receive numerous e-mails from enthusiastic newly licensed therapists thanking me for helping them to pass their licensing exams—they all say that the organization of the book made the difference. So, spending some time with this text should better prepare you for the big exams in your future (and if you have already passed these, you should be all the more impressed with yourself for doing it the hard way).

Lay of the Land

This book is organized into three parts:

Part I: **Introduction to Family Therapy Theories** provides an introduction to competencies, research, ethics, and the philosophical foundations of the field.

Part II: **Family Therapy Theories** covers the major schools of family therapy:
- Systemic theories: MRI, Milan, and strategic
- Structural family therapies: Structural family therapy and functional family therapy
- Experiential family therapies: Satir's human growth model and emotionally focused couples therapy
- Intergenerational and psychodynamic theories
- Cognitive–behavioral and mindfulness-based family therapies
- Solution-based therapies
- Postmodern therapies: Collaborative and narrative therapies

Part III: **Case Documentation** details the five steps to competent therapy described at the beginning of this chapter:

- Case conceptualization
- Clinical assessment
- Treatment planning
- Evaluating progress
- Progress notes

Anatomy of a Theory

The theory chapters in Part II are organized in a user-friendly way to maximize your ability to use the book to support you when developing case conceptualizations, writing treatment plans and progress notes, and designing interventions with clients. Theory chapters follow this outline:

ANATOMY OF A THEORY

In a Nutshell: The Least You Need to Know

The Juice: Significant Contributions to the Field

Rumor Has It: The People and Their Stories

The Big Picture: Overview of the Therapy Process

Making Connections: The Therapeutic Relationship

The Viewing: Case Conceptualization

Targeting Change: Goal Setting

The Doing: Interventions

Scope It Out: Cross-Theoretical Comparison

Putting It All Together:

- Case Conceptualization and Treatment Plan Template
- Treatment Plan Template for Individuals with Depression/Anxiety Symptoms
- Treatment Plan Template for Couples/Families with Conflict

Tapestry Weaving: Working with Diverse Populations

- Ethnic, Racial, Gender, and Cultural Diversity
- Sexual Identity Diversity

Research and Evidence Base

Online Resources

Reference List

Case Example: Vignette with a complete set of clinical paperwork described in Part III, including case conceptualization, clinical assessment, treatment plan, and a progress note

In a Nutshell: The Least You Need to Know: The chapters begin with a brief summary of the key features of the theory. Although it may not be the absolute least you need to know to get an A in a theory class or help a client, it is the basic information you should have memorized and are able to quickly articulate at any moment to help you keep your theories straight.

The Juice: Significant Contributions to the Field: In the next section, I use the principle of primacy (first information introduced) to help you remember one of the most significant contributions of the theory to the field of family therapy. In most cases, well-trained clinicians who generally use another approach to therapy are likely to be skilled and use this particular concept because it has shaped standard practice in the field. This section is your red flag to remember a seminal concept or practice for the theory. Feedback from students indicates this is often one of their favorite sections. (I only hope that isn't because they skim the rest of the chapter; but, of course, *you* would never think of such a thing.)

Rumor Has It: The People and Their Stories: In this section, you can read about the developers of the theory and how their personal stories shaped the evolution of the ideas. And, yes, some of the rumors are juicier than others. As the focus of this text is how therapy theories are actually used in contemporary settings, I have deemphasized the history and development of the theory, but you will find brief summaries of such history here.

The Big Picture: Overview of the Therapy Process: The big picture provides an overview of the flow of the therapy process: what happens in the beginning, middle, and end, and how change is facilitated across these phases.

Making Connections: The Therapy Relationship: All approaches start by establishing a working relationship with clients, but each approach does it differently. In this section, you will read about the unique ways that therapists of various schools build relationships that provide the foundation for change.

The Viewing: Case Conceptualization: The case conceptualization section will identify the signature theory concepts that therapists from each school use to identify and assess clients and their problems. This really is the heart of the theory and where the real differences emerge. *I encourage you to pay particularly close attention to these.* For this third edition, you will find theory-specific case conceptualization forms at www .masteringcompetencies.com. You can also read more about case conceptualization in Chapter 13.

Targeting Change: Goal Setting: Based on the areas assessed in the case conceptualization and the overall therapy process, each approach has a unique strategy for identifying client goals that become the foundation for the treatment plan.

The Doing: Interventions: Probably the most exciting part for most new therapists, the doing section outlines the common techniques and interventions for each theory. In some cases, a section for techniques used with special populations is included if these are notably different than those in standard practice.

Scope It Out: Cross-Theoretical Comparison: In Chapter 3, I introduce Karl Tomm's IPscope for conceptualizing interpersonal patterns. This approach helps therapists identify several different types of interpersonal patterns and facilitates easy comparison with other theories in the book. I will introduce each theory using this common language to help you quickly grasp the big picture and compare it to other theories.

Putting It All Together: Case Conceptualization and Treatment Plan Templates: After graduation, you will probably thank me most for this section, which provides templates for theory-specific case conceptualization and treatment plans that can be used for addressing depression, anxiety, or trauma with individual clients and conflict with couples and families. These plans tie everything in the chapter together (just imagine a little bow on top).

Tapestry Weaving: Working with Diverse Populations: This section reviews specific approaches for working with diverse populations using the theories covered in the chapter. Each chapter includes sections on ethnic and sexual identity diversity issues.

Research and Evidence Base: Finally, the chapters end with a brief review of the research and evidence base for each theory to offer a general sense of empirical foundations for the theory. In some cases, influential evidence-based treatments (see Chapter 2 for a definition) are highlighted.

Try It Yourself: Throughout the chapter you will find opportunities to "try it for yourself" and apply a concept to yourself or with a partner.

Questions for Personal Reflection and Class Discussion: At the end of each chapter, you will find questions to help you meaningfully engage the material.

Online Resources: A list of web pages and web documents are included for those who want to pursue specialized training or conduct further research on the theory.

Reference List: Many students pass right over reference lists and forget all about them. But if you have to do an academic paper or literature review on any of these theories, this should be your first stop. In this case, I had several hundred books and articles go through my 12-by-12-foot office while writing the editions of this book. Thus, you can certainly shorten the time it takes to locate key resources by pursuing these before you hit the library yourself. (Oh, I forgot, no one steps foot in these places anymore; I meant "surf" the library's web page while still wearing your bunny slippers.)

Case Example: Finally, each chapter ends with a case vignette, case conceptualization, clinical assessment, treatment plan, and progress note to give you a sense of how the theory looks in action and how to put down on paper. The details for how to complete these forms are in Chapters 11–15.

Voice and Tone

Finally, I should mention that the voice and tone of this textbook is a bit different from that of your average college read. Hopefully, you have noticed by now that I am talking right at ya. I also like to add some humor and have some fun while I write. Why? Well, first, I have more fun writing this way. But, more importantly, I want to engage you as if you were one of my students or supervisees learning how to apply these ideas for the first time. Family therapies are relationship-based practices, one in which the parties construct knowledge together. So, it's hard for me to write about these ideas as a detached, faceless author, thereby perpetuating the myth of objectivity in knowledge construction (you'll better understand why I'm worried about this after reading about the philosophical foundations of family therapy in Chapter 3). So, as I write, I'm imagining you as a real person, eager to learn about how to use these ideas to help others. I am going to try to reach out to you, answer questions I imagine you have, and periodically tap you on the shoulder to make sure you are still awake ☺

Suggested Uses for This Text

Suggestions for Thinking about Family Therapy Theories

As you read the chapters in this book, you are going to be tempted to identify which ones you like the best and deemphasize the ones to which you are less attracted. This may seem like a great idea at first, but here are some points to consider:

Favorite vs. Useful: The theories that the average therapist finds personally useful are probably not the same ones that the average client of a new therapist is likely to find useful. Many therapists are psychologically minded, meaning that they enjoy thinking about the inner world and how it works. However, most new therapists begin working in lower-fee clinics that serve diverse, multiproblem clients and families, many (but not all) of whom are not psychologically minded because they are often struggling with issues of survival and/or come from cultural traditions that place less value on analysis and understanding of the inner world. So, the theory you find most useful to you personally may not be a good fit for your first client.

Appreciative: The theories in this book are not casually chosen. They have become part of the standard cannon of theories because generations of therapists have found them helpful. Each has wisdom worthy of study. The one lesson I have learned over the years is that the more theories therapists understand, the better able they are to serve their clients because their understanding of the human condition and its concomitant problems is broader. Thus, I recommend approaching each theory with an attitude of searching for its most wide and useful parts. I facilitate this for you in the "Juice" section of each chapter, which identifies the one concept I believe has near universal utility from the particular theory.

Common Threads: Family therapy theories are ironic: in one sense they are very different and inform distinct and mutually exclusive behaviors and attitudes. However, the better you understand one, the better you understand them all. In fact, some therapists, the common factors proponents, argue that theories are generally equally effective because they are simply different modes for delivering the same factors (Miller et al., 1997; you will read more about this in Chapter 2). So, it is quite possible that commonalities across theories are *more important* than their differences.

Suggestions for Using This Book to Learn Theories

First, I recommend that you set aside an hour or two to read about a single theory from beginning to end (from the "In a Nutshell" to "Putting It All Together") to help get the full sense of the theory. Some chapters have a couple theories in one, so for these, it is fine to read the chapter in chunks. In addition, some learners may find it helpful to scan the treatment plan (either the template or example at the end of the chapter) or some other section first to provide a practical overview; that said, I have tried to organize the ideas in the way most people seem to prefer. But I encourage you to discover what works best for you, as different learners have different strategies that work best for them. When you are done with a chapter, you might want to try completing a case conceptualization and treatment plan for yourself (you may have to make up a problem if you are nearly perfect) or someone else to get a sense of how this would work.

Finally, I strongly recommend that either after reading the chapter or after going to class you take good old-fashioned notes. Yes, I mean it. I recommend that you type up (or if you prefer, handwrite) a complete outline of the key concepts in your own words. Why do I advocate such painful torture? When we read long, dense books such as this one, we all fade in and out of alert attentiveness to what we are reading—often lapsing into more interesting fantasies or less interesting to-do lists—and—gasp!—sometimes even skim large sections of the text (no, I am not surprised or offended). The only way to make sure that you really understand the concepts you read about is to put them in your own words and organize them in a way that makes sense to you. If you need to take culminating exams or plan to pursue licensure, you will have to log the concepts in this book into your long-term memory, which requires more than cramming for a final exam. If you are new to graduate and professional school, I am sorry to be the bearer of the sad news: this is not like undergraduate study, where forgetting everything you learned the week after finals was generally not a problem. Being a mental health professional requires that you master and build upon what you learn. You will be expected to know what is in this book for the entire time you are active in the profession (seriously—and if you think that is bad, just wait until you get to a class on diagnosis—you'll have to memorize an even longer book). So, if your former study habits included all-night cramming, gallons of espresso (or other favorite caffeine-delivery system), and minimal recall after the exam, you might want to try my note-taking tip or some other strategy as you move forward.

Suggestions for Using This Book to Write Treatment Plans

I want to emphasize that the treatment plan format, templates, and examples in this book are just that: formats, templates, and examples. They do not represent the only approach or the only right approach. They are simply a solid approach based on the common standards and expectations. You most likely will work at a counseling agency or institution that uses another format, but the same general rules (those in Chapter 15) will still apply. That is why understanding the principles of how to write good goals and interventions is more important than memorizing the format.

Furthermore, don't use the templates and examples too rigidly. Feel free to modify the goal statements and techniques to fit the unique needs of your client. I have provided some relatively specific goals as an example of what might work and encourage you to radically tailor these for each client's unique needs. You will notice that treatment plans in the case study do not rigidly follow the templates; I encourage you to do the same.

Suggestions for Use in Internships and Clinical Practice

When working as an intern or licensed mental health professional, this book can be useful for teaching yourself theories and techniques in addition to learning how to complete clinical documentation. You will likely find that when you work with new populations and problems, you may be interested in considering how other therapy models might approach these situations. This book is designed to be a prime resource that can be quickly scanned to identify other possibilities. Alternatively, you might have a colleague or supervisor who uses a theory with which you are not familiar. You can use this book to quickly review that theory and keep from looking uneducated. In addition, this book is written to help you appreciate and find common ground across theories, which can be of particular benefit when working in a "mixed theory" context. However, to actually learn to practice any of these theories well, I strongly urge you to take advanced training from experts in that approach.

Suggestions for Studying for Licensing Exams

Licensing exams are not designed to be unnecessarily tricky or scary, they simply ensure that you have the necessary knowledge to practice therapy without supervision *and not harm anybody.* And they are a vocabulary test. If you have honestly engaged in your classes, done your homework, avoided cramming for tests and papers, and made it a priority to get decent supervision, you should have a strong foundation for taking your licensing exam. You should already have in your possession books (such as this) that cover all of the content to be studied for the exam. If your exam is to be taken upon finishing a lengthy post-master's internship, you should use the entire two- to four-year period to read as many books as possible on the theories and materials covered by the exam (that means no novels for a few years).

I do not recommend that all of my students take long, expensive "review courses" because such courses are not necessary for those who are proactive in mastering the material on the exam long before they sign up to take it. If you start studying only after you are approved to take the test, you are starting about two to four years too late—and then, yes, you will need to take a crash course. My basic suggestion for studying for a mental health licensing exam is this: read an original text on each major theory during your post-degree internship, use the *Diagnostic and Statistical Manual of Mental Disorders* (DSM), and keep up with laws and ethics; and then buy the practice exams (without the study guides) and take them until you consistently get 5% above the required passing score (e.g., 75% if the passing score is 70%). If you find that you are weak in a particular area, such as theory or DSM, use a text such as this, which is designed with the license review in mind. Once you consistently get 75%, you are ready—with the most learning and the least expense—to take the test.

Suggestions for Faculty to Measure Competencies and Student Learning

This book is specifically designed to help faculty and supervisors simplify and streamline the onerous task of measuring student competencies as required by the various accreditation bodies. The forms and scoring rubrics for assessing student learning using counseling, psychology, social work, and family therapy competencies are available on the book's web page for instructors (see login.cengage.com). On this website, instructors will also find free online lectures, PowerPoint slides, sample syllabi, and a test bank. This text may be used as the primary or secondary text in a family therapy theories class or as a primary text in a prepracticum or practicum/fieldwork class. Because of its combination of solid theory and practical skills, it can easily be used across more than one class to develop students' abilities to conceptualize theory and complete clinical documentation, skills that are not likely to be mastered in a single class.

When designing a class to measure competencies and student learning using these treatment plans and case conceptualizations, I recommend initially going over the scoring rubrics with students so that they understand how these are used to clearly define what needs to be done and the expectations for the final product. I have found that is most helpful to provide two to three opportunities to practice case conceptualization and treatment planning over a semester to provide feedback and enable students to improve and build upon these skills in a systematic fashion. Specifically, I have a small group present a case conceptualization and treatment plan with each theory studied based on a video the class watches on the theory; that way they have enough information to actually conceptualize the client dynamics and treatment. Then the entire class can see an example and discuss the thought process of developing the plan. A later or final assignment for the class can be to independently develop a treatment plan for a case (either one assigned by the instructor, from a popular movie, personal life, or actual client). By the end of a semester, with these activities, students will have developed not only competence but also confidence in their case conceptualization and treatment planning abilities.

QUESTIONS FOR PERSONAL REFLECTION AND CLASS DISCUSSION

1. How would you define "competent" therapy and what specific behaviors do you associate with competency?
2. Describe why you think each of these are common threads to competency: diversity, research, law and ethics, and person-of-the-therapist.
3. What learning and study strategies works best for you? Based on the description in this text, what do you think is the best way for you to learn the material in this text?

Students will find digital forms, online lectures, and numerous useful resources for the text on the Cengage website (www.cengagebrain.com) and the author's websites (www.dianegehart.com and www.masteringcompetencies.com). These include:

- **MindTap:** Go to MindTap® for digital study tools and resources that complement this text and help you be more successful in your course and career. There's an interactive eBook plus videos of client sessions, skill-building activities, quizzes to help you prepare for tests, apps, and more—all in one place. If your instructor didn't assign MindTap, you can find out more about it at CengageBrain.com.
- Online lectures: MP4 recordings of yours truly discussing content of select chapters
- Digital forms for all assignments: case conceptualization, clinical assessment, treatment plan, and progress note
- Links to related websites and readings

MindTap

Go to MindTap® for digital study tools and resources that complement this text and help you be more successful in your course and their careers. There's an interactive eBook plus videos of client sessions, skill-building activities, quizzes to help you prepare for tests, apps, and more—all in one place.

Forms, Scoring Rubrics, and Other Teaching Resources

Instructors will find numerous resources for the book on the Cengage website (login.cengage.com) and the author's websites (www.dianegehart.com and www.masteringcompetencies.com). These include:

- Digital forms for all assignments: case conceptualization, clinical assessment, treatment plan, and progress note
- Online lectures by the author
- Sample syllabi for how to use this book in a theory class, prepracticum skills class, or practicum class [Cengage only]
- PowerPoint slides for all chapters [Cengage only]
- Scoring rubrics for each assignment correlated to each profession's competencies: counseling, family therapy, psychology, and social work [Cengage only]
- Test bank [Cengage only]

Marriage and Family Therapy Core Competencies

Nelson, T. S., Chenail, R. J., Alexander, J. F., Crane, R. Johnson, S. M., & Schwallie, L. (2007). The development of the core competencies for the practice of marriage and family therapy. *Journal of Marital and Family Therapy*, 33, 417–438.

Counselor Education Competencies (Marriage, Couple, and Family Counseling

www.cacrep.org

Social Work Competencies: National Association of Social Workers

www.socialworkers.org

Clinical Psychology Competencies

http://www.apa.org/ed/graduate/competency.aspx

REFERENCES

Gehart, D. (2011). The core competencies in marriage and family therapy education: Practical aspects of transitioning to a learning-centered, outcome-based pedagogy. *Journal of Marital and Family Therapy, 37,* 344–354.

Killen, R. (2004). *Teaching strategies for outcome-based education.* Cape Town, South Africa: Juta Academic.

Lebow, J. (2006). *Research for the psychotherapist: From science to practice.* New York: Routledge.

McDonough-Means, S. I., Kreitzer, M. J., & Bell, I. R. (2004). Fostering a healing presence and investigating its mediators. *Journal of Alternative and Complementary Medicine, 10,* S25–S41.

Miller, S. D., Duncan, B. L., & Hubble, M. (1997). *Escape from Babel: Toward a unifying language for psychotherapy practice.* New York: Norton.

Monk, G., Winslade, J., & Sinclair, S. (2008). *New horizons in multicultural counseling.* Thousand Oaks, CA: Sage.

Nelson, T. S., Chenail, R. J., Alexander, J. F., Crane, R. Johnson, S. M., & Schwallie, L. (2007). The development of the core competencies for the practice of marriage and family therapy. *Journal of Marital and Family Therapy, 33,* 417–438.

Sprenkle, D. H. (2002). Editor's introduction. In D. H. Sprenkle (Ed.), *Effectiveness research in marriage and family therapy* (pp. 9–25). Alexandria, VA: American Association for Marriage and Family Therapy.

Weimer, M. (2002). *Learner-centered teaching: Five key changes to practice.* New York: Jossey-Bass.

2

Research and Ethical Foundations of Family Therapy Theories

Learning Objectives

After reading this chapter and a few hours of focused studying, you should be able to:

- Identify the major streams of research in couple and family therapy.

- Describe the difference between **evidence-based practice** and **evidence-based treatments.**

- Identify presenting issues for which couple or family therapy approaches are identified as the theory of choice.

- Identity legal and ethical issues that are unique to working with couples and families.

Lay of the Land

This chapter covers two key foundational elements of competent family therapy practice: the evidence base and ethics. The evidence-base section is divided into four major sections:

1. Evidence-based practice
2. **Common factors** research

3. Evidence-based treatments
4. Review of the marriage and family therapy (MFT) evidence base

The ethics section covers legal and ethical issues that are particularly salient when working with couples and families. I have invited a colleague, Ben Caldwell, to write this section. He quotes legal and ethical codes by memory, with numbers, and in far more detail than most listeners would prefer. I should also warn you that he rarely offers the black-and-white answers we all hope for. Even so, I am sure even seasoned therapists will learn a thing or two from this section.

Research and the Evidence Base

In the twenty-first century, all therapists are expected to be well versed in the evidence base for the treatments they use and the problems they treat, in much the same way that we expect our medical doctors to use only procedures and drugs that have been well researched for our particular medical condition. This may or may not come as a surprise to you, but in many ways, mental health therapists have not been well versed in the evidence base for their field, especially as compared with other medical professions. (FYI: we are considered by most as *medical* professionals.) For many years, it has been as if researchers and clinicians spoke two different languages, with little communication between them. In some cases, the research has been too specific or too vague to be useful to the average practitioner. In other cases, therapists work from philosophical positions that do not value research, instead focusing on the individual needs of a particular client. The good news is that translation efforts over the past two decades have made becoming an evidence-based practitioner easier than you might imagine. This chapter covers three strands of research that inform daily practice of family therapy in contemporary practice—evidence-based practice, common factors, and evidence-based treatments—and also introduces you to an excellent resource for quick and easy review of the MFT evidence base.

The Minimum Standard of Practice: Evidence-Based Practice

More commonly used in the medical field, *evidence-based practice* uses research findings to inform clinical decisions for the care of individual clients. In a nutshell, evidence-based practice refers to knowing the evidence base related to a specific client's problem and contextual issues and using that information to make treatment decisions. For example, the research literature is very clear that systemic–structural family therapy approaches are the treatment of choice for adolescents with conduct and substance abuse disorders. Even if you are not formally trained in one of these approaches (see Chapters 4 and 5 to start your training), because the evidence base is so strong, ethically you should use this knowledge to inform your treatment decisions. Think of it this way: If you were this child's parent, would you want to take your child to a therapist who has his or her own way of doing things based on theory and experience, or to one who uses research on best practices to decide how best to help your child? You'd need a really strong referral to choose the first option.

Every therapist should strive to be an evidence-based practitioner. Many would consider it an ethical obligation, because the evidence base is quickly redefining standard practice (see the "Ethics" section below). Patterson and colleagues (2004) describe five steps of evidence-based practice for family therapists:

Step 1: Develop an answerable question to focus the search for information: What treatments are most effective for teens who cut to relieve emotional pain?

Step 2: Search the literature for the best empirical evidence to answer the question: Search digital databases such as PsychInfo and scholar.google.com using the keywords *adolescents, self-harm,* and *treatment.*

Step 3: Evaluate the validity, impact, and applicability of the research to determine its usefulness in this case: Is the study randomized? Were there comparison groups? What was the treatment effect size? Were the findings clinically relevant?

Step 4: Determine whether the research findings are applicable to the current client's situation: What are the potential benefits and risks of applying these findings with this client? Do I need to consider any diversity factors, such as age, ethnicity, class, or family system?

Step 5: After implementing the evidence-based practice (EBP), evaluate the effectiveness in this client's individual case: How did the client respond? Were there signs of improvement, no change, or signs of worsening?

Becoming an evidence-based practitioner requires a willingness to continually learn and adapt one's practice to integrate the latest findings in the field. It also requires therapists to be responsive to their client's individual needs—even if researchers indicate that a particular approach works for most clients with a specific condition, you need to evaluate whether it works for yours; if it doesn't, you need to adjust your approach. Essentially, it comes down to making a more informed decisions so that you are optimally efficient. As research becomes more clinician-friendly and relevant, I anticipate that therapists will have a far closer relationship to their evidence base.

Heart of the Matter: Common Factors Research

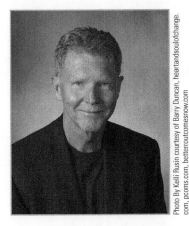

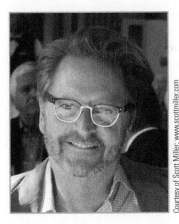

Over the past decade, professional literature has been abuzz over the "common factors debate" (Blow, Sprenkle, & Davis, 2007; Sprenkle & Blow, 2004; Sprenkle, Davis, & Lebow, 2009). Common factors proponents contend that the effectiveness of therapy has more to do with the key elements found in all theories than with the unique components of a specific theory. To simplify the argument even further: the similarities matter more than the differences. This position is supported by meta-analyses (analyses of several research studies) of outcome studies in the field: when research studies control for confounding variables (such as therapist loyalty, comparison group, or measures of outcome), there is little evidence to support the superiority of one theory over another, both in psychotherapy in general (Lambert, 1992; Wampold, 2001) and in family therapy specifically (Shadish & Baldwin, 2002).

Within the common factors community, some (Miller, Duncan, & Hubble, 1997) emphasize the common factors while minimizing the role of theory, whereas others take a more moderate approach (Sprenkle & Blow, 2004), maintaining that theories are still important because they are the *vehicles through which* therapists deliver the common factors, and because specific models may have an added benefit in certain contexts. Sprenkle and Blow (2004) point out that the common factors approach does not require therapists to relinquish therapeutic models but instead to understand their purpose differently. Rather than providing the "answer" to the client's problems, common factor proponents propose that using a structured treatment inspires confidence from clients in the therapeutic process, allowing therapists to coherently actualize common factors. From this perspective, a therapeutic model is better understood as a tool that increases therapist effectiveness rather than the "one and only true path" that resolves the client's problem.

Lambert's Common Factors Model

The most frequently cited common factors model is grounded in the work of Michael Lambert (1992). After reviewing outcome studies in psychotherapy, Lambert estimated that outcome variance (the degree to which change is attributed to a specific variable) could be attributed to four factors:

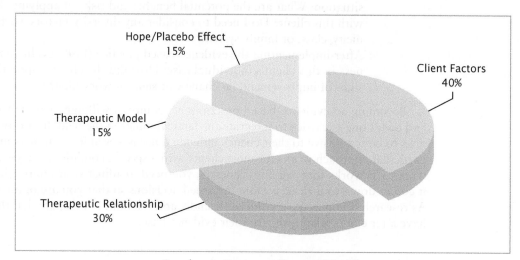

Lambert's Common Factors Model

LAMBERT'S COMMON FACTORS MODEL

- **Client Factors:** An estimated 40%; includes client motivation and resources
- **Therapeutic Relationship:** An estimated 30%; the quality of the therapeutic relationship as the *client* evaluates it
- **Therapeutic Model:** An estimated 15%; the therapist's specific model for treatment and the techniques used
- **Hope/Placebo Effect:** An estimated 15%; the client's level of hope and belief that therapy will help

Often these percentages are cited as facts, but although they are well-informed estimates based on a careful analysis of existing research, the numbers were not generated through an actual research study. Rather than exact percentages, they should be considered general trends in the research that inspire therapists to critically reconsider how they can help clients.

Wampold's Common Factors Model

Wampold (2001) conducted a meta-analysis similar to Lambert's, but compared only studies that included two or more actual therapy models (rather than comparing a model to the generic "treatment as usual" or a no-treatment control group). He presents evidence for the following:

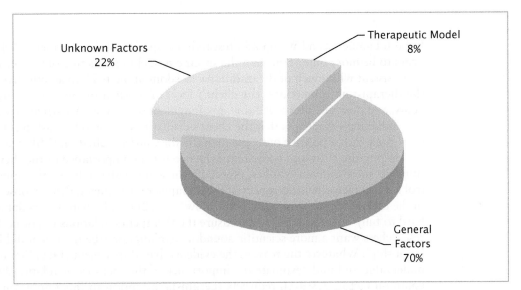

Wampold's Common Factors Model

WAMPOLD'S COMMON FACTORS MODEL

- **Therapeutic Model:** 8%; the unique contributions of a specific theory (compare with 15% in Lambert's model)
- **General Factors:** 70%; therapeutic alliance, expectancy, hope
- **Unknown Factors:** 22%; variance that is not related to known variables

Wampold's research further underscores that common elements across theories contribute more to positive therapeutic outcomes than the unique elements of a specific theory. Thus, research across theories continually indicates that general or common factors have the greatest impact on outcome; although this result may be due to the limits of research (Sprenkle & Blow, 2004) or other factors, it is the best information to date on the subject.

Client Factors

Lambert's (1992) research, which has been made most accessible to clinicians in the work of Miller and colleagues (1997), emphasizes the importance of activating client resources, such as encouraging clients to create and use support networks and increasing client motivation and engagement in the therapeutic process. Tallman and Bohart (1999) propose that most theories work equally well because of the client's ability to adapt and utilize whatever techniques and insights the therapist may offer; the therapeutic process effectively becomes a Rorschach (ink blot test) that the client uses to create change.

Miller et al. describe two general categories of client factors:

1. *Client characteristics* include the client's motivation to change, attitude about therapy and change, commitment to change, personal strengths and resources (cognitive, emotional, social, financial, spiritual), and duration of symptoms.
2. *Extratherapeutic factors* include social support, community involvement, and fortuitous life events.

Therapeutic Relationship

In both Lambert's and Wampold's research, the quality of the therapeutic relationship appears to be more important than the specific model in predicting outcome, a finding that is consistent with much of the traditional wisdom in the field. In an effective relationship, the therapist accommodates the client's level of motivation, works toward the client's goals, and demonstrates a genuine, nonjudgmental attitude. A particularly interesting—and humbling—finding is that the client's evaluation of the relationship is more strongly correlated with a positive outcome than the therapist's evaluation (Miller et al., 1997).

Despite the clear and consistent evidence for the importance of the therapeutic relationship, most outcome studies, especially those on evidence-based therapies, try to control for and factor out the impact of the therapist on treatment, thereby obscuring the role of the therapist in effective treatment (Blow et al., 2007). Perhaps this is done because it is hard to fully operationalize and measure the therapeutic relationship, or perhaps because researchers want a more scientific-sounding explanation (the treatment did it, not the relationship). Whatever the reason, the evidence-based treatment (EBT) literature seems to undervalue and underestimate the importance of the therapeutic relationship. However, common factors research redirects therapists' attention to this important component. Therapists wanting to closely attend to relationship variables can use measures such as the Session Rating Scale (see Chapter 14) to monitor the relationship on a weekly basis.

Therapeutic Model: Theory-Specific Factors

Theory-specific factors are what the therapists say and do to facilitate change while following their therapeutic model. These factors are what therapists and third-party payers consider important. However, as Lambert's research and estimations indicate, technique may not be as important as is typically assumed, actually being only half as important as the therapeutic relationship. However, it is still an influential factor over which therapists have significant control.

Hope and the Placebo Effect: Expectancy

Hope and expectancy, or the *placebo* effect, refer to clients' belief that therapy will help them resolve their problem. Lambert's (1992) emphasis on this factor heightens therapists' awareness of an often-neglected aspect of the therapeutic process, at least in the research literature (Blow et al., 2007). With this awareness, therapists can more consciously work to instill hope, which is particularly critical in the initial sessions.

Diversity and the Common Factors

Common factors can be particularly useful when working with a diverse—whether culturally, sexually, linguistically, or in ability—patient population because diversity always implies unique client resources and challenges, particularly for the therapeutic relationship, choice of approach, and strategies for instilling hope. For example, although gay, lesbian, bisexual, and transgendered clients are often ostracized in the general community, many have extensive informal and formal social support networks; the same is true of many ethnic groups and disabled or chronically ill people. Thus, the societal challenge is partially offset by unique resources. Therapists can help clients leverage these resources to better manage the often daunting challenges of being different from the majority.

Similarly, with diverse clients, the task of creating a therapeutic relationship in which the client feels accepted rather than judged requires more mindfulness and thoughtfulness because the therapist may not be aware of all the dynamics and traditions of these groups. Education on local diverse communities is of course necessary, but humility and admitting that you do not know the answer is often more important because it cultivates respect and openness (Anderson, 1997). When therapists proceed with curiosity and a willingness to learn, they often discover distinct and effective means for instilling hope from within the client's culture and primary community, further strengthening the therapeutic relationship.

The natural question that follows from the common factors debate is: Do we still need theory? As noted by Sprenkle and Blow (2004), some therapists lean toward the "dodo bird verdict," suggesting that theory matters very little. The more moderate stance of Sprenkle and Blow emphasizes that "the models are important because they are the vehicles through which the common factors do their work" (2004, 126).

Following this moderate position, theory still plays a critical role for new and seasoned clinicians, but not the role one might initially expect it to play. Rather than providing a system to help clients alleviate their symptoms and resolve their problems, a theory is a *tool* that helps the therapist to help the client. *Thus, theory may be most relevant for the therapist—not the client.*

Theory gives therapists a system for interpreting the information they get about clients so that they can say and do things that will be useful. It also helps therapists know how best to relate and respond to clients. Without theory, it is easy to get lost in a sea of information, emotion, and challenging behaviors. Theory gives therapists a systematic way of dealing with the wide range of difficulties clients bring. Thus, choosing a theory involves identifying a one that makes sense to the therapist and is useful to the therapist in navigating the "wild ride" that is psychotherapy. That said, future research may identify specific circumstances in which certain models work better for certain clients (Sprenkle & Blow, 2004).

Show Me Proof: Evidence-Based Therapies

Just in case you thought the debate was over, there is yet another thread in the theory debate that is pulling therapists in the apparently opposite direction from the common factors research: empirically supported treatments, often referred to as "evidenced-based therapies." These therapeutic models, which were developed through research and randomized trials (Sprenkle, 2002), should not be confused with evidence-based *practice* (see above), although EBTs are sometimes referred to as evidence-based practices to keep us all thoroughly confused (this is one instance where the plural refers to something quite different from the singular).

When therapists, licensing boards, or funding institutions refer to therapy models as "evidence-based," they are generally referring to a set of standards that a 1993 task force of the American Psychological Association (APA) established for what was initially called *empirically validated treatments (EVTs)* and later called *empirically supported treatments (ESTs)*, the change underscoring that a treatment is always in the process of being further studied and refined (American Psychological Association, 1993; Chambless et al., 1996). The APA established several categories for describing empirically supported therapies, and others have developed similar categories.

Empirically Supported Treatments and Their Kin: Empirically Supported Treatment Criteria

ESTs meet the following criteria (Chambless & Hollon, 1998; Sprenkle, 2002):

- Subjects are randomly assigned to treatment groups.
- In addition to the group that receives the treatment being studied, there must also be *one* of the following:
  - A no-treatment control (usually subjects are on a waiting list)
  - An alternative treatment (for comparison; may be an unspecified approach: "treatment as usual")
  - A placebo treatment
- Treatment is significantly better than the no-treatment control and at least equally as effective as an established alternative.
- Treatment is based on a written treatment manual with specific criteria for including or excluding clients.

- A specific population with a specific problem is identified.
- Researchers use reliable and valid outcome measures with appropriate statistical measures.

Criteria for Additional Forms of Evidence-Based Treatments

In addition to the criteria for empirically supported treatments, criteria have been set for other EBTs:

- Efficacious treatments: Meeting more stringent criteria, these treatments must meet the requirements for EBTs and must also undergo two independent investigations (studies conducted by someone who is not closely involved in the development of the treatment or invested in its outcome) (Chambless & Hollon, 1998; Sprenkle, 2002).
- Efficacious and specific treatments: Meeting the highest standards, these treatments must meet the criteria for efficacious treatments and must also be *superior* to alternative treatments in at least two independent studies (Chambless & Hollon, 1998; Sprenkle, 2002).

EST Pros and Cons

The advantages of ESTs are the following:

1. They have greater scientific support.
2. They have written manuals to guide treatment and are highly structured.
3. They target a specific population with a specific problem.

The disadvantages of ESTs are these:

1. They have limited applicability because they target a specific and therefore limited population.
2. They are expensive: therapists need highly specific training in the model and also need to be trained in a number of models to function effectively in most work environments.

Meta-Analytically Supported Treatments (MASTs)

A meta-analysis is a quantitative research method that combines results from multiple studies, generally by examining the effect size or the outcome variance attributed to the treatment. Using meta-analytic studies, Shadish and Baldwin (2002) developed the following criteria for MASTs to broaden the type of research that can be used to establish efficacy while maintaining rigorous scientific standards:

- Effect sizes from more than one study of the treatment must be combined meta-analytically.
- All studies must be randomized comparisons of the treatment to a no-treatment control group.
- Meta-analysis must indicate a statistically significant effect size and a significant test.
- Meta-analysis must use sound methods (e.g., aggregating effect sizes).

Real-World Applications of ESTs and MASTs

In 2002, Shadish and Baldwin identified 24 family therapy theories that fit the criteria for a MAST, whereas only 5 met the criteria for an EST. This difference existed primarily because ESTs require: (a) a written treatment manual and (b) a narrowly defined population with a specific problem; however, MASTs allow for other forms of training and more general populations to demonstrate efficacy. The findings of the APA's 2005 follow-up report on ESTs highlight the necessity for more broadly defined standards for EBTs such as MASTs (Woody, Weisz, & McLean, 2005). This survey indicated that although a higher percentage of ESTs were taught in the classroom, clinical training in ESTs dropped significantly from 1993 to 2003. When asked to identify the reasons, supervisors cited "uncertainty about how to conceptualize training in ESTs, lack of time, shortage of trained supervisors, inappropriateness of established ESTs for a given population, and philosophical opposition" (Woody et al., 2005, 9). Arguably, all but perhaps the last of these obstacles are clearly linked to the exact things that make ESTs unique: written treatment manuals and a narrowly defined population. Thus, although promising, ESTs have some practical limitations at this time, especially for the general practitioner.

Research in Perspective

Therapists need to keep the EBT movement in perspective. Almost all research indicates that any therapy is better than no treatment at all: that is one of the major ideas behind the common factors movement (Miller et al., 1997; Sprenkle & Blow, 2004). The EBT approach refines what we know and aims to develop better and more specific therapies; however, this does not mean that nothing in the field has ever been researched or studied. A more fair and realistic assessment is that family therapy and mental health therapies have an established history of meaningful research, and our ability to do research more precisely continually increases. Research courses have been part of family therapy curricula from the beginning and are increasingly valued and expanded. A research orientation is not new; however, our ability to conduct more meticulous and useful studies is improving.

Perhaps it is useful to reflect on the broader picture. More than in many other mental health disciplines, family therapy theories were developed through observational research (Moon, Dillon, & Sprenkle, 1990). Teams of therapists observed sessions through one-way mirrors, developed hypotheses about what might work, tested these hypotheses, and then refined them as they went along. Rather than trying to prove a theory, these therapist-researchers were using outcomes to inform the development of a new frontier in mental health: working with couples and families. This type of research is rigorous in a different dimension than ESTs; namely, it can be usefully applied in everyday work settings by persons with standard training. According to Shadish and Baldwin (2002), many family therapy approaches that draw from this tradition fit the criteria for MASTs: these treatments worked for decades and have been refined and designed to target specific populations in EBTs, many of which are highlighted in this book.

Try It Yourself

Either by yourself or with a partner, describe your thoughts on common factors research vs. evidence-based treatments. Which do you think is more clinically useful? How do you imagine using both to inform distinct elements of your practice?

Review of the MFT Evidence Base

Finally, I want to let you know about academic gold mines that makes grad students and their faculty particularly giddy when they discover them: reviews of the evidence base. These publications do much of the heavy lifting for you by summarizing the evidence base for specific populations. Because couple and family therapy is a very specific area of focus, there are several excellent options available, including an extensive series of reviews in the *Journal of Marital and Family Therapy,* a set of reviews in the *Journal of Family Therapy,* and Lebow's (2006) user-friendly guide to research for psychotherapists. Finally, Christensen (2010) outlines a unified protocol for couples therapy based on the evidence base, the first of its kind for relational work.

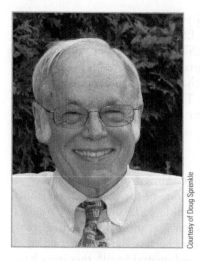

Courtesy of Doug Sprenkle

2012 Journal of Marital and Family Therapy Review

In January 2012, the American Association for Marriage and Family Therapy published the 38th volume of the *Journal of Marital and Family Therapy* (JMFT) (Sprenkle, 2012). You may not have had the best relationships with journal articles up to this point in your education—that is common. But I think this one is going to change all that. In a nutshell, this edition of JMFT includes 12 articles in which experts in the field summarize the entire evidence base for you. It is an academic's fantasy come true. This is the third of such reviews of the MFT evidence base, making it the only mental health discipline I know of to have such a concise and easily accessible review of the associated research (and trust me, I have looked). This single resource can make evidence-based practice with couples, families, and children a breeze.

The areas of research reviewed include:

- Conduct disorder and delinquency with adolescents (Baldwin et al., 2012; Henggeler & Sheidow, 2012)
- Child and adolescent disorders (Kaslow et al., 2012)
- Affective disorders (e.g., mood disorders; Beach & Whisman, 2012)
- Treatment of couple distress (Lebow et al., 2012)
- Treatment of couples experiencing interpersonal violence (Stith et al., 2012)
- Relationship education for nondistressed couples (Markman & Rhoades, 2012)
- Family psychoeducation for severe mental illness (Lucksted et al., 2012)
- Family therapy for drug abuse (Rowe, 2012)
- Couple and family interventions for health problems (Shields et al., 2012)
- Client perceptions of MFT (Chenail et al., 2012)

2014 Journal of Family Therapy Review

A pair of articles in the *Journal of Family Therapy,* which is published by the Association for Family Therapy and Systemic Practice in the Great Britain, reviews the evidence base for using systemic family therapy to treat both child and adult concerns (Carr, 2014a, 2014b). Carr presents an overview of a wide range of presenting issues for which systemic approaches are used alone or in conjunction with other methods. Highlights of this review include:

- Infancy: Family therapy has been effectively used to address a range of infant concerns, including sleep, feeding, and attachment problems, with family therapy often having better outcomes than treatment as normal for these conditions.
- Child abuse and neglect: Family therapy has been demonstrated to reduce physical abuse and neglect significantly better than comparison treatments, with only 19% of parents in family treatment having a repeated report of abuse, as compared with 49% with standard treatment. Similarly, treating sexual abuse victims with models like trauma-focused cognitive–behavioral therapy (Cohen, Mannarino, & Deblinger, 2006), which includes a strong family component, were also more effective than treatment as usual.
- Childhood conduct problems and attention-deficit/hyperactivity disorder (ADHD): Family therapy is perhaps the most-studied areas with the most robust evidence base in the field, and it is consistently identified as the treatment of choice for children with conduct issues and attention-deficit disorders. For example, family therapists have developed four specific EBTs for conduct disorder, including functional family therapy (covered in Chapter 5), which are found to be superior to treatment as usual. For ADHD, systemic family interventions that target parenting practices are essential to effective treatment with or without medications. In addition, researchers have found that medication stops having a therapeutic effect after approximately 3 years, after which, the only treatment associated with behavioral improvement is family therapy.

- Adolescent substance misuse: Family therapy is more effective than other types of interventions, including cognitive–behavioral therapy, motivational interviewing, psychoeducation, and other forms of individual and group therapy.
- Childhood emotional problems: Family therapy is effective for treating childhood anxiety and depression, including related issues of school refusal, self-harm, and obsessive–compulsive disorder, and more effective in maintaining posttreatment improvements.
- Adolescent eating disorder: Family therapy is extremely effective for treating adolescents diagnosed with eating disorders, with no more than 10 to 15% having symptoms 6 years later. Furthermore, outpatient family-based treatment is far superior in reducing relapse rates as well as being significantly less expensive than inpatient treatment.
- First episode of psychosis in adolescents: Multifamily groups and family psychoeducation have been found to be very effective in preventing relapse in adolescents having a psychotic episode for the first time.
- Childhood somatic and physical health problems: In clinical trials, family therapy was found to be very effective for treating a range of physical health conditions, including recurrent abdominal pain, poorly controlled asthma, and poorly controlled diabetes.
- Couple relationship distress: Couples therapy, particularly evidenced-based approaches, such as emotionally focused couple therapy (see Chapter 6) and integrative behavioral couples therapy (see Chapter 8), are extremely effective in improving relational distress; 70% of couples experience moderate to significant benefit.
- Psychosexual problems: Psychosexual problems respond well to couples therapy to address these concerns, which include erectile disorder and sexual pain disorder, with 73% faring better than wait-listed controls.
- Interpersonal partner violence: In contrast to older treatment recommendations, emerging research indicates that mild-to-moderate intimate partner violence with family-only batterers responds better to couple-based programs rather than traditional batterer group programs. However, conjoint therapy is not appropriate for couples with batterers who have more severe abuse or more severe mental health issues, including antisocial or borderline personality disorder.
- Adult anxiety: Although individual cognitive–behavioral therapies are commonly used for anxiety, family-based treatments are particularly effective for three of the most severe adult anxiety disorders: posttraumatic stress disorder, obsessive–compulsive disorder, and agoraphobia with panic disorder.
- Adult mood disorders: One of the most common mental health issues, family therapy is more effective than no treatment, as effective as individual treatment in all cases, and *more* effective than individual therapy for persons who have relational distress. Simply stated: if a person reports that there is relational distress while depressed, couple or family therapy is indicated.

  - Adult alcohol misuse: Couples and family treatments are regularly used in treating persons with alcohol disorders, especially to help prevent future relapse, which is particularly high for this population.
  - Chronic physical illness: Families dealing with the chronic physical illness of a member experience tremendous stress. Family interventions, including career support groups, lead to better physical and mental health for both patients and their families.

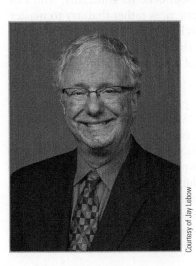

Courtesy of Jay Lebow

Lebow's Review of Evidence Base

In perhaps the most engaging and fun (really, it's true) review of literature in the field, Lebow (2006) reviews the entire field of psychotherapy. His review highlights the fact that contemporary family therapy approaches, particularly the evidence-based ones such as emotionally focused therapy or functional family therapy, are often the treatment of choice, which is clearly outlined in the list above. Some highlights about couples and family therapy from his extensive review include:

- Difficult-to-engage clients: Researchers have found that family therapy is one approach for engaging clients who are reluctant or resistant to psychotherapy, which often includes persons diagnosed with alcohol or substance abuse problems, psychotic disorders, or conduct issues.

- Marriage preparation and enrichment programs for nondistressed couples: Researchers have found that marital preparation and enrichment programs are very effective in helping reduce future couple distress and divorce, with 66% of couples better off than those who do not participate in such a program. In addition, researchers have found that these programs result in significant changes in behavior in addition to increasing relationship satisfaction.

- Happy marriage: Although there is a fair amount of debate about what makes for happy couples, researchers do agree that the following are critical elements: (a) criticism, defensiveness, contempt, and stonewalling can be damaging to relationships, especially when frequent, and (b) maintaining a high ratio of positive-to-negative experiences in the relationship.

- Effects of divorce: After the first 1 to 2 years of divorce, members of most divorced families return to the same functioning, symptom, and happiness levels of nondivorced families. Overall, rates of problems in divorced families is only 10 to 15% higher than in intact families. High conflict, whether in a marriage or a divorce, is the most significant risk factor, with some arguing that it is more detrimental than divorce itself.

- Blended families: Divorce rates are higher for second marriages—60%, vs. 50% for first-time marriages. Like the transition after divorce, the transition period for blended families is typically difficult, especially in the first 2 years.

- Therapies that do not work: In general, psychotherapy is beneficial for the vast majority of clients. However, researchers have found that three things do not work: (a) group therapy for adolescents with conduct and substance abuse issues, which nonetheless are frequently used in treatment programs and mandated by courts; (b) the Rorschach assessment, which seems to accurately identify only those with active psychosis; and (c) critical incident stress debriefing, which for many increases rather than reduces symptoms after trauma.

Unified Protocol for Couples Therapy

Christensen (2010) reviewed the evidence base for couples therapy to identify commonalities across EBTs models to create a unified protocol, which up to this point had been done only for a handful of emotional disorders. Unified protocol benefits clinicians, who can more easily focus on the fundamental practices rather than try to master multiple approaches, as well as researchers, who can more efficiently design research on the key elements of change. Christensen proposes the following elements for a unified protocol for couples therapy:

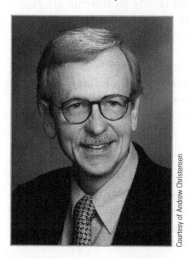

Courtesy of Andrew Christensen

- Provide contextualized, dyadic, objective conceptualization of problems: The first principle is to provide a systemic recontextualization of the couple's problems. As you will see in Part II of this text in the "Scope It Out" section, each couple and family therapy theory has its own approach to doing this, but they all do it. For couples, most approaches help couples see how the reciprocal behaviors of each partner reinforce the negative behavior in the other partner to create a negative interaction cycle. Most approaches have specific ways to reframe this interaction to reduce blaming one's partner and instead to have a more gentle and empathetic explanation for the behavior of each.

- Modify emotion-driven, dysfunctional, and destructive interactional behavior: The next principle is to reduce destructive behaviors, which includes physical abuse and sexual coercion in the extreme and more commonly involves verbal abuse, yelling, and interrupting. Couples therapists have many strategies for modifying these more destructive behaviors, including structured time-outs, in-session enactments, and outside referrals for individual therapy for serious abuse situations.
- Elicit avoided, emotion-based private behavior: Couples therapists also help couples to address avoided issues, such as a growing sense of alienation, lack of physical contact, or substance misuse. In most cases, therapists access these avoided and private emotions by identifying more vulnerable emotions—such as loss, hurt, or rejection—related to the couples negative interactions.
- Foster productive communication: Most evidence-based couples therapy approaches help couples to improve their communication, which is the presenting problem for most couples when they come to therapy. This process typically involves developing skills in both expression and listening, which can be done directly as psychoeducation or more indirectly through coaching a couple through a difficult discussion.

Try It Yourself

Either by yourself or with a partner, identify the findings in the couple and family therapy evidence base that most surprise you? Excite you? Concern you?

Legal and Ethical Issues in Couple and Family Therapy

Benjamin E. Caldwell, Psy.D.

I know, for many of you, when you hear the phrase "legal and ethical issues," you brace yourself for cautionary tales of what you had better not do if you don't want the licensure police to come beating down your door.

This section is not like that. I promise. I will start with a brief overview of professional practice standards for psychotherapists (you may already be familiar with these; if not, there are a handful of excellent texts fully devoted to those standards). Then I will talk about some of the particularly challenging areas of legal and ethical decision-making for therapists working with couples and families. Finally, I will discuss technology, suicide, and whether a therapist can refuse to treat clients who identify as lesbian, gay, bisexual, transgender, and questioning (LGBTQ)—three controversial issues that are reshaping professional standards in family therapy today.

Lay of the Land: More than Just Rules

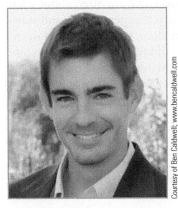

Courtesy of Ben Caldwell; www.bencaldwell.com

Here is my one (and only, I promise) paragraph of fearmongering. People can sue you, or file a complaint against you to your licensing board, any time for any reason. They can sue you for looking at them funny. They can complain about you for breathing too loudly (or too quietly). They can sue you for not suing them first. If you base your entire practice on trying to never get sued or to never get a complaint, you are trying to control something that is beyond your control. Now, whether someone will *win* that lawsuit or whether a board will *do* anything about that complaint—that is another story. You can and should take reasonable steps to protect yourself, including knowing your state's laws, maintaining professional liability insurance, and consulting with colleagues, supervisors, and attorneys whenever necessary. But doing all of those things does not make you ethical. They are like a football player's shoulder pads: They are great for protection from injury, but they do not make you a great football player.

The fact is, being an ethical professional is about much more than simply knowing and following the rules. It is true that rules-based (and, as is often the case, fear-based) teaching about law and ethics does help you to know what the rules are—at least, until the rules change. But being an ethical professional is about knowing what to do when the legal and ethical rules governing our field *do not* tell you specifically what to do. There are times when those rules are not clear, or when they appear to contradict themselves. In those situations, simply knowing the rules will only leave a therapist confused and anxious, hoping that they do not do the wrong thing. It is in those instances when your character as a professional is most revealed. Being an ethical professional means engaging in a thoughtful and careful decision-making process that results in the best outcomes for your clients, within the accepted standards of the field.

Those accepted standards are largely consistent across mental health professions. This section is not meant to be a replacement for a full law and ethics course or textbook, and it is not meant to cover the full scope of the legal and ethical issues in psychotherapy. (For a complete textbook focused on the legal and ethical issues in couple and family work, I would recommend Wilcoxon, Remley, and Gladding's *Ethical, Legal and Professional Issues in the Practice of Marriage and Family Therapy*.) Instead, this section is meant to offer particular guidance on those issues most relevant to—or most different in—couples and family therapy. Working with more than one person on a therapeutic issue raises unique concerns, and it is these concerns I will emphasize. A brief, broader overview is necessary to set the stage, but if you are already familiar with general professional ethics in psychotherapy, you can safely skip this part and pick up at the section on "Specific Legal and Ethical Concerns in Couple and Family Work."

The Big Picture: Standards of Professional Practice

Practicing any form of therapy in a professional manner means understanding three levels of rules that govern professional behavior:

* Laws
* Ethics
* Standard of care

Laws

First, there are laws. Laws are either set by government, in the form of legislation and regulation; or by judges, whose rulings in some cases establish specific responsibilities for professionals. *Tarasoff v. California Board of Regents,* which established a therapist's responsibility to intervene when a client poses an immediate danger to an identifiable victim, is an example of case law impacting psychotherapists. Laws are often about what you *must* do (like pass a licensing exam in order to practice independently) and *must not* do (like insurance fraud or sleeping with clients). They do not have exceptions, except those also spelled out in law. For example, you must maintain confidentiality *except* when a client is a threat to themselves or others and in other instances defined in state and federal law. (Regulations are a subset of laws. Instead of being set by a state legislature, regulations are often set by licensing boards through state administrative processes. They do, however, hold the power of law.)

Laws trump everything else. If a law and an ethical responsibility set different standards for professional behavior with regard to a particular issue, the therapist should follow the higher standard. But if a law directly contradicts an element of an ethical code, the therapist must abide by the law, in whatever manner allows for the most adherence to the ethical code possible.

Ethics

The second level of standards that govern professional behavior is ethics. Each of the major professional associations in mental health publishes a code of ethics that serves to guide responsible professional behavior. Counselors and psychologists have ethics codes published by the American Counseling Association (ACA; www.counseling .org) and the American Psychological Association; APA; (www.apa.org), respectively. In family therapy, the American Association for Marriage and Family Therapy (AAMFT; www.aamft.org), the California Association of Marriage and Family Therapists (CAMFT; www.camft.org), and the International Association of Marriage and Family Counselors (IAMFC; www.iamfconline.org) each publishes their own code of ethics. These codes go beyond the rules of the law, and they define in more detail the expectations for family therapists. However, no ethical code can be expected to offer specific guidance on every possible scenario a therapist will encounter. Being an ethical practitioner is about much more than knowing the codes; it is also about understanding ethical *reasoning* so that you can make the best choice of what to do when the legal and ethical rules are not clear.

There are a handful of biomedical ethical principles (Beauchamp & Childress, 2009; Veatch, Haddad, & English, 2014) that may be used when weighing the ethics of decisions in mental health work:

- *Fidelity* refers to keeping promises and upholding loyalty. This can be challenging in couples and family work, where family members may attempt to get the therapist to take sides in their internal struggles.
- *Justice* refers to treating people fairly, bearing in mind that fair treatment does not always mean equal treatment.
- *Autonomy* refers to the right of clients to make their own decisions and act independently. In family therapy, it is particularly important that a therapist respect a client's right to make his or her own decisions regarding romantic relationships, such as choosing to cohabit, separate, divorce, or marry and regarding child care, including custody and visitation.
- *Beneficence* refers to the therapist's obligation to actively work to benefit clients. If a couple or family does not appear likely to benefit from ongoing treatment with a therapist, the clients should be referred to another therapist.
- *Nonmaleficence* refers to avoiding harm to clients or others.
- *Veracity* refers to providing accurate, complete, and objective information to clients and others. This includes information about diagnosis, possible risks and benefits of treatment, and the progression of treatment.

None of these principles are absolute, and each must be appropriately balanced with the other principles. For example, while it might do a great deal of good for every client who posed even a moderate risk of violence to be hospitalized (maximizing beneficence), involuntary hospitalization poses such a high cost to autonomy that we reserve it only for the most immediately high-risk patients.

When ethical guidelines for handling a particular situation are unclear or appear to contradict, it is generally recommended that mental health professionals return to these general principles to assess the risks and benefits of their options. Several different models of ethical decision-making exist for precisely this purpose (e.g., Corey et al., 2015; Kitchener, 1986; Koocher & Keith-Spiegel, 2007; Tarvydas, Vazquez-Ramos, & Estrada-Hernandez, 2015), and some of these models have been specifically applied to a family therapy context (Wilcoxon et al., 2012). As part of that process, you may find it helpful to engage in a process of scoring possible courses of action on how well they would uphold these principles (Caldwell & Stone, in press).

Standard of Care

Finally, the third level of standards governing professional behavior is called the *standard of care*. California's definition of "reasonable suspicion" of child abuse, which triggers a therapist's mandated reporting responsibility, is one effort to define the standard of care in law:

> *For purposes of this article, "reasonable suspicion" means that it is objectively reasonable for a person to entertain a suspicion, based upon facts that could cause a reasonable person in a like position, drawing, when appropriate, on his or her training and experience, to suspect child abuse or neglect. "Reasonable suspicion" does not require certainty that child abuse or neglect has occurred nor does it require a specific medical indication of child abuse or neglect; any "reasonable suspicion" is sufficient. (California Penal Code 11166(a)(1))*

In essence, the standard says, "If another therapist would suspect child abuse with the information and training you have, you should suspect it too." This is what it means to have a standard of care: It is what most people at the same professional level are doing. Case documentation (described in Chapters 11 to 15) works on a similar principle: While legal and ethical standards do not tend to specify what should be in progress notes, therapists tend to follow standard formatting and include similar content, because that is what their peers do. Even in elements of therapy for which there is no legal or ethical standard, failing to live up to the standard of care is seen as inadequate professional behavior.

There is no single place for family therapists to look for a standard of care in writing. However, if you are unclear about the standard of care on any specific issue, the wise thing to do is consult with the colleagues and supervisors you most respect. They can best inform you what others in the profession are doing.

Specific Legal and Ethical Concerns in Couples and Family Work

Handling legal and ethical issues in couples and family work can be tremendously complex. The therapist is tasked with making decisions that will uphold the interests of multiple family members, whose interests sometimes conflict with one another.

Several areas specific to couples and family work have rules that differ from those for individual therapy. These include identifying the patient, documentation, confidentiality, communicating with other systems, working with minors, child abuse reporting, and intimate partner violence.

Who Is Your Patient?

Perhaps the most difficult challenge in couples and family work is identifying who exactly it is you are treating. In individual therapy, it is easy to identify your patient: Look at the person sitting in front of you. Couples and families, however, come to therapy with complex complaints. In some instances, they identify one member of the family as the problem who has brought them to you. In other instances, they say that the entire relationship or entire family is struggling. Who is the therapist treating? The most recent version of the *AAMFT Code of Ethics* (AAMFT, 2015) acknowledges this concern, without a specific directive on how to address it. The code simply requires marriage and family therapists to "find an appropriate balance" between conflicting goals within the family system.

The question is not just academic. How you answer it will have an impact on how you organize your treatment plan, how you document the case, how you handle conflict between family members, and even how payment takes place. Indeed, it is likely to reflect your underlying philosophy when it comes to couples and family work.

Therapists who specialize in treating couples and families often view themselves as treating the entire system as a unit. These therapists usually label themselves as "relational" or "systemic" in their work. Accordingly, they will keep a single file for the entire family, even if different combinations of family members are present at specific sessions. The treatment plan will be focused on systemic goals involving relationship or family functioning, goals that usually are agreed upon by all members of the couple or family attending therapy. Relational therapists do not ignore individual functioning, but rather they consider it in its interpersonal context.

Documentation

In treating the family as a unit, the therapist is likely to be keeping a single file on the entire family. That would mean one treatment plan for the entire family and one progress note per session, no matter how many family members attended. That also means that under most state laws, the consent of every family member in treatment would be needed to release records to any individual family member requesting them.

If you are treating an individual, and other family members sometimes join in therapy to support the individual's progress toward their treatment goals, then it makes the most sense to document the session as part of the individual client's existing file, noting the involvement of the others. In this case, only the individual receiving treatment needs to consent to the release of their records.

Some work settings require therapists doing couples or family work to keep a separate and distinct file for each participant in the therapy. While this does allow for detailed recording of each person's behavior—something that can get lost when a single progress note is written for a session involving several family members—it also means that the therapist will spend significant additional time documenting each session and needs to be thoughtful about how to document family interactions in an individual's file. In this instance, each individual could consent to the release of their own records, but they could not request the release of other family members' files. (State laws on this may vary, so it is of course important to be familiar with the laws of your state.)

Confidentiality

Confidentiality is both a legal and ethical requirement for psychotherapists, and most of the time it is fairly straightforward: You cannot share what clients tell you. (My treatment contract for many years has included the line, "The therapy office is like Las Vegas. What you say here, stays here.") There are exceptions to this spelled out in the law: Therapists are required to break confidentiality to report child abuse and when necessary to stop clients who pose an imminent danger to themselves or others. There are many other exceptions to confidentiality spelled out in state and federal laws, and it is important that your clients be made aware of both the general rule of confidentiality and its specific exceptions.

Confidentiality becomes more complex when working with couples and families. Consider a married couple where one partner is having an affair. If that partner tells you about the affair during a phone call and then tells you something like "I really want to make my marriage work, but I am not ready to end the affair yet. Please don't tell my spouse," what should the therapist do? Revealing the secret could lead the couple to give up on treatment and possibly their marriage. Keeping the secret, however, would mean colluding with the partner having the affair—and if the other partner found out later that you had known about the affair and kept it secret, that partner would likely feel betrayed.

If you are treating a couple or family, it is vital to have a policy around the holding of secrets. Two schools of thought have emerged around what the ideal secrets policy is:

1. A *"no secrets" policy.* This policy allows the therapist to communicate anything learned from any individual in the family to any of the other individuals in the family at any time. In short, it says that the therapist will not hold a secret for one family member. Holding secrets creates power imbalances in the therapy room and could require that a therapist "play dumb" about such important issues as affairs or substance use. Refusing to hold secrets means that any such information, if it comes to the therapist, can be dealt with in the therapy setting.

2. A *limited-secrets policy.* While family therapists typically do not advocate holding *all* secrets, there are many who will agree to hold *some* information in individual confidence. Doing so allows for a more thorough and trustworthy assessment process. For example, a couples therapist may see each partner individually during the assessment stage of therapy with plans to work with the couple together afterward. By assessing individually, and being willing to hold secrets from that assessment, a therapist can encourage clients to be more honest about relational issues they may not feel

comfortable discussing in front of their partner. Affairs, substance use, trauma history, and domestic violence are all examples of subjects that clients may be more honest about individually than in front of their loved ones.

The codes of ethics for family therapists do not say what a therapist's policy about secrets should be, but it is reasonable to conclude that a therapist working with couples and families should: (1) have a policy with regard to secrets; (2) inform clients of what the policy is, preferably in writing at the beginning of treatment; and (3) stick to that written policy.

Try It Yourself

Either by yourself or with a partner, describe your thoughts about maintaining confidentiality with couples and families? Should therapists ever see a member of couple or family separately?

Communicating with Other Systems

Family therapists often handle issues with regard to divorce, custody, parenting, and family functioning and as a result often have connections with other systems, such as schools and court systems. In some cases, it may be outside system that hires and pays the therapist, again raising the question of who, exactly, the "client" is. The therapist may be required to submit regular progress reports to the court, for example, on treatment goals for which the clients had little to no say.

All family members should be made aware as early as possible in therapy of the nature of the relationship the therapist has with third parties involved in the treatment. All family members should be informed about what information will be shared, with whom, and for what reasons.

Working with Minors

Even if you intend to do individual therapy, working with minors will make you a family therapist. Family members typically must give consent for the minor to receive treatment, they often want to be included in the therapy process, and they usually have a right to access treatment records. (Each of these varies a bit from state to state, so again, be sure you are familiar with your state's laws.)

State laws differ as to when a minor can consent on their own for therapy. Generally speaking, someone under the age of 18 cannot enter therapy without the consent of their parents. However, some states make exceptions to this. In California, for example, minors age 12 or older can independently consent for therapy if the therapist determines that the minor is mature enough to participate intelligently in treatment.

Whether it is part of an individual or family process, any work you do with a minor on their own should come with clear boundaries. Bear in mind here that family members may have conflicting motivations. Parents who are fearful for their child's well-being may want you to tell them everything that happens in an individual meeting with the child. The child, meanwhile, often will prefer a safe place to explore difficult emotional issues *without* the sense that their parents are always peering in. Many therapists resolve this conflict through a written agreement that defines what information will stay between the therapist and the minor and what information will be shared with the family. (As you may have guessed, this would be common among therapists using a "limited secrets" policy.) For example, if a minor is struggling to navigate peer relationships at school, the minor may not want the therapist to share that information with their parents—and it can be argued that the greater good is served by the therapist holding that information.

The child gets a safe place to be honest about their struggles, and the parents are not harmed by not having that information. On the other hand, if a minor is engaging in drug or alcohol use, or otherwise endangering their physical health, that information would be shared with the parents. Again, whatever policy the therapist chooses to employ when it comes to secrets, the policy should be clear and in writing, and the therapist should abide by it.

Child Abuse Reporting

In working with children and families, a therapist sometimes will suspect that child abuse has taken place. Sometimes this will arise directly from what clients tell the therapist; other times, the therapist makes this assessment based on physical or behavioral evidence of abuse. While state laws vary, psychotherapists typically must report physical abuse, sexual abuse, and neglect to local authorities so that the victim, as well as other potential victims, can be protected. It is vital to be aware of your state's rules for what must be reported, to whom, and how quickly once the therapist learns of the abuse.

Therapists who work with adolescents and their families should be particularly aware of their state's laws with regard to the reporting of consensual sexual activity among minors. States may differentiate between consensual sexual activity that qualifies as criminal and activity that qualifies as abusive (e.g., in some states there are some instances of statutory rape that would be considered criminal but not abusive). Since abuse *must* be reported, but criminal activity that is not abuse usually *cannot* be reported, every therapist must remain keenly aware of their state's current laws. The age of your client, the age of their partner, the nature of their relationship (e.g., whether an older partner appears to be exploiting a younger one), and the specific activities they have engaged in all may be relevant to the question of whether their relationship can be considered abusive.

Intimate Partner Violence

Several researchers have suggested that couples therapists should more thoroughly assess all couples entering therapy for current and past intimate partner violence (IPV). Without thorough assessment, such violence often goes unreported. Among couples seeking outpatient counseling, 36 to 58% have experienced male-on-female violence, and 37 to 57% have experienced female-on-male violence, in the past 12 months (Jose & O'Leary, 2009). Recent or ongoing violence can be a major impediment to successful couples therapy, and is considered a contraindication for emotionally focused therapy (Johnson, 2004), which is one of the best-validated approaches to couples work.

Generally speaking, a therapist cannot break confidentiality to report IPV on its own. If children have witnessed violence between their parents, however, the situation becomes more complex, as does the therapist's responsibility to protect the children involved. In California, when children have witnessed domestic violence, a therapist can (but is not required to) report this to law enforcement as emotional abuse. Be sure you know your state's laws on child abuse reporting before filing a report based on witnessing violence in the home.

The treatment of IPV for those convicted of a first or second offense raises specific ethical questions, particularly with regard to weighing potential risks against potential benefits of treating couples together. At present, treatment is often through court-mandated, gender-specific group therapy (Babcock, Green, & Robie, 2004). Such treatments appear to have small but meaningful impacts on recidivism (Stith et al., 2012). However, they also suffer from high dropout rates and often draw recidivism data from arrest reports. This makes their measure of recidivism subject to underreporting.

For a therapist who treats couples, inevitably some of their clients will have a history of IPV. Other couples enter therapy with active, ongoing violence. There has been debate in the literature for years about how these couples should be treated. That debate follows many of the issues noted above, particularly with regard to balancing the chance of benefit for couples with the risk of harm. Some consider the risk of harm too great to engage in any couples- or family-based treatment for at least several months after the last violent incident, noting concerns that some aggressors may become more violent when treated for IPV in a couples context. Others cite conflicting publications that support seeing couples together when their violence history has been low-level and mutual (e.g., Bograd & Mederos, 1999). Depending on where you practice, there may be state, county, or agency rules governing the treatment of domestic violence, particularly if one partner has been convicted of IPV.

Current Legal and Ethical Issues in Couples and Family Work

Professional standards change over time. Ideally, as a professional, you will take an active role in those changes. The AAMFT Code of Ethics (AAMFT, 2015) calls on family therapists to take an active role in developing or changing laws and regulations regarding family therapy to ensure such rules are in the public interest (Preamble). Often the changes in professional standards come about as a result of new forms of treatment or changes in the larger populations we serve. There are three specific issues that are currently reshaping the professional standards for couple and family therapy: technology, suicide, and therapist refusals to treat clients who identify as LGBTQ.

Technology

As videoconferencing and related technology have become more sophisticated, therapists have begun to utilize technology to provide services to clients who may not be able to come in to the office. Clients who live in rural areas without adequate health care services can be particularly helped by phone or videoconference therapy, as can clients with specific language needs that cannot be met by providers close to them.

Providing therapy services by phone or Internet is a challenging undertaking with individuals; with couples and families, it becomes even more challenging. Much of the information a therapist gathers in working with a couple and family has to do with the interaction between clients in session. When the couple or family can be seen only through a computer screen—or, if the therapy is taking place by phone, when the couple or family cannot be seen at all—it becomes much more difficult for a therapist to assess the dynamics being acted out. It may be for this reason that research on therapy that takes place by phone or videoconference has so far focused almost exclusively on individual therapy (Barak et al., 2008).

For therapists who do wish to attempt couples or family work by phone or Internet, there are several things to be aware of. First, a therapist's license authorizes them to work only in the state where they are licensed. A therapist licensed in Texas, for example, could not do telephone therapy with a couple in New York; the therapist would likely be seen as practicing in New York without a license.[1] Second, therapists providing phone- or Internet-based services must abide by additional ethical requirements, including: (1) ensuring that electronically provided therapy is appropriate, considering the clients' needs and abilities; (2) informing clients about the potential risks and benefits of the technology being used; (3) ensuring the security of the connection, to protect privacy and confidentiality; and (4) ensuring that the therapist has appropriate training and experience in using the technology. These requirements are present in both the AAMFT and ACA codes of ethics. The ACA code goes further, requiring that therapists also plan with clients for

Footnote

1. There have not yet been many test cases on this issue, though there is at least one instance of this rule being enforced. Christian Hageseth III, a psychiatrist in Colorado, prescribed antidepressant medication to a teenage patient in California through an Internet pharmacy (the psychiatrist and the patient never met). The antidepressant triggered thoughts of suicide in the patient, who ultimately killed himself. California pressed charges against the psychiatrist for practicing in California without a license, and Hageseth received jail time (Sorrel, 2009).

what to do if the connection is lost or a crisis occurs. Finally, there are no well-established protocols for couples and family therapy aided by technology, though as of this writing the AAMFT was working on such a document.

Technology is also impacting couples and family work in a very different way: By changing how couples and families relate to one another. While electronic communication allows families to maintain connection more easily over great distances, it also is frequently used to facilitate affairs and risky sexual behavior. The negative impacts of online activities are an increasingly common reason given by couples who seek therapy in my practice. However, the negative impacts of online relationships on couples and families are only beginning to be understood from a research perspective (Hertlein & Webster, 2008).

Suicide

Few topics trigger the integration of personal and professional values more than suicide. Social attitudes on the issue appear to be evolving. As states including Washington, Oregon, California, and Vermont have legalized the practice of assisted suicide over the past several years and other states have considered the possibility, concerns have arisen about what a family therapist's responsibilities would be if confronted with a client who is weighing taking their own life. In the states where assisted suicide is legal, it typically requires that the patient have been diagnosed as terminally ill without reasonable hope of recovery. Suicide is then allowed, with the understanding that it allows for the patient to die with dignity on their own terms and avoids what may otherwise be painful and costly medical interventions that would not significantly prolong life or improve quality of life.

Even in states where assisted suicide is not allowed, some patients engage in a conscious and planned effort to take their own life before an illness overtakes them. Sandra Bem, a well-known psychologist, killed herself in May 2014 rather than continuing to suffer the deterioration that she knew would come with Alzheimer's disease. Her story was detailed in the *New York Times* (Henig, 2015), and cases like it pose a moral dilemma for therapists who may be confronted with a client who has planned their death. Simply put, is suicide always wrong? Does it always demand that a therapist intervene to stop it? Particularly for family therapists, does it change things at all if the person has discussed their plan with family, as Bem did, and has the family's support?

The most recent ACA code of ethics (ACA, 2014) directly addresses this issue. However, the current family therapy codes do not, leaving many family therapists without clear guidance on how to proceed. Family therapists generally take reasonable steps to prevent a threatened suicide, and it may be difficult for a therapist to support a client who is planning to take his or her own life. Some may worry that by failing to stop a planned suicide, the therapist would be violating the standard of care in the field or that they may even be seen as complicit in the act.

Under the 2014 ACA Code of Ethics, counselors have the *option,* but not the requirement, to maintain the confidentiality of terminally ill clients planning to take their own lives. Standard B.2.b of the ACA Code reads:

> *Counselors who provide services to terminally ill individuals who are considering hastening their own deaths have the option to maintain confidentiality, depending on applicable laws and the specific circumstances of the situation and after seeking consultation or supervision from appropriate professional and legal parties.* (ACA, 2014, p. 7)

Again, however, family therapists' codes do not provide guidance on this issue. Such situations require a family therapist to be abundantly clear not just on their professional values but also on their personal morals and how the two intertwine. A case involving someone planning to take his or her own life is one that is likely to require a great deal of consultation.

Refusal to Treat LGBTQ Clients

At least three court cases have come about in the past several years with regard to psychotherapists who said they were unwilling to treat gay and lesbian clients. These have led to a broader discussion in the field about where a therapist's obligations to serve clients end and their right to practice based on their own values begins.

It is generally accepted that family therapy cannot be value-free. All therapists bring their values into the therapy room. Indeed, a value for helping the larger community through promoting healthy relationships is often part of why someone becomes a family therapist. In the interest of autonomy, therapists are usually taught to understand clients through the lens of the clients' values. The CAMFT code of ethics calls on therapists to be aware of their own personal values and not impose those values upon their clients. Similar clauses can be found in the ethics codes of APA, ACA, and the National Association of Social Workers.

In the court cases, however, therapists have asserted that their values with regard to sexuality preclude them from treating gay and lesbian clients. Julea Ward, a counseling student at Eastern Michigan University (EMU), refused to treat a lesbian client, and worked with her supervisor to ensure the client could be treated by another therapist at the same agency who did not share her conflict. EMU felt that her refusal to treat the client was discriminatory and told Ward she must complete a remediation plan. She refused to do so, and was expelled from the program as a result. She then sued the university. Jennifer Keeton, a student at Augusta State University, filed a similar lawsuit after also being told she must complete a remediation plan to ensure she would not impose her values with regard to sexuality on her clients. She had not refused to treat specific clients, but had made many statements in her classes that made it clear she would not work with gay or lesbian clients. Finally, Marcia Walden was suspended and soon fired after she refused to treat a Centers for Disease Control and Prevention (CDC) employee's same-sex relationship. Walden, who was working for a CDC contractor, had referred the case to a colleague who did not share Walden's opposition to same-sex relationships.

These cases each present strong examples of situations in which an ethical code can appear to be contradictory. On one hand, nondiscrimination clauses in all professional ethical codes in mental health suggest that clients cannot be turned away simply on the basis of their sexual orientation. On the other hand, competence clauses, also present in all professional ethical codes in mental health, require that therapists not work with clients that the therapist is not qualified to treat. If a therapist does not feel qualified to treat gay and lesbian clients, which clause becomes more important?

The court cases have yet to provide clear case law for therapists to follow, though they have generally sided against the therapists involved. The Keeton and Walden cases were dismissed by federal courts in 2012. Ward's case was settled in 2015, with EMU providing Ward a payment but not admitting any wrongdoing or changing any policies.

Partly in response to those cases, legislators in several states have pursued "conscience clause" laws that would allow therapists to refuse treatment to clients based on the therapist's beliefs, even if those beliefs are discriminatory (Caldwell, 2013). Most notably, in 2016 Tennessee passed a law specific to counselors and therapists that allows for treatment refusals based on any sincerely held belief, whether religious in nature or not, even if discriminatory. It is important to remember, however, that even where refusals to treat gay and lesbian clients may be *legal*, that does not mean that doing so is *ethical*. Any counselor or therapist who violates the antidiscrimination clause in their profession's **code of ethics** is still subject to disciplinary action.

Conclusion

Even with the best preparation and knowledge, therapists working with couples and families will face situations that leave them unsure of how to proceed. Laws are typically made in reaction to events that have already taken place, so they are not going to cover every new situation that may emerge. Ethical codes are similarly imperfect, and a standard of care does not exist for every situation. Thankfully, as a professional therapist, you have a number of resources available that can help you with difficult decision-making.

If you face legal or ethical questions in your work with couples and families, it is always better to ask questions *before* acting than after. As noted above, a number of good models of ethical decision-making are available to assist in your process of figuring out what to do next. Consulting with supervisors and colleagues can help give you a good idea of what other professionals would do in similar situations. Consulting with an attorney will help determine your legal responsibilities; your professional liability insurance carrier is likely to offer free legal consultation, and your professional association may provide the same. For questions about your ethical responsibilities, most professional associations have an ethics committee or ethics consultant who can provide advice to members.

QUESTIONS FOR PERSONAL REFLECTION AND CLASS DISCUSSION

1. How might a therapist create hope—one of the key common factors—for clients?
2. Why do you think the quality of therapeutic relationship might have more impact than specific techniques?
3. Do you think therapists should have to demonstrate their effectiveness? How do you think they should approach this?
4. What do you think about the emphasis on EBTs by third-party payers?
5. What issues do you think will be the most challenging when maintaining confidentiality with couples and families? How might you address that?
6. What do you think will be your personal challenge with working with a person who is having suicidal thoughts? With taking a child abuse report?
7. What are your thoughts about the pros and cons of online therapy? For what situations or populations might it be a good option? For which clients might it be a bad choice?
8. What are your thoughts on therapists being able to refuse clients based on their personal beliefs with the possibility that clients will experiences this as a significant abandonment or even trauma?

ONLINE RESOURCES FOR RESEARCH

American Psychological Association Documents on ESTs:
www.apa.org/divisions/div12/journals.html

Common Factors Research: Miller's and Duncan's sites:
http://scottdmiller.com
http://heartandsoulofchange.com

Substance Abuse and Mental Health Services Administration (SAMHSA) Registry of Evidence-Based Practices:
http://www.nrepp.samhsa.gov

Go to MindTap® for an eBook, videos of client sessions, activities, digital forms, practice quizzes, apps, and more—all in one place. If your instructor didn't assign MindTap, you can find out more information at CengageBrain.com.

ONLINE RESOURCES FOR LAW AND ETHICS

American Association for Marriage and Family Therapy Code of Ethics:
http://www.aamft.org/imis15/content/legal_ethics/code_of_ethics.aspx

American Association for Marriage and Family Therapy Legal and Ethical Resources (membership required):

http://www.aamft.org/iMIS15/Professional/MFT_Resources/Legal_and_Ethics/Content/Legal_Ethics/Legal_Ethics.aspx

American Counseling Association Code of Ethics:
http://www.counseling.org/resources/codeofethics/TP/home/ct2.aspx

American Psychological Association Code of Ethics:

http://www.apa.org/ethics/code/index.aspx

Ben Caldwell's blog on research and policy issues in psychotherapy:

http://www.psychotherapynotes.com

California Association of Marriage and Family Therapists Code of Ethics:

http://www.camft.org/AM/Template.cfm?Section=Code_of_Ethics&Template=/CM/HTMLDisplay.cfm&ContentID=11235

CPH and Associates (a professional liability insurance carrier) "Avoiding Liability Bulletin":

http://cphins.com/legalresources/bulletin

National Association of Social Workers Code of Ethics:

http://www.socialworkers.org/pubs/code/code.asp

Student Press Law Center information on the Jennifer Keeton case, including a link to the ruling:

http://www.splc.org/news/newsflash.asp?id=2403

REFERENCES

American Association for Marriage and Family Therapy. (2015). *AAMFT Code of Ethics*. Alexandria, VA: AAMFT.

American Counseling Association. (2014). *2014 ACA Code of Ethics*. Alexandria, VA: ACA.

American Psychological Association. (1993, October). *Task force on promotion and dissemination of psychological procedures: A report adopted by the Division 12 Board*. Retrieved from http://www.apa.org/divisions/div12/journals.html

Anderson, H. (1997). *Conversations, language, and possibilities: A postmodern approach to therapy*. New York: Basic Books.

Babcock, J. C., Green, C. E., & Robie, C. (2004). Does batterers' treatment work? A meta-analytic review of domestic violence treatment. *Clinical Psychology Review, 23*(8), 1023–1053.

Baldwin, S., Christian, S., Berkeljon, A., & Shadish, W. (2012). The effects of family therapies for adolescent delinquency and substance abuse: A meta-analysis. *Journal of Marital and Family Therapy, 38*, 281–304.

Barak, A., Hen, L., Boniel-Nissim, M., & Shapira, N. (2008). A comprehensive review and a meta-analysis of the effectiveness of internet-based psychotherapeutic interventions. *Journal of Technology in Human Services, 26*(2/4), 109–160.

Beach, S., & Whisman, M. (2012). Affective disorders. *Journal of Marital and Family Therapy, 38*, 201–219.

Beauchamp, T. L., & Childress, J. F. (2009). *Principles of biomedical ethics* (6th ed.). New York: Oxford University Press.

Blow, A. J., Sprenkle, D. H., & Davis, S. D. (2007). Is who delivers the treatment more important than the treatment itself? *Journal of Marital and Family Therapy, 33*, 298–317.

Bograd, M., & Mederos, F. (1999). Battering and couples therapy: Universal screening and selection of treatment modality. *Journal of Marital and Family Therapy, 25*(3), 291–312.

Caldwell, B. E. (2013). Whose conscience matters? *Family Therapy Magazine, 12*(5), 20–27.

Caldwell, B. E., & Stone, D. J. (in press). Using scaling to facilitate ethical decision-making in family therapy. *American Journal of Family Therapy*.

Carr, A. (2014a). The evidence base for couple therapy, family therapy and systemic interventions for adult-focused problems. *Journal of Family Therapy, 36*(2), 158–194. doi:10.1111/1467-6427.12033

Carr, A. (2014b). The evidence base for family therapy and systemic interventions for child-focused problems. *Journal of Family Therapy, 36*(2), 107–157. doi:10.1111/1467-6427.12032

Chambless, D. L., & Hollon, S. D. (1998). Defining empirically supported therapies. *Journal of Consulting and Clinical Psychology, 66,* 7–18.

Chambless, D. L., Sanderson, W. C., Shoham, V., Johnson, S. B., Pope, K. S., Crits-Christoph, P., Baker, M., Johnson, B., Woody, S. R., Sue, S., Beutler, L., Williams, D. A., & McCurry, S. (1996). An update on empirically validated treatments. *Clinical Psychologist, 49*(2), 5–18.

Chenail, R., George, S., Wulff, D., Duffy, M., Scott, K., & Tomm, K. (2012). Clients' relational conceptions of conjoint couple and family therapy quality: A grounded formal theory. *Journal of Marital and Family Therapy, 38,* 241–264.

Christensen, A. (2010). A unified protocol for couple therapy. In K. Hahlweg, M. Grawe-Gerber, D. H. Baucom, K. Hahlweg, M. Grawe-Gerber, & D. H. Baucom (Eds.), *Enhancing couples: The shape of couple therapy to come* (pp. 33–46). Cambridge, MA: Hogrefe.

Cohen, J. A., Mannarino, A. P., & Deblinger, E. (2006). *Treating trauma and traumatic grief in children and adolescents.* New York: Guilford

Corey, G., Corey, M. S., Corey, C., & Callanan, P. (2015). *Issues and ethics in the helping professions* (9th ed.). Stamford, CT: Cengage Learning.

Henggeler, S., & Sheidow, A. (2012). Empirically supported family-based treatments for conduct disorder and delinquency in adolescents. *Journal of Marital and Family Therapy, 38,* 30–58.

Henig, R. M. (2015, May 14). The last day of her life. *New York Times Magazine.* Retrieved from http://www.nytimes.com/2015/05/17/magazine/the-last-day-of-her-life.html

Hertlein, K. M., & Webster, M. (2008). Technology, relationships, and problems: A research synthesis. *Journal of Marital and Family Therapy, 34,* 445–460.

Johnson, S. M. (2004). *The practice of emotionally focused couple therapy: Creating connection* (2nd ed.). New York: Guilford.

Jose, A., & O'Leary, K. D. (2009). Prevalence of partner aggression in representative and clinic samples. In K. D. O'Leary & E. M. Woodin (Eds.), *Psychological and physical aggression in couples: Causes and interventions* (pp. 15–35). Washington, DC: American Psychological Association.

Kaslow, N., Broth, M., Smith, C., & Collins, M. (2012). Family-based interventions for child and adolescent disorders. *Journal of Marital and Family Therapy, 38,* 82–100.

Kitchener, K. S. (1986). Teaching applied ethics in counselor education: An integration of psychological processes and philosophical analysis. *Journal of Counseling and Development, 64,* 306–310.

Koocher, G. P., & Keith-Spiegel, P. (2007). *Ethics in psychology and the mental health professions: Standards and cases.* New York: Oxford University Press.

Lambert, M. (1992). Psychotherapy outcome research: Implications for integrative and eclectic therapists. In J. C. Norcross & M. R. Goldfried (Eds.), *Handbook of psychotherapy integration* (pp. 94–129). New York: Wiley.

Lebow, J. (2006). *Research for the psychotherapist: From science to practice.* New York: Routledge.

Lebow, J., Chambers, A., Christensen, A., & Johnson, S. (2012). Research on the treatment of couple distress. *Journal of Marital and Family Therapy, 38,* 145–168.

Lu!cksted, A., McFarlane, W., Downing, D., & Dixon, L. (2012). Recent developments in family psychoeducation as an evidence-based practice. *Journal of Marital and Family Therapy, 38,* 101–121.

Markman, H., & Rhoades, G. (2012). Relationship education research: Current status and future directions. *Journal of Marital and Family Therapy, 38,* 169–200.

Miller, S. D., Duncan, B. L., & Hubble, M. (1997). *Escape from Babel: Toward a unifying language for psychotherapy practice.* New York: Norton.

Moon, S. M., Dillon, D. R., & Sprenkle, D. H. (1990). Family therapy and qualitative research. *Journal of Marital and Family Therapy, 16,* 357–373.

Patterson, J. E., Miller, R. B., Carnes, S., & Wilson, S. (2004). Evidence-based practice for marriage and family therapies. *Journal of Marital and Family Therapy, 30,* 183–195.

Rowe, C. (2012). Family therapy for drug abuse: Review and updates 2003–2010. *Journal of Marital and Family Therapy, 38,* 59–81.

Shadish, W. R., & Baldwin, S. A. (2002). Meta-analysis of MFT interventions. In D. H. Sprenkle (Ed.), *Effectiveness research in marriage and family therapy* (pp. 339–370). Alexandria, VA: American Association for Marriage and Family Therapy.

Shields, C., Finley, M., Chawla, N., & Meadors, P. (2012). Couple and family interventions in health problems. *Journal of Marital and Family Therapy, 38,* 265–280.

Sorrel, A. L. (2009). Doctor gets jail time for online, out-of-state prescribing. *American Medical News,* June 8, 2009.

Sprenkle, D. (Ed.). (2012). Intervention research in couple and family therapy [Special edition]. *Journal of Marital and Family Therapy, 38*(1).

Sprenkle, D. H. (Ed.). (2002). Editor's introduction. In D. H. Sprenkle (Ed.), *Effectiveness research in marriage and family therapy* (pp. 9–25). Alexandria, VA: American Association for Marriage and Family Therapy.

Sprenkle, D. H., & Blow, A. J. (2004). Common factors and our sacred models. *Journal of Marital and Family Therapy, 30,* 113–129.

Sprenkle, D. H., Davis, S. D., & Lebow, J. (2009). *Beyond our sacred models: Common factors in couple, family, and relational psychotherapy.* New York: Guilford.

Stith, S., McCollum, E., Amanor-Boadu, Y., & Smith, D. (2012). Systemic perspectives on intimate partner violence treatment. *Journal of Marital and Family Therapy, 38,* 220–240.

Tallman, K., & Bohart, A. C. (1999). The client as a common factor: Clients as self-healers. In M. A. Hubble, B. L. Duncan, & S. D. Miller (Eds.), *The heart and soul of change: What works in therapy* (pp. 91–131). Washington, DC: American Psychological Association.

Tarvydas, V., Vazquez-Ramos, R., & Estrada-Hernandez, M. (2015). Applied participatory ethics: Bridging the social justice chasm between counselor and client. *Counseling and Values, 60*(2), 218–233.

Veatch, R. M., Haddad, A. M., & English, D. C. (2014). *Case studies in biomedical ethics.* New York: Oxford University Press.

Wampold, B. E. (2001). *The great psychotherapy debate: Models, methods, and findings.* Mahwah, NJ: Erlbaum.

Wilcoxon, S. A., Remley, T. P., & Gladding, S. T. (2012). *Ethical, legal, and professional issues in the practice of marriage and family therapy* (updated 5th ed.). Upper Saddle River, NJ: Pearson.

Woody, S. R., Weisz, J., & McLean, C. (2005). Empirically supported treatments: 10 years later. *Clinical Psychologist, 58,* 5–11.

3

Philosophical Foundations of Family Therapy Theories

Learning Objectives

After reading this chapter and a few hours of focused studying, you should be able to:

- Describe the foundational assumptions of systemic theory.

- Provide an overview of Karl Tomm's approach to conceptualizing interaction patterns in therapy.

- Outline the basic assumptions of postmodern approaches used in family therapy.

- Identify the four major philosophical schools in family therapy.

Lay of the Land

Before exploring the various models of family therapy, I want to briefly introduce you to their philosophical foundations. The two closely related philosophical traditions that inform family therapy approaches are **systems theory** and **social constructionism**, the latter a particular form of **postmodernism**. To some degree or another, all schools of family therapy have been influenced by these two theories, with traditional therapies drawing more heavily from systemic theory and more recent ones from social constructionist theory.

Systemically Influenced Family Therapies and Theories

- Systemic and strategic theories: Mental Research Institute (MRI), Milan, strategic therapies (see Chapter 4)
- Structural family therapy and functional family therapy (see Chapter 5)

- Experiential family therapy theories: Satir's human growth model, and emotionally focused couples therapy (see Chapter 6)
- Intergenerational theories: Bowen's intergenerational and psychoanalytic therapies (see Chapter 7)
- Cognitive–behavioral family therapies (see Chapter 8)
- Early solution-based therapies (see Chapter 9)

Social Constructionist Family Therapies

- Later solution-based therapies (see Chapter 9)
- Narrative therapy (see Chapter 10)
- Collaborative therapy (see Chapter 10)

In this chapter, I introduce key philosophical concepts in the field that are the foundations for the applied theories in Part II. For many readers, these concepts seem disembodied on the initial reading and become clearer only after reading about applied theories in Part II. If that is the case for you, I recommend you reread this. It may suddenly make sense rather than haunt you.

Here's a bird's eye view of the chapter:

- Systemic foundations: First, you will be introduced to the classic systemic theories upon which the original family therapy approaches were originally built in the 1960s.
- Social constructionist foundations: Next, you will learn about the social constructionist and postmodern philosophical foundations that significantly shaped the field in the 1980s and 1990s.
- Contemporary systemic framework: Then I present a comprehensive—and arguably streamlined—21st-century model for conceptualizing systems that draws from both systemic and postmodern concepts that was developed by Karl Tomm and his colleagues (2014).
- Contemporary approach to gender and culture in family therapy: I will also review the contemporary approaches of feminist and diversity awareness that address limits of traditional systemic approaches; these issues will also be addressed more specifically in each of the chapters in Part II of the book.
- Choosing your theory: The last portion of this chapter will address the question of how to approach choosing a theoretical orientation for those entering the profession.

Systemic Foundations

Rumor Has It: The People and Their Stories

> *The concepts that constitute Communication or Interactional [Systems] Theory emerged not from any one individual, but, rather were the product of the interaction between the members of what has become known as the Palo Alto Group [the Bateson team]."—Weakland (1988, p. 58)*

The Macy Conferences

Not so long ago (1940), in a place not so far away (New York City), Josiah Macy (of Macy's department store fame) assembled an unexpected configuration of scholars and researchers to discuss how groups of things operate to form a system (Segal, 1991). This series of conferences in the early 1940s, the Macy Conferences, gave birth to *general*

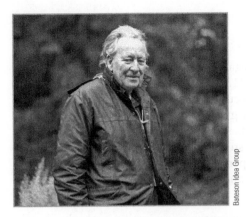

Bateson Idea Group

systems theory and *cybernetic systems theory,* which describe how biological, social, and mechanical systems operate. Rather than being developed by a single person, these ideas emerged from interactive dialogue and shared research of numerous experts and scholars on the cutting edge of their fields. Their theories led to a new approach to psychotherapy—family therapy—which is not simply a modality (i.e., working with a family vs. an individual) but, rather, a unique philosophical view of human behavior.

Gregory Bateson

Gregory Bateson, who participated in the Macy Conferences with his then-wife Margaret Mead, was a British anthropologist who explored cybernetic theory by studying intertribal interactions in New Guinea and Bali (Bateson, 1972, 1979, 1991; Mental Research Institute, 2002). Bateson's elegant and thoughtful articulations of cybernetic theory influenced numerous disciplines, including communications, anthropology, and family therapy. As part of his research on human communications, he assembled what was later known as the *Bateson group:* Don Jackson, Jay Haley, William Fry, and John Weakland. For 10 years, he studied communication in families with members diagnosed with schizophrenia, provided consultation on cybernetic theory, and introduced team members to the trance work of Milton Erickson. The result was the *double-bind theory of schizophrenia* (Bateson, 1972), which reconceptualized psychotic behavior as an attempt to meaningfully respond in a family system characterized by double-bind communications. Bateson's prior anthropological research helped the team view problematic human behavior as a function of larger social systems rather than being purely intrapsychic.

Heinz von Foerster

Another participant at the Macy Conferences, Heinz von Foerster was born in Austria and originally studied physics before developing his theories on cybernetic systems, second-order cybernetics, and radical constructivism, a postmodern theory that describes how an individual constructs his or her reality (Mental Research Institute, 2002). His work also contributed to the philosophical foundation for systemic therapies.

Milton Erickson

Trained in medicine as a psychiatrist, Erickson was a master therapist, well known for his brief, rapid, and creative interventions and considered by many to be the father of modern hypnosis (Erickson & Keeney, 2006; Mental Research Institute, 2002). The early MRI team consulted with Erickson as it developed its brief approach to family therapy. Erickson's clinical innovations, brief approach, and emphasis on possibilities are reflected in its therapies. Erickson's work was also highly influential in the development of solution-based therapies (see Chapter 9).

Bradford Keeney

A family therapist, Keeney studied with Bateson in exploring the implications of the cybernetics of cybernetics, or second-order cybernetics, which acknowledges the role of the observer (e.g., the therapist) on what is observed (Keeney, 1983, 1985). In his more recent anthropological work, he has studied shamanism and the cybernetic (i.e., holistic) worldviews of native cultures, most notably the Kalahari Bushmen (Keeney, 1994, 1997, 1998, 2000a, 2000b, 2001a, 2001b, 2002a, 2002b, 2003). He has also used concepts from improvisational theater to develop *improvisational therapy* (Keeney, 1990) and, with his colleague Wendell Ray, has also developed *resource-focused therapy,* a strength-focused, systemic approach (Ray & Keeney, 1994).

Systemic Theoretical Concepts

General Systems Theory

Von Bertalanffy (1968), an Austrian biologist, began work on the ideas of **general systems theory** in the mid-1920s (Rambo & Hibel, 2013). Von Bertalanffy's general systems theory was one of the foundational theories discussed at the Macy Conferences, which were attended by rocket scientists building self-guided missiles, anthropologists studying intertribal interactions in Bali, and ecologists studying the interactions between species. These researchers discovered that, whether studying mechanical parts, social groups, or animals, they were noticing that systems operated using the same basic principles. General systems theory included the following concepts:

- The whole is greater than the sum of its parts.
- Systems can be viewed in terms of hierarchy, executive organization, and subsystems.
- Systems strive toward self-preservation and therefore its members work in service of the system as well as themselves.

Cybernetic Theory: Homeostasis and Self-Correction

Closely related to general systems theory and originally developed by computer engineer Norbert Weiner, **cybernetic theory** describes how systems maintain balance or homeostasis through self-correction (Rambo & Hibel, 2013). Anthropologist Gregory Bateson (1972) pioneered the study of social systems using cybernetic theory, which has had the most influence on the field of family therapy. The term *cybernetic* means "steerman" in Greek, which hints at the functional principles of cybernetic systems: they are *self-correcting* and therefore able to "steer" their own course; in contrast, a computer, for example, needs an outside entity to steer it (Bateson, 1972). What does a cybernetic system steer toward? **Homeostasis,** which in the case of families refers to the unique set of behavioral, emotional, and interactional norms that create stability for the family or other social group. Despite what the name might imply, homeostasis is not static but *dynamic.* Much like a gymnast constantly moving to maintain her balance on a beam, systems must be constantly in flux to maintain stability. In all living systems, it takes work to maintain balance, whether in mood, habits, weight, or overall health. The key to maintaining stability is the ability to self-correct, which requires feedback.

Negative and Positive Feedback

You can pretty much guarantee that the concepts of *negative* and *positive feedback* will be included on any multiple-choice test about family therapy. Why? Because the disciplinary use of the terms are the opposite of their colloquial use. So remember, the questions about negative and positive feedback are always *trick questions*—that is, if you haven't studied. Here's how to remember their definitions:

NEGATIVE VERSUS POSITIVE FEEDBACK

Negative feedback: System is outside acceptable homeostatic conditions = let's steer back to homeostasis. In most cases, any behavior outside homeostatic norms is quickly corrected with negative feedback to maintain systemic homeostasis.

Positive feedback: When negative feedback is not working to steer the system back to "normal," a positive feedback may be used to resolve the crisis in another way, introducing new behaviors and possibly a new homeostasis. In virtually all cases, the initial systemic response to positive feedback is negative feedback to get back to homeostasis.

> But sometimes the crisis is so severe that the positive feedback cannot be corrected, and the system must then reorganize its homeostatic norms.

Negative feedback is let's get back to "more of the same" feedback (Bateson, 1972; Watzlawick, Bavelas, & Jackson, 1967). Whenever behaviors stray outside the boundaries of a couple or family's homeostasis, **negative feedback** mechanisms kick in to try to bring things back to normal. For example, when a child's behavior is outside the expected norm, a parent may yell or criticize in an attempt to get the child's behavior back to acceptable parameters. If the parent is unsuccessful, a **positive feedback** loop might be created. Positive feedback involves escalating behavior that leads to a new homeostasis, which in this example might be physical violence or involving a parent who is rarely involved or any other action that might lead to a new homeostasis. In either case, the trigger could be due to what is generally considered bad news (death of a loved one, a fight with a spouse, a problem at work) or good news (graduation from college and needing to find a job, getting married and starting a new household, moving to a new city for a job). Both good and bad news can trigger negative or positive feedback loops, which result in one of two options: (a) return to former homeostasis, or (b) create a new homeostasis.

In most cases, a system initially responds to challenges to homeostasis with negative feedback by trying to get back to its former homeostasis as quickly as possible. After a fight, most couples quickly want to make up and "get back to normal." After a death, most talk about how getting back to normal will take a while, depending on how significant the deceased person was to their lives. However, sometimes it is not possible to get back to the "old normal," and a new normal needs to be created. The new norm or homeostasis is also referred to as "second-order change."

First- and Second-Order Change

Second-order change is when a system restructures its homeostasis in response to positive feedback and the rules that govern the system fundamentally shift (Watzlawick, Weakland, & Fisch, 1974). *First-order change* refers to when the system returns to its previous homeostasis after positive feedback. In first-order change, the roles can reverse (e.g., a former distancer could start pursuing), but the underlying family structure and rules for relating stay essentially the same: someone is pursuing someone. This type of first-order shift is frequent in the early stages of couples therapy when partners shift between being the pursuer and the distancer. For example, at the beginning of therapy, the woman asks for more closeness from her husband, and he asks for more space. As therapy progresses, the roles may shift. Although the problem may appear to be resolved, functionally there has been no shift in the rules that regulate intimacy in the relationship; the partners have just changed roles, so it looks and feels different. A second-order shift with this couple would involve reducing the overall pursuer–distancer pattern and increasing each person's ability to tolerate more togetherness and more distance.

It is also important to remember that second-order change is not always necessary in therapy; it depends on the client's situation. In therapy, first-order solutions make logical sense; second-order solutions seem odd and illogical because they are introducing new rules into the system. Here's a clinical confession: in actual practice the distinction between first- and second-order change is often difficult to discern. I sometimes like to say, "That was 1.5-order change." Perhaps that is because most of us change in small shifts. However, the concept of first- and second-order change enables the therapist to ask whether roles have merely shifted or whether there has been a fundamental change in the ability to negotiate more intense intimacy and tolerate greater independence.

"One Cannot Not Communicate"

The early work of the Bateson team resulted in the classic text by Watzlawick et al. (1967), *Pragmatics of Human Communication,* in which its members proposed the following axiom: "One cannot not communicate." In addition to blatantly ignoring high school English teachers' rules about double negatives, this axiom seems to contradict the most common problem presented by couples and families: "We can't (or don't) communicate." So, where did this claim come from? The Bateson team learned from its research with schizophrenic family members that even schizophrenic attempts to not communicate (e.g., nonsense, immobile states, etc.) still send a message, often communicating a desire to not communicate. Since all behavior is a form of communication, and it is impossible to not be engaged in some form of behavior (at least while we are alive), it follows that we are always communicating. As we all know, silence speaks volumes, as does nonsense, withdrawal, or a frozen pose; thus, even the most creative attempts to not communicate send a message. More commonly, the claim "we just can't communicate" means that one person doesn't like what the other has to say and that the two are unable to reach agreement, at which point it is helpful to examine the anatomy of the communicated messages—namely, the **report-and-command aspects of communication**.

Communication: Report and Command (Metacommunication)

Each communication has two components—*report* (content) and *command* (relationship)—that help therapists conceptualize communication and, more importantly, miscommunication. The report is the content: the literal meaning of the statement. The command is the **metacommunication**, or the communication about how to interpret the communication (Watzlawick et al., 1967). The command aspect always *defines the relationship* between two people. For example, the same piece of advice (content), such as "You might want to wear sunscreen today," can be accompanied by a command that defines either a peer–peer relationship or a one-up–one-down relationship. This is where miscommunication, double-bind communication, and arguments come in.

ELEMENTS OF A COMMUNICATED MESSAGE

Communicated message = **Report:** data, information (primarily verbal)
  + **Command:** defining relationship (primarily nonverbal)

The concept of report and command helps explain why couples, families, friends, co-workers, and basically any two humans can have elaborate, drawn-out arguments over taking out trash, toilet seat lids, cat litter, toothpaste, and the recalled order of events at last night's party. These arguments, although appearing to be over "little things," are really about *how the relationship is being defined* in relation to the little things; thus, they are about a big thing, namely, how to define each person's role in the relationship.

When arguing over trash and cat litter, couples are usually disagreeing with each other's message at the command (relationship) level, not the content. It often helps to move the discussion directly to the metacommunication level, communicating about the command aspect of the communication, which, in the case of household chores, may include power dynamics or perceived caring. By directly discussing the metacommunication aspects (e.g., when the wife tells her husband to take out the trash, he feels that she is treating him like a child), the couple can clarify these relational issues, at which point the content issues are usually quickly resolved. Since every communication, verbal or nonverbal, has both report and command functions, the process of "getting meta" is infinite, because the partners can then talk about the metacommunication (command) aspect of the first metacommunication.

Psychoeducation note: Although psychoeducation is not a traditional systemic technique, spending a minute or so teaching clients about this issue can help some clients better understand what is going on in their arguments if it fits with your theoretical orientation.

Double Binds

The **double-bind theory** goes back to the Bateson group's (that consisted of Jackson, Haley, Fry, and Weakland) earliest research on families with a member diagnosed with schizophrenia (Bateson, 1972). Watzlawick et al. (1967) identify the following ingredients of a double-bind communication:

1. Two people are in an *intense relationship* that has high survival value, such as a familial relation, a friendship, a religious affiliation, a doctor–patient relationship, a therapist–client relationship, or a relationship between an individual and his or her social group.
2. Within this relationship, a message is given that is structured with: (a) a primary injunction (e.g., a request or order) and (b) a simultaneous secondary injunction that contradicts the first, usually at the metacommunication level.
3. The receiver of the contradictory injunctions has the sense that he or she *cannot escape* or step outside the cognitive frame of the contradictions, either by metacommunicating (e.g., commenting on the contradiction) or by withdrawing, without threatening the relationship. The receiver is made to feel "bad" or "mad" for even suggesting there is a discrepancy.

Common examples are the commands "love me" or "be genuine," in which one person orders another to have spontaneous and authentic feelings. In their research, the MRI team noticed that this type of communication characterized families who had a member diagnosed with schizophrenia. A common exchange in these families was a mother who gave her child a cold, distant hug (command aspect communicates distance) and then said, "Why are you never happy to see me?" (report aspect suggests closeness). No matter how the child responds, the mother can prove him or her wrong. Thus, the "logical" response is a *nonresponse* or *nonsense response,* which characterizes schizophrenic behavior, such as word salad (spoken words that have no real meaning), loose associations (tangentially relating words or topics), or catatonic behavior (rigid, repetitive behavior that has no interactive meaning).

Although the double-bind theory does not account entirely for how schizophrenia develops or who develops it, it is still useful for clinicians working with families that get stuck—whether or not there is a member diagnosed with schizophrenia. Common examples of double binds in families that present for therapy are the following:

- Someone asks a partner or child to spontaneously "show love" in a specific manner (bring flowers, do chores), but when the person shows love in the way requested, the partner or parent says, "That does not count because I had to ask you to do it." This becomes a double-bind situation, with no way for the person to show genuine feeling.
- A very strict parent makes all the child's decisions but says, "I trust you to make good decisions." When the child tries to comment on the incongruency, the parent reverts to "But I *do* trust you."

Identifying the double bind is the therapist's first step at intervening in these destructive patterns.

Symmetrical and Complementary Relationships

Originating in Bateson's (1972) anthropological work, the distinction between symmetrical and complementary relationships is frequently used to understand family interactions.

In **symmetrical relationships**, the parties have "symmetrical" or evenly distributed abilities and roles in the system: an equal relationship (Watzlawick et al., 1967). Conflict in symmetrical systems generally takes the form of two equals fighting until there is a winner: each is viewed and experienced as a relative equal, and the outcome is not predictable. In family relationships, symmetrical dynamics are often seen in couples and similar-aged siblings.

In contrast, in **complementary relationships**, each party has a distinct role that balances or complements the other, often resulting in a form of hierarchy. Conflict in these relationships is less frequent because there are clearly defined, separate roles. Complementary dynamics often become a problem with couples when their roles become exaggerated or rigid. Examples of common complementary dynamics include pursuer–distancer, emotional–logical, visionary–planner, and easygoing–organized. These dynamics can provide a counterbalance that is enjoyable and helpful, especially early in the relationship; however, often these roles become exaggerated and rigid, creating a feeling of being "stuck." Often by the time clients present for therapy, each person appears to have individual psychiatric symptoms or deeply ingrained personality traits; at this point it is quite difficult for anyone to still see the roles that each person has taken on as part of the systemic dance. The family therapist's task is to see these rigid complementary roles as part of the larger system rather than as fixed personality structures. It is then much easier to have hope for change and to be creative in making change.

The Family as a System

The defining feature of systemic approaches is viewing the family as a **system**, an entity in itself, with the whole greater than the sum of its parts (Watzlawick et al., 1967). What does this really mean? Systemic therapists view the interactional patterns of the family as a sort of "mind" or organism that is not controlled by any single member or outside entity, such as a therapist. This view results in several surprising propositions:

- **No single person orchestrates the interactional patterns.** The rules that govern family interactions are not consciously constructed; instead, they emerge through an organic process of interaction, feedback (reaction), and correction until a norm or homeostasis is formed. In fact, many of the early arguments in a relationship serve as feedback to shape the emerging relationship's homeostatic norms. In most cases, this whole process occurs with minimal metacommunication about how the relational rules are being formed.
- **All behavior makes sense in context.** Because all behavior is a form of communication, it makes sense in the context in which it is expressed, within the rules of that particular system. Thus, even the seemingly nonsensical communication of schizophrenia makes sense in the larger family system.
- **No single person can be blamed for family/relational distress.** Because no one consciously creates the rules, but rather patterns are mutually negotiated through ongoing interactions, it follows that no single person can be fully blamed for family problems. Although individuals do have moral and ethical obligations in cases of abuse, the interactions "make sense" within the broader relational context and rules.
- **Personal characteristics are dependent on the system.** Although a member may display certain characteristics or tendencies, these are not inherent personality characteristics that exist independently of the system; rather, they emerge from the interactional patterns in the system. Thus, even when a family reports, "Suzie has always been like this" (e.g., angry, helpful, forgetful), the therapist takes this to be a statement more about the rules (possible rigidity) of the system than a truth about Suzie.

Epistemology

The proposition "I see you" or "You see me" is a proposition which contains within it what I am calling "epistemology." It contains within it assumptions about how we get information, what sort of stuff information is, and so forth . . . certain propositions about the nature of knowing and the nature of the universe in which we live and how we know about it.—Bateson (1972, p. 478)

Bateson's ideas about **epistemology** are foundational to all systemic family therapies. In the strict philosophical sense, *epistemology* is the study of knowledge and the process of knowing. From his cybernetic investigations, Bateson concluded that most of the propositions that humans assume to be true are erroneous; they *appear* true because they capture one dimension of an interactional sequence, but they rarely include the broader awareness of how observer and observed reciprocally reinforce and impact each other. Thus, a wife's complaint that her husband is cold and indifferent does not take into account how their ongoing series of interactions has impacted each of their behaviors and frames for interpretation. Family therapists pay careful attention to the family's epistemology, the operating premises that underlie their actions and cognitions (Keeney, 1983).

Second-Order Cybernetics

A later distinction in systemic literature, **second-order cybernetics**, refers to applying systemic principles to the observing system, which in family therapy is the therapeutic system (therapist observing the family system). In the process of observing another system, a new observer–observed system is created: a second-order (or second-level) system. The therapist is no longer a neutral, unbiased observer, but is rather an active participant in creating what is observed.

The cocreation process happens in several different ways. First, a therapist's descriptions reveal *more about the therapist* than about the family, in that any description reflects what information the therapist deems most valuable and useful. Second, *how* a therapist interacts with or treats a family significantly impacts the actions and attitudes of the family while in the therapist's presence. A therapist who engages a family in a detached, professional manner will elicit different behaviors than one who uses a playful, low-key style. Which is more "real"? Neither, or more accurately, both. Each response is a "natural, honest" response for the family system *in the context* of a particular professional. Therapists who maintain an awareness of second-order cybernetic principles remain continually attuned to how their behavior is shaping that of the client and how their descriptions of clients reflect their own values. This attention to the cocreation of the therapist–client reality became the focus of social constructionist therapists.

The Spirit of Systemic Therapists

Systemic therapists are known for their ability to see the big picture at all times. Even when a client presents with an individual issue, such as depression or anxiety, systemic therapists always view it within the larger relational contexts in which the symptom makes sense. In addition, they are known for their *irreverent* (see Chapter 4 for more details) attitude toward problems: whether the symptoms are conflict, feeling blue, drinking, psychosis, or an eating disorder, the systemic therapist is never flustered and never views one as more "serious" than another or more an "individual" than a "family" problem. Instead, all behavior is simply a means of communicating that makes sense within a particular relational system, with each person in the system doing the best he or she can. Thus, they always refrain from blaming one member of the family for a problem. This is perhaps the most difficult shift in perspective for new therapists.

Systemic therapists are able to stay focused on the interconnection of meaning and communication, on the dance between people, rather than get lost in the labeling and unidirectional thinking of individual pathology. They carefully attend to how behavior is always shaped by complex webs of relations within the family, community, and larger society. They view much of what the average person might consider an "individual problem" as part of a much larger set of interactions, of which the problem is only a small part. Their nonpathologizing, nonblaming view offers clients a refreshing and often liberating new way to think about a situation. Above all, they are pragmatic, always considering whether their interventions were useful or not, and if not, figuring out what interventions might be useful.

Social Constructionist Foundations

Social constructionist philosophy is a particular strand of postmodern philosophy, which has influenced a wide range of disciplines, including art, theater, music, architecture, literature studies, cultural studies, and philosophy. Because their systemic foundations had already conceptualized reality from a relational perspective, family therapists were the first mental health professionals to embrace postmodern philosophy. Of the various postmodern schools—constructivist, social constructionist, structuralist, and poststructuralist—social constructionism has been the most influential in the development of new psychotherapy models, such as solution-focused, collaborative, and narrative therapies (see Chapters 9 and 10).

Side by Side: Comparing Systemic and Social Constructionist Theories

The move from a systemic view (particularly the second-order cybernetic perspective) to a social constructionist perspective can be seen as a natural evolution and continuation of systemic concepts, which describe how social interactions shape a person's experience of reality. Although the vocabulary and metaphors change, the emphasis on relationships and the relational construction of reality do not. The earliest writings in family therapy explored how people construct their lived reality through interpersonal relations (Bateson, 1972; Fisch, Weakland, & Segal, 1982; Jackson, 1952, 1955; Watzlawick, 1977, 1978/1993, 1984; Weakland, 1951), laying the foundation for postmodern approaches. In fact, many of the original approaches that began systemically, such as Milan therapy and the MRI approach (see Chapter 4), over time evolved into a more constructionist form. Thus, systemic and postmodern therapies have more shared views than differences, especially when compared with other nonrelational psychotherapies.

Systemic and social constructionist theories share the following assumptions:

- A person's lived reality is relationally constructed.
- Personal identity and an individual's symptoms are related to the social systems of which they are a part.
- Changing one's language and description of a problem alters how it is experienced.
- Truth can be determined only within relational contexts; an objective, outsider perspective is impossible.

Despite these and other similarities, there are notable differences that can be traced to a shift in metaphor. Systems theory uses a *systems* metaphor: a family is a system, a group of individuals who coordinate meaning and their understanding of the world. Social constructionist therapies use a *textual* metaphor: people narrate their lives to create meaning using the social discourses available to them. In addition, social constructionist therapies emphasize the role of the therapist in the coconstruction of the client's reality, much like systemic therapists' attention to second-order cybernetic dynamics, resulting in a different approach to relating to clients and their problems. Furthermore, constructionist therapists use clients' language and stories differently than systemic therapies to create interventions.

Rumor Has It: The People and Their Stories

Kenneth Gergen

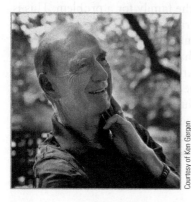

Courtesy of Ken Gergen

A social psychologist, Ken Gergen first introduced social constructionist ideas to the mental health professions in a 1985 article in *American Psychologist*. His work has laid the foundation for the development of social constructionist therapy approaches, most notably collaborative therapy (Anderson, 1997; Anderson & Gehart, 2007; Anderson & Goolishian, 1992) and to a lesser degree narrative therapy (Freedman & Combs, 1996; White & Epston, 1990). His work has included detailed applications of social constructionism to psychological and social issues (Gergen, 1999, 2001) and to postmodern ethics (McNamee & Gergen, 1999). His most recent work is on positive aging (Gergen & Gergen, 2007).

Sheila McNamee

Working with Gergen, Sheila McNamee, a communications theorist, has been a leader in translating social constructionist ideas to therapy (McNamee & Gergen, 1992), including an in-depth exploration of ethical issues (McNamee & Gergen, 1999). She has also been at the forefront of developing social constructionist pedagogy (McNamee, 2007).

John Shotter

John Shotter's social constructionist work focuses on how people coordinate joint action through shared meanings and understanding (Shotter, 1993). His work emphasizes the ethics of mutual accountability in social relationships (Shotter, 1984).

Michel Foucault

Rejecting philosophical labels such as a *postmodernist, structuralist,* and *poststructuralist,* Michel Foucault (1972, 1979, 1980) was a prolific social critic and philosopher who described how power and knowledge shape individual realities in a given society. A significant influence on Michael White's narrative therapy (see Chapter 10), Foucault's work introduces the political and social justice ramifications of language and power in therapy.

Ludvig Wittgenstein

An Austrian philosopher, Wittgenstein's philosophy of language (1973) is highly influential in postmodern therapies, notably solution-focused brief therapy and collaborative therapy (see Chapters 9 and 10). He describes language as inextricably woven into the fabric of life and argues that language cannot be meaningfully removed from its everyday use, as it commonly is in philosophical and theoretical discussions.

Mikhail Bakhtin

A Russian critic and philosopher, Bakhtin worked on dialogue and concepts of identity, emphasizing that the self is *unfinalizable* (can never be fully known) and that self and other are inextricably intertwined (Baxter & Montgomery, 1996).

Postmodern Theoretical Concepts

Skeptical of Objective Reality

Postmodernists are skeptical about the possibility of identifying an objective reality, such as x is a healthy behavior and y is not (Gergen, 1985). They describe reality as "mute" (Gergen, 1998), meaning that events and things in life do not come with prepackaged meanings, such as marriage is good, fat is ugly, and cars are bad. Instead, meaning is constructed by communities of people.

Reality Is Constructed

Postmodernists view all "truths" and "realities" as *constructed* (you will notice and perhaps be irritated by the frequent use of quote marks to emphasize that a concept is a construction, not a truth). Language and consciousness are necessary to develop meanings and to determine the value of an object or thing (Gergen, 1985; Watzlawick, 1984). Different postmodern schools emphasize and analyze different levels of reality construction;

however, they principally recognize that the construction of reality is a complex process that involves all of the following levels:

- Linguistic level—poststructuralism and philosophy of language: Focuses on how words shape our reality rather than being a reflection of it, a premise shared by all forms of postmodern thinking.
- Personal level—constructivism: Focuses on how reality is constructed within an individual organism; most closely associated with later developments of MRI and Milan therapies (Watzlawick, 1984).
- Relational level—social constructionism: Focuses on how reality is created in immediate relationships (Gergen, 1985, 1999, 2001); most closely associated with collaborative therapy.
- Societal level—critical theory: Focuses on how reality is constructed at the larger, societal level; most closely associated with narrative therapy, which draws heavily on the work of Foucault (1972, 1979, 1980).

Reality Is Constructed through Language

Postmodernists generally agree that reality is constructed primarily through language. Language is not neutral: words have real effects in our lives (Gergen, 1985). Most importantly for therapeutic purposes, words are the primary medium for: (a) fashioning our identities and (b) identifying what is a problem and what is not (Anderson, 1997; Gergen, 2001). For example, a person can interpret the same set of events (e.g., losing one's cool) as "having a bad day" or "being a bad person"; each has dramatically different implications for identity and the definition of the problem. This level of reality construction, used in all postmodern therapies, is emphasized by poststructuralists and constructivists.

Reality Is Negotiated through Relationships

The meanings we attribute to life experiences are not developed alone but rather in relationships, with immediate friends and family and more broadly with society and the subcultures of which we are a part (Gergen, 1985). The meaning a person gives to a particular behavior, haircut, job, family relation, sex act, or religious view is always embedded in a web of "local" (immediate) relationships as well as the larger societal dialogue about the particular issue. Thus, how a person views premarital sex, lying, or disciplining children develops through and within the multiple layers of outer dialogues. Postmodern therapists help clients untangle the dialogues around problems so that clients can determine those with which they choose to affiliate. This level of reality construction is emphasized in theories that emphasize social constructionism and critical theory.

Shared Meanings Coordinate Social Action

Shared meanings and values are needed to coordinate social action, or more simply, to get along with others (Gergen, 2001; Shotter, 1993). Without agreed-upon meanings on what is polite and what is rude or what is good and what is bad, it would be impossible for humans to live together—there would be total chaos. Instead, groups of people coordinate meanings and values: we call this "culture."

Tradition, Culture, and Oppression

We cannot make sense of our lives outside of tradition or culture, which refers not only to ethnicity and nationality, but also to any small or large group that has a set of norms. Cultural traditions create a framework for: (a) making meaning of our individual lives and (b) successfully coordinating our actions with others. Culture provides a set of values that its members can use to interpret their lives, knowing whether they are living a "good" life. In addition, culture provides a framework for safely and effectively interacting with others, allowing for the shared meanings necessary for marriage, family life, commerce, recreation, and religion. However, selecting certain goods and values over others inevitably labels certain behaviors and qualities as bad and undesirable. If a culture values productivity, it views taking time to relax negatively; if a culture values family, it deemphasizes individuality. Thus, all cultures are by their very nature oppressive (Gergen, 1998), because—by definition—they must identify certain behaviors as acceptable and others as unacceptable. The degree to which a culture is oppressive is directly correlated with its ability to be reflexive.

Reflexivity and Humanity

Any given culture remains *humane* to the extent that it is **reflexive,** able to examine its effects on others and to question and doubt its values and meanings (Gergen, 1998). Within any group of people, there are some people for whom the dominant cultural norms fit and others for whom they do not. The extent to which a culture listens and responds to the minority voices within it is the extent to which that culture maintains its humanity, growing and expanding to reduce the oppressive forces that are inescapable if humans are to live with one another.

Social Constructionism, Postmodernism, and Diversity

Postmodern philosophy, with its suspiciousness about singular "truths," has profoundly affected most current therapies because it heightens awareness of diversity issues. Postmodernists challenge the concept that norms cannot be fairly established because these norms are created by one group within the society and do not fairly capture the lived experience of others in that society, and even less so the reality of other groups or cultures. This is readily seen with gender, socioeconomic status, age, culture, religion, and other factors. Postmodernism proposes that the behaviors, thoughts, and feelings of a white, middle-aged, Protestant male from the Northeast cannot be assumed to be the same as those of an adolescent son of Southeast Asian immigrants who are semi-migrant farmers in California's Central Valley. They both have their own reality and truth and their respective norms and definitions of a good life; therapists must meet each with this fact in mind.

The Postmodern Spirit

It is difficult to capture the spirit or general sense of postmodernists, but I am going to try. As you might imagine, they would say that such an attempt will fail before beginning because words are always contextualized by their user's reality and can convey only that reality, not the essence of what is described. As such, the shift to a postmodern epistemology involves an ongoing awareness of how each moment of reality is constructed, how each person gives unique meaning to lived experience. When this realization infuses your view of the world—this may sound dramatic, but I think it is fair to say—your life and relationships will never be the same again.

Simply keeping the fluid nature of meaning and reality in the foreground changes how you view and relate to others and any life experience. When your partner is upset about something that seems innocuous to you, you soften and become curious about how your partner is interpreting that event. When a client shares a fear or viewpoint that seems odd or surprising, you become intensely interested in how she came to that understanding of her life and listen to her story, fascinated with how meaning evolved. If ever a couple or family appears in your office with entirely different perspectives on the same situation, this seems only natural to you, and you help them weave together these unique perspectives. Furthermore, you will no longer be able to maintain convictions and opinions like you used to—instead, you will hold all of your views more tentatively, always open to their evolving further.

One of the greatest mistakes I see new therapists make is trying to use postmodern techniques without fully adopting the true spirit of postmodernism. As you might imagine, these therapists are not very effective. Postmodern therapists are masters at seeing possibilities, hope, and strengths where other do not. Their assumptions make them optimists extraordinaire.

If you experienced some of the above ideas as a bit complex or difficult to quickly grasp, you are not alone (I can hear a sigh of relief as I type). Contemporary systemic therapists have developed—arguably—more streamlined approaches for working systemically that you are likely to find more user-friendly, especially in session and actual practice.

Tomm's Interpersonal Patterns (IP)

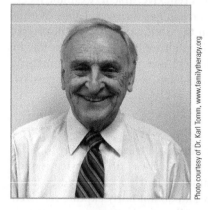

Photo courtesy of Dr. Karl Tomm, www.familytherapy.org

A pioneer of family therapy, Karl Tomm has been evolving his approach to working with families for more than three decades at the University of Calgary. Early in his work with families, he came under pressure from funding sources to provide individual mental health diagnoses using the *Diagnostic and Statistical Manual of Mental Disorders* (DSM) to justify use of public funds (see Chapter 12). After some difficult negotiation, he arranged instead to provide "systemic" diagnoses to support continued funding for the Family Therapy Program and its associated clinic that served the community (Tomm et al., 2014). The result is an elegant and easy-to-use (or at least easier-to-use— I'll let you be the judge) approach to systemic conceptualizing of interpersonal patterns (Tomm et al., 2014). In Chapter 4 on systemic therapies, I will describe how to apply Tomm's approach therapy, which has both systemic and postmodern influences, in more detail. In this chapter, I introduce his work as a contemporary approach to conceptualizing systemic dynamics.

Tomm refers to his approach to conceptualizing systemic dynamics as *the IPscope,* a "scope" for observing all forms of interpersonal patterns (IP). Not an actual object but a heuristic (something that enables one to learn), the **IPscope** is a cognitive instrument that therapists can use to assist in observing individuals, couples, families, and larger systems by focusing on the interpersonal patterns that organize their behaviors. Specifically, the IPscope is used to identify interpersonal patterns between two or more people that are: (a) recurrent and relatively stable, (b) mutually reinforcing, and (c) a complementarity, typically involving a coupling of two paired behaviors, feelings, attitudes, etc., such as pursuing and distancing or criticizing and defending. Tomm and his colleagues do not consider the patterns identified using the IPscope as capturing an essential "truth" about a person or relationship, but rather they are "serviceable fictions" or tools that help the therapist to facilitate treatment (Tomm et al., 2014). They use the IPscope to conceptualize interpersonal processes at three levels:

- Couple/family relationships: As one might expect, the IPscope is used to identify relational patterns in couples and families.
- External systems: The IPscope, can also be used to identify patterns with external systems, including extended family, community, school, peer groups, ethnic groups, religious organizations, lesbian, gay, bisexual, transgender, and questioning (LGBTQ) communities, etc.
- Intrapersonally: These patterns are also used to describe intrapsychic patterns within a person, including patterns that may characterize a way of thinking (such as depression or anxiety) as well as relating to our internalized images of the significant others. These internalized relationship patterns have real effects in the outside world. Often, after imagining a response, we preemptively respond, forgetting that the other person has not done the egregious (or use any adjective) act in reality. In fact, many of us have more arguments with the imagined others in our heads than with the actual people in the real world. This gives me hope; we can probably influence these internal representations of others more than the real others.

As illustrated in the following figure, these three levels of patterns occur simultaneously and affect one another.

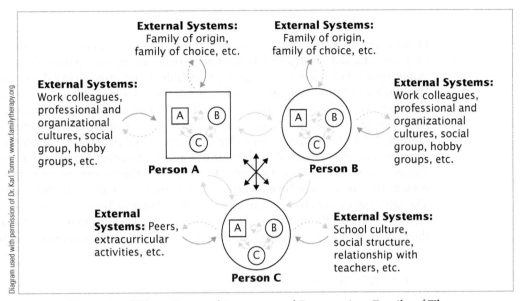

Diagram of Three Types of Interpersonal Patterns in a Family of Three.

Identify Interpersonal Patterns

Tomm and his colleagues describe several basic guidelines for identifying interpersonal patterns:

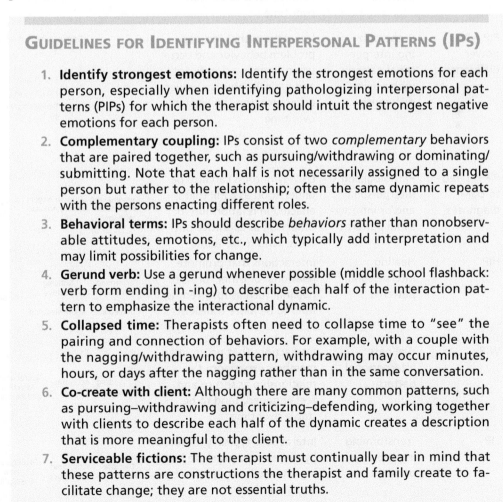

GUIDELINES FOR IDENTIFYING INTERPERSONAL PATTERNS (IPs)

1. **Identify strongest emotions:** Identify the strongest emotions for each person, especially when identifying pathologizing interpersonal patterns (PIPs) for which the therapist should intuit the strongest negative emotions for each person.

2. **Complementary coupling:** IPs consist of two *complementary* behaviors that are paired together, such as pursuing/withdrawing or dominating/submitting. Note that each half is not necessarily assigned to a single person but rather to the relationship; often the same dynamic repeats with the persons enacting different roles.

3. **Behavioral terms:** IPs should describe *behaviors* rather than nonobservable attitudes, emotions, etc., which typically add interpretation and may limit possibilities for change.

4. **Gerund verb:** Use a gerund whenever possible (middle school flashback: verb form ending in -ing) to describe each half of the interaction pattern to emphasize the interactional dynamic.

5. **Collapsed time:** Therapists often need to collapse time to "see" the pairing and connection of behaviors. For example, with a couple with the nagging/withdrawing pattern, withdrawing may occur minutes, hours, or days after the nagging rather than in the same conversation.

6. **Co-create with client:** Although there are many common patterns, such as pursuing–withdrawing and criticizing–defending, working together with clients to describe each half of the dynamic creates a description that is more meaningful to the client.

7. **Serviceable fictions:** The therapist must continually bear in mind that these patterns are constructions the therapist and family create to facilitate change; they are not essential truths.

Types of Interpersonal Patterns

Historically, when systemic practitioners discussed interactional or interpersonal patterns, they were almost always referring to negative interpersonal patterns that included the symptomatic behavior. For example, a **pathologizing interpersonal pattern** in Tomm's approach would include pursuing/distancing, as described above. Tomm expanded this idea to include identifying multiple other forms of interactional patterns that can be useful in therapy, which include healing, wellness, and transformative interpersonal patterns (Tomm, 2014). In addition, sociocultural interpersonal patterns, which can be positive or negative, are also identified as they inform and shape other patterns. Therapists identify clients' various interpersonal patterns to distinguish the interaction patterns related to the presenting problem and then identify patterns that are likely to promote desired change. The table below summarizes the interpersonal patterns Tomm and his colleagues use to facilitate therapy. Fair warning: At first it may seem like acronym soup, but once you get the hang of it, it is a surprising useful shorthand for discussing systemic dynamics.

IPSCOPE TYPOLOGY OF PATTERNS

	TYPE OF INTERPERSONAL PATTERN	DESCRIPTION	DIAGRAM
PIP	Pathologizing interpersonal patterns	Interactions that include the problem behavior, such as conflict; tend to be stable over time	Distancing/Pursuing Defending Criticizing
PIP with power difference	Pathologizing interpersonal patterns with power difference	Interactions that include problem behavior and occur when there is a significant and typically abusive power difference; tend to be stable over time	Domineering/Submitting Submitting; Dismissing/Acquiescing
PIP related to DSM diagnoses	Pathologizing interpersonal and/or intrapersonal patterns	DSM symptoms can also be understood as a PIP that is enacted in relationship to others OR as cognitive patterns; tend to be stable	Denying Free Expression of Anger/ Turning Anger Inward Against the Self Criticizing Self Criticizing Other
HIP	Healing interpersonal patterns	Interactions that promote relational or other forms of healing, such as forgiveness; tend to be more transient	Performing More Acts of Competence Noticing Positive and Acknowledging Forgiving Apologizing
WIP	Wellness interpersonal patterns	Interactions that occur when members experience the relationship as secure and feel engaged; tend to be stable over time	Setting Limits/ Accepting Limits Appreciating Affection and Respect Showing Affection and Respect
TIP	Transforming interpersonal patterns	Interactions typically initiated by therapist to promote healing and wellness; tend to be more transient	Disclose Experience/ Ask About Experience Distinguishing New Possibilities Reflexive Questions

IPSCOPE TYPOLOGY OF PATTERNS *(continued)*

	Type of Interpersonal Pattern	Description	Diagram
DIP	Deteriorating interpersonal patterns	Interactions that occur when there is a shift from wellness to symptomatic interactions; tend to be more transient	Failing to Learn — Withholding Information — Self-Conscious and Awkward Performing — Scrutinizing Performance
SCIP	Sociocultural interpersonal patterns	Interaction patterns between a person or system and dominant discourses; unlike the others, these generally take the form of Belief/Action	Belief: Patriarchal Entitlement — Action: Males Exercising Dominance; Belief: Egalitarian Gender Relations — Action: Males and Females Sharing Power

Pathologizing Interpersonal Patterns (PIPs)

Traditional family therapy approaches focused their conceptualizations on identifying the problem or PIPs, which are interactions that increase negativity or suffering in one or both persons who are interacting. These patterns are typically related directly to the presenting problem. Tomm and colleagues' (2014) approach also recognizes power differences in these dynamics, such as those seen in abusive relationships; this is a significant component of his approach when working with couples and families in which there are problematic issues with power and influence. In such circumstances, the therapist must intervene differently because the person in the "lower" position typically has less influence over the dynamic and may be at greater risk for retaliation during the change process. This approach also allows for the conceptualization of clinical DSM symptoms as a type of PIP that may be enacted with others or primarily enacted in the clients' internal world.

Healing Interpersonal Patterns (HIPs)

A **HIP** is considered an "antidote" for a particular PIP by bringing forth positive behaviors that either preclude or contradict some elements of the PIP (Gaete, Sametband, & Sutherland, 2014). These healing interactions typically facilitate forgiveness or insight that enable the parties to avoid or minimize future PIP interactions.

Wellness Interpersonal Patterns (WIPs)

Characterizing the majority of interactions in healthy relationship, a **WIP** bringing forth competence, positivity, and intimacy, such as giving affection and appreciating affection (Tomm, 2014).

Transforming Interpersonal Patterns (TIPs)

Similar to a HIP, a **TIP** is any interaction that facilitates moving from a PIP to a WIP. Most therapeutic interventions can be considered TIPs, as can between-client behaviors, such as asking about concerns and disclosing concerns (Tomm, 2014).

Deteriorating Interpersonal Patterns (DIPs)

DIPs are behaviors that typically lead to slip into a PIP, such as scrutinizing performance and self-conscious performing (Tomm, 2014). These can be initiated by the client or inadvertently, and hopefully unintentionally, by a therapist who has not carefully assessed the interpersonal patterns.

Sociocultural Interpersonal Patterns (SCIPs)

SCIPs describe beliefs, values, and societal discourses that inform interpersonal interaction patterns (St. George & Wulff, 2014) and may have a negative or a beneficial effect. For example, each culture defines specific gender roles that shape how we interact in both same-sex and opposite-sex relationships. Within a couple, each partner may have different gender-role expectations, which likely leads to conflict and possibly a PIP, such as a husband with patriarchal beliefs that lead to attempts to dominate and a wife with feminist beliefs that lead to her resisting his attempts to control. Therapists can identify the SCIPs that reinforce the PIP as well as work with the clients to identify alternative, viable SCIPs that could facilitate HIPs and WIPs, such as egalitarian beliefs about gender relations.

In the following figure, you can see how these various patterns interconnect. You can see a clear progress from PIPs to HIPs and then to WIPs with TIPs moving toward wellness and DIPs moving away from wellness. The SCIPs affect all interaction patterns, both those related to wellness and those related to pathology. Part of the therapeutic process is to identify SCIPs associated with pathology and help clients identify new discourses that will promote a greater sense of wellness.

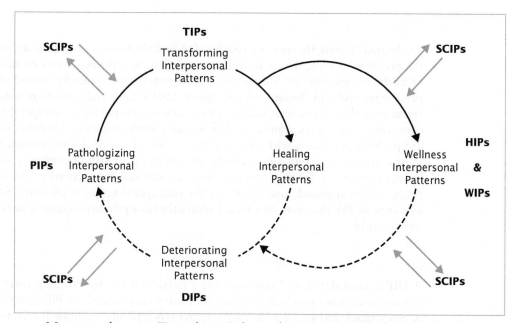

Movement between IPs within a Relationship System with Influence of SCIPs.

If your head is starting to spin with the various IPs, you may find the PIP–HIP–WIP dance helpful in remembering how they are all related. As silly as it sounds, I encourage you to actually stand up right now and follow along because such multisensory techniques actually facilitate learning:

- **PIP:** Start standing at the PIP: this is where therapy begins.
- **HIP:** Take one step to right for the HIP: this is the early and middle phases of therapy, where the therapist facilities change.
- **WIP:** Take another step to the right for the WIP: this is the late phase of therapy and hopefully the predominant pattern after therapy.

- DIP: Then circle back from the HIP to the PIP for the DIP: this is when there are setbacks or early signs of setback.
- TIP: Now circle forward and around to the HIP for the TIP: this is how the therapist facilitates the process from PIP to WIP or actions taken by clients that move toward WIPs.
- SCIP: For the finale, do one more circle but with jazz hands this time for the SCIP.

If you overcame SCIPs that label such an activity as unnecessary for learning because it is not academic enough and instead aligned with SCIPs that privilege evidence-based learning and/or plain fun and you stood up and did this, chances are you won't trip on IPs from this point forward. Instead, you will be happily skipping through systemic case conceptualization, which is the strength of this model.

COMPARISON OF INTERPERSONAL PATTERNS ACROSS FAMILY THERAPY MODELS

	CASE CONCEPTUALIZATION	GOAL SETTING (WIP)	INTERVENTIONS: FACILITATING CHANGE	PRIMARILY USED IP = X OPTIONAL = (x)			
				PIP	HIP	WIP	SCIP
Systemic–strategic	Track and identify function of PIP focusing on behavioral interactions	WIPs conceptualized as virtually any interactional pattern that does NOT create symptoms in individuals or relationships (e.g., abuse)	Use directives or other TIPs that interrupt rather than correct PIP, thereby unbalancing the system and creating opportunities for system to self-reorganize with WIPs	X	(x)	X	(x)
Structural	Map PIP focusing on boundaries, hierarchy, and roles; may also track HIPs and SCIPs	WIPs conceptualized as clear boundaries and hierarchy and meeting developmental needs of all	Use enactments and related TIPs to directly guide family on how to enact WIPs	X	(x)	X	(x)
Functional Family Therapy	Identify relational and hierarchical function of PIP; identify effect of SCIPs	WIPs conceptualized as developmentally appropriate relational bonds and hierarchy as well as WIPs with broader sociocultural network	Use systemic reframing and psycho-education TIPs to create HIPs and WIPs	X	X	X	X
Satir Model	Track and sculpt PIP with focus on emotional dynamics of interactional patterns and each person's internal PIPs	WIPs conceptualized as congruent communication and self worth	Sculpt PIP and WIPs; communication coaching to create HIPs and WIPs	X	X	X	(x)
Emotionally focused therapy	Stage 1: Identify PIP with primary attachment and secondary emotions	WIPs conceptualized as ability to maintain secure attachment	Stage 2: TIPs to facilitate HIPs Stage 3: TIPs to solidify WIPs	X	X	X	(x)

(continued)

COMPARISON OF INTERPERSONAL PATTERNS ACROSS FAMILY THERAPY MODELS (continued)

	CASE CONCEPTUALIZATION	GOAL SETTING (WIP)	INTERVENTIONS: FACILITATING CHANGE	PRIMARILY USED IP = X OPTIONAL = (x)			
				PIP	HIP	WIP	SCIP
Bowen intergenerational therapy	Identify intergenerational PIPs with focus on differentiation and anxiety	WIP conceptualized as differentiation process and ability to manage anxiety	TIPs that promote insight into PIP to promote WIPs	X	(x)	(x)	(x)
Psychodynamic	Identify family of origin and current PIPs, which are conceptualized as interlocking pathologies (e.g., defense mechanisms and object relations)	WIP conceptualized as ego-directed action rather than use of defenses and capacity for intimacy without loss of self	TIPs that provide insight into PIPs to promote WIPs	X	(x)	(x)	(x)
Cognitive–behavioral family therapy	Identify behaviors and thoughts that trigger and reinforce PIP	WIP conceptualized in terms of behaviors and cognitions that do not cause symptoms or relational distress	TIPs that educate client on specific WIPs to replace PIPs or cognitive techniques to enable clients to "discover" better ways for themselves	X	(x)	X	(x)
Solution-based therapies	Identify and behaviorally define WIPs; may inquire about PIPs	WIP defined as client's preferred solution	TIPs to identify small steps to enact WIPs	(x)	(x)	X	(x)
Narrative therapy	Identify relationship between PIPs, WIPs, and SCIPs	WIP defined as client's preferred narrative with conscious choice of one's positioning in relation to dominant discourses	TIPs to reconstruct SCIPs to create HIPs; restory identity and problem narratives to create WIPs	X	X	X	X
Collaborative therapy	Identify each person's construction of PIPs; may include SCIPs	WIPs conceptualized as identity narratives in which client has strong sense of agency in relation to problem	Transform PIPs through dialogic conversation (TIP) to "dissolve" the problem (HIPs) and co-create WIPs; being public to address value differences and influence in external systems	X	X	X	X

HIP = healing interpersonal pattern; PIP = pathologizing interpersonal pattern; SCIP = sociocultural interpersonal pattern; TIP = transformative interpersonal pattern (can be on part of therapist, client, or other); WIP = wellness interpersonal pattern.

Using Tomm's IPscope to Compare Family Therapy Models

Shortly after Tomm et al.'s (2014) book came out, I adopted it for my class on systemic therapy. I initially introduced the IPscope to my students as another systemic model for use with clients. However, as the semester progressed, we found ourselves continuing to talk about PIPs, HIPs, and WIPs. For example, when I was teaching Satir's sculpting intervention (see Chapter 6), I explained that first you sculpt each person's experience of the PIP and then go back and have each sculpt the WIP. Similarly, when we got to Bowen's intergenerational theory (see Chapter 7), we noticed that he was tracking PIPs that repeat from one generation to the next. When discussing solution-focused therapies (see Chapter 9), everyone pointed out that this is the only theory that does not routinely map out PIPs; instead, they carefully map out WIPs. My students loved it and seemed to grasp the similarities and differences between theories much more clearly.

In the above table, I provide a brief, broad-strokes comparison of how each family therapy model (covered in Part II of this text) addresses IPs in the processes of: (a) case conceptualization, (b) goal setting, and (c) facilitating the change process. As you read through Part II of the book, you may want to refer back to this table to help you make distinctions between the different theories. Even without understanding the specifics of these theories, you can quickly note some interesting patterns. First, all theories except solution-focused therapy routinely assess the PIP. You may also observe that most therapy models do not characteristically facilitate HIPs; instead, most focus on WIPs. The table also illustrates how only three theories have built SCIPs into the foundation of the theory; for most, factoring the influence of sociocultural issues have been an add-on in recent years. To facilitate your learning, this table is available for download from the Cengage website as well as www.masteringcompetencies.com. In Part II of this book, each chapter will contain a "Scope It Out" section that describes the theories in the chapter using the common language of the IPscope to facilitate your understanding of each theory as well as your ability to more easily compare theories in the text.

Contemporary Approach to Power, Gender, and Culture in Family Therapy

Although rarely acknowledged consciously, gendered cultural norms provide each couple and family with blueprints for how to do and be a couple or family. All people draw from these often-unspoken cultural guidelines to create expectations for self and others as wife, husband, mother, father, eldest child, adult child, etc. Without such culturally defined norms, humans would struggle (more than they already do) to create meaningful relationships because they would not have shared understandings to coordinate their behaviors (Shotter, 1984, 1993). Although these norms enable people to more efficiently harmonize relational behavior, they can be limiting and problematic in other ways. Cultural norms also significantly shape our attitudes toward nonheterosexual relationships, extended family members, and broader social networks (Tomm et al., 2014). However, as you can see from the table, clearly identifying the influence of cultured gender and sex-role norms has not been standard in our field.

Feminists and social-justice advocates have long directed the attention of family therapists to these issues (Knudson-Martin & Mahoney, 1996; Walsh, 1989; Walters et al., 1988). They point out that early systemic family therapy approaches using general and cybernetic models were based on the assumption that there is by default equally shared power and influence between members of heterosexual couples. In fact, Karl Tomm's IPscope is one of first approaches for diagramming gender and cultural power dynamics in systemic therapy, both with the PIP that illustrates a power difference and with SCIPs (St. George & Wulff, 2014; Tomm et al., 2014).

Research studies consistently find that despite widely espoused egalitarian ideals, contemporary heterosexual couples nonetheless tend to replicate cultured gendered patters of inequity and invisible male power (Coontz, 2005; Knudson-Martin, 2013; Knudson-Martin & Mahoney, 1996). Even more worrisome, many of these couples *believe* they have an egalitarian relationship because they say that is what they want, but functionally there is a significant disparity in power, influence, workload, and needs being met (Knudson-Martin, 2013). In fact, researchers have found that many heterosexual couples—both the men and the women—describe unequal relationships as "fair" because of the belief that men have more entitlements than women.

Contemporary researchers have found that both men and women have a greater sense of personal well-being and marital satisfaction in egalitarian relationships (Knudson-Martin, 2013). Mental health professionals in general and family therapists specifically rarely raise the issue of gendered power as part of treatment; this may be because they are part of the same culture that functionally reinforces male power at the same time as it espouses egalitarian rhetoric. Yet there are many benefits to shared power for couples. For example, when they perceive equality, couples have more direct communication by both parties, rather than one using indirect communication; this results in a greater sense of intimacy and relationship satisfaction (Knudson-Martin, 2013). In contrast, in unequal relationships, both men and women report higher levels of anxiety and depression. One reason for this may be that for a couple to experience emotional intimacy, the subordinate person must have self-worth validated and this struggle for affirmation may override the bids for intimacy. Along these lines, Mirgain and Cordova (2007) found that a person's sense of safety in being vulnerable with one's partner mediated a person's marital satisfaction and emotional skills, consistent with early family therapy assertions that unequal balance impedes relational intimacy because neither the dominant nor the submissive partner is in a safe enough position to be emotionally vulnerable. Gottman (1999) found that men's ability to accept influence is the single best predictor of divorce, with 80% of such marriages with this dynamic ending in divorce. In his updated work on the subject, Gottman (2011) clarifies that a man's ability to "be influenced" by his female partner must involve emotional attunement, the ability to intentionally attend to the emotions of one's partner and respond appropriately. This attunement creates the sense of trust that was the missing element in his early model of the sound marital house (see Chapter 8).

One might assume that the goal of helping couples create egalitarian relationships may be culturally insensitive to clients with more traditional cultural or religious values, but research findings indicate this is not the case (Knudson-Martin, 2013). Many couples in traditional cultures have relationships with shared power and influence. For example, in one study with couples from Iran, even though the legal system gives men significant authority over their wives, many couples nonetheless had mutually supportive and satisfying relationships (Moghadam, Knudson-Martin, & Mahoney, 2009). Similarly, in Singapore both male and female partners reported egalitarian relationship processes; in fact, it may be possible that such collectivist cultural values may make equality more likely in heterosexual relationships (Quek & Knudson-Martin, 2008). Likewise, in a study of Chinese Americans, who often have strong ties to their traditional collectivist culture as well as dominant cultural values, researchers found that couples existed along a spectrum balancing more traditional values of structural harmony with more "we-centered" egalitarian couple priorities (Quek et al., 2010). Although same-sex relationships can have power imbalances, they tend to be more egalitarian because partners are generally more intentional in defining their respective roles (Knudson-Martin, 2013; Jonathan, 2009).

Knudson-Martin (2013) notes that in some cases when couples present for therapy it may appear as though the female has more power, but often this is due to a temporary power shift. For example, if the woman has had an affair, expresses a desire to end the relationship, or has recently expressed significant anger, it may seem that the power dynamics are reversed. In such cases, the therapist should take a careful relationship history to understand the full context and history of the power dynamics. Furthermore, Knudson-Martin (2015) adds that their team rarely sees cases in which the female partner dominates the male in ways and to the degree comparable to domination by men because they do enter the relationship with the social position and power to do so.

Finally, it is important to note that therapists have been part of the problem. Chen-Feng and Galick (2015) reviewed videos of outpatient therapy with heterosexual couples conducted by therapists specializing in couples and family therapy. Their analysis revealed that the majority of therapists appeared to be unintentionally reinforcing gender discourses, specifically the following three:

1. men should be the authority,
2. women should be responsible for the relationship, and
3. women should protect men from shame.

Therapist reinforcement of these discourses was subtle. No therapist said anything directly about which gender should do what. Instead, the bias was revealed by whose experiences were validated and stories tracked, to whom questions were directed, who answered certain questions, who was asked to change and how, and how the presenting problem was defined. Some common patterns they identified included:

- Reinforcing male privilege: Men's concerns were rarely questioned and readily identified as a valid problem to be addressed, sometimes even before the women's perspective was expressed.
- Expecting women to accommodate: When discussing change, therapists regularly expected women to accommodate men's needs, often without asking the woman about what she needed from the man or asking the man to do a similar level of accommodating.
- Protecting men from shame: Even when the husband had been unfaithful, women regularly described a dynamic in which "the relationship is fine" if the woman refrains from voicing her concerns or needs. Therapists consistently ignored such remarks by women, reinforcing rather than challenging this problematic power imbalance.

In summary, like their clients, therapists struggle to identify gender inequities and need intentional, focused training to learn to see problematic gendered cultural discourses that limit couples' ability to create the egalitarian relationships they desire.

Socioemotional Relationship Therapy

Knudson-Martin and Huenergardt (2010; Knudson-Martin, 2013) have developed a model that therapists can use to increase mutual support in couple relationships: **socioemotional relationship therapy**. Rather than attempt to prescribe or force a particular form of "egalitarian" relationship, therapists using this approach instead facilitate dialogues and conditions that enable the couple to experience relating to each other from equal positions

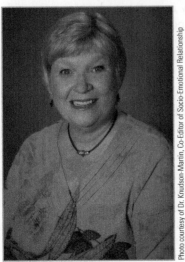

from within their particular cultural values. Therapists facilitate this process by providing leadership that actively counters gendered power imbalances and invites couples to explore and experience alternative gender discourses, enabling them to enact their egalitarian ideals. Through this process, each couple defines what mutual support looks like in their relationship and within their cultural norms, creating the potential for greater intimacy and relational satisfaction.

The sociocultural relationship therapy model is based on the following principles (Knudson-Martin & Huenergardt, 2015; Knudson-Martin et al., 2015):

- Sociocultural context, identity, and relationships: Sociocultural contexts and their inherent power differentials structure both a person's identity and their relational processes.
- Emotion, power, and social identity: Emotion is inextricably connected to one's sociopolitical context and one's societal and power positions. Rather than simply emerging from within, emotions

inherently involve a neurobiological response to a social situation of some kind (Knudson-Martin & Huenergardt, 2015).

- Power is relational: Power is relational and revealed in the degree to which each partner can influence the other. In couple relationships, power dynamics are revealed by who attends to whose emotions, who feels entitled to have needs met, and who typically accommodates.
- Mutually supportive relationships: Relationships should be mutually supportive to each partner, as such relationships foster both individual and relational health.
- Active intervention: Therapists must consciously and actively intervene in societal-based power disparities.

Socioemotional relationship therapy identifies four ways in which couples can orient to one another that form the *circle of care* that characterizes mutual support in egalitarian relationships (Knudson-Martin & Huenergardt, 2015):

- Shared relational responsibility: **Relational responsibility** requires both partners to be accountable for how their actions affect others and the relationship. This involves both practical matters, such as sharing the daily chores of living, as well as taking care of the emotional needs of family members. In addition, it involves both partners caring for the relationship itself: noticing and taking action to ensure that the relationship is strong and healthy.
- Mutual vulnerability: Mutual vulnerability involves each person being willing to be open and honest and have the courage to take the emotional risk that is inherent in intimate relationships. This also involves a readiness to open oneself to self-examination, especially in response to the concerns of one's partner.
- Mutual attunement: Mutual attunement refers to each partner attending to the emotional life and needs of the other; it creates a sense of mutual support.
- Mutual influence: Mutual influence refers to each partner allowing the other to influence personal thoughts, feelings, and behaviors. This willingness to be influenced by one's partner must come from mutual attunement, rather than a sense of obligation, fear, or superiority.

Implications for Practice

When working with clients using a socioemotional approach, therapists attend to power processes that are present in the interactions between: (a) each partner's personal emotional experience, (b) societal and cultural discourses about gender, and (c) the couple's interaction patterns (Knudson-Martin, 2013; Knudson-Martin & Mahoney, 2009). In particular, therapists carefully avoid cultural messages that place the burden of relational responsibility and vulnerability on women; instead, they engage the more powerful, typically male partner to initiate relational connection. They use a three-phase process with seven competencies to help couples increase mutual support in their relationships; these phases include: (a) establish an equitable foundation for therapy, (b) interrupt the flow of power, and (c) facilitate alternative experiences (Knudson-Martin & Huenergardt, 2015).

- Phase I: Establish an equitable foundation for therapy
    - Competency 1: Identify couple's enactment of cultural discourses. Therapists using a socioemotional approach begin by listening for how the couple enacts societal and gendered discourses and explore each partner's personal values, beliefs, and experiences related to these discourses.
    - Competency 2: Attune to underlying sociocultural emotion. The therapist creates a therapeutic context in which both partners feel understood and validated. During this process, the therapist affirms each partner's sociocultural identity and the emotions that arise from it, such as a sense of feeling abandoned or not respected. However, although therapists genuinely emotionally attune to each person's experience, they thoughtfully avoid organizing therapy around the dominant partner's emotional reality. Thus, just because a husband may feel his wife does not attend to his needs enough, this does not automatically result in making this a goal of treatment. First,

the therapist explores the gendered and culturally informed expectations that inform the husband's perception, typically exploring whether the expectation of having one's needs attended to by one's partner applies equally in the relationship.

- **Competency 3: Identify relational power dynamics.** The therapist then identifies power processes in the couple relationship and makes these visible to the couple, highlighting how these dynamics relate to the presenting problem and presenting goals for therapy. For example, after identifying the emotional and contextual expectations from the more powerful partner, the therapist inquires of the less powerful partner whether she experiences what he is asking for, such as attending to the partner's needs in the example above. The therapist might ask the wife, "Do you receive the type of attentiveness to your needs that he is wanting from you? If not, do you ever ask? If not, what stops you?" With questions such as these and observations of how partners respond to each other in session, the therapist explores the mutuality of care and rights in the relationship, which reveals the relative balance of power in the relationship and the unique power exchanges for the couple. During this process the therapist is careful to validate the reality of the more powerful partner but still hold him accountable. Without consciously choosing to conceptualize the dynamics between heterosexual couples with a socioemotional lens, most therapists using standard therapy models use the husband's definition of the problem ("my wife ignores my needs") to set the goals of therapy. However, in doing so, a therapist would be inadvertently reinforcing a gendered power imbalance.

- **Phase II: Interrupt the flow of power**
  - **Competency 4: Facilitate relational safety.** The therapist begins this process by having the more powerful partner take the lead in being emotionally vulnerable and initiate reconnection in the relationship. This includes asking the more powerful partner to identify relational needs as well as highlighting the need for safety for the less powerful partner.
  - **Competency 5: Foster mutual attunement.** The therapist fosters **attunement** within the couple by encouraging the more powerful partner to initiate attuning to his partner's emotions and encouraging the partners to avoid gender-stereotyped behavior that impedes attunement. Quite often, the female partner responds to the male's vulnerability by enacting culturally prescribed gender behavior by rushing in to take care of the man's emotions. The therapists bring the couple's attention to such patterns and then helps them find an alternative way in which they can reciprocate attunement and care.

- **Phase III: Facilitate alternative experience**
  - **Competency 6: Create a relationship model based on equality.** When therapists use a socioemotional approach to identify a power imbalance, they act to not only identify it but also to introduce a viable alternative to the gender-stereotyped norms, a process that involves having the clients envision relational equality, explore the potential consequences of such mutuality, and recognize and reinforce actions that created the mutuality.
  - **Competency 7: Facilitate shared relational responsibility.** Beginning with the more powerful partner, therapists facilitate equal engagement in maintaining and supporting the relationship so that there is a sense of mutual attunement, influence, and vulnerability. This enables couples to address other issues in their relationship from an equitable and mutually supportive foundation.

Try It Yourself

Either by yourself or with a partner, share your thoughts on socioemotional relational therapy. Do you agree with the definition of *circle of care* as a way to create an egalitarian relationship? Do you have any personal experience that relates to this model?

Rock–Paper–Scissors and Other Strategies for Choosing a Theory

What theory should I use? Which is the best? Which is the best for me? Do I have to pick a theory? What if I like them all? Can't I just be eclectic? These are some of the first questions that students ask as they begin to study family therapy theories. The answers are more complex than one would imagine, leaving honest instructors and supervisors no option but to respond with maddening "both/and" or "yes-and-no" answers (trust me, they do not do this just to torture students for recreation and sport—it really is an honest answer). But let me give you a hint: philosophical foundations are part of the answer.

How to Choose: Dating versus Marrying

Much like parents' advice to their teenage children, in the first few years, I recommend that you casually "date" a theory before you decide to settle down. I am always surprised by new therapists who feel this tremendous pressure to find the "perfect" or "right" theory for them immediately—much like teenagers who are convinced that their first love will be their lifelong partner: it's possible, just not the most common scenario. You might want to "play the field" for a while to learn what is out there and what works best for you.

Fortunately, theory dating generally ends better than romantic dating. After dating a theory, you are almost always forever enriched with new skills and knowledge, which is only sometimes true in the romantic realm. In addition, the breakup part is almost always gentler. Thus, you can decide to try out a new theory every semester of your training or every year or so in your practice. After dating even two or three, your skill set and knowledge base will have grown significantly. You will have also learned more about who you are and your style as a therapist. At that point, you may find that it is time to settle down with one more than with the others. When that happens, you are ready to define your philosophy.

Defining Your Philosophy

Once you have spent a few years dating, you may find that you are ready to settle down with one theory. Just as in love, there should be an engagement period, during which you clearly define your commitment and get to know your new partner—and family of origin—more intimately. In the case of theory dating, this involves pursuing advanced training in your theory of choice, usually by going to intensive seminars or working with a supervisor who specializes in your theory. Just as in marriage, in which a commitment to one person entails a commitment to an entire family, once you decide to commit to a theory, you are also committing to the broader philosophy that is the theory's foundation. I believe that therapists who are clear about their philosophy of what it means to be human (ontology) and how people learn and change (epistemology) are best positioned to handle the variety of problems with which skilled therapists must learn to work. If you master only the techniques (system of doing), then you are less well prepared for handling the variety of issues that highly competent therapists must master.

Although there are many ways to define the philosophical foundations of family therapies, I find it simplest to begin by considering four major categories: modernist, humanistic, systemic, and postmodern. Each has its own approach to defining truth, reality, the therapeutic relationship, and the therapist's role in the change process. The following table summarizes their differences.

OVERVIEW OF PHILOSOPHICAL SCHOOLS

	MODERNIST	HUMANISTIC	SYSTEMIC	POSTMODERN
Truth	Objective truth	Subjective truth	Contextual truth	Multiple, coexisting truths
Reality	Objective; observable	Subjective; individually accessible	Contextual; emerges through systemic interactions; no one person has unilateral control	Coconstructed through language and social interaction; occurs at individual, relational, and societal levels
Therapeutic relationship	Therapist as expert; hierarchical	Therapist as empathetic other	Therapist as participant in therapeutic system	Therapist as non-expert; co-constructor of meaning
Therapist's role in change process	Teaching and guiding clients in better ways of being and interacting	Creating a context that supports natural self-actualization process	"Perturbing" system, allowing system to reorganize itself; no direct control of system	Facilitating a dialogue in which client constructs new meanings and interpretations

Modernism

Modernism is founded on the logical-positivist assumptions of an external, knowable "truth." In modernist approaches, the therapist assumes an unequivocal role as expert, which is more common in individual and family forms of cognitive–behavioral and psychodynamic therapies (see Chapters 7 and 8; e.g., Dattilio & Padesky, 1990; Ellis, 1994; Scharff & Scharff, 1987).

Modernist Assumptions

- The therapist is an expert who assumes the primary responsibility for identifying pathology, problems, and goals, often assuming the role of teacher or mentor.
- Theory and research are the primary sources of information for identifying problems and diagnosing.
- The therapist uses theory and research to select treatment approaches; clients are expected to adapt to the selected treatment.

Two family therapy schools fit this category: psychodynamic and cognitive–behavioral therapies. Although broadly grounded in modernist assumptions about knowledge, each theory has its own unique position on the primary source of truth, the means through which it is best identified, and how best to define the therapeutic relationship.

MODERNIST THERAPIES

	PSYCHODYNAMIC THERAPIES	COGNITIVE–BEHAVIORAL THERAPIES
Primary source of objective truth	Therapist's analysis of client dynamics based on theory	Measurable, external variables
Means of identifying truth	"Reality check"; comparing client experience against external perceptions, events, etc.	Scientific experimentation; therapist's definition of "reality" and/or social norms (identified through research)
Therapeutic relationship	Hierarchical; therapist indirectly leads client toward goals	Educational; therapist is straightforward in directing client toward goals

Humanism

Humanistic therapies (see Chapter 6) are founded on a phenomenological philosophy that prioritizes the individual's subjective truth. They include Carl Rogers's (1951) client-centered therapy, Fritz Perl's gestalt therapy (Passons, 1975), Virginia Satir's (1972) communication approach, Carl Whitaker's symbolic–experiential therapy (Whitaker & Keith, 1981), and Sue Johnson's emotionally focused therapy (Johnson, 2004).

Humanistic Assumptions

- By nature, humans are essentially good.
- All people naturally tend toward growth and strive for self-actualization, a process of becoming authentically human.
- The primary focus of treatment is the subjective, internal world of clients.
- Therapeutic interventions target emotions with the goal of promoting catharsis, the release of repressed emotions.
- A supportive, nurturing environment promotes therapeutic change.

The work of Virginia Satir and Carl Whitaker most clearly illustrates this philosophical stance, which in family therapy is always combined with a systemic perspective that accounts for the effect of family dynamics on an individual's emotional inner life. Although Satir's and Whitaker's approaches are based on the same philosophical traditions, their therapeutic approaches have dramatically different styles and assumptions, including the best ways to address self-actualization, change, confrontation, and the therapist's use of self (referring to how therapists use their personhood in session).

HUMANISTIC THERAPIES	SATIR'S COMMUNICATION APPROACH	WHITAKER'S SYMBOLIC–EXPERIENTIAL APPROACH
Means of promoting self-actualization	Emotionally safe and nurturing environment	Affective confrontation; "perturbing" the system
Change	Structured experiential exercises; role modeling	In vivo interactions with the therapist
Style of confrontation	Gentle, educational	Direct, affective
"Authentic" use of self	Genuine caring for the client	Unedited and honest sharing of emotions and thoughts

Systemic Therapy

Rather than a formal philosophical school, systemic therapies are grounded in *general systems theory,* which stresses that living systems are open systems, connected with and embedded within other systems (von Bertalanffy, 1968), and *cybernetic systems theory,* which emphasizes a system's ability to self-correct to maintain homeostasis (Bateson, 1972). The latter is more influential in the development of specific therapeutic models, such as the MRI's brief, problem-focused approach (Watzlawick et al., 1974), strategic therapy (Haley, 1976; Madanes, 1981), and the Milan team's systemic approach (Boscolo et al., 1987). Systems theories emphasize *contextual* truth, truth generated through repeated interpersonal interactions that set a "norm" and rules for behavior.

Systemic Assumptions

- One cannot *not* communicate; all behavior is a form of communication.
- An individual's behavior and symptoms always make sense in the person's broader relational contexts.

- All behaviors, including unwanted symptoms, serve a purpose within the system, allowing the system to maintain or regain its homeostasis or feeling of "normalcy."
- No one individual unilaterally controls behavior in a system. Thus, no one person can be blamed for problems in a couple or family relationship; instead, problematic behavior is viewed as emerging from the interactions between members of the system.
- Therapeutic change involves alternating the interaction patterns within the system.

Within the field of systemic family therapy, Bateson's (1972) distinction between first-order and second-order cybernetics had a significant impact on how therapists worked with families. With **first-order cybernetics,** the therapist is an objective, neutral observer describing the family as an outsider. Such therapy relies on assessment instruments and the therapist's perception of the family system. *Second-order cybernetic* theory applies the rules of first-order cybernetics on itself, positing that the therapist cannot be an objective, outside observer but instead creates a new system with the family: the observer–observed or therapist–family system. This second-order system is subject to the same dynamics as the first, including the drive to maintain homeostasis and rules for relating that are mutually reinforced. Second-order cybernetic theory maintains that whatever the therapist observes in the family reveals more about the therapist's values and priorities than about the family's because any description exposes what the therapist pays attention to and what the therapist ignores or misses. Second-order cybernetics laid the foundation for the transition to postmodern therapy, specifically constructivism in the MRI and Milan schools (Watzlawick, 1984).

In general, all systems therapists are influenced by both first- and second-order cybernetic theory. In practice, therapists generally emphasize one level of systems analysis or another. Broadly speaking, strategic and structural therapies were based on first-order theory, and the MRI and Milan approaches gravitated toward second-order and later constructivist approaches.

- *First-order cybernetic approaches* lean toward the modernist tendency to find a more objective form of truth. Therapists who practice systemic therapies with a first-order orientation use more assessment instruments of family functioning and rely heavily on the therapist's perception of the system to guide practice.
- *Second-order cybernetic approaches* lean more toward a postmodern approach to truth (see next section). Their focus is on how the therapist and client coconstruct a second-order system, which has its own unique set of rules for establishing truth.

SYSTEMIC THEORIES

	FIRST-ORDER CYBERNETICS	**SECOND-ORDER CYBERNETICS**
Level(s) of analysis	Family system	Family system (level 1) and therapist–family system (level 2)
Target of interventions	Correcting interactional sequences	"Perturbing" or interrupting interactional sequences
Therapist's role	Tends to appear as a knowledgeable expert	Cocreator of therapeutic system
Focus of assessment	Behavioral sequences	Meaning-making systems (epistemology)

Postmodern Therapy

Postmodern therapies are based on the premise that objective truth can never be fully known because it must always pass through subjective and intersubjective filters.

Postmodern Assumptions

- The human mind does not have access to an outside reality independent of human interpretation; objectivity is not humanly possible.
- All knowledge and truth are culturally, historically, and relationally bound and therefore intersubjective: constructed within and between people.
- What a person experiences as "real" and believes to be "true" is shaped primarily through language and relationships.
- Language and the words used to describe one's experiences significantly affect how one's identity is shaped and experienced.
- The identification of a "problem" is a social process that occurs through language, both at the immediate local level and at the broader societal level.
- Therapy is a process of co-constructing new realities related to the client's personal identity and relationship with the problem.

Within family therapy, three schools of postmodernism are particularly influential (Anderson, 1997; Hoffman, 2002; Watzlawick, 1984):

- **Constructivism:** Constructivists focus on the construction of meaning within the individual organism, on how information is received and interpreted.
- **Social constructionism:** Social constructionists focus on how people cocreate meaning in relationships. They emphasize how truth is generated at the local (immediate) relational level.
- **Structuralism and poststructuralism:** Structuralists and poststructuralists focus on analyzing how meanings are produced and reproduced within a culture through various practices and discourses.

POSTMODERN PHILOSOPHICAL FOUNDATIONS

	CONSTRUCTIVISM	SOCIAL CONSTRUCTIONISM	STRUCTURALISM AND POSTSTRUCTURALISM
Level of reality construction	Individual organism	Local relationship	Societal, political
Associated theories	Later MRI and Milan theories	Collaborative therapy; reflecting teams	Narrative therapy; feminist and culturally informed therapies
Focus of interventions	Recasting interpretations with new language	Dialogues that highlight multiple meanings and interpretations	Deconstruction and questioning of dominant discourses (popular knowledge)
Therapist's role	Facilitate alternative interpretations	Non-interventional; facilitate dialogical process	Help identify external and historical influences

Dancing with Others Once You Marry

Once you commit yourself to a theory and philosophical stance, it ironically becomes much easier to dance with others. As you master one theoretical approach and deepen your understanding of its underlying philosophical assumptions, you are able to understand other theories at a greater depth. This is perhaps where the common factors come in. Similar principles seem to be at play in all theories, and the more intimate you are with one theory the better able you are to identify these factors in others. It is also the case that you can see more clearly the subtle differences in outcome from philosophical assumptions, word choices, and interventions that differ across theories.

As therapists become more aware of the set of philosophical assumptions underlying their theory, whichever school that might be, they learn to skillfully adapt and integrate ideas from other approaches in a way that is philosophically consistent with their own approach. Therapists who are "eclectic" or "integrative" in a way that is not grounded in a single philosophical set of assumptions will confuse their clients. One week, such a therapist might use a modernist approach and is an expert who has answers and knows the best way to approach the problem. The next week, the therapist might try to use a postmodern approach, in which the client is expected to be the expert and participate more as an equal. The following week, the therapist might then shift to systemic ideas that emphasize the importance of context in defining the problem. As you might well imagine, a client working with this therapist is going to be very confused, because each week the client is required to relate differently to the therapist and to assume a different level of participation. The therapist is also sending contradictory messages as to what is the measuring stick for "truth," progress, and direction. However, if the therapist is able to keep the philosophical assumptions consistent throughout therapy—What is our measuring stick for truth? What are our roles?—then the therapist can adapt concepts and techniques from other approaches without sending conflicting messages to the client, thus effectively incorporating a wider range of practices within a coherent approach to therapy.

Try It Yourself

Which broad theoretical school are you most attracted to? Which resonates least with you? What prior life experiences or personality characteristic may account for this?

QUESTIONS FOR PERSONAL REFLECTION AND CLASS DISCUSSION

1. Does the idea of a family being a system with its own homeostasis resonate with you and your life experiences?
2. Describe a complementary relationship in your life.
3. Describe a double-bind situation in your life.
4. Describe the dynamics of your family of origin. What were the basic homeostatic behaviors and roles for each person? When there was positive feedback, what were the forms of negative feedback used to restore balance and "normalcy" to the family?
5. Social constructionists describe how we attribute meaning to events and things in our world. Provide an example from your life.
6. Social constructionists describe how societal discourses shape individual identity. Provide an example from your life.
7. Karl Tomm's system for identifying interpersonal includes healing and wellness patterns. How might this be a useful distinction in couple and family therapy?
8. Socioemotional relationship therapy is designed to enable couples to address power imbalances and create a more equitable relationship. What benefits and challenges do you see with this approach?

ONLINE RESOURCES

Ken Gergen's web page:
www.swarthmore.edu/SocSci/kgergen1/web/page.phtml?st=home&id=home

Mental Research Institute:
www.mri.org

John Shotter's web page:
http://pubpages.unh.edu/~jds

The Taos Institute:
Explores social constructionist practices in a wide range of disciplines.
www.taosinstitute.org

Go to MindTap® for an eBook, videos of client sessions, activities, digital forms, practice quizzes, apps, and more—all in one place. If your instructor didn't assign MindTap, you can find out more information at CengageBrain.com.

REFERENCES

Anderson, H. (1997). *Conversations, language, and possibilities: A postmodern approach to therapy.* New York: Basic Books.

Anderson, H., & Gehart, D. (Eds.). (2007). *Collaborative therapy: Relationships and conversations that make a difference.* New York: Brunner/Routledge.

Anderson, H., & Goolishian, H. (1992). The client is the expert: A not-knowing approach to therapy. In S. McNamee & K. J. Gergen (Eds.), *Therapy as social construction* (pp. 25–39). Newbury Park, CA: Sage.

Bateson, G. (1972). *Steps to an ecology of mind.* San Francisco, CA: Chandler.

Bateson, G. (1979). *Mind and nature: A necessary unity.* New York: Dutton.

Bateson, G. (1991). *A sacred unity: Further steps to an ecology of mind.* New York: Harper/Collins.

Baxter, L. A., & Montgomery, B. M. (1996). *Relating: Dialogues and dialectics.* New York: Guilford.

Boscolo, L., Cecchin, G., Hoffman, L., & Penn, P. (1987). *Milan systemic family therapy.* New York: Basic Books.

ChenFeng, J. L., & Galick, A. (2015). How gender discourses hijack couple therapy—And how to avoid it. In C. Knudson-Martin, M. A. Wells, S. K. Samman, C. Knudson-Martin, M. A. Wells, & S. K. Samman (Eds.), *Socio-emotional relationship therapy: Bridging emotion, societal context, and couple interaction* (pp. 41–52). New York: Springer Science + Business Media. doi:10.1007/978-3-319-13398-0_4

Coontz, S. (2005). *Marriage, a history: From obedience to intimacy or how love conquered marriage.* New York: Viking.

Dattilio, F. M., & Padesky, C. A. (1990). *Cognitive therapy with couples.* Sarasota, FL: Professional Resources Exchange.

Ellis, A. (1994). *Reason and emotion in therapy* (rev. ed.). New York: Kensington.

Erickson, B. A., & Keeney, B. (Eds.). (2006). *Milton Erickson, M.D.: An American healer.* Sedona, AZ: Leete Island Books.

Fisch, R., Weakland, J., & Segal, L. (1982). *The tactics of change: Doing therapy briefly.* New York: Jossey-Bass.

Foucault, M. (1972). *The archeology of knowledge,* translated by A. Sheridan-Smith. New York: Harper and Row.

Foucault, M. (1979). *Discipline and punish: The birth of the prison.* Middlesex, UK: Peregrine Books.

Foucault, M. (1980). *Power/knowledge: Selected interviews and other writings.* New York: Pantheon Books.

Freedman, J., & Combs, G. (1996). *Narrative therapy: The social construction of preferred realities.* New York: Norton.

Gaete, J., Sametband, I., & Sutherland, O. (2014). Can I give you a TIP? Inviting healing conversations in practice. In K. Tomm, S. St. George, D. Wulff, & T. Strong (Eds.), *Patterns in interpersonal interactions: Inviting relational understandings for therapeutic change* (pp. 103–123). New York: Routledge.

Gergen, K. J. (1985). The social constructionist movement in modern psychology. *American Psychologist, 40,* 266–275.

Gergen, K. J. (1998, January). *Introduction to social constructionism.* Workshop presented at the Texas Association for Marriage and Family Therapy Annual Conference, Dallas, TX.

Gergen, K. (1999). *An invitation to social construction.* Newbury Park, CA: Sage.

Gergen, K. (2001). *Social construction in context.* Newbury Park, CA: Sage.

Gergen, M., & Gergen, K. (2007). Collaboration without end: The case of the Positive Psychology Newsletter. In H. Anderson & D. Gehart (Eds.), *Collaborative therapy: Relationships and conversations that make a difference* (pp. 391–402). New York: Brunner/Routledge.

Gottman, J. M. (1999). *The marriage clinic: A scientifically based marital therapy.* New York: Norton.

Gottman, J. M. (2011). *The science of trust.* New York: Norton.

Haley, J. (1976). *Problem-solving therapy: New strategies for effective family therapy.* San Francisco, CA: Jossey-Bass.

Hoffman, L. (2002). *Family therapy: An intimate history.* New York: Norton.

Jackson, D. (1952, June). The relationship of the referring physician to the psychiatrist. *California Medicine, 76*(6), 391–394.

Jackson, D. (1955). Therapist personality in the therapy of ambulatory schizophrenics. *Archives of Neurology and Psychiatry, 74,* 292–299.

Johnson, S. M. (2004). *The practice of emotionally focused marital therapy: Creating connection* (2nd ed.). New York: Brunner-Routledge.

Jonathan, N. (2009). Carrying equal weight: Relational responsibility and attunement among same-sex couples. In C. Knudson-Martin & A. R. Mahoney (Eds.), *Couples, gender and power: Creating change in intimate relationships* (pp. 79–104). New York: Springer.

Keeney, B. (1983). *Aesthetics of change.* New York: Guilford.

Keeney, B. (1985). *Mind in therapy: Constructing systematic family therapies.* New York: Basic Books.

Keeney, B. (1990). *Improvisational therapy: A practical guide for creative clinical strategies.* New York: Guilford.

Keeney, B. (1994). *Shaking out the spirits: A psychotherapist's entry into the healing mysteries of global shamanism.* Barrytown, NY: Station Hill.

Keeney, B. (1997). *Everyday soul: Awakening the spirit in daily life.* New York: Riverhead Books.

Keeney, B. (1998). *The energy break: Recharge your life with autokinetics.* New York: Golden Books.

Keeney B. (2000a). *Gary Holy Bull: Lakota Yuwipi man.* Stony Creek, CT: Leete's Island Books.

Keeney, B. (2000b). *Kalahari Bushmen.* Stony Creek, CT: Leete's Island Books.

Keeney, B. (2001a). *Vusamazulu Credo Mutwa: Zulu High Sanusi.* Stony Creek, CT: Leete's Island Books.

Keeney, B. (2001b). *Walking Thunder: Diné medicine woman.* Stony Creek, CT: Leete's Island Books.

Keeney B. (2002a). *Ikuko Osumi: Japanese master of Seiki Jutsu.* Stony Creek, CT: Leete's Island Books.

Keeney, B. (2002b). *Shakers of St. Vincent.* Stony Creek, CT: Leete's Island Books.

Keeney, B. (2003). *Ropes to God.* Stony Creek, CT: Leete's Island Books.

Knudson-Martin, C. (2013). Why power matters: Creating a foundation of mutual support in couple relationships. *Family Process, 52*(1), 5–18. doi:10.1111/famp.12011

Knudson-Martin, C. (2015). When therapy challenges patriarchy: Undoing gendered power in heterosexual couple relationships. In C. Knudson-Martin, M. A. Wells, & S. K. Samman, (Eds.), *Socio-emotional relationship therapy: Bridging emotion, societal context, and couple interaction* (pp. 15–26). New York: Springer Science + Business Media. doi:10.1007/978-3-319-13398-0_2

Knudson-Martin, C., & Huenergardt, D. (2010). A socio-emotional approach to couple therapy: Linking social context and couple interaction. *Family Process, 49,* 369–386.

Knudson-Martin, C., & Huenergardt, D. (2015). Bridging emotion, societal discourse, and couple interaction in clinical practice. In C. Knudson-Martin, M. A. Wells, & S. K. Samman (Eds.), *Socio-emotional relationship therapy: Bridging emotion, societal context, and couple interaction* (pp. 1–13). New York: Springer Science + Business Media. doi:10.1007/978-3-319-13398-0_1

Knudson-Martin, C., Huenergardt, D., Lafontant, K., Bishop, L., Schaepper, J., & Wells, M. (2015). Competencies for addressing gender and power in couple therapy: A socioemotional approach. *Journal of Marital and Family Therapy, 41*(2), 205–220.

Knudson-Martin, C., & Mahoney, A. R. (1996). Gender dilemmas and myth in the construction of marital bargains: Issues for marital therapy. *Family Process, 35*(2), 137–153. doi: 10.1111/j.1545-5300.1996.00137.x

Knudson-Martin, C., & Mahoney, A. R. (2009). *Couples, gender, and power: Creating change in intimate relationships.* New York: Springer.

Madanes, C. (1981). *Strategic family therapy.* San Francisco, CA: Jossey-Bass.

Mirgain, S. A., & Cordova, J. V. (2007). Emotion skills and marital health: The association between observed and self-reported emotion skills, intimacy, and marital satisfaction. *Journal of Counseling and Clinical Psychology, 26*, 983–1009.

Moghadam, S., Knudson-Martin, C., & Mahoney, A. (2009). Gendered power in cultural contexts part III: Couple relationships in Iran. *Family Process, 48*, 41–54.

McNamee, S. (2007). Relational practices in education: Teaching as conversation. In H. Anderson & D. Gehart (Eds.), *Collaborative therapy: Relationships and conversations that make a difference* (pp. 313–336). New York: Brunner/Routledge.

McNamee, S., & Gergen, K. J. (Eds.). (1992). *Therapy as social construction.* Newbury Park, CA: Sage.

McNamee, S., & Gergen, K. J. (1999). *Relational responsibility: Resources for sustainable dialogue.* Newbury Park, CA: Sage.

Mental Research Institute. (2002). *On the shoulders of giants.* Palo Alto, CA: Author.

Passons, W. R. (1975). *Gestalt therapies in counseling.* New York: Holt, Rinehart, and Winston.

Quek, K. M., & Knudson-Martin, C. (2008). Reshaping marital power: How dual-career newlywed couples create equality in Singapore. *Journal of Social and Personal Relationships, 25*(3), 511–532. doi:10.1177/0265407508090871

Quek, K. M., Knudson-Martin, C., Rue, D., & Alabiso, C. (2010). Relational harmony: A new model of collectivism and gender equality among Chinese American couples. *Journal of Family Issues, 31*(3), 358–380. doi: 10.1177/0192513X09351162

Rambo, A., & Hibel, J. (2013). What is family therapy? Underlying premises. In A. Rambo, C. West, A. Schooley, & T. V. Boyd (Eds.), *Family therapy review: Contrasting contemporary models* (pp. 3–8). New York, NY: Routledge.

Ray, W. A., & Keeney, B. (1994). *Resource focused therapy.* London: Karnac Books.

Rogers, C. (1951). *Client-centered therapy.* Boston, MA: Houghton Mifflin.

Satir, V. (1972). *Peoplemaking.* Palo Alto, CA: Science and Behavior Books.

Scharff, D., & Scharff, J. S. (1987). *Object relations family therapy.* New York: Aronson.

Segal, L. (1991). Brief therapy: The MRI approach. In A. S. Gurman & D. P. Knishern (Eds.), *Handbook of family therapy* (pp. 171–199). New York: Brunner/Mazel.

Shotter, J. (1984). *Social accountability and selfhood.* Oxford, UK: Blackwell.

Shotter, J. (1993). *Conversational realities: Constructing life through language.* Thousand Oaks, CA: Sage.

St. George, S., & Wulff, D. (2014). Braiding socio-cultural interpersonal patterns into therapy. In K. Tomm, S. St. George, D. Wulff, & T. Strong (Eds.), *Patterns in interpersonal interactions: Inviting relational understandings for therapeutic change* (pp. 124–142). New York: Routledge.

Tomm, K. (2014). Introducing the IPscope: A systemic assessment tool for distinguishing interpersonal patterns. In K. Tomm, S. St. George, D. Wulff, & T. Strong (Eds.), *Patterns in interpersonal interactions: Inviting relational understandings for therapeutic change* (pp. 13–35). New York: Routledge.

Tomm, K., St. George, S., Wulff, D., & Strong, T. (2014). *Patterns in interpersonal interactions: Inviting relational understandings for therapeutic change.* New York: Routledge.

von Bertalanffy, L. (1968). *General system theory: Foundations, development, applications.* New York: George Braziller.

Walsh, F. (1989). Reconsidering gender in the marital quid pro quo. In M. McGoldrick, C. Anderson, & F. Walsh (Eds.), *Women in families: A framework for family therapy* (pp. 267–285). New York: Norton.

Walters, M., Carter, B., Papp, P., & Silverstein, O. (1988). *The invisible web: Gender patterns in family relationships.* New York: Guilford.

Watzlawick, P. (1977). *How real is real?: Confusion, disinformation, communication.* New York: Random House.

Watzlawick, P. (1978/1993). *The language of change: Elements of therapeutic conversation.* New York: Norton.

Watzlawick, P. (Ed.). (1984). *The invented reality: How do we know what we believe we know?* New York: Norton.

Watzlawick, P., Bavelas, J. B., & Jackson, D. D. (1967). *Pragmatics of human communication: A study of interactional patterns, pathologies, and paradoxes.* New York: Norton.

Watzlawick, P., Weakland, J., & Fisch, R. (1974). *Change: Principles of problem formation and problem resolution.* New York: Norton.

Weakland, J. (1951). Method in cultural anthropology. *Philosophy of Science, 18,* 55.

Weakland, J. (1988, June 10). Personal interview with Wendel A. Ray. Mental Research Institute, Palo Alto, CA.

White, M., & Epston, D. (1990). *Narrative means to therapeutic ends.* New York: Norton.

Whitaker, C. A., & Keith, D. V. (1981). Symbolic-experiential family therapy. In A. S. Gurman & D. P. Kniskern (Eds.), *Handbook of family therapy* (pp. 187–224). New York: Brunner/Mazel.

Wittgenstein, L. (1973). *Philosophical investigations* (3rd ed.), translated by G. E. M. Anscombe. New York: Prentice Hall.

PART II

Couple and Family Therapy Theories

4

Systemic and Strategic Therapies

Learning Objectives

After reading this chapter and a few hours of focused studying, you should be able to:

- **Theory:** Describe the following elements of systemic–strategic family therapy:
  - Process of therapy
  - Therapeutic relationship
  - Case conceptualization
  - Goal setting
  - Interventions

- **Case Conceptualization and Treatment Plan:** Complete theory-specific case conceptualizations and treatment plans for systemic–strategic using templates that are provided.

- **Research:** Provide an overview of significant research findings for systemic–strategic therapies and describe key elements of the following evidence-based treatment: multisystemic and brief strategic family therapy.

- **Diversity:** Analyze strengths, limitations, and appropriate applications for using systemic–strategic approaches with clients in relation to their social location/diverse identities, including but not limited to ethnic, racial, and/or sexual/gender identity diversity.

- **Cross-Theoretical Comparison:** Compare how systemic–strategic therapies utilize interpersonal patterns (IPs) with other approaches described in this book.

> *Through time, you learn how to look at a system and appreciate it for what it is.*
> *Never expect the system to be different. It's important for the therapist and for*
> *the trainee to train themselves to see the system, to be interested in it,*
> *to appreciate this kind of a system without wanting to change it.*
> —Boscolo, Cecchin, Hoffman, & Penn, 1987, p. 152)

Lay of the Land

Chapter 3 outlined the systemic foundations of various kinds of therapy, especially the contributions of the Bateson group. This chapter discusses these therapies in more detail. Three teams of therapists developed what are broadly considered to be systemic or strategic theories:

- Mental Research Institute (MRI; a.k.a. the Palo Alto group): After the Bateson team concluded their groundbreaking research on family dynamics with schizophrenia, Richard Fisch and Don Jackson worked together to found the Mental Research Institute, which has since served as the most influential training center in family therapy, inspiring Jay Haley's strategic work (which he conceptualized prior to the MRI approach), the Milan team's systemic approach, Virginia Satir's human growth model (see Chapter 6), and solution-focused brief therapy (see Chapter 9). The Brief Therapy Project at the MRI was designed to find the quickest possible resolution to client complaints, typically relying on action-based interventions (Watzlawick & Weakland, 1977; Watzlawick, Weakland, & Fisch, 1974; Weakland & Ray, 1995).

- Milan Systemic Therapy: After joining together to further Selvini Palazzoli's work with families who have anorectic or schizophrenic children, Mara Selvini Palazzoli, Gianfranco Cecchin, Giuliana Prata, and Luigi Boscolo formed the Milan team. Early in their work, they studied at the MRI and returned to Italy to design a therapeutic model that embodied the cybernetic systems theory of Bateson (1972, 1979; see Chapter 3). This model is called "Milan systemic therapy," or "long-term brief therapy." Milan therapists closely attend to how client language shapes family dynamics (Selvini Palazzoli, Cecchin, Prata, & Boscolo, 1978).

- Strategic Therapy: One of the original associates at the MRI, Jay Haley developed his own form of systemic therapy with his then-wife, Cloe Madanes. Their approach focuses on the use of power and, in their later work, love in family systems (Haley, 1976).

- Tomm's IPscope: Introduced in Chapter 3, Karl Tomm and colleagues (2014) have developed a contemporary systems approach that tracks not only systemic processes related to the presenting problem but also to healing, wellness, and change. The conceptualization piece of this approach is clearly systemic but many of the interventions have strong postmodern influences.

Systemic–Strategic Family Therapy
In a Nutshell: The Least You Need to Know

Using what most therapists consider the classic family therapy method, systemic family therapists conceptualize the symptoms of individuals within the larger network of their family and social systems while maintaining a nonblaming, nonpathologizing stance toward all members of the family. Systemic therapies are based on **general systems theory** and **cybernetic systems theory**, which propose that families are living systems characterized by certain principles, including **homeostasis**, the tendency to maintain a particular range of behaviors and norms, and **self-correction**, the ability to identify when the system has gone too far from its homeostatic norm and then to self-correct to maintain balance (see Chapter 3). Systemic therapists rarely attempt linear, logical solutions to "educate" a family on better ways to communicate—this is almost never successful. Instead, they tap into the systemic dynamics to effect change. They introduce small, innocuous, yet highly meaningful alterations to the family's interactions, allowing the family to naturally reorganize in response to the new information. Because this method effects change quickly, systemic therapies were the original *brief therapies*. Karl Tomm's (Tomm, St. George, Wulff, & Strong, 2014) contemporary systemic approach, the IPscope model, also incorporates sociocultural interpersonal patterns and more postmodern interventions.

The Juice: Significant Contributions to the Field

If you remember anything from this chapter, it should be the ideas discussed below.

Systemic Reframing: Juice from MRI

Reframing is a central technique that is found in most forms of systemic family therapy, such as structural therapy (see Chapter 5) and experiential family therapy (see Chapter 6). The MRI team approached reframing from a constructivist position that is summarized in the following propositions (Watzlawick et al., 1974):

1. We experience the world through our categorizations of objects, people, and events ("If my husband does not bring flowers or offer other romantic gestures, he does not really love me").
2. Once an object, person, or event is categorized, it is very difficult to see it as part of another category ("Our relationship must be in trouble if he has stopped being romantic").
3. Reframing uses the same "fact" that supports one categorization to support another categorization; once a person sees things using this second perspective, it is difficult to see the original situation in the same way (e.g., "My husband's drop in romance may mean that he has become more comfortable and authentic in the relationship rather than playing courting games; it could be a sign of deepening commitment").

The basic component of reframing is finding an alternative yet equally plausible explanation (categorization) for the same set of facts. Of course, the key is identifying the client's current worldview and finding an equally viable frame for the problem behavior from the client's perspective. Reframing in systemic family therapies typically involves considering the role of the symptom in the broader relational system, often highlighting how it helps maintain balance (homeostasis) in the relationship. Unlike in cognitive–behavioral therapies, clients are not expected to literally believe or adopt the proposed reframe; instead, it is hoped that the reframe will be "news that makes a difference," allowing clients to generate useful understandings. For example, with certain couples it makes sense to reframe their arguments as a way to build passion and maintain connection in their relationship. Such a reframe is offered to a couple without expectation that it will have a specific effect, because the system is considered a unique entity that will make its own meaning. If the couple does not find the reframe helpful, perhaps not responding or disagreeing with it, the therapist uses this information to better understand their worldview and then identify other potentials for reframing the problem.

Circular Questions: Juice from Milan

Regardless of which therapeutic model one chooses to practice, **circular questions** are perhaps one of the most useful techniques when working with more than one person in the room. Such questions help: (a) assess and (b) make overt the overall dynamics and interactive patterns in the system, thereby reframing the problem for all participants without the therapist having to verbally provide a reframe, as already described in Systemic

Reframing (Selvini Palazzoli et al., 1978; Selvini Palazzoli, Boscolo, Cecchin, & Prata, 1980). For example, I once had a family come to me complaining about a child's "anger problem." After they described the child's "problem" behavior, I inquired about how the rest of the family responded to the child's anger. The mother reported that she responded by getting frustrated and often yelled, and the father sharply corrected the child. As they listened to themselves describe their responses, both conceded that they responded to his anger with anger; they also noted that the younger sister disappeared into another room or somehow disengaged because of the intensity. As the parents began to look at their half of the interaction pattern, it became clear that anger was highly "contagious" for the three of them, while it evoked anxiety in the daughter. These questions allowed the family to view their "son's anger problem" in the context of the broader interaction pattern, thus opening new options for relating.

Specific forms of circular questions (Cecchin, 1987) include the following:

- Behavioral sequence questions: Therapists use these questions to trace the entire sequence of behaviors that constitute the problem: "After John got mad, what did mom do? What did dad do? What did his sister do?" And after the response, "What did John do next?" The therapist follows the sequence of interactions until homeostasis is restored.
- Behavioral difference questions: Therapists use behavioral difference questions when clients start labeling people and assuming that a particular behavior is part of a person's inherent personality. For example, if a child claims, "My mom's a nag," the therapist would ask, "What does she do that makes her a nag?" The description of problem behavior, "tells me to do things," is then compared with others: "How does your dad ask you to do things? Your teacher? How do *you* ask others to do things?"
- Comparison and ranking questions: Comparison and ranking questions are useful for reducing labeling and other rigid descriptions in the family: "Who is the most upset when Jackie has an episode? Who is the least affected? Who is the most helpful during these times? The least helpful?"
- Before-and-after questions: When a specific event has occurred, before-and-after questions can be useful in assessing how the event affected the family dynamics: "Did you and your mother fight more or less after your dad got sick?"
- Hypothetical circular questions: Hypothetical questions are used to offer a scenario and have family members describe how each is likely to respond: "If mom were suddenly placed in the hospital, who would be most likely to be at her bedside? The least likely?"

Try It Yourself

Find a partner and take turns asking circular questions related to a current life problem. In what ways do these questions change how you view or define the problem?

Directives: Juice from Strategic Therapy

Directives are the most basic of strategic techniques (Madanes, 1991); however, they are also the most frequently misunderstood by new therapists. In essence, directives are directions for the family to complete a specific task, usually between sessions but sometimes within the session. The tasks are rarely "logical" or linear solutions to the problem; instead they somehow "perturb" the system's interaction patterns to create new interactions (Haley, 1987). Thus, if a couple is arguing, the therapist will *not* ask them to set the timer so that each person speaks for 5 minutes followed by the other summarizing or responding for the next 5 minutes. That would be a logical or linear directive such as those found in cognitive–behavioral family therapy (see Chapter 8). Nor will the therapist ask the couple to simply stop or learn a communication technique; the assumption is that if they could do this, they would have already done so. Instead, the therapist asks them to argue but to change one or two key elements, such as the place, timing, or turn-taking style. A directive may be to have their "normal" argument while fully clothed in the bathtub or to have it after rearranging furniture to simulate a courtroom.

Directives get people out of their ruts with the *smallest change possible*. When these directives work, clients generally experience a simultaneous shift in emotions, insight, and behavior. I like to compare it to a chocolate–vanilla swirl soft serve ice cream: the changes are perfectly synchronized and come fully integrated together. From the clients' perspective, directives jolt them out of their usual life patterns, and generally the clients know exactly how to shift themselves to make the necessary changes. Unlike insight in traditional psychodynamic therapy, directives create visceral aha moments because clients are in the midst of the action that needs to change. It is a bit like sudden enlightenment in the Zen tradition—hence, I like to think of systemic therapists as the Zen Masters and Mistresses of the field.

IPscope: Juice from Calgary

See Chapter 3 for a complete description.

Rumor Has It: The People and Their Stories

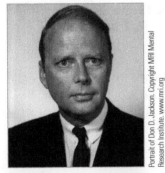

The Clinical MRI Team

Don Jackson

A brilliant clinician and founder of the MRI in 1958, Jackson was a principal figure in family therapy, especially in the development of concepts such as family homeostasis, family rules, relational quid pro quo, conjoint therapy, interactional theory, and, along with others at MRI, the double-bind theory (MRI, 2002; Watzlawick, Bavelas, & Jackson, 1967); he also was one of the first to question the myth of normality (Jackson, 1967).

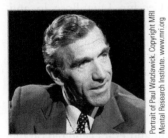

Paul Watzlawick

Born in Austria, Paul Watzlawick was a communications theorist who co-founded the Brief Therapy Center at the MRI with Weakland and Fisch, with a goal of developing an ultrabrief approach to therapy (Watzlawick, 1977, 1978/1993, 1984, 1990). In his later writings, Watzlawick explored implications of radical constructivism for therapy and human communication in cleverly titled books such as *How Real Is Real?* (1977), *The Invented Reality* (1984), *Ultra Solutions: How to Fail Most Successfully* (1988), and *The Situation Is Hopeless but Not Serious: The Pursuit of Unhappiness* (1993).

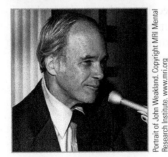

John Weakland

Originally trained as a chemical engineer, Weakland joined the Bateson group and helped to articulate the application of communication theory, emphasizing the importance of basing theory on concrete and observable behaviors rather than inferences or constructs, which are not observable (MRI, 2002). Along with Haley, Weakland integrated Erickson's work at the MRI with the Brief Therapy Project.

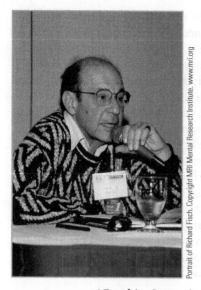

Richard Fisch

After initially proposing the creation of the MRI, Richard Fisch was appointed by Jackson to be the director of the new Brief Therapy Project, which was inspired by Erickson's brief hypnotic work; the goal was to develop a highly teachable form of brief psychotherapy (Watzlawick et al., 1974). Thus, Fisch spearheaded the development of the therapy model for which the MRI is most famous, studying how to influence others with words and indirect influence (Fisch & Schlanger, 1999; Fisch, Weakland, & Segal, 1982; MRI, 2002).

Wendel Ray

Former director and senior research fellow at the MRI, Wendel Ray has been instrumental in ushering systemic therapies into the 21st century, working with Bradford Keeney (see Chapter 3) to develop *resource-focused therapy,* a strength-based systems therapy (Ray & Keeney, 1994); with Milan team colleagues to further develop systemic concepts, such as *irreverence, cybernetics of prejudices,* and *eccentricity* (Cecchin, Lane, & Ray, 1992); and with colleagues at the MRI on theoretical and archival work (Weakland & Ray, 1995). He also serves as the Hammond Endowed Professor of Education and Professor of Family Systems Theory at the University of Louisiana at Monroe.

Barbara Anger-Diaz and Karin Schlanger

Barbara Anger-Díaz and Karin Schlanger train therapists in brief therapy with Latino families; training and therapy are conducted in Spanish at the Latino Brief Therapy and Training Center at the MRI.

Giorgio Nardone

Working closely with Watzlawick in his later works (Nardone & Watzlawick, 1993), Giorgio Nardone founded the Centro di Terapia Strategica in Arezzo, Italy, and the Brief Strategic and Systemic World Network. Founded in 2003, the latter brings together strategic and systemic therapy practitioners from around the world.

The Milan Team

The Milan team included Mara Selvini Palazzoli, Gianfranco Cecchin, Luigi Boscolo, and Giuliana Prata and was founded in 1967 by Selvini Palazzoli, who was studying anorexia in Italy at the time (Campbell, Draper, & Crutchley, 1991). They met weekly without pay, seeing families and studying the work of Bateson and the MRI group and frequently inviting Watzlawick for consultations. The team developed a unique approach that focused on meaning and ritual. In 1979, the team separated along interest and gender lines: Selvini Palazzoli and Prata, primarily researchers, wanted to continue their investigation into treating families with psychotic members, while Cecchin and Boscolo worked together on clinical and training applications. The later work of Selvini Palazzoli and Prata centered on the *invariant prescription* (discussed later in this chapter), while Cecchin and Boscolo explored Keeney's *second-order cybernetics* (1983) and related works, attending to language and the construction of meaning through multiple descriptors and eventually moving toward a more postmodern, social constructionist stance (see Chapter 10). Lynn Hoffman and Peggy Penn, featured in Chapter 10 worked closely with Boscolo and Cecchin.

Strategic Therapists
Jay Haley and Cloe Madanes

Jay Haley, one of the original members of the Bateson team, student of Milton Erickson, and cofounder of the Brief Therapy Project at MRI, developed his own systemic

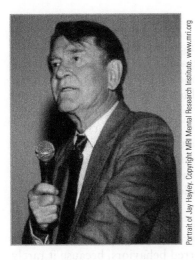

Portrait of Jay Hayley. Copyright MRI Mental Research Institute. www.mri.org

approach, strategic therapy (Haley, 1963, 1973, 1976, 1980, 1981, 1984, 1987, 1996; Haley & Richeport-Haley, 2007; MRI, 2002). He and his wife, Cloe Madanes (1981, 1990, 1991, 1993), founded the Family Therapy Institute in Washington, D.C. Their approach is based on the concepts of hierarchy, power, and love, and uses *directives* for interventions.

Eileen Bobrow

Eileen Bobrow founded and directs the Strategic Family Therapy and Training Center at the MRI, which prior to her arrival focused primarily on the Brief Therapy Model developed at the MRI.

Jim Keim

A research fellow at the MRI, Jim Keim (1998) uses strategic therapy to work with families with children diagnosed with oppositional defiant disorder and conduct disorder.

Tomm's IPscope
Karl Tomm

A psychiatrist by training and pioneer of family therapy, Karl Tomm founded the Calgary Family Therapy Centre at the University of Calgary in 1973. For nearly four decades, he has developed and refined his approach for working with families, which draws from both second-order cybernetic concepts as well as contemporary postmodern

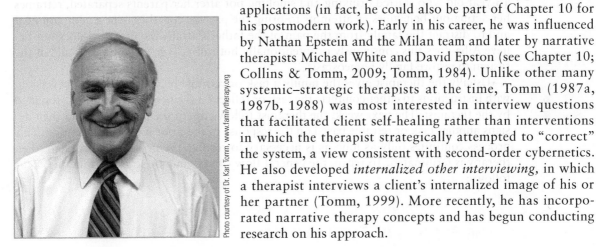

Photo courtesy of Dr. Karl Tomm, www.familytherapy.org

applications (in fact, he could also be part of Chapter 10 for his postmodern work). Early in his career, he was influenced by Nathan Epstein and the Milan team and later by narrative therapists Michael White and David Epston (see Chapter 10; Collins & Tomm, 2009; Tomm, 1984). Unlike other many systemic–strategic therapists at the time, Tomm (1987a, 1987b, 1988) was most interested in interview questions that facilitated client self-healing rather than interventions in which the therapist strategically attempted to "correct" the system, a view consistent with second-order cybernetics. He also developed *internalized other interviewing,* in which a therapist interviews a client's internalized image of his or her partner (Tomm, 1999). More recently, he has incorporated narrative therapy concepts and has begun conducting research on his approach.

Sally St. George

A professor of family therapy, Sally St. George works with Karl Tomm at the University of Calgary. She and Dan Wulff have been instrumental in developing practices for working with sociocultural interpersonal patterns (SCIPs) and conducting research on the IPscope.

Dan Wulff

A professor of social work and a colleague of Tomm at the University of Calgary, Dan Wulff has worked with St. George to develop practices for working with SCIPs as well as conducting research on the IPscope.

Tom Strong

A professor of counseling psychology and also a colleague of Tomm, Tom Strong (I imagine that gets a bit confusing) focuses his research on the counseling change process as well as social constructionist theories.

The Big Picture: Overview of Treatment

Systemic and strategic therapies focus solely on resolving the presenting problem, with the therapist imposing no other goals or agendas. Therapists see the presenting problem not as an individual problem but as a relational one, specifically an *interactional* one (Cecchin, 1987; Haley, 1987). Neither an individual nor a relationship is considered "dysfunctional"; instead, the problem is viewed as part of the interactional sequence of behaviors that have emerged through repeated exchanges, with no one person to blame.

The early stages of all three approaches involve getting a clear, behavioral description of the interaction sequence surrounding the problem, beginning with the initial exchange prior to the escalation of symptoms and ending with the interaction sequence that returns the system to homeostasis. Once the therapist has identified the interactional behavioral patterns and meanings associated with the problem, he or she uses one of many potential interventions to interrupt, not correct, this sequence. Much the way a school of fish cannot be shepherded but only interrupted and allowed to regroup, systemic and strategic therapists do not try to linearly instruct clients in preferred behaviors, because it rarely if ever works (Haley, 1987). Instead, they interrupt the problem sequence of behaviors, allowing the family to reconfigure itself around the new information that has been introduced to the system. For example, if a parent and child complain of frequent arguments, the therapist does not try to educate them in better communication. Instead, the therapist interrupts the sequence by reframing the child's defiance as a veiled attempt to remain close to the parent because the child fears the transition to college, or the therapist may ask parent and child to ritualize the process with hats symbolizing their positions. For example, in the case study at the end of this chapter, the therapist working with Alba, a 16-year-old who started drinking and smoking pot after her parents separated, reframes her acting-out behaviors as attempts to bring the parents together over a common goal and to distract the family from the pain of the father's affair; the therapist does not believe Alba does this consciously or intentionally but rather is following the "pull" of the system to restore family homeostasis.

Usually the therapist gives the family a task or reframe before they leave the session, with instructions to either complete the task or reflect on the new interpretation presented by the therapist. The next week, the therapist follows up on the prior week and then designs another task or reframe based on the response to the prior week's intervention. This process continues only as long as is necessary to resolve the presenting problem; then therapy is terminated. To recap, the general flow of systemic or strategic therapies is as follows:

THE PROCESS OF SYSTEMIC THERAPY

- **Assess the interactional sequence and associated meanings:** The therapist identifies the interactional behavior sequences that constitute the problem, including the actions and reactions of everyone in the system and the associated meanings.

- **Intervene by interrupting the interactional sequence:** Using a reframing technique or a task, the therapist interrupts the sequence (avoids trying to fix or repair the sequence), allowing the family to reorganize itself in response to the perturbation. *Note: The differences between MRI, strategic, and Milan therapies are primarily seen in the preferred method of interrupting the interactional sequence.*

- **Evaluate outcome and client response:** After the intervention, the therapist assesses the family's response and uses this information to design the next intervention.

- **Interrupt the new pattern:** The therapist then interrupts the new pattern with another intervention. This continues—interrupt behavioral sequence, allow family to reorganize and respond, and intervene again—until the problem is resolved.

Making a Connection: The Therapeutic Relationship

Respecting and Trusting the System

Systemic therapists respect the family as a system, as an entity that has its unique epistemology, or way of knowing and understanding the world. They have a deep, abiding trust that the system can reorganize itself without the therapist forcing change. Instead, the therapist provides opportunities for the family to reorganize itself. The symptoms are never seen as indicators of individual pathology but rather as the by-product of family interactional sequences that have served a purpose.

Adapting to Client Language and Viewpoint

In the first meeting, the therapist tries to establish a positive, trusting relationship with the client (Nardone & Watzlawick, 1993; Watzlawick, Weakland, & Fisch, 1974). One approach is to adapt to the clients' language, communication style, and worldview, speaking logically with clients who focus on reason and more intensely with clients who have a more emotional manner of expression. First and foremost, the therapist respectfully engages with the client's representational framework or epistemology, including beliefs, values, and language. This is the inverse of traditional psychoanalysis, in which the patient must adapt to the language and viewpoint of the therapist.

Neutrality

In 1978 (Selvini Palazzoli et al.; Selvini Palazzoli et al., 1980), the Milan team first described their therapeutic stance as one of **neutrality**, which has been one of the most misunderstood concepts related to their work (Boscolo et al., 1987). For the Milan team, neutrality connoted not only nonpartiality toward particular family members or problem descriptions but also multipartiality, the willingness to honor all perspectives.

In one sense, neutrality refers to the *pragmatic effect* the therapist has on the family, not the therapist's own feelings (Cecchin, 1987). Thus if, at the end of the session, the family cannot identify which "side" the therapist took, then the therapist has had the effect of being neutral. However, during the session, the therapist often appears to take a side by asking questions that align with a certain person's view of the problem; the therapist must counterbalance this by asking questions that align with each of the other perspectives so that at the end the therapist is viewed as neutral.

Neutrality also implies not becoming attached to particular meanings, descriptions, or outcomes (Boscolo et al., 1987). The Milan team carefully avoided buying into any one description of the problem, *including their own*. Neutrality extended to their own hypotheses and ideas about the family, and they avoided "falling in love" with their own ideas. Later, Cecchin et al. (1992) characterized this form of neutrality as a form of *irreverence* (discussed in next section) that allows for broad maneuverability. When therapists do not rigidly adhere to a particular problem description, they can see more possibilities for intervention rather than focusing on the single solution that fits with their preferred hypothesis.

Irreverence

The concept of irreverence was not highlighted until later in the literature (Cecchin et al., 1992), but—when properly understood—it clearly captures the therapist's relationship to the *problem* (not the client). The magic of this approach is derived from the therapist's irreverent relationship with problems.

What is there to be irreverent about? Systemic therapists are irreverent regarding the "catastrophic" appearance of problems. They do not give in to the appearance that a person has a "personality flaw," "illness," "unresolved childhood issue," or other deep, troubling problem, even though problems appear that way, especially to those who live with them. But the systemic therapist knows that appearances are deceiving because problems are intimately connected with the relational and broader social context. In a different context, a person's problem behaviors would be different. The context and problem are always influencing each other. The art of irreverence is to not honor the problem as a mighty foe and assume it has more power than it does. Its power is entirely dependent on its context. With experience, the therapist is able to see through the appearance of a "big, horrible" problem and instead see that the person, problem, and context form a fluid dance—and experience teaches that by changing only a few steps in the dance, the problem shifts, diminishes, and eventually disappears.

Irreverence is felt in the therapist's confidence and unpanicked response to problem issues. It is driven not by disrespect but rather by *fearlessness*. Whatever problem the client brings—whether the loss of a child or a teen's drama of the week—the therapist remains fearless, maintaining a deep sense of calm and faith in systemic processes, knowing that the problems are never as insurmountable as they appear and that systems are inherently self-correcting. Irreverence does not imply lack of empathy or sensitivity. Rather, it allows the therapist to maintain an openness, creativity, and flexibility to provide maximum benefit to the client. In this chapter's case study, the therapist's irreverence toward 16-year-old Alba's decision to start drinking and smoking pot after her parents separated keeps the therapist from being overly panicked about the acting-out behaviors and enables her and the whole family to focus on the issue: Alba's sense of betrayal and loss. By not overreacting to the drinking and drugs—but not ignoring them either—the therapist gives them less power and creates space for more critical issues.

Maneuverability

Maneuverability refers to the therapist's freedom to use personal judgment in defining the therapeutic relationship (Nardone & Watzlawick, 1993; Segal, 1991; Watzlawick et al., 1974). Therapists may choose to maintain an expert position or a one-down stance (see next section), depending on what would be most helpful to the family. Similarly, the therapist may be more distant or more emotionally engaged, depending on the circumstances. Furthermore, the therapist may choose to be disliked by the client or be the "bad guy" in order to achieve the desired change in the family system, always attuned to whatever role might be most beneficial for the family.

The One-Down Stance, or Helplessness

The one-down stance is used to increase clients' motivation, often paradoxically by claiming, "I'm not sure if I am able to handle such a problem" (Segal, 1991). This move is often helpful with clients who act as if their situation is hopeless; when the therapist takes the hopeless stance, the client is motivated to find hope. Systemically this works because in most systems there is a counterbalance: if one person is hopeless, the other feels compelled to be hopeful to maintain a balance. This same dynamic is also observed between couples in crisis: generally one person will manage the crisis, allowing the other one to more fully feel the panic and trauma.

Beyond serving this paradoxical purpose, the one-down stance also expresses a certain attitude toward the family system. Systemic therapists view the system as an entity with its own rules and integrity that must be respected, much like a mountain climber must respect the awesome forces of nature or the sailor an ocean. Like a family system, nature and the ocean are not things the therapist can control; instead, there is a deep respect for their power and ways. Thus, the one-down stance is a sincere and genuine position for a systemically trained therapist.

Social Courtesy

Haley (1987) describes the initial stage of therapy as the social stage, a time during which the therapist engages in casual social conversation, about the weather or traffic, to make clients comfortable and reduce their sense of shame: "the model for this stage is the courtesy behavior one would use with guests in the home" (p. 15). Before discussing the problem, the therapist ensures that all members have been properly greeted. During this first social stage, the therapist is assessing interactions and mood (Haley & Richeport-Haley, 2007).

Collaboration

Influenced by second-order cybernetics and social constructionist theories, contemporary systems therapists adopt a more collaborative relationship with clients (Tomm et al., 2014). Rather than assume a strategic posture by trying to directly effect change, contemporary systemic therapists use reflexive questions designed to facilitate client self-healing. in which the therapist and client co-create new meanings and action (Gaete, Sametband, & Sutherland, 2014; Tomm, 1987a).

The Viewing: Case Conceptualization and Assessment

Interactional Patterns

When systemic or strategic therapists view a family, they focus on the **interactional patterns** between people (Boscolo et al., 1987; Watzlawick et al., 1974). To illustrate this focus to new therapists, I have a "family of four" grab hold of a bright yellow rope to form a circle. Then I have them "dance" and move about in various patterns. Initially, the audience's eyes naturally focus on the movement of the dancers, our default, socialized habit of viewing interactions. I then have the family do the dance again, asking the audience to focus exclusively on the yellow rope and how it moves as it traces the interactional patterns of distance and closeness. This is a very gross and incomplete metaphor for how a systemic therapist looks at a family, but I think it helps get the point across: the focus is always on the yellow rope—the interaction—or what Milan therapists call the "game" (Boscolo et al., 1987). Often, English speakers think that the Milan term *family game* implies manipulation and ill intent, meanings the term may have in English. However, that is not the connotation of *game* in the systemic context, which focuses on the relational rules for how the family interacts, rules that are not consciously created but rather naturally emerge from the family interaction pattern.

Family interactions can be hard to detect, especially early in training. The trick is tracing the homeostatic dance (how A responds to B and B in turn responds to A), which involves identifying the earliest triggers or signs of the problem and tracing the increase in tension until the problem or symptom occurs; then continuing to track the interactions until things go back to homeostasis again (everyone seems to forget this last step, which often provides the most useful information for intervention). When observing a family interacting, therapists can assess the dance patterns by focusing less on the content of the conversation and more on the metacommunication (see Chapter 3) and interactions (movement of the rope). Whether action-based or language-based, virtually all interventions used by traditional systemic–strategic therapists have a single intention: interrupt the negative interaction patterns that include the presenting problem or symptom. These interaction patterns can be roughly illustrated as shown here:

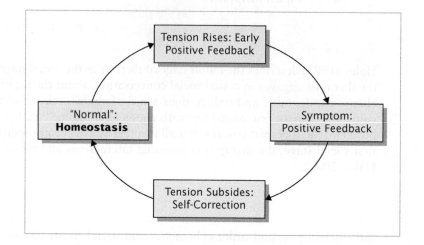

For example, if a couple is arguing about how to discipline a defiant child, the therapist will not focus on solving the problem with the child but rather on how the parents communicate: Does each share opinions, thoughts, and feelings? How does each respond to the other's divergent opinion? What strategies does each use to convince the other? Does one person get the last word? How do they get back to "normal"? By focusing on the interactional pattern or couple game for negotiating this type of problem, the therapist can identify where they are stuck.

IDENTIFYING THE INTERACTIONAL SEQUENCE

1. **Homeostasis (normality):** Can you describe what things are like when things feel "normal" and "okay"? What are things like before the tension starts?

2. **Start of tension:** Can you tell me how things usually begin? Who does what, and how do others respond? How does the first respond back?

3. **Escalation and symptom:** Can you describe the escalation that leads to [specify the client's specific symptom]? Who does what, and how does each person in the household respond?

4. **Return to homeostasis:** Describe how things get back to normal.

Try It Yourself

Find a partner and use the above questions to assess the interactional sequence for a relational problem.

In addition to observing actual interactions, it is often necessary to ask circular questions to assess the interactional sequence; these questions can be used with individuals, couples, or families. For example, with the couple having trouble with the defiant child, the therapist would ask: "What is happening just before the problem incident? What is each person saying and doing? How does the child respond? How does each parent and anyone else involved respond to the defiance? How does the child respond to this? How do the parents respond to the child next?" and so on, until family homeostasis is restored.

QUESTIONS FOR ASSESSING FAMILY INTERACTIONS

To develop a concrete description of the interactional pattern, Nardone and Watzlawick (1993, p. 30) recommend that therapists answer the following questions:

- What are the patient's usual, observable behavior patterns?
- How does the patient define the problem?
- How does the problem manifest itself?
- In whose company does the problem appear, worsen, disguise itself, or not appear?
- Where does it usually appear?
- In what situations?
- How often does the problem appear, and how serious is it?
- What has been done and is currently being done (by the patient alone or by others) to resolve the problem?
- Whom or what does the problem benefit?
- Who could be hurt by the disappearance of the problem?

IPscope

Introduced in Chapter 3, contemporary systemic therapists conceptualize use the **IPscope** to identify several interpersonal interaction patterns, which include not only those associated with the problem pathologizing interpersonal patterns (PIPs) but also wellness (WIPs), healing (HIPs), sociocultural (SCIPs), transformative (TIPs), and deteriorating (DIPs) interpersonal patterns. By tracking these multiple interaction patterns, therapists can conceptualize not only the problem but also the most likely interactions that will address the problems, which can serve to guide the therapy process. See Chapter 3 for detailed discussion.

"More of the Same" Solutions

When tracking interactional patterns, MRI therapists also focus on identifying "**more of the same**" **solutions**—that is, solutions that perpetuate the problem (Watzlawick et al., 1974). For example, if the parents always respond to a child's defiance with some form of lecture and verbal punishment, this would be a "more of the same" solution that is not working for the family. This "attempted solution" (i.e., verbal punishment) would be identified as the interactional behavior sequence that maintains the problem. After identifying the more-of-the-same behaviors and logic system (e.g., bad behavior is corrected with punishment), the therapist then identifies a behavior that represents a 180-degree shift in logic (e.g., cooperative behavior that is motivated by a strong emotional bond).

More-of-the-same solutions can further be described as mishandling the problem in one of three ways (Watzlawick et al., 1974):

- Terrible simplifications (action is necessary but none is taken): The client or family attempts to solve the problem by *denying* it: this solution is common with addictions, marital problems, and problematic family dynamics.
- The utopian syndrome (action is taken when it is not necessary): The client or family tries to change something that is either unchangeable or nonexistent: this solution is common with depression, anxiety, procrastination, perfectionism, and unrealistic demands on a relationship or a child.
- Paradox (action is taken at the wrong level): Either a first-order solution is attempted for a problem that necessitates a second-order solution (e.g., parents are unable to adjust parenting techniques as child matures) or a second-order solution is attempted for a first-order problem (e.g., when people demand attitude or personality changes

and are not content with behavioral changes). This solution is common with schizophrenia, relational impasses, domestic violence, and abuse.

The Tyranny of Linguistics

When assessing families, the Milan team paid particular attention to the family's word choices and expressions. They were mindful of how language, particularly descriptions of self and others, shape lived reality; they called this the "**tyranny of linguistics**" (Selvini Palazzoli et al., 1978). For example, the statements "I am depressed" and "He's an angry person" are global labels that create little space for noticing numerous moments throughout the day when other feelings and identities may be experienced. Instead, Milan therapists encourage descriptions of a person's *action*: times when I "do" depression or when he is "doing" anger. This subtle shift of words suddenly opens new opportunities for how people experience themselves while also allowing for descriptions of times when the depression is not as strong or a person is not angry.

For Milan therapists, positive labels, such as "intelligent" or "good," are as limiting and problematic as negative descriptors. Like negative descriptions, positive labels obscure the relational context that shapes them (Boscolo et al., 1987). Both positive and negative descriptors are avoided in favor of interactional behavioral descriptions.

Strategic Conceptualization

Madanes (1991) identifies five ways to think about a problem in strategic therapy; these dimensions can be used to conceptualize the role of a symptom in the family system or in an individual's broader social world. One or more of these is used, depending on the case.

- Involuntary versus voluntary: Clients generally present by viewing the problem as involuntary; strategic therapists instead view the symptoms as voluntary, with the exception of organic illness. For example, they see arguing, worrying, or being depressed as behaviors or solutions clients choose.
- Helplessness versus power: Although symptomatic people appear helpless, their symptoms also generate significant power, allowing them to make otherwise unreasonable demands, receive more care and attention, or excuse otherwise unacceptable behavior. For example, agoraphobia can be seen as an attempt to keep the family close.
- Metaphorical versus literal: Symptoms may be viewed as a metaphor for another problem sequence of behaviors in the system. For example, a child's defiance can be seen as a metaphor for the same defiance the husband feels but does not express toward the mother; or bingeing can be seen as a metaphor for rejecting the mother's attempt to overnurture the child.
- Hierarchy versus equality: Therapists may conceptualize the presenting problem as a demand for more or less hierarchy, depending on the family's set of circumstances. For example, caving in to a child's tantrums allows the child to be at the top of the power hierarchy.
- Hostility versus love: Many family interactions—rejecting a lover because one feels unworthy, disciplining a child, pursuing a partner for sex or communication—can be viewed as motivated by either hostility or love. Strategic therapists may use either interpretation, depending on the therapeutic situation. For example, a husband's constant pursuit of sex may be a sign of love and caring *or* a power move because he feels he has none, depending on the situation. Similarly, a wife's refusal of sex could be motivated by love for husband (e.g., only wanting sex when she really has feelings) or family (e.g., gives too much and is too tired) *or* a power move to gain control because she feels she has none.

Try It Yourself

Find a partner and use the above questions to reframe a relationship problem you have had using one of these strategic conceptualizations.

Strategic Humanism

The latest developments in strategic therapy emphasize increasing the family's ability to love and nurture rather than dominate and control, which is consonant more generally with the evolution of the field of family therapy (Madanes, 1993). Thus, case conceptualizations focus more on the family's unsuccessful attempts to show love rather than on their attempts to control one another. For example, Jim Keim's (1998) work with oppositional children aims to increase parental nurturing behaviors to help them reestablish a more effective hierarchy, highlighting that a nurturing parent can be as much of an authority as a disciplinarian; once some authority has been reestablished in the nurturing realm, Keim instructs parents to begin enforcing behavioral rules.

The Observation Team

The hallmark of the art of systemic or strategic viewing has always been the **observation team**. Early in the development of these ideas, teams would sit behind a one-way mirror to observe the therapist working with the family. The team could see the systemic dance more rapidly and completely because the person in the room very quickly falls in sync with the family system and has a more difficult time seeing the entire dance. Anyone who has spent time behind a mirror and in front of it knows that you are always smarter behind it. The distance created by not being part of the interactional dance of the family increases one's ability to see the dance more clearly and quickly. Arguably the main reason family therapists still train with a mirror is to develop the ability to see the system's dynamics. This is not to say that a therapist in the room can't see the system's dynamics; it is just harder and takes more practice to do so.

Targeting Change: Goal Setting

Symptom-free Interaction Patterns

Systemic therapists help the family to develop a new set of interaction patterns (i.e., homeostasis), a new game or dance that does not include symptoms (or any subsequent symptoms; Boscolo et al., 1987). Stated yet again, the goal is to create a family homeostasis that is problem-free—or at least does not involve facing the same problem over and over again (Watzlawick et al., 1974).

No Theory of Health

Unlike many earlier schools of therapy, such as psychodynamic or humanistic, systemic therapy does not have a predetermined definition of "healthy family functioning" that the therapist uses to define therapeutic goals. As already stated, therapists do not have a theory of health that defines how the family should look at the end of therapy. Instead, it is believed that the family system (not individual members) will reorganize itself from within to find a "functional," symptom-free interaction pattern in response to the *perturbations* or disruptions introduced by the therapist.

The Problem Is the Attempted Solution (MRI Therapy)

Goals in the MRI brief therapy approach are developed using the following four-step procedure (Watzlawick et al., 1974):

1. Define the problem: Use concrete, behavioral terms to describe the actions and reactions of all involved. For example, "My son is always defiant" is not a well-defined problem; a preferred problem description is "When I ask my son to do something, he says 'no' and when I push further he starts yelling and cursing; that's when I give in."

2. Identify attempted solutions: The therapist may ask, "How have you attempted to deal with this problem?" and listens for patterns in the various **attempted solutions** (e.g., threats that are not carried out, negotiating with the child).
3. Describe the desired behavioral change: MRI therapists take great care to develop concrete, behavioral goals that meaningfully focus clients' and therapists' attention in useful directions. The goals must be realistic, specific, and time-limited.
   - Realistic: Therapists need to be careful to avoid utopian goals, such as "Every time I ask my son to do something, he will obey." Instead, the therapist helps the client develop the more realistic goal of "increasing the frequency with which my son politely carries out my first request."
   - Specific: Goals describe clear behaviors and interactions rather than vague intentions, such as "communicate better." As Watzlawick says, "It is the vagueness of goals that make their attainment impossible" (Watzlawick et al., 1974, p. 112).
   - Time-limited: MRI brief therapists prefer to set a clear time limit for a specified goal, such as "within 4 weeks."
4. Develop a plan: MRI therapists use two basic systemic principles:
   - The target of change is the *attempted solution*.
   - The tactic of change is to use the *client's own language* to speak directly to the client's view of reality.

Thus, the plan is never linear or directive psychoeducation on how to " better communicate." Such plans and interventions are used in cognitive–behavioral therapy (see Chapter 8, not systemic therapy). In dramatic contrast, an MRI systemic approach targets the attempted solution rather than the presenting problem; again, this differs from solution-based therapies, which target the preferred solution (see Chapter 9). Thus, rather than target a child's tantrums by teaching parents how to employ positive and negative reinforcement, systemic therapists identify the class of solutions used by the parents and develop an intervention that represents a 180-degree shift. If the parents respond by becoming embarrassed and giving in, the therapist designs an intervention in which the parents are emotionally unaffected and consistent in carrying out consequences. On the other hand, if the parents typically respond with strict, harsh punishment, the therapist suggests an emotionally engaged and gentle approach.

Strategic Goals

The main goal of therapy is to get people to behave differently and so to have different subjective experiences. —Haley, 1987, p. 56

Strategic therapy does not have a predefined set of long-term goals for individual or family functioning, other than to promote a change that alters people's subjective experiences (mood, thoughts, and behaviors). Madanes (1990, 1991) conceptualizes all problems brought to therapy as stemming from an existential dilemma between love and violence, because these two experiences tend to be closely correlated in human affairs. Thus, the ultimate strategic goal is to help clients find ways to love without dominating, intruding upon, or harming the other. This goal may be achieved by doing the following (Madanes, 1991):

- Correcting the couple or family hierarchy (either increasing or decreasing it)
- Reducing intrusion or increasing engagement by changing a parent or partner's level of involvement
- Reuniting family members
- Changing who is helpful and how, including empowering children to be appropriately helpful
- Repenting for an injustice and forgiving
- Increasing the expression of compassion and unity

The Doing: Language-Based Interventions

Systemic Reframing; Circular Questions (see Juice)

This intervention is described in detail in "The Juice" section, above.

The Hypothesizing Process (Milan Therapy)

*The construction of hypotheses is a continuous process, coevolving with the family's movement. The act of **hypothesizing** is best described using the concepts of cybernetic feedback loops, for as the family's response to the question modifies or alters one hypothesis, another is formed based on the specifics of that new feedback. This continuous process of hypothesis construction requires the therapist to reconceptualize constantly, both as an interviewer and team member.— Boscolo et al., 1987, p. 94*

The process of generating a hypothesis, emphasized in the Milan approach, continues throughout therapy and generally has the following two phases:

1. Hypothesizing for conceptualization: This is the behind-the-mirror process of developing and revising hypotheses that the therapist and team use to guide their "viewing" and provide an overall focus and direction for therapy.
2. Hypothesizing as intervention: When the therapist and team believe it will benefit the family, the hypothesis they have been developing behind the mirror is shared verbally with the family as an in-session intervention.

As already discussed, a hypothesis usually defines the role of the symptom in maintaining the family's homeostasis (Boscolo et al., 1987). For example, a teen's delinquent behavior may serve to bring the parents closer together; without the child's "problem" behavior, the couple might experience other difficulties that would be harder for the family to manage. Hypotheses can also highlight how the family wants to simultaneously keep things the same and change, two counterbalancing forces. When therapists deliver hypotheses to the family, the purpose is to "create news of a difference" and shift how they think about the problem, thus creating new possibilities for change. Hypotheses need to be worded so that they are different from how the family is currently viewing the situation yet not so different that they react against it. Instead, hypotheses need to be *plausible* in the family's current worldview (Watzlawick et al., 1974).

The Milan team identified three common types of hypotheses (Boscolo et al., 1987):

- Hypotheses about alliances: These describe alliances and coalitions: who is on whose team.
- Hypotheses about myths and premises: These identify unrealistic or problematic myths and premises that are contributing to the problem (myths of the perfect marriage, ideal child, etc.).
- Hypotheses that analyze communication: These track problematic communication patterns, such as double binds.

Positive Connotation: The Milan Reframe

Milan therapists originally developed **positive connotations** to not contradict themselves when prescribing **paradoxical interventions** (Selvini Palazzoli et al., 1978). Therapists use positive connotation to respect both the family's fear of change and their request for change. They interpret the behavior of each member of the family positively, as having an underlying benevolent motivation (Boscolo et al., 1987). A common positive connotation is reframing a child's problematic behavior as a way to keep the parents together and reframing the parents' arguments about how to handle this behavior as a way to show their dedication to the family and each other. Perhaps the most important outcome of positive connotation is the effect it has on the therapist, enabling the therapist to view members of the system less judgmentally and with greater hope.

Try It Yourself

Create a positive reframe for a relational problem experienced by you or a friend.

The Therapeutic Double Bind and Counterparadox (MRI and Milan, respectively)

The MRI therapeutic double bind is used to undo a double-bind message in a family or relationship; similarly, the Milan counterparadox is used to therapeutically respond to the paradoxes, or double binds, that families and couples create for themselves (Selvini Palazzoli et al., 1978; Watzlawick et al., 1967). The difference between a problem-generating double bind and a therapeutic double bind is simple: in the problem-generating form, no matter what you do, you are wrong; there is no escape. In a therapeutic double bind or counterparadox, no matter what you do, you do something different, something that moves you in a new direction.

A common double bind is when one party demands that the other spontaneously display love and affection. For example, a wife may demand that her husband spontaneously express his love in more romantic ways: flowers, candlelight dinners, and gifts. If he does what she asks, she can say that he only did it because she asked and that it wasn't spontaneous; if he does not do anything romantic, then she can say he obviously doesn't care because he didn't follow through. Either way he loses. A therapeutic double bind would be to have him show his romantic side in any way other than the specific ways his wife demands. If he follows this directive literally, he will initiate new romantic behavior in the system; if he does not follow the instructions and instead chooses to use one of his wife's suggestions, then he is doing so without the command to do so. If you think it is tough to design such an intervention on your own, you are right—that is why the early family therapists preferred to work in teams. They could then more quickly assess the family's double binds and identify helpful therapeutic paradoxes.

Invariant Prescriptions (Milan Therapy)

One of the Selvini Palazzoli's earliest therapeutic innovations and the focus of her long-term research, the **invariant prescription** is just what it sounds like: an intervention that is not varied across families (Selvini Palazzoli, 1988). Used primarily with families whose children are labeled anorexic or schizophrenic, the intervention severs covert coalitions between a parent and a child. Parents are instructed to arrange to go on a date (or other outing) and to not tell the children where they are going or why. The desired effect is to create a secret between the parents, ending inappropriate coalitions by creating a clear boundary between the parents as a unified team and the symptomatic child. The child loses the status of being a special confidant of the one parent, lessening his/her emotional burden and resulting in fewer problem symptoms. Although originally designed for severe pathology such as anorexia and psychosis, this intervention is also effective with modern parents who overemphasize transparent and open communication with their children to the extent that the children use this information to "manipulate" them. The therapist in this chapter's case study uses a variation of this technique with 16-year-old Alba, who is acting out after her parents separate; the invariant prescription helps restore the parental alliance so that Alba does not feel the "systemic pull" to act out to get her parents to work together.

Dangers of Improvement (MRI and Strategic Therapy)

A technique used by MRI and strategic therapists, the *dangers of improvement* involves asking clients to identify potential problems that might arise if the problem were resolved (Segal, 1991). For example, if a child becomes more independent in doing homework and getting chores done, what will the mother and father do to feel that they are parenting their child? If a couple suddenly stops arguing, how will they keep the flame of passion alive in their relationship? If a person stops being depressed and starts socializing again, how will he protect his solitude and quiet time? These questions undermine unrealistic and utopian worldviews that not only created the current problem but are also likely to be the source of new problems to come.

Restraining, Going Slow

Restraining or the directive to *go slow* is another common systemic and strategic intervention that carries a paradoxical flavor (Segal, 1991). When therapists restrain or instruct clients to go slow, they warn clients to avoid changing too fast and encourage them to take change slowly. This has a paradoxical effect similar to a therapeutic double bind in that if the client complies, change will happen and the client will be better prepared for the setbacks that characterize most attempts at change. On the other hand, if the client has a rebellious response, he or she will attempt to rebel against slowness by working harder toward desired change. In either case, the change process is supported and "immunized" against setbacks.

Deconstructive TIPs (Transforming Interpersonal Patterns)

Using Tomm's IPscope approach, Gaete and colleagues (2014) distinguish between two types of transforming interpersonal patterns (TIPs) that therapists can use to facilitate change: deconstructive and constructive TIPs. Deconstructive TIPs involve asking clients questions that invite them to reconsider their assumptions related to the problem. Typically, this process involves questioning their individualistic perspective and moving toward a more relational view of the situation. Therapists can do this by asking questions that help clients explore how their behavior and responses may—unintentionally—perpetuate the pathologizing interpersonal pattern (PIP), such as "what do you think your partner is thinking when you begin to raise the issue?" In addition, therapists can explore sociocultural patterns (SCIPs) that may help clients to shift assumptions that fuel the PIP. For example, a therapist could ask about the division of labor for a dual-career couple and explore gender discourses that may be reinforcing an unfair division of labor. Furthermore, circular questions and systemic reframing can also be used to deconstruct meanings that perpetuate the PIP. When working with a relationship in which there is a significant power difference, the therapist begins deconstructive TIPs by directing questions at the more powerful person, which is similar to the socioemotional relational therapy methods described in Chapter 3. Regardless of the exact method, therapists using the IPscope are careful to track the interpersonal pattern related to the TIP to ensure that their action has the intended helpful effect. If not, the therapist addresses this issue with the clients respectfully, directly, and immediately and with the attitude that the therapist will work to correct the misunderstanding.

The Doing: Action-Oriented Interventions

Directives (MRI and Strategic Therapy; also See Directives in Juice Section Above)

Used in both strategic and MRI approaches, directives are behavioral tasks that the therapist gives to clients to alter their interaction patterns. Haley (1987) identifies two general types of directives: straightforward and indirect. **Straightforward directives** are used when the therapist has the power and influence to get people to do what is asked; **indirect directives** are used when the therapist has less authority in the eyes of the client. Indirect directives generally take the form of paradoxical or metaphorical tasks.

Technically, straightforward directives mean giving good advice, but Haley is quick to admonish against them: "Giving good advice means the therapist assumes that people have rational control of what they are doing. To be successful in the therapy business, it may be better to drop that idea" (Haley, 1987, p. 61). Therefore, most straightforward directives aim to change the way the family interacts by introducing *new action*. Often therapists are tempted to ask clients to stop doing something; Haley warns against this also: "If the therapist tells someone to stop usual behavior, he must usually go to an extreme or get other family members to cooperate and change their behavior" (p. 60). Thus, most strategic directives *resequence* interaction patterns by requesting small behavioral or contextual changes, such as having the other parent discipline a child who has broken house rules or asking a couple to add a 10-second pause between exchanges in a fight. These smaller changes are much easier to accomplish. The differences between straightforward and indirect directives are outlined in the following table.

THERAPEUTIC DIRECTIVES

	STRAIGHTFORWARD DIRECTIVES	INDIRECT DIRECTIVES
Type of task	• Do something different: alter behavioral sequence • Stop a behavior (rarely used) • Good advice; psychoeducation (rarely if ever used)	• Paradoxical tasks • Metaphorical tasks
Type of therapeutic relationship	• Therapist has influence; well accepted as expert	• Therapist less well accepted as expert
Type of problem	• Client able to feel control over small behaviors requested as part of task	• Client feels he or she has very little control

Straightforward Directives

Haley maintained that "the best task is one that uses the presenting problem to make a structural change in the family" (1987, p. 85). Designing straightforward directives involves several steps:

1. Assess the situation: The therapist identifies the interaction sequence of behaviors that constitute the presenting problem; for example, the child comes home after curfew, the father angrily enforces a harsh punishment, and the mother defends the child to the husband and does not enforce the punishment.
2. Target a small sequence change: The therapist finds one small behavioral change in the sequence that the family can reasonably make that would alter the problem sequence; for example, have the mother enforce the curfew, or have the daughter propose a "fair" punishment for breaking curfew.
3. Motivate the family: Haley (1987) emphasizes the importance of motivating the family *before* the task is issued. For straightforward tasks this is usually done by appealing to the shared goal: begin by first talking about how everyone wants the problem behavior to stop: "Everyone agrees that they want the arguing at home to stop."
4. Give precise, doable instructions for the directive: When describing the task, the therapist needs to be extremely precise—when, where, how, who, on which day of the week—while accounting for weekend changes in schedules, weekday homemaking tasks, and special events during the week that the task is assigned. Tasks should be clearly *given* rather than suggested: "Next week, when Susan comes in late from curfew or breaks any other house rule, mom, I want you to enforce the consequences, and dad, you are not to be part of the discussion with Susan and your wife. If you need to discuss what happened, you will discuss it with your wife alone."

5. Review the task: The therapist asks the family members to repeat their parts: "Just to review and make sure we all understand, can each of you tell me what you are going to do this week?"

6. Request a task report: The following week, the therapist asks the family how it went. Generally, one of three things happens: (a) they did it, (b) they didn't do it, or (c) they partially did it (Haley, 1987). If clients completed the task, they are congratulated. If they partially did the task, the therapist does not excuse them too quickly because that would send a message that undermines the therapist's authority. If they failed to attempt the task, Haley uses two responses, one nice and one not so nice. In the nice response, the therapist says, "I must have misunderstood you or your situation to ask that of you—otherwise you would have done it" (1987, p. 71). In the not-so-nice approach, the therapist emphasizes that the family has missed an opportunity to make changes for their own good and that this is a failure and a loss for them (not that they disappointed the therapist); the therapist does not ask them to redo the task even if they say they want to. Instead, the therapist uses this experience to increase motivation for the next task.

Indirect Directives: Paradoxical Interventions (MRI, Milan, and Strategic Therapies)

Perhaps the most misunderstood of strategic and systemic interventions, *paradoxical intervention,* also called *symptom prescription,* involves instructing clients to engage in the problem behavior in some fashion, such as by assigning a couple to argue from 7:00 to 7:15 on Tuesday and Thursday. Symptom prescription and other paradoxical interventions are "paradoxical" because they do not follow linear logic—at least at first blush. You will know when it is time to use one of these because when it is appropriate to use paradox it will not seem paradoxical—at least in the mind of the therapist—it will be the only logical, obvious action to take. Paradox makes sense with two general types of problems: (a) when making any other therapeutic changes disrupts the family's current level of stability or (b) when the problem seems "uncontrollable" from the client's perspective: I can't keep myself from worrying, nagging, eating, fighting, etc.

Paradox with Families That Avoid Change

When family members stabilize around one member being the problem, they are often resistant to the therapist's attempts to change that perception because it may create more discomfort than they are currently experiencing; in these situations paradox can be useful (Haley, 1987). The therapist may restrain or caution against certain changes: "Perhaps you need to argue to keep your passion strong; if you stopped, things might get worse." Or the therapist might choose to paradoxically encourage relapse to prevent it (Haley, 1976). Paradoxical tasks are difficult to deliver because the therapist must communicate several messages at once:

- I want to help you resolve your problem.
- I am sincerely concerned about you.
- I think you can be normal, but perhaps you cannot be.

When paradox is successful, change is usually spontaneous.

Paradox with Uncontrollable Symptoms

If clients have symptoms that they claim they absolutely cannot control, it makes sense to use *symptom prescription* as an intervention. Symptom prescription changes the *context* of the problem behavior. If the context changes, the *meaning* of the behavior must change. When the meaning changes, thoughts, feelings, and subsequent behaviors automatically change also. A common example is using paradox for worrying, which is particularly difficult to treat because it is a cognitive and emotional process that often has few associated behaviors. When clients are given the directive to set an egg timer and worry for 10 minutes at a particular time in the day, worrying radically changes from a vague, free-floating experience to a consciously chosen activity that they can voluntarily start and, most often they quickly discover, can also stop at will. When the context is changed, the meaning and experience of worrying change, often creating significant movement on a symptom that seemed totally out of the client's control.

Indirect Directives: Metaphorical Tasks (Strategic Therapy)

Inspired by Milton Erickson's trance work and therapeutic style, the metaphoric task is used when it is not appropriate to explicitly address a problem (Haley, 1987). Haley believes that metaphors need to be acted on, not just talked about, to create change. Metaphoric tasks involve four stages:

1. The therapist identifies an area of the client's life with dynamics similar to those of an area the therapist wants to change (e.g., discussing adopting a pet with a child who has been adopted).
2. The therapist uses a story or conversation to discuss how adoption works (e.g., what happens when the dog gets sick).
3. The therapist takes a position about how things should change in the metaphoric area (e.g., child is ready to adopt first pet).
4. A task is usually assigned in the metaphoric area (e.g., child's parents are encouraged to help him adopt a pet).

Pretend Techniques (Strategic Therapy)

"Fake it 'til you make it" sums up the spirit of **pretend techniques**, used principally by strategic therapists. In these techniques, clients are asked to "pretend" they have achieved their goal for a designated period of time (from minutes to days) to help make their desired changes. When they fake a behavior, even for a short period of time, often there is a genuine change in perspective, feeling, or behaviors. For example, when a couple is asked to fake being in love for an evening, they often feel those genuine feelings return. Systemically, this technique works by triggering old, preferred interaction patterns that are already there or, if this is an entirely new behavior, by creating new interaction sequences that are now available within the system. In either case, brief periods of pretending introduce new interactional sequences, creating new options for behavioral, emotional, and cognitive change.

Ordeals (Strategic Therapy)

Inspired by the work of Milton Erickson, **ordeals** are often used in strategic therapy when the client feels helpless in controlling a symptom such as overeating, smoking, nail biting, and drinking. They are based on a simple premise: "If one makes it more difficult for a person to have a symptom than to give it up, the person will give up the symptom" (Haley, 1984, p. 5). Rather than try to develop linear, logical means for stopping the behavior (that would be a cognitive–behavioral approach), the strategic therapist allows the symptom with a twist: the client must complete another task, an "ordeal," before or after the symptom.

The ordeal need not be directly related to the undesired activity, but it often has a metaphoric relation to it. For example, if a person is trying to reduce his/her "emotional eating" to soothe difficult emotions, the ordeal would target the behavior and internal tension in either a linear or logical way (e.g., engage in a favorite hobby, write in a journal) or in an indirect or nonlogical way (e.g., perform a random act of kindness for a stranger or loved one, clean the house). In most cases, ordeal therapy is less about creating a horrific, unappealing ordeal to stop undesired behavior and more about shaking up or perturbing the systemic pattern so that new behavioral sequences can evolve. To return to the family dance metaphor, the ordeal isn't a behavioral deterrent or punishment as much as a new piece of furniture in the middle of the dance floor that forces the system to make changes to navigate around it. As the system adjusts to this rather small and innocuous twist, it must change to create new steps and is able to do so with less fear and resistance than if it were told to stop dancing its favorite (or at least best-rehearsed) dance.

Constructive Transforming Interpersonal Patterns (TIPs)

Constructive transforming interpersonal patterns (TIPs) involve therapists and clients actively working together to identify and enact healing interpersonal patterns (HIPs) and wellness interpersonal patterns (WIPs; Gaete et al., 2014). Therapists can identify what might constitute healing or wellness patterns in at least two ways: (a) by listening carefully to what clients say spontaneously, and (b) by directly asking for their clients' thoughts. For example, if when discussing the PIP, a client naturally offers a description of how he would prefer to interact ("I wish I could be more emotionally attuned to her"), the therapist can start with this description and follow up with questions about what that might look like to begin identifying what type of interactional pattern would have meaning for the couple.

Internalized-Other Interviewing

Arguably a systemic version of the classic Gestalt empty chair technique, Tomm (1999) developed **internalized-other interviewing** to help clients generate a more relational perspective associated with the presenting problem and help in generating HIPs. As described in Chapter 3, Tomm conceptualizes relationships not just with physical others but also with our internal representations of these others. For many of us, we spend as much relating to the image of our partners, parents, children and friends as we do to the actual people. This internalized-other interview can be helpful in multiple ways, including generating compassion for and understanding of the other's reality, identifying assumptions and inaccuracies that may be fueling the PIP, and inspiring greater relational responsibility. The therapist begins by asking clients about their willingness to participate in the interview and then speaking to the client literally *as if* the client is the other (e.g., using his/her name, second person "you"). The therapist also emphasizes that the client is speaking from his/her internalized other rather than trying to pretend to be the other person; this is particularly important if the other person is in the room. The questions asked during internalized-other interviewing are designed to help the client explore the interactional patterns in greater depth. For example, clients may ask the internalized other, "When your partner (the client who is speaking) shuts down and will not continue the conversation, what is that like for you? Which part of this did you share with your partner? What didn't you share? Why?" Through this process, clients begin to develop new perspectives that help move toward WIPs and HIPs. Tomm cautions that this approach can make clients feel very vulnerable, and therapists should be compassionate and gentle during the process (Tomm, 1999; Tomm, Hoyt, & Madigan, 1998). He also notes that this process can be challenging if the client misunderstands and tries to be the literal other or if the client gives the answers he/she wishes the other person would say.

Burnham (2000) recommends the following steps to this interview process:

Internalized-Other Interviewing

1. Choose the person, problem, or emotion to be explored.
2. Introduce internalized-other interviewing and describe how it could be helpful to the client's specific situation.
3. Begin by "grounding" the person being interviewed in the identity of the other by using the other's name and asking nonthreatening questions about daily life, job, etc.
4. Move on to ask questions about how the internalized other experiences the problem situation, including how he/she experiences the client speaking in these interactions.

This process can be used in multiple ways, including interviewing:

- Multiple internalized others within one person
- The same internalized other in several people
- The internalized other of the other
- A problem, belief, emotion, or diagnosis as an internalized other

Scope It Out: Cross-Theoretical Comparison

Using Tomm's IPscope described in Chapter 3 (Tomm et al., 2014), this theory approaches the conceptualization of systemic, interpersonal patterns as discussed below.

Case Conceptualization

The quintessential systemic approach, classic systemic–strategic therapists conceptualize their work by focusing almost exclusively on pathologizing interpersonal patterns (PIPs). Systemic–strategic therapists begin tracking the PIP by mapping the behavioral sequence that constitutes the pattern, following the interactions from the beginning of symptoms (positive feedback) back to homeostasis, carefully tracking each person's role in the system. Then they step back and identify the more basic complementary pattern, which they can do by identifying "more of the same solutions," strategic conceptualization of power and love, the tyranny of linguistics, or another method for systemically conceptualizing the fundamental dynamic. Obviously, therapists using Tomm's IPscope approach conceptualize treatment using all possible IPs.

Goal Setting

Systemic–strategic therapists do not use a theory of health to guide their work. Instead, they trust that in response to their interventions or "perturbing" of the system, the system will create WIPs that are most appropriate and work best for them. Essentially, their goal is for the client or family to no longer have PIPs, and virtually any WIP that allows for all members to be symptom-free is an acceptable goal. For therapists working primarily from Tomm's IPscope, their focus is typically on identifying potential HIPs, which are targeted during the working phase of therapy and then finally they set their goals on stabilizing WIPs for the closing phase.

Facilitating Change

Whether action-based or language-based, virtually all interventions or transformative interpersonal patterns (TIPs) used by traditional systemic—strategic therapists have a single intention: interrupt the PIP. The fundament TIP between therapist and client could be described as shown here:

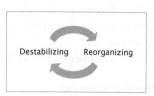

All interventions are intended to destabilize the PIP in some way, either by introducing new interpretations (e.g., a reframe) or new behaviors (e.g., directives). These destabilizing TIPs require the client/family to respond to something new, thereby organizing their interpretations or behavior in a new way. This process continues until WIPs are stabilized and PIPs are no longer enacted. Therapists using Tomm's IPscope facilitate change by using deconstructive (e.g., challenging client constructions of the problem, etc.) and constructive (e.g., identifying new action) TIPs to help clients enact HIPs and WIPs.

Putting It All Together: Systemic–Strategic Case Conceptualization and Treatment Plan Templates

Areas for Theory-Specific Case Conceptualization: Systemic–Strategic

When conceptualizing client cases, contemporary systemic–strategic therapists typically use the following dynamics to inform their treatment plan. You can download a digital version of the theory-specific case conceptualization on MindTap or at www.masteringcompetencies.com.

Pathologizing Interpersonal Pattern

Describe dynamic of primary PIP (**PIPs; A ⇆ B**):

☐ Pursuing/Distancing ☐ Criticizing/Defending ☐ Controlling/Resisting ☐ Other:___
Describe Start of Tension: _____
Describe Conflict/Symptom Escalation: _____
Describe Return to "Normal"/Homeostasis: _____

What is the metacommunication (how is each attempting to define the relationship) in this interaction? _____

Family Life Cycle

Identify client's phase of family life cycle; include all that apply:

- Single adult
- Committed couple
- Family with young children
- Family with adolescent children
- Divorce
- Blended family
- Launching children
- Later life

Describe struggles with mastering developmental tasks in one or more of the following stages.

Attempted Solutions

List attempted solutions that DIDN'T work:

Complementary Roles

Complementary patterns between _____ and _____:

- Pursuer/distancer
- Overfunctioner/underfunctioner
- Emotional/logical
- Good/bad parent

Hypothesis: Role of Symptom in System

Hypothesize the homeostatic function of presenting problem. How might the symptom serve to maintain connection, create independence/distance, establish influence, reestablish connection, or otherwise help create a sense of balance in the family?

Sociocultural Patterns

Describe how sociocultural factors and issues of power and marginalization inform the problem interaction cycle (e.g., cultural, gender, immigration status, economic class, sexual/gender orientation, religion, ability).

TREATMENT PLAN TEMPLATE FOR INDIVIDUAL WITH DEPRESSION/ANXIETY: SYSTEMIC–STRATEGIC

You can download a blank treatment plan (with or without measures) at www.Cengage .com/MindTap (MindTap account required) or www.masteringcompetencies.com. The following treatment plan template can be used to help you develop individualized treatments for use with individuals with depressive or anxiety symptoms.

Systemic–Strategic Treatment Plan: Client Goals with Interventions

Early-Phase Client Goal

1. Increase possibilities for reframing and systemically viewing the problem to reduce depressed mood/anxiety.
   a. Reframe problem in relational context to shift meaning of symptoms.
   b. Circular questions to enable client to see systemic interaction cycle and client's role in it.

Working-Phase Client Goals

1. Reduce client's sense of seeming helplessness related to [presenting symptoms] to reduce depression and anxiety.
   a. Paradoxical tasks that exaggerate helplessness and reveal hidden benefits.
   b. Deliver hypothesis to client that reframes symptoms from a systemic perspective, highlighting how each person's behavior is contextualized by other's.

2. Reduce and disrupt frequency of pathologizing interpersonal and intrapersonal patterns to reduce depression and anxiety.
   a. Circular questions to identify differences, see behavioral sequences, and consider hypothetical situations to shift meaning associated with problem behaviors and how they fit into relational patterns.
   b. Paradoxical behavioral prescriptions that require client to enact particular depression symptoms at specific times to interrupt problem behavior sequence.

3. Increase frequency of wellness interpersonal and intrapersonal patterns to reduce depression and anxiety.
   a. Directives that instruct client to make a small but meaningful alternation to symptom pattern.
   b. Behavioral prescription that represents a 180-degree shift to attempted solutions.

Closing-Phase Client Goals

1. Increase effectiveness of relational interaction patterns with partner/family to reduce potential for relapse of depression and anxiety.
   a. Rituals that reinforce new patterns
   b. Behavioral prescription to have client slightly but meaningfully alter his/her half of problem interactions with others.

Treatment Tasks

1. Develop working therapeutic relationship using theory of choice.
   a. **Respect and trust the system** while **adapting client language** and maintaining therapeutic **maneuverability**.

2. Assess individual, relational, community, and broader cultural dynamics using theory of choice.

a. Assess the interactional sequence(s) related to the problem, including rise of tension, symptom, return to homeostasis, metacommunication, and complementary patterns; identify stage of family life cycle.

b. Conceptualize problem using one or more systemic–strategic frames, such as more-of-the-same solutions, voluntariness, helplessness, hierarchy, love, etc.

3. Identify needed referrals, crisis issues, collateral contacts, and other client needs.

a. *Crisis assessment intervention(s):* Address crisis issues such as self-harm, suicidal ideation, substance use, risky sexual behavior, etc.

b. *Referral(s):* Connect client with **resources** in client's **community** that could be supportive; make collateral contacts as needed.

TREATMENT PLAN TEMPLATE FOR COUPLE/FAMILY CONFLICT: SYSTEMIC–STRATEGIC

You can download a blank treatment plan (with or without measures) at www .cengagebrain.com or www.masteringcompetencies.com. The following treatment plan template can be used to help you develop individualized treatments for use with couples and families who report relational distress.

Systemic–Strategic Treatment Plan: Client Goals with Interventions

Early-Phase Client Goal

1. Increase possibilities for systematically viewing relational conflict and each person's role in it to reduce conflict.

   Interventions:

   a. Strategic reframing that recharacterizes each person's role in the interaction as having an ultimate, underlying motivation of love.

   b. Circular questions to enable clients to see systemic interaction cycle and each person's role in it.

Working-Phase Client Goals

1. Reduce frequency of and disrupt pathologizing interpersonal patterns to reduce conflict.

   Interventions:

   a. Circular questions to identify differences, see behavioral sequences, and consider hypothetical situations to shift meaning associated with problem behaviors and how they fit into relational patterns.

   b. Behavioral prescriptions that interrupt conflict by altering the where, when, how, and who of the conflict.

2. Increase frequency of wellness interpersonal patterns that enable couple/family to [identify specific problem: such as solve problems effectively] to reduce sense of emotional isolation.

   Interventions:

   a. Directives that instruct client to make a small but meaningful alternation to symptom pattern.

   b. Ordeal therapy that alters sequence of behaviors related to couple/family conflict.

3. Increase frequency of wellness interpersonal patterns that enable couple/family to [identify specific problem: such as experience intimacy] to reduce sense of emotional isolation.

   Interventions:

   a. Directives that instruct client to make a small but meaningful alternation to symptom pattern.

b. Metaphorical tasks that make overt the covert power associated with being symptomatic.

Closing-Phase Client Goals

1. Increase ability to see how **love** motivates own and other's behaviors in the relationship to increase sense of wellbeing and connection.
   a. **Reframe problem interactions** focusing on how love motivates interactions, even problem interactions.
   b. **Directives/metaphorical tasks** designed to highlight the hidden motivation of love.

2. Increase ability to [complete developmental tasks] for **family life stage** to reduce chance of relapse.
   a. **Directives** designed to rebalance independence and interdependence based on stage of family life.
   b. **Pretend techniques** to help master new developmental challenges.

Treatment Task

1. Develop working therapeutic relationship using theory of choice.
   a. **Respect and trust the system** while **adapting client language** and maintaining therapeutic **maneuverability**.

2. Assess individual, relational, community, and broader cultural dynamics using theory of choice.
   a. Assess the interactional sequence(s) related to the problem, including rise of tension, symptom, return to homeostasis, metacommunication, and complementary patterns; identify stage of family life cycle.
   b. Conceptualize problem using one or more systemic–strategic frames, such as more-of-the-same solutions, voluntariness, helplessness, hierarchy, love, etc.

3. Identify needed referrals, crisis issues, collateral contacts, and other client needs.
   a. *Crisis assessment intervention(s):* Address crisis issues such as psychological abuse, intimate partner violence, hidden affair, self-harm, suicidal ideation, substance use, etc.
   b. *Referral(s):* Connect client with **resources** in client's **family and community** that could be supportive; make collateral contacts as needed.

Tapestry Weaving: Diversity Considerations

Ethnic, Racial, and Cultural Diversity

Because systemic and strategic family therapies do not rely on a theory-based definition of health and normalcy, they adapt relatively easily to different cultural groups and subpopulations: "Since in strategic family therapy a specific therapeutic plan is designed for each problem, there are no contraindications in terms of patient selection and suitability" (Madanes, 1991, p. 396). Furthermore, drawing on systemic and constructivist foundations, these therapies aim to work from *within* the client's worldview; when this is successfully achieved, the therapist adapts the language and interventions to the client's values and beliefs.

Of particular interest, two groups of systemic therapists have systematically adapted and used the approach with Latino/Hispanic clients. The Latino Brief Therapy Center at the MRI uses the nonnormative and nonpathologizing principles of the model to guide its work, creating unique meaning and interventions with each client, rather than rely on cultural stereotypes of the extremely diverse Latino community (Anger-Díaz, Schlanger, Rincon, & Mendoza, 2004). Similarly, Brief Strategic Family Therapy, an evidence-based approach that uses elements of systemic and structural family therapies (see Chapter 5 for a detailed description), was developed specifically to treat Hispanic youth with high-risk behaviors and substance use issues; the approach has also been found to be effective with African American youth (Robbins, Horigian, Szapocznik, & Ucha, 2010; Santisteban et al., 1997).

In addition to these specific treatment approaches, McGoldrick, Giordano, and Garcia-Preto (2005) provide descriptions of how systemic ideas and approaches can be modified to meet the needs families from 46 different ethnicities, an invaluable resource when working with cultural groups other than one's own (and perhaps your own; read and see). Although these descriptions must be general and do not capture the unique lived experience of a particular client who may be in front of you at a given moment, they can give the therapist a clue about how best to understand and engage the client (and most clients appreciate you having at least a clue about their background as well as giving them room to share their own unique experience and beliefs). The case study at the end of this chapter illustrates how a systemic approach can be used with a second-generation Catholic Mexican American family whose teenage daughter has begun smoking pot and drinking.

Sexual and Gender Identity Diversity

Because of its nonpathologizing and nonnormative assumptions and its attention to larger systemic dynamics, systemic therapies have been widely used with clients who identify as lesbian, gay, bisexual, transgendered, or questioning (LGBTQ). Butler (2009) identifies five principles for adapting systemic therapy approaches for these clients.

1. *Understanding heterosexism:* Therapists need to be aware that gender and sexual minorities have *daily* experiences of being marginalized, judged, and ignored and rarely see their reality reflected in advertisements, movies, and other social forums.
2. *Therapist self-reflectivity:* Heterosexual therapists need to engage in personal self-reflection of their experience of being privileged and having their sexual and gender orientations generally approved by society.
3. *Locating your position, transparency, and self-disclosure:* Based on the work of feminist therapists, Butler recommends disclosing one's gender and sexual orientation when working with LGBTQ clients. Such openness allows for frank discussions about areas of similarity and differences, helping to address issue of power and hierarchy. However, too much self-disclosure can be nonproductive.
4. *Client as expert, and therapist as curious.* Drawing upon collaborative therapy principles (see Chapter 10), therapists should assume a curious stance, viewing clients as the experts in their lives and lifestyles.
5. *Connecting to wider systems:* Finally, therapists should consider the larger social systems of which their LGBTQ clients are a part and encourage them to seek positive, supportive communities.

Butler (2009) also discusses how therapists need to adjust their approach with LGBTQ couples. First, therapists should be aware that sex, gender roles, monogamy, family of origin, family of choice, and expartners generally have very different meanings with these couples. Furthermore, gender roles are thought to have more impact than sexual orientation per se in these relationships, with internalized gender roles often greatly restricting same-sex relationships and being a particular issue in couples with a transgendered partner. Therapists can help couples to deconstruct their gender-role expectations and assumptions in ways that strengthen the partnership. Finally, therapists should keep in mind that the family life cycle looks different for most LGBTQ individuals, couples, and families (Golden, 2009).

Adolescents Coming Out to Family

Another common issue that family therapists address is adolescents coming out to their families (Butler, 2009). First and foremost, therapists should be aware that gay, lesbian, bisexual, and transgendered youth have higher rates of suicidality, substance abuse, self-harm, depression, anxiety, and school issues, so it is important to monitor the adolescent's safety and address these issues. Before coming out, most adolescents are generally able to accurately predict their parents' responses based on casual comments about sexuality over the years. Therapists can use DeVine's (1984) stage theory for the family's process of coming out to help families negotiate this transition.

- *Subliminal awareness:* The child's sexuality is suspected and sometimes provoked by inquiries about dating and same-sex friendships.
- *Impact:* The child announces his/her sexuality and suspicions are confirmed.
- *Adjustment:* The family struggles to maintain its old homeostasis, while the child is expected to hide or deny his/her sexuality.
- *Resolution:* The family comes to accept the child's sexuality identity.
- *Integration:* The family shifts their values related to gender and sexual norms.

Many parents whose child comes out report a "loss" of their dreams of having a wedding or grandchildren, and much of their initial response may actually reflect the personal losses they are projecting. Therapists can help redirect parents to focus on their child's real needs at this time while also developing a more hopeful view of their future family life.

Transgendered Youth

There is little research or literature to guide therapists when working with transgendered persons, especially youth. However, unlike gay, lesbian, and bisexual youth, transgendered youth often cannot hide their difference, and thus it is more likely to be a point of family discussion, whether the child wants it public or not (Coolhart, Baker, Farmer, Malaney, & Shipman, 2013). The majority of transgendered youth (59%) report negative parental reactions to their gender identity, at least initially, with those who are more gender-nonconforming reporting greater conflict with parents (Grossman, D'Augelli, Howell, & Hubbard, 2005). However, parental acceptance is important for transgendered individuals and is correlated with adult life satisfaction and self-esteem (Erich, Tittsworth, Dykes, & Cabuses, 2008).

Coolhart and colleagues (2013) outline an assessment tool for therapists working with transgendered youth and their family. They recommend working with the family of transgendered youth whenever possible, attending to systemic dynamics. The assessment tool consists of questions that cover the following nine domains:

- *Early awareness and family context:* These questions address the general family structure and history as well as both parents' and youth's early gender experiences. For example: "Please provide additional information about how your family's context in terms of racial, ethnic, and national communities interfaces with beliefs about variant expressions of gender and sexuality" (p. 16).
- *Parents' attunement with youth's affirmed gender:* These questions address how the parents and family have responded to the youth's transgender identity. For example: "When your child disclosed (or you discovered) their transgender identity, what was this experience like for you individually, as a couple, and as a family as a whole?" (p. 17).
- *Current gender expression:* These questions address the youth's current preference for expressing gender. For example: "Have you dressed privately in clothing typically associated with your affirmed gender? When did you first begin to dress in private? How did it feel when you first began to dress in private? Did anyone else know? If so, what was their reaction?" (p. 17).
- *School context:* These questions explore the youth's experience and possible harassment at school related to gender identity. For example: "What is your current gender expression at school? Are you 'out' to any of your friends?" (p. 18).
- *Sexual relationships/development:* These questions are typically asked of the youth in private and address sexual orientation, abuse, and activity. For example: "How do

you identify your sexual orientation? Have you ever experienced or witnessed sexual or physical abuse?" (p. 19).

- *Current intimate relationship(s):* If the youth is involved in a current relationship, the therapist inquires about the relationship and the partner's knowledge of the youth's gender identity and possible interest in transitioning.
- *Physical and mental health:* These questions assess for physical and mental health issues that may need addressing, including the potential for self-harm and substance abuse.
- *Support:* These questions aim to identify sources of support for the family and youth, including family, friends, church, neighbors, support groups, Internet connections, etc.
- *Future plans/expectations:* This last set of questions explores whether the youth has plans for gender transition, hormone therapy, surgery, children, etc.

Research and the Evidence Base

Systemic therapy began as a research project: the Bateson team began by studying communication in families with members diagnosed with schizophrenia. The tradition of observational research has been integrated into required standard training in systemic and strategic models in the form of observation teams. There has not been a lot systematic research on outcomes of specific systemic models—such as strategic, Milan, or MRI—however, there is consistent and growing research on the effectiveness of evidence-based systemic approaches for specific conditions, such as adolescent substance abuse, adolescent conduct issues, depression related to relationship distress, severe mental illness, and couples distress (Sprenkle, 2012). These evidence-based treatments use key theoretical concepts and techniques from systemic family therapies and apply them to a specific population.

Systemic therapies are quickly emerging as a leading force in the realm of evidence-based treatments. Numerous empirically supported treatments incorporate key elements of systemic and strategic therapies, including:

- Multisystemic Family Therapy (Henggeler et al., 1998; see "Clinical Spotlight" in this chapter)
- Brief Strategic Family Therapy (structural ecosystemic therapy, structural ecodevelopmental preventive interventions; see Clinical Spotlight in this chapter; Szapocznik & Williams, 2000)
- Ecosystemic Structural Therapy (see Chapter 5; Lindblad-Goldberg, Dore, & Stern, 1998)
- Multidimensional Family Therapy (Liddle, Dakof, & Diamond, 1991)
- Functional Family Therapy (see Chapter 5)
- Emotionally Focused Couples Therapy (see Chapter 6)

Although each of these approaches is unique, they all incorporate identifying the problem interaction sequence and in some way interrupting or altering it and using one or more systemic or strategic techniques to address the needs of a specific population.

Clinical Spotlight: Multisystemic Therapy

Multisystemic therapy (MST) was developed in the 1970s to treat serious juvenile offenders (Multisystemic Therapy Services, 1998). A family-based treatment model, MST draws from strategic, structural, socioecological, and cognitive–behavioral therapy models. In addition, MST also places significant emphasis on the adolescent's and family's broader social network, removing offenders from problematic social networks, improving school and/or vocational performance, and developing a strong support network for the child and the family (Henggeler, 1998; Henggeler & Borduin, 1990; Multisystemic Therapy Services, 1998).

Goals

The overarching goals of MST include the following:

- Decrease antisocial behavior and other clinical problems
- Improve functioning in family relations
- Improve functioning in school and/or work contexts
- Minimize out-of-home placements, including incarceration, residential treatment, and hospitalization

Case Conceptualization

When conceptualizing treatment, MST therapists consider risks and protective factors in the following domains: individual, family, peer, school, and neighborhood and community (Multisystemic Therapy Services, 1998).

	RISKS	PROTECTIVE FACTORS
Individual	Positive attitude toward antisocial behavior, psychological symptoms, hostility, low intellectual functioning and verbal skills	Intelligence, eldest child, easygoing personality, prosocial values, problem-solving skills
Family	Lack of parental supervision, ineffective or inconsistent discipline, lack of emotional expression, conflict, parental difficulties	Connection to parents and family, supportive family, strong parental relationship
Peer	Association with socially deviant peers, poor relational skills, few prosocial friends	Connections with prosocial friends
School	Poor performance, little interest, little support	Committed to education, goals, acceptable performance
Neighborhood and community	High family mobility, criminal subculture, disorganized	Involvement in religious or social organizations, strong support network

Principles of Intervention

1. Finding the fit: The therapist assesses how the adolescent's problems fit systemically within the broader family, peer, school, and community culture.
2. Focus on positives and strengths: Therapeutic interactions emphasize strengths and potential strengths, in both the individual adolescent and the family.
3. Increasing responsibility: Interventions aim to increase responsible behavior with all family members, promoting parental involvement and helping teens accept responsibility for their choices.
4. Focus on the present, on action, and on clarity: Interventions are action-oriented and present-focused, and they target specific, easily defined problems that are easily tracked and measured, such as achieving a specific grade point average or adhering to a curfew.
5. Targeting sequences: Consistent with its systemic foundation, sequences of behaviors are the target of change; these sequences can be between family members or with peers and the larger social systems.

6. Developmentally appropriate: Interventions are developmentally appropriate for youth, promoting step-by-step advancement of the competencies and skills needed for success as an adult.
7. Continuous effort: Interventions, by design, require daily or weekly effort from the family.
8. Evaluation and accountability: Rather than blame the family if an intervention does not work, MST continually assesses the effectiveness of interventions and adjusts as necessary to ensure success.
9. Generalization: Treatment is designed to help the adolescent and family generalize their skills and abilities to solve problems in other life areas.

Clinical Spotlight: Brief Strategic Family Therapy

Drawing on structural and strategic therapies, Jose Szapocznik and his colleagues at the Center for Family Studies developed brief strategic family therapy (BSFT) to address drug abuse problems with Cuban youth in Miami (Szapocznik & Williams, 2000; Szapocznik, Hervis, & Schwartz, 2003). Expanded and adopted to treat African Americans and other Hispanic populations, this therapy is recognized as an evidence-based approach; a complete manual is available through the National Institute for Drug Abuse website (Santisteban et al., 1997; Szapocznik et al., 2003). BSFT is based on three central concepts: *systems, structure* (patterns of interaction), and *strategy*.

Goals

Brief strategic family therapy has two goals:

- Reduce or eliminate child drug use
- Change family interactions that are supporting the problem behaviors (youth drug use)

Case Conceptualization

In comparison with other evidence-based approaches, BSFT focuses primarily *within* family dynamics, using structural and strategic family therapy concepts (Santisteban, Suarez-Morales, Robbins, & Szapocznik, 2006; Szapocznik et al., 2003):

- Structure and organization: The therapist uses traditional structural concepts, such as subsystems, hierarchy, leadership, and coalitions, to assess the structure, organization, and flow of information in the family.
- Resonance: Using the structural therapy concepts of boundaries, the therapist assesses emotional resonance within the broader context of cultural norms: enmeshed (high resonance) and disengaged (low resonance).
- Developmental stage: The therapist uses the family's ability to adapt its structure to support members in their current life stage of development (e.g., increasing autonomy as children grow).
- Life context: The therapist assesses the effects of the family's broader social life, such as extended family, community, school, peers, and courts.
- Identified patienthood: The more the family believes the identified patient is to blame for all its problems, the more difficult it is to treat the family.
- Conflict resolution: The therapist assesses the family's style of conflict resolution:
  - Denial: Conflict is not allowed to emerge: "We have no problems."
  - Avoidance: When conflict arises, it is quickly stopped or covered up, such as by procrastinating, minimizing, or postponing difficult conversations.
  - Diffusion: When the problem is brought up, the subject is switched to another problem topic, often as a personal attack against the person who raised the issue.

- Conflict emergence without resolution: Conflict occurs but no resolution is reached.
- Conflict emergence with resolution: The family is able to resolve the conflict.

Principles of Intervention

Interventions are deliberately chosen to target the aspects of family interactions that are most likely to achieve the desired outcome.

- *Joining:* The therapist uses structural family therapy, joining, to connect with the family system.
- *Enactments:* Structural enactments are used to assess family functioning and restructure family interactions.
- *Working in the present:* Interventions target current interactions with minimal focus on the past.
- *Reframing negativity:* Therapists reframe negative interpretations to promote caring and concern within the family.
- *Reversals:* Therapists may coach one or more family members to do or say the *opposite* of what is typically done or said.
- *Working with boundaries and alliances:* Standard structural techniques are used to either loosen or strengthen boundaries to better meet developmental needs.
- *Detriangulation:* The therapist may remove a third, less powerful person from a conflict between two others.
- *Opening closed systems:* Systems in which open conflict is not allowed must be "opened" to allow effective expression and resolution of differences.

QUESTIONS FOR PERSONAL REFLECTION AND CLASS DISCUSSION

1. Identify a personal characteristic of yours that has a strong systemic component (i.e., you are this way more in one relationship than another or has been exaggerated over the years due complementarity with a partner).
   - Does this characteristic feel like it is an inherent characteristic of "you" or does it feel "situational"?
   - Can you identify a characteristic of another person that seems "inherently in the individual" but may have more of a systemic basis to it?
   - Would you agree that to some extent all behavior is shaped by broader systemic and social dynamics? Why or why not?
2. What would "joining the system" look like in your family of origin?
3. Are you ready to "trust the system" to reorganize itself in a way that is best for itself? Why or why not?
4. Where are you currently in the family life cycle? How are approaching the tasks of balancing independence and interdependence?
5. Trace a problem interaction cycle in your life from "normal" through the rise in tension and symptom and back to "normal" again.
6. How do cultural communities function as a system in a person's life?
7. How do culture and gender play out in your family system?
8. How might the experience of being marginalized due to same-sex orientation affect a person's boundaries with:
   - A partner?
   - A supportive family of origin?
   - A nonsupportive family of origin?
   - Supportive friends?

ONLINE RESOURCES

Brief Strategic and Systemic World Network

www.bsst.org

Mental Research Institute

www.mri.org

Multisystemic Therapy

www.mstservices.com

Strategic Therapy: Jay Haley

www.jay-haley-on-therapy.com/html /strategic_therapy.html

Strategic Therapy: Cloe Madanes

www.cloemadanes.com

Strategic Therapy: Eileen Bobrow

www.briefstrategicfamilytherapy.com

Systemic Therapy: Wendel Ray

www.wendelray.com

Go to MindTap® for an eBook, videos of client sessions, activities, digital forms, practice quizzes, apps, and more—all in one place. If your instructor didn't assign MindTap, you can find out more information at CengageBrain.com.

REFERENCES

*Asterisks indicate recommended introductory readings.

Anger-Díaz, B., Schlanger, K., Rincon, C., & Mendoza, A. B. (2004). Problem-solving across cultures: Our Latino experience. *Journal of Systemic Therapies*, *23*(4), 11–27. doi:10.1521/jsyt.23.4.11.57837

*Bateson, G. (1972). *Steps to an ecology of mind*. San Francisco, CA: Chandler.

Bateson, G. (1979). *Mind and nature: A necessary unity*. New York: Dutton.

*Boscolo, L., Cecchin, G., Hoffman, L., & Penn, P. (1987). *Milan systemic family therapy*. New York: Basic Books.

Burnham, J. (2000). Internalized-other interviewing: Evaluating and enhancing empathy. *Clinical Psychology Forum*, *140*, 16–20.

Butler, C. (2009). Sexual and gender minority therapy and systemic practice. *Journal of Family Therapy*, *31*(4), 338–358. doi:10.1111/j.1467-6427.2009.00472.x

Campbell, D., Draper, R., & Crutchley, E. (1991). The Milan systemic approach to family therapy. In A. S. Gurman & D. P. Knishern (Eds.), *Handbook of family therapy* (pp. 325–362). New York: Brunner/Mazel.

*Cecchin, G. (1987). Hypothesizing, circularity, and neutrality revisited: An invitation to curiosity. *Family Process*, *26*(4), 405–413.

Cecchin, G., Lane, G., & Ray, W. (1992). *Irreverence: A strategy for therapist survival*. London: Karnac Books.

Collins, D., & Tomm, K. (2009). Karl Tomm: His changing views on family therapy over 35 years. *Family Journal*, *17*(2), 106–117.

Coolhart, D., Baker, A., Farmer, S., Malaney, M., & Shipman, D. (2013). Therapy with transsexual youth and their families: A clinical tool for assessing youth's readiness for gender transition. *Journal of Marital And Family Therapy*, *39*(2), 223–243. doi:10.1111/j.1752-0606.2011.00283.x

DeVine, J. L. (1984). A systemic inspection of affectional preference orientation and the family of origin. *Journal of Social Work and Human Sexuality*, *2*, 9–17.

Erich, S., Tittsworth, J., Dykes, J., & Cabuses, C. (2008). Family relationships and their correlations with transsexual well-being. *Journal of GLBT Family Studies*, *4*(4), 419–432. doi:10.1080/15504280802126141

Fisch, R., & Schlanger, K. (1999). *Brief therapy with intimidating clients*. New York: Jossey-Bass.

*Fisch, R., Weakland, J., & Segal, L. (1982). *The tactics of change: Doing therapy briefly*. New York: Jossey-Bass.

Gaete, J., Sametband, I., & Sutherland, O. (2014). Can I give you a TIP? Inviting healing conversations in practice. In K. Tomm, S. St. George, D. Wulff, & T. Strong (Eds.), *Patterns in interpersonal interactions: Inviting relational understandings for therapeutic change* (pp. 103–123). New York: Routledge.

Goldberg, A. E. (2009). Lesbian, gay, and bisexual family psychology: A systemic, life-cycle perspective. In J. H. Bray, & M. Stanton (Eds.), The Wiley-Blackwell handbook of family psychology (pp. 576–587). Wiley-Blackwell. doi:10.1002/9781444310238.ch40

Grossman, A. H., D'Augelli, A. R., Howell, T. J., & Hubbard, S. (2005). Parents' reactions to transgender youths' gender nonconforming expression and identity. *Journal of Gay and Lesbian Social Services, 18*(1), 3–16.

Haley, J. (1963). *Strategies of psychotherapy.* New York: Grune and Stratton.

Haley, J. (1973). *Uncommon therapy: The psychiatric techniques of Milton H. Erickson, M.D.* New York: Norton.

Haley, J. (1976). *Problem-solving therapy: New strategies for effective family therapy.* San Francisco, CA: Jossey-Bass.

Haley, J. (1980). *Leaving home: The therapy of disturbed young people.* New York: McGraw-Hill.

Haley, J. (1981). *Reflections on therapy.* Chevy Chase, MD: Family Therapy Institute of Washington, DC.

Haley, J. (1984). *Ordeal therapy.* San Francisco, CA: Jossey-Bass.

*Haley, J. (1987). *Problem-solving therapy* (2nd ed.). San Francisco, CA: Jossey-Bass.

Haley, J. (1996). *Learning and teaching therapy.* New York: Guilford.

Haley, J., & Richeport-Haley, M. (2007). *Directive family therapy.* New York: Hawthorne.

Henggeler, S. W. (1998). *Multisystemic therapy.* Charleston, NC: Targeted Publications Group. Retrieved from www.addictionrecov.org/paradigm/P_PR_W99/mutisys_therapy.html.

Henggeler, S. W., & Borduin, C. M. (1990). *Family therapy and beyond: A multisystemic approach to treating the behavior problems of children and adolescents.* Pacific Grove, CA: Brooks/Cole.

Henggeler, S. W., Schoenwald, S. K., Borduin, C. M., Rowland, M. D., & Cunningham, P. B. (1998). *Multisystemic treatment of antisocial behavior in children and adolescents.* New York: Guilford.

Jackson, D. D. (1967). The myth of normality. *Medical Opinion and Review, 3,* 28–33.

*Keeney, B. (1983). *Aesthetics of change.* New York: Guilford.

Keim, J. (1998). Strategic family therapy. In E. Dattilio (Ed.), *Case studies in couple and family therapy* (pp. 132–157). New York: Guilford.

Liddle, H. A., Dakof, G. A., & Diamond, G. (1991). Adolescent substance abuse: Multidimensional family therapy in action. In E. Daufman & P. Kaufman (Eds.), *Family therapy of drug and alcohol abuse* (pp. 120–171). Boston, MA: Allyn and Bacon.

Lindblad-Goldberg, M., Dore, M., & Stern, L. (1998). *Creating competence from chaos.* New York: Norton.

Madanes, C. (1981). *Strategic family therapy.* San Francisco, CA: Jossey-Bass.

Madanes, C. (1990). *Sex, love, and violence: Strategies for transformation.* New York: Norton.

Madanes, C. (1991). Strategic family therapy. In A. S. Gurman & D. P. Knishern (Eds.), *Handbook of family therapy* (pp. 396–416). New York: Brunner/Mazel.

Madanes, C. (1993). Strategic humanism. *Journal of Systemic Therapies, 12*(4), 69–75.

McGoldrick, M., Giordano, J., & Garcia-Preto, N. (2005). *Ethnicity and family therapy* (3rd ed.). New York: Guilford.

Mental Research Institute. (2002). *On the shoulders of giants.* Palo Alto, CA: Author.

Multisystemic Therapy Services. (1998). *Multisystemic therapy.* Retrieved from www.mstservices.com/text/treatment.html.

*Nardone, G., & Watzlawick, P. (1993). *The art of change: Strategic therapy and hypnotherapy without trance.* San Francisco, CA: Jossey-Bass.

Ray, W. A., & Keeney, B. (1994*). Resource focused therapy.* London: Karnac Books.

Robbins, M. S., Horigian, V., Szapocznik, J., & Ucha, J. (2010). Treating Hispanic youths using brief strategic family therapy. In J. R. Weisz & A. E. Kazdin (Eds.), *Evidence-based psychotherapies for children and adolescents* (2nd ed.) (pp. 375–390). New York : Guilford.

Santisteban, D. A., Coatsworth, J. D., Perez-Vidal, A., Mitrani, V., Jean-Gilles, M., & Szapocznik, J. (1997). Brief structural/strategic family therapy with African American and Hispanic high-risk youth. *Journal of Community Psychology, 25*(5), 453–471. doi:10.1002/(SICI)1520-6629(199709)25:5<453::AID-JCOP6>3.0.CO;2-T

Santisteban, D. A., Suarez-Morales, L., Robbins, M. S., & Szapocznik, J. (2006). Brief Strategic Family Therapy: Lessons learned in efficacy research and challenges to blending research and practice. *Family Process, 45*(2), 259–271. doi: 10.1111/j.1545-5300.2006.00094.x

Segal, L. (1991). Brief therapy: The MRI approach. In A. S. Gurman & D. P. Knishern (Eds.), *Handbook of family therapy* (pp. 171–199). New York: Brunner/Mazel.

Selvini Palazzoli, M. (Ed.). (1988). *The work of Mara Selvini Palazzoli.* New York: Aronson.

*Selvini Palazzoli, M., Boscolo, L., Cecchin, G., & Prata, G. (1980). Hypothesizing-circularity-neutrality: Three guidelines for the conductor of the session. *Family Process, 19*(1), 3–12.

Selvini Palazzoli, M., Cecchin, G., Prata, G., & Boscolo, L. (1978). *Paradox and counterparadox: A new model in the therapy of the family in schizophrenic transaction.* New York: Aronson.

Sprenkle, D. (Ed.). (2012). Intervention research in couple and family therapy [Special edition]. *Journal of Marital and Family Therapy, 38*(1).

Szapocznik, J., & Williams, R. A. (2000). Brief strategic family therapy: Twenty-five years of interplay among theory, research and practice in adolescent behavior problems and drug abuse. *Clinical Child and Family Psychology Review, 3*(2), 117–135.

Szapocznik, J., Hervis, O. E., & Schwartz, S. (2003). *Brief strategic family therapy for adolescent drug abuse* (NIH Publication No. 03-4751). NIDA Therapy Manuals for Drug Addiction. Rockville, MD: National Institute on Drug Abuse.

Tomm, K. (1984). One perspective on the Milan systemic approach: I. Overview of development, theory and practice. *Journal of Marital and Family Therapy, 10*(2), 113–125. doi:10.1111/j.1752-0606.1984.tb00001.x

Tomm, K. (1987a). Interventive interviewing: I. Strategizing as a fourth guideline for the therapist. *Family Process, 26*(1), 3–13. doi:10.1111/j.1545-5300.1987.00003.x

Tomm, K. (1987b). Interventive interviewing: II. Reflexive questioning as a means to enable self-healing. *Family Process, 26*(2), 167–183. doi:10.1111/j.1545-5300.1987.00167.x

Tomm, K. (1988). Interventive interviewing: III. Intending to ask lineal, circular, strategic, or reflexive questions? *Family Process, 27*(1), 1–15. doi:10.1111/j.1545-5300.1988.00001.x

Tomm, K. (1999). Co-constructing responsibility. In S. McNamee & K. J. Gergen, & Associates (Eds.) *Relational Responsibility: Resources for Sustainable Dialogue* (pp. 129–137). Thousand Oaks, CA: Sage.

Tomm, K., Hoyt, M., & Madigan, S. (1998). Honoring our internalized others and the ethics of caring: A conversation with Karl Tomm. In M. Hoyt (Ed.), *The handbook of constructive therapies* (pp. 198–218). Philadelphia, PA: Brunner-Routledge.

Tomm, K., St. George, S., Wulff, D., & Strong, T. (2014). *Patterns in interpersonal interactions: Inviting relational understandings for therapeutic change.* New York: Routledge.

Watzlawick, P. (1977). *How real is real? Confusion, disinformation, communication.* New York: Random House.

Watzlawick, P. (1978/1993). *The language of change: Elements of therapeutic conversation.* New York: Norton.

Watzlawick, P. (Ed.). (1984). *The invented reality: How do we know what we believe we know?* New York: Norton.

Watzlawick, P. (1988). *Ultra solutions: How to fail most successfully.* New York: Norton.

Watzlawick, P. (1990). *Munchhausen's pigtail or psychotherapy and "reality" essays and lectures.* New York: Norton.

Watzlawick, P. (1993). *The situation is hopeless but not serious: The pursuit of unhappiness.* New York: Norton.

Watzlawick, P., Bavelas, J. B., & Jackson, D. D. (1967). *Pragmatics of human communication: A study of interactional patterns, pathologies, and paradoxes.* New York: Norton.

Watzlawick, P., & Weakland, J. H. (1977). *The interactional view: Studies at the Mental Research Institute, Palo Alto, 1965–1974.* New York: Norton.

*Watzlawick, P., Weakland, J., & Fisch, R. (1974). *Change: Principles of problem formation and problem resolution.* New York: Norton.

Weakland, J., & Ray, W. (Eds.). (1995). *Propagations: Thirty years of influence from the Mental Research Institute.* Binghamton, NY: Haworth.

Systemic Case Study: Adolescent Substance Use and Divorce

The Fernandez family has brought their daughter, Alba (16), to an outpatient community mental health clinic because she has begun drinking and smoking pot on the weekends with a new group of friends. Up to this point, she had been a good student who was active in numerous school activities. Her parents separated six months ago after Alba's mother Irma discovered that her husband Tom was having an affair. When the affair was discovered, Tom refused to end the relationship. Irma kicked him out, but is torn about following through with the divorce because she comes from a devout Catholic family that disapproves of divorce even under these circumstances. Alba's younger brother, Jesse (14), is an honor student who tries to stay out of the conflict between Alba and the parents.

After meeting with the family, a systemic family therapist developed the following case conceptualization.

STRATEGIC SYSTEMIC CASE CONCEPTUALIZATION

For use with individual, couple, or family clients

Date: 6/19/16   **Clinician:** Maria Sanchez, MFT Trainee   **Client/Case #:** 4001

Introduction to Client & Significant Others

Identify significant persons in client's relational/family life who will be mentioned in case conceptualization:

Adults/Parents: Select identifier/abbreviation for use in rest of case conceptualization

AF1:   Female Age: 36 Hispanic/Latino Married heterosexual Occupation: Department Store Clerk Other: Catholic

AM1:   Male Age: 34 Hispanic/Latino Married heterosexual   Occupation: Insurance Agent Other: Son of Immigrants from Mexico, Catholic

Children/Adult Children: Select identifier/abbreviation for use in rest of case conceptualization

CF1:   Female Age: 16 Hispanic/Latino Grade: 10th School: Green Field Highschool Other identifier: Active in multiple school activities, including music and soccer

CM1:   Male Age: 14 Hispanic/Latino Grade: 8th School: Valley Middle School Other identifier: Honor Student

Others: Identify all: _____

Presenting Concerns

Describe each significant person's description of the problem, focusing on OBSERVABLE behaviors:

AF1:   Couple separated six months ago due to AM34's affair; AF36's family is very disapproving but AF36 refuses to stay together; primary concern is CF16's recent alcohol/drug use.

AM1:   Fell in love with another woman; feels bad about effects on family but is not sure what else to do; primary concern is the children and CF16's drug use.

CF1:   Angry about parent's likely divorce; feels father abandoned family; sees "partying" as normal and thinks she is entitled because of the stress her parents caused her.

CM1:   Sees father as weak for affair and frustrated with mother's anxiety over religious issues. Disappointed in parents but copes by staying focused on school.

Broader System: Description of problem from extended family, referring party, school, legal system, etc.:

Extended Family: AF Family of Origin: Views divorce from religious perspective and believes couples should work things out. AM Family of Origin: Understanding of divorce given the distant marriage that AM34 parents had.

Mrs.Gomez: School Counselor: Concerned that CF16 is starting down dangerous path in reaction to parents' separation.

Name: _____

Background Information

Trauma/Abuse History (recent and past): AF reports one incident of sexual abuse as child (7 yr) by neighbor; AM report that in the early years of his youth, his family was very poor, often not having housing or enough to eat.

Substance Use/Abuse (current and past; self, family of origin, significant others): AM34's father was an alcoholic, as is his brother, which has resulted in numerous distant relationships in his family.

(continued)

Background Information *(continued)*

parents are concerned that CF16 may develop substance abuse issues that run on AM34's side of the family. CF16 regularly partakes in alcohol and pot but has only tried the harder drugs a couple of times. Since the separation, CF16 started hanging out for longer hours with friends, getting connected with a crowd that regularly uses alcohol and pot and has periodic access to heroin and methamphetamines.

Precipitating Events (recent life changes, first symptoms, stressors, etc.): Six months prior, the CF16 and CM14 were both exceling academically and socially, and they report things at home were relatively calm. However, six months ago, AF36 discovered AM34 was having an affair; AM34 refused to end it. AF36 asked him to leave and she stayed in the home with the children. They have filed for divorce but are not actively moving the process along. Both children were very surprised and disappointed in father. Parents bickered frequently but seemed to be committed in the relationship. Since the separation, CM14 has been quieter than usual, focusing on his studies. Neither of the children is enthusiastic about seeing their father, often choosing to go with friends or engaging in school activities during their scheduled visits.

Related Historical Background (family history, related issues, previous counseling, medical/mental health history, etc.): The couple had sought marital counseling two years prior for their arguing; things improved for awhile but later returned to about the same level of conflict. AF36 comes from a very religious family, her oldest brother is a Catholic priest and her younger brother is cut off from the family because he is in a same-sex relationship.

Interactional Patterns

Primary Pathologizing Interpersonal Pattern (PIPs; A ⇆ B): *Describe dynamic of primary PIP:*

☐ Pursuing/Distancing   ☐ Criticizing/Defending   ☒ Controlling/Resisting   ☐ Other: _____

Describe Start of Tension: CF 16 gets caught drinking.

Describe Conflict/Symptom Escalation: AF36 begins yelling and lecturing and sets a harsh punishment she does not follow through on. When AM34 hears about what happens the next day, he tries having a long talk with CF16 about her choices, focusing on the detrimental effects on her future and ignoring her emotional reasons for "escaping."

Describe Return to "Normal"/Homeostasis: After a day or two of distance, AF softens and reconnects with CF; within a couple of weeks the pattern repeats.

What is the metacommunication in this interaction? *The metacommunication seems to be about power and control: CF16's behavior communicates wanting more independence and separation on one level, while the parents are also trying to assert their power and influence.*

Family Life Cycle

Check all that apply:

☐ Single Adult
☐ Committed Couple
☐ Family with Young Children
☒ Family with Adolescent Children
☒ Divorce
☐ Blended Family
☐ Launching Children
☐ Later Life

Describe struggles with mastering developmental tasks in one or more of these stages: Ever since having children, the couple had difficulty maintaining a strong emotional bond. They are now experiencing the shift to family with adolescents, which is a significant shift toward independence and less interdependence, at the same time they are experiencing divorce, another transition that increases independence and separation. AF36 feels as though she has primary responsibility for raising the children, while AM34 reports feeling disconnected from family life.

Attempted Solutions

Attempted Solutions that DIDN'T work:

1. Parents lecturing CF16 has not reduced her drinking and drug use.
2. AF36 setting harsh but unenforced consequences not working; stalling on moving forward with the divorce may not be as effective as hoped.
3. _____

Complementary Roles

Complementary Patterns between AF36 *and* AM34:

☒ Pursuer/distancer
☐ Overfunctioner/underfunctioner
☐ Emotional/logical
☐ Good/bad parent
☐ Other: _____

Example of pattern: Historically, AF36 pursued AM34 for connection and engagement, similar dynamic during separation.

Hypothesis: Role of Symptom in System

Hypothesized homeostatic function of presenting problem: How might the symptom serve to maintain connection, create independence/distance, establish influence, reestablish connection, or otherwise help create a sense of balance in the family? CF16's acting out serves the purpose of drawing the parents together to manage her; it also distracts all members of the family from the pain of the separation and disapproval (and potential cut off) from AF36's family of origin.

Social Location

Describe how sociocultural factors and issues of power and marginalization inform the problem interaction cycle (e.g., cultural, gender, immigration status, economic class, sexual/gender orientation, religion, ability): AF36's cultural, religious, and family background reinforce the idea that divorce is a sin, which is creating significant internal struggle for her because a part of her believes it is unwise to remain in a relationship with a man who will not leave his mistress. This view seems to increase the stress of the potential divorce for all family members, possibly informing CF16's acting out and CM14's withdrawal. Additionally, the couple seems to have had an imbalanced and stereotypically gendered division of household and parenting tasks, which lead AF to feel overwhelmed by her job and domestic tasks and AM to disconnect from family life. Although AF reports no physical abuse, she did not feel she could influence him significantly, especially to participate equally in domestic chores. AM is currently embracing a more traditional and detached father role, which has only been exacerbated by the affair.

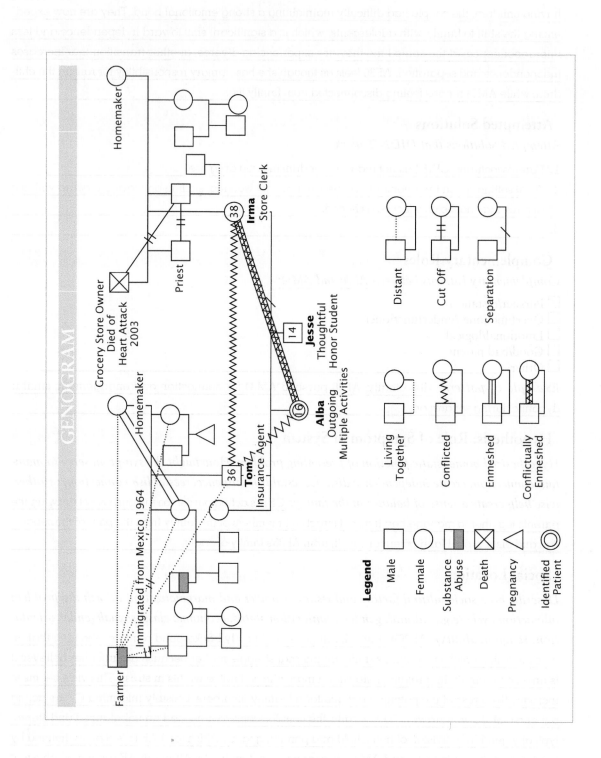

CLINICAL ASSESSMENT

Clinician: Maria Sanchez, MFT Trainee	Client ID #: 4001	Primary configuration: ☐ Individual ☐ Couple ☒ Family	Primary Language: ☒ English ☒ Spanish ☐ Other: _____

List client and significant others

Adult(s)

Adult Female   Age: 36   Hispanic/Latino   Partnered heterosexual   Occupation: Department Store Clerk   Other identifier: Catholic

Adult Male   Age: 34   Hispanic/Latino   Partnered heterosexual   Occupation: Insurance Agent   Other identifier: Child of Immigrant Parents (Mexico)

Child(ren)

Identified Patient: Child Female   Age: 16   Hispanic/Latino   Grade: 10th   School: Typical High School Other identifier: Active in Extracurriculars (soccer, music)

Child Male   Age: 14   Hispanic/Latino   Grade: 8th   School: Typical Middle School   Other identifier: Honor Student

Others: _____

Presenting Problem(s)

		Complete for children:
☐ Depression/hopelessness	☐ Couple concerns	☒ School failure/decline performance
☐ Anxiety/worry	☒ Parent/child conflict	
☒ Anger issues	☐ Partner violence/abuse	☐ Truancy/runaway
☒ Loss/grief	☒ Divorce adjustment	☐ Fighting w/peers
☐ Suicidal thoughts/attempts	☐ Remarriage adjustment	☐ Hyperactivity
☐ Sexual abuse/rape	☐ Sexuality/intimacy concerns	☐ Wetting/soiling clothing
☒ Alcohol/drug use	☒ Major life changes	☐ Child abuse/neglect
☐ Eating problems/disorders	☐ Legal issues/probation	☐ Isolation/withdrawal
☐ Job problems/unemployed	☐ Other: _____	☐ Other: _____

Mental Status Assessment for Identified Patient

Interpersonal	☐ NA	☒ Conflict ☐ Enmeshment ☐ Isolation/avoidance ☐ Harassment ☐ Other: _____
Mood	☐ NA	☐ Depressed/Sad ☐ Anxious ☐ Dysphoric ☒ Angry ☒ Irritable ☐ Manic ☐ Other: _____
Affect	☐ NA	☒ Constricted ☐ Blunt ☐ Flat ☐ Labile ☐ Incongruent ☐ Other: _____
Sleep	☐ NA	☐ Hypersomnia ☐ Insomnia ☒ Disrupted ☒ Nightmares ☐ Other: _____
Eating	☐ NA	☒ Increase ☐ Decrease ☐ Anorectic restriction ☐ Binging ☐ Purging ☐ Other: _____
Anxiety	☒ NA	☐ Chronic worry ☐ Panic ☐ Phobias ☐ Obsessions ☐ Compulsions ☐ Other: _____
Trauma symptoms	☒ NA	☐ Hypervigilance ☐ Flashbacks/intrusive memories ☐ Dissociation ☐ Numbing ☐ Avoidance efforts ☐ Other: _____

(continued)

Mental Status Assessment for Identified Patient (*continued*)

Psychotic symptoms	☒ NA	☐ Hallucinations ☐ Delusions ☐ Paranoia ☐ Loose associations ☐ Other: _____
Motor activity/ speech	☐ NA	☐ Low energy ☐ Hyperactive ☒ Agitated ☐ Inattentive ☐ Impulsive ☐ Pressured speech ☐ Slow speech ☐ Other: _____
Thought	☐ NA	☐ Poor concentration ☐ Denial ☒ Self-blame ☐ Other-blame ☐ Ruminative ☐ Tangential ☐ Concrete ☐ Poor insight ☒ Impaired decision-making ☐ Disoriented ☐ Other: _____
Sociolegal	☐ NA	☐ Disregards rules ☒ Defiant ☐ Stealing ☐ Lying ☐ Tantrums ☐ Arrest/ incarceration ☐ Initiates fights ☐ Other: _____
Other symptoms	☐ NA	_____

Diagnosis for Identified Patient

Contextual Factors considered in making diagnosis: ☒ Age ☒ Gender ☒ Family dynamics ☒ Culture ☒ Language ☒ Religion ☐ Economic ☐ Immigration ☐ Sexual/gender orientation ☐ Trauma ☐ Dual diagnosis/comorbid ☐ Addiction ☐ Cognitive ability ☐ Other: _____

Describe impact of identified factors on diagnosis and assessment process: Used teen-friendly language with CF using gender and ethnic similarity to connect; considered current family dynamics when assessing CF mood and behavior; although Spanish is spoken with extended family, CF identifies English as her primary language and prefers to speak in English in session; the family speaks English together at home. Family's religious beliefs and intergenerational history of addiction also considered as part of assessment.

DSM-5 Level 1 Cross-Cutting Symptom Measure (optional): Elevated scores on: (free at psychiatry.org) ☒ I Depression ☐ II Anger ☐ III Mania ☒ IV Anxiety ☒ V Somatic ☐ VI Suicide ☐ VII Psychosis ☒ VIII Sleep ☐ IX Memory ☐ X Repetitive ☐ XI Dissociation ☐ XII Personality ☒ XIII Substance ☐ Not administered

DSM-5 Code	**Diagnosis with Specifier** *Include Z/T-Codes for Psychosocial Stressors/Issues*
1. F43.23	1. Adjustment Disorder w Disturbance of Mood and Conduct, Acute
2. F10.10	2. R/O Alcohol use disorder
3. F12.10	3. R/O Cannabis use disorder
4. _____	4. _____
5. _____	5. _____

List Specific DSM-5 Criterion Met for Diagnosis

1. Stressor: parents separated; father moved out; father had affair
2. Began drinking and smoking pot on weekends with friends; incidents of drinking/driving or severe intoxication
3. Grades have dropped from 3.5 to 2.75 GPA
4. More arguing and defiance at home
5. Will continue to monitor substance used to rule out misuse disorders

Medical Considerations

Has patient been referred for psychiatric evaluation? ☐ Yes ☒ No
Has patient agreed with referral? ☐ Yes ☐ No ☒ NA
Psychometric instruments used for assessment: ☐ None ☒ Cross-cutting symptom inventories ☐ Other: _____

Client response to diagnosis: ☒ Agree ☐ Somewhat agree ☐ Disagree ☐ Not informed for following reason: _____

Current Medications (psychiatric & medical) ☒ NA

1. _____ ; dose _____ mg; start date: _____
2. _____ ; dose _____ mg; start date: _____
3. _____ ; dose _____ mg; start date: _____
4. _____ ; dose _____ mg; start date: _____

Medical Necessity: *Check all that apply*

☒ Significant impairment ☒ Probability of significant impairment ☒ Probable developmental arrest

Areas of impairment:

☒ Daily activities ☒ Social relationships ☒ Health ☐ Work/school ☒ Living arrangement ☐ Other: _____

Risk and Safety Assessment for Identified Patient

Suicidality	**Homicidality**	**Alcohol Abuse**
☒ No indication/denies	☒ No indication/denies	☐ No indication/denies
☐ Active ideation	☐ Active ideation	☐ Past abuse
☐ Passive ideation	☐ Passive ideation	☒ Current; freq/amt: 2–3 beers/week
☐ Intent without plan	☐ Intent without means	**Drug Use/Abuse**
☐ Intent with means	☐ Intent with means	☐ No indication/denies
☐ Ideation in past year	☐ Ideation in past year	☐ Past use
☐ Attempt in past year	☐ Violence past year	☒ Current drugs: Marijuana
☐ Family or peer history of completed suicide	☐ History of assaulting others	Freq/amt: 1–2/week
	☐ Cruelty to animals	☐ Family/sig. other use

Sexual & Physical Abuse and Other Risk Factors

☐ Childhood abuse history: ☐ Sexual ☐ Physical ☐ Emotional ☐ Neglect
☐ Adult with abuse/assault in adulthood: ☐ Sexual ☐ Physical ☐ Current
☐ History of perpetrating abuse: ☐ Sexual ☐ Physical ☐ Emotional
☐ Elder/dependent adult abuse/neglect
☐ History of or current issues with restrictive eating, binging, and/or purging
☒ Cutting or other self-harm: ☐ Current ☒ Past: Method: 1–2 times 6 mo ago
☐ Criminal/legal history: _____
☐ Other trauma history: _____
☐ None reported

Indicators of Safety

☐ NA
☒ At least one outside support person
☒ Able to cite specific reasons to live or not harm
☐ Hopeful
☒ Willing to dispose of dangerous items
☐ Has future goals

☒ Willingness to reduce contact with people who make situation worse
☐ Willing to implement safety plan, safety interventions
☐ Developing set of alternatives to self/other harm
☒ Sustained period of safety: 6 mo
☐ Other: _____

Elements of Safety Plan

☐ NA
☒ Verbal no harm contract
☐ Written no harm contract
☒ Emergency contact card
☒ Emergency therapist/agency number
☐ Medication management:

☒ Plan for contacting friends/support persons during crisis
☐ Specific plan of where to go during crisis
☒ Specific self-calming tasks to reduce risk before reach crisis level (e.g., journaling, exercising, etc.)
☐ Specific daily/weekly activities to reduce stressors
☐ Other: _____

Legal/Ethical Action Taken: ☒ NA ☐ Action: _____

(continued)

Case Management

Collateral Contacts
- Has contact been made with treating *physicians or other professionals*: ☐ NA ☒ Yes ☐ In process. Name/Notes: _____
- If client is involved in mental health *treatment elsewhere*, has contact been made? ☐ NA ☒ Yes ☐ In process. Name/Notes: Divorce group at school
- Has contact been made with *social worker*: ☒ NA ☐ Yes ☐ In process. Name/Notes: _____

Referrals
- Has client been referred for *medical assessment*: ☒ Yes ☐ No evidence for need
- Has client been referred for social services: ☒ NA ☐ Job/training ☐ Welfare/Food/Housing ☐ Victim services ☐ Legal aid ☐ Medical ☐ Other: _____
- Has client been referred for *group* or other support services: ☒ Yes: Divorce group at school ☐ In process ☐ None recommended
- Are there anticipated *forensic/legal* processes related to treatment: ☐ No ☒ Yes; describe: Custody hearings

---

Support Network
- Client social support network includes: ☐ Supportive family ☐ Supportive partner ☒ Friends ☒ Religious/spiritual organization ☐ Supportive work/social group ☐ Other: _____
- Describe anticipated effects treatment will have on others in support system (Children, partner, etc.): Addressing CF's issues may increase the focus on CM and need for a divorce.
- Is there anything else client will need to be successful? Parents may benefit from individual therapy.

Expected Outcome and Prognosis
☒ Return to normal functioning ☐ Anticipate less than normal functioning ☐ Prevent deterioration

Client Sense of Hope: 5 Moderate hope

Evaluation of Assessment/Client Perspective
How were assessment methods adapted to client needs, including age, culture, and other diversity issues?
Used adolescent-friendly language and humor. Considered Mexican American and Catholic religious beliefs when assessing family's response to divorce.

Describe actual or potential areas of client–clinician agreement/disagreement related to the above assessment:
CF sees her "partying" as normal; parents see it as abuse. As she is still functioning fairly well at school and keeping up with most major commitments and relationships, does not qualify for abuse at this point in time, but is likely to if trend continues.

_____ , _____ _____
Clinician Signature   License/Intern Status   Date

_____ , _____ _____
Supervisor Signature   License   Date

TREATMENT PLAN

Date: 06/20/2016   **Case/Client #:** 4001

Clinician Name: Maria Sanchez, MFT Trainee   **Theory:** Systemic

Modalities planned: ☐ Individual Adult ☐ Individual Child ☐ Couple ☒ Family ☐ Group: _____
Recommended session frequency: ☒ Weekly ☐ Every two weeks ☐ Other: _____
Expected length of treatment: 6 months

Treatment Plan with Goals and Interventions

Early Phase Client Goal

1. Increase family's ability to systemically view the problem and their complementary roles to reduce CF16's need to drink and smoke to distract family from the issues they are avoiding.

   Measure: Able to sustain responsible alcohol/substance use behavior for period of 2 ☐ wk ☒ mo with no more than 1 mild episode of intoxication.

   a. Use positive connotation of CF16 drinking as her way of sacrificing self and grades in order to distract parents from their pain; highlight cultural traditions of female sacrifice for family.

   b. Circular questions to reframe CF16's drinking: Who does her drinking hurt the most in the present? Who will be hurt by it most in the long run? If she were to stop partying, who would be the most surprised? The least? What positive/negative effects would this have on the family?

Working Phase Client Goals

1. Increase effectiveness of the parental coalition in relating to children to reduce the need for CF16 to act out to get them on the same team.

   Measure: Able to sustain effective parenting for period of 2 ☐ wk ☒ mo with no more than 2 mild episodes of defiance.

   a. Use variation of invariant prescription in which parents clearly communicate alliance by maintaining secrets from kids; relate to Mexican American cultural traditions.

   b. Directives to AM34 that increase emotional connection with children, such as a ritual greeting or good-bye during visits and for AF36 to increase consistency, such as writing a "house citation" instead of verbally disciplining.

2. Decrease CF16's systemic role of sacrificing herself to maintain family homeostasis and increase her freedom to attend to the developmental task of increased independence to reduce poor decision making and increase her motivation for success at school.

   Measure: Able to sustain motivation for period of 2 ☐ wk ☒ mo with no more than 2 mild episodes of poor choices.

   a. Circular questions that reveal how her acting out is helping everyone but her in the family

   b. Paradoxical "go slow" injunctions for her not to stop all the bad behavior too soon—so that parents have a reason to keep delaying the divorce

(continued)

Treatment Plan with Goals and Interventions (*continued*)

Closing Phase Client Goals

1. Increase <u>family's ability to emotionally and practically navigate separation and divorce</u> to reduce <u>CF16 substance misuse.</u>

   Measure: Able to sustain low conflict and effective problems solving for period of 3 ☐ wk ☒ mo with no more than 2 mild episodes of conflict or CF acting out.

   a. <u>Circular questions to safely communicate about feelings, plans, desires, related to separation and divorce and identify possibilities for proceeding</u>

   b. <u>Directives that instruct client to make a small but meaningful alternation to symptom pattern</u>

2. Increase <u>father's emotional connection to children</u> to reduce <u>children's anger toward father.</u>

   a. <u>Rituals to facilitate reparation of betrayal due to affair between AM34 and family members</u>

   b. <u>Reframing to help AM and children adjust to new roles.</u>

Treatment Tasks

1. Develop working therapeutic relationship using theory of choice.

   Relationship building approach/intervention:

   a. <u>Respect and trust the family system while adapting their language and maintaining therapeutic maneuverability. Maintain neutrality and use client language to build relationship with all members.</u>

2. Assess individual, relational, community, and broader cultural dynamics using theory of choice.

   Assessment strategies:

   a. <u>Assess the problem interactional sequence(s), including rise of tension, symptom, return to homeostasis, metacommunication, and complementary patterns; assess role of all members in the household</u>

   b. <u>Identify more-of-the-same solutions, including terrible simplifications, utopian syndrome, and paradox. Circular questions to assess family meaning system and roles of each.</u>

3. Identify needed referrals, crisis issues, collateral contacts, and other client needs.

   a. *Crisis assessment intervention(s):* <u>Refer CF16 for medical/psychiatric evaluation due to alcohol/substance use; contact school counselor.</u>

   b. *Referral(s):* <u>Family doctor, school counselor</u>

Diversity Considerations

Describe specifically how treatment plan, goals, and interventions were adapted to address each area of diversity (note: identify specific ethnicity, e.g., Italian American rather than White):

Age: <u>Treatment plan adapted to CF16 and CF14 age by using humor and "realness" to establish and maintain rapport.</u>

Gender/Sexual Orientation: Mexican vs. American gender role identities considered with interventions for reestablishing parental coalition; want to avoid unfair division of labor and burden within cultural traditions.

Race/Ethnicity Religion/Class/Region: Respect Catholic religious beliefs and Mexican American cultural values toward divorce and parenting and used cultural/religious background to develop appropriate reframes and interventions.

Other factors: Assess CF's school and peer environments to better understand motivation for substance use as well as culturally viable options for avoiding substance use.

Evidence-Based Practice (Optional)

Summarize evidence for using this approach for this presenting concern and/or population: There is an extensive evidence base for using systemic–strategic approaches with families and adolescents with substance abuse, including functional family therapy, multidimensional family therapy, multisystemic family therapy, and brief strategic family therapy. Virtually all evidence-based treatments for adolescent substance abuse have a significant systemic–strategic. Additionally, these approaches, particularly brief strategic, have been researched and shown to be effective with Latino families.

Client Perspective (Optional)

Has treatment plan been reviewed with client X Yes ☐ No; If no, explain: _____

Describe areas of Client Agreement and Concern: Both parents state that they believe the other person is the "real" problem, but are willing to come to conjoint family sessions for their daughter's sake. AF prefers harsher punishments for CF than AM.

_____, _____   _____ _____, _____ ____

Therapist's Signature   Intern Status   Date   Supervisor's Signature   License   Date

PROGRESS NOTE

Date: 06/20/2016 **Time:** 6:00 ☐ am/☒ pm **Session Length:** ☐ 45 min. ☒ 60 min. ☐
Other: _____ minutes

Present: ☒ Adult Male ☒ Adult Female ☒ Child Male ☒ Child Female ☐ Other: _____

Billing Code: ☐ 90791 (eval) ☐ 90834 (45 min. therapy) ☐ 90837 (60 min. therapy) ☒ 90847
(family) ☐ Other: _____

Symptom(s)	Duration and Frequency Since Last Visit	Progress
1: CF drinking	Report 1 beer, No Marijuana	Maintained
2: Conflict w/AM	Kids went on weekly visit, "ok time"	Progressing
3: Triangulation	Kids report no incidents of triangulation	Significantly Improved

Explanatory Notes on Symptoms: CF reports drinking only once with friends at weekend party after a
school event. Mother does not suspect other incidents this week.

In-Session Interventions and Assigned Homework

Followed up on last week's directives; used circular questions to make overt divorce tensions that
are being played out on kids. Developed plan to alter CF ordeal of writing e-mail to parents before going out to include "responsibility (safety) plan" for night; altered AM directive for special
greeting to include "secret handshake"; continued invariant prescription with a closed parent-
only meeting at the end of the session.

Client Response/Feedback

Family hopeful about progress and actively help develop assignments for week. CF responds well
to defiance-based, paradoxical messages

Plan

☒ Continue with treatment plan: plan for next session: Follow up on assigned tasks for week;
monitor substance use.
☐ Modify plan: _____

Next session: Date: 6/27 Time: 6:00 ☒ am/☐ pm

Crisis Issues: ☒ No indication of crisis/client denies ☐ Crisis assessed/addressed: describe below
CF denies heavy alcohol or drug use; parents report there is no indication of this; deny cutting.

_____, _____ _____
Clinician's Signature   License/Intern Status   Date

◇◇◇◇◇◇◇◇◇◇◇◇◇◇◇◇◇◇◇◇◇◇◇◇◇◇◇◇◇◇◇◇◇◇◇◇

Case Consultation/Supervision ☐ Not Applicable
Notes: Supervisor encouraged focusing on interrupting family dynamics and moving toward raising
the issue of divorce and how things will work in future.

Collateral Contact ☐ Not Applicable

Name: <u>Christopher Abounayan, School Counselor</u>   Date of Contact: 6/19 Time: <u>2:00:</u> ____

☐ am/☒ pm ☒ Written release on file: ☐ Sent/☐ Received ☐ In court docs ☐ Other: _____

Notes: <u>Counselor reports grades slightly up; no other reported problems.</u>

_____ ,   _____   _____
Clinician's Signature   License/Intern Status   Date

_____ ,   _____   _____
Supervisor's Signature   License   Date

5

Structural Family Therapies

Learning Objectives

After reading this chapter and a few hours of focused studying, you should be able to:

- **Theory:** Describe the following elements of structural family therapy and functional family therapy:

  - Process of therapy
  - Therapeutic relationship
  - Case conceptualization
  - Goal setting
  - Interventions

- **Case conceptualization and treatment plan:** Complete a theory-specific case conceptualizations and treatment plans for structural family therapy and functional family therapy using templates that are provided.

- **Research:** Provide an overview of significant research findings for structural family therapies and describe key elements of the following evidence-informed treatments: ecosystemic structural family therapy and intensive structural therapy.

- **Diversity:** Analyze strengths, limitations, and appropriate applications for using structural approaches with clients in relation to their social location/diverse identities, including but not limited to ethnic, racial, and/or sexual/gender identity diversity.

- **Cross-theoretical comparison:** Compare how structural family therapy and functional family therapy utilize interpersonal patterns (IPs) with other approaches described in this book.

> *Training in family therapy should therefore be a way of teaching techniques whose essence is to be mastered, then forgotten. After this book is read, it should be given away, or put in a forgotten corner. The therapist should be a healer: a human being concerned with engaging other human beings, therapeutically, around areas and issues that cause them pain, while always retaining great respect for their values, areas of strength, and esthetic preferences. The goal in other words is to transcend technique.*
> —Minuchin & Fishman, 1981, p. 1

Lay of the Land

Primarily associated with the work of Salvador Minuchin and his colleagues at the Philadelphia Child Guidance Center, structural therapy is considered by many to be a quintessential family therapy approach. The key elements of this model are included in several evidence-based treatments, including ecosystemic structural therapy and functional family therapy. This chapter presents structural family therapy and the following related approaches:

- Ecosystemic structural therapy: Developed by the current director of the Philadelphia Child Guidance Center, Marion Lindblad-Goldberg, this approach places greater emphasis on the broader social systems and incorporates several new elements, including attachment, trauma, and emotional regulation.
- Intensive structural therapy: The former director of training at the Philadelphia Child Guidance Center, Charles Fishman (2012) has developed intensive structural therapy, an approach that directly addresses how broader social contexts maintain dysfunctional family structure. This approach has been used extensively with anorexic adolescents and their families (Fishman, 2006).
- Functional family therapy: An evidence-based approach for working with youth experiencing conduct and substance abuse issues, functional family therapy (FFT) draws heavily on structural family therapy concepts for case conceptualization and intervention. In addition, however, many of the interventions are more characteristic of cognitive–behavioral approaches (see Chapter 8). The integrative nature of FFT poses challenges for textbook authors; ultimately, I chose to put it in this chapter because it will likely help you better understand the more complex theoretical foundations of structural family therapy. Feel free to evaluate the wisdom of this choice after reading Chapter 8. By the way, if you have ever wondered what professors chat about after hours at professional conferences, they often debate exciting topics, such as should FFT go in the structural or cognitive–behavioral therapy chapter, and then go to bed by ten. They call that a fun evening.

Structural Family Therapy

In a Nutshell: The Least You Need to Know

As the name implies, structural therapists map family structure—boundaries, hierarchies, and subsystems—to help clients resolve individual mental health symptoms and relational problems (Minuchin & Fishman, 1981). After assessing family functioning, therapists aim to restructure the family, realigning boundaries and hierarchies to promote growth and resolve problems. They are active in sessions, staging enactments, realigning chairs, and questioning family assumptions. Structural family therapy focuses on strengths, never seeing families as dysfunctional but rather as people who need assistance in expanding their repertoire of interaction patterns to adjust to their ever-changing developmental and contextual demands.

The Juice: Significant Contributions to the Field

If you remember a thing or two from this chapter, they should be the following:

Juice 1: Boundaries, or Rules for Relating

Boundaries are one of the few family therapy terms that have trickled into the vernacular; this term is used so often that your clients come in talking about them. At first glance, the term seems two-dimensional, and much like Goldilocks, you are tempted to sum things up by saying they are too rigid, too weak, or just right. However, as you begin to work with the idea of boundaries, you quickly learn that boundaries are far more complex than they initially appear. But let's start with the simple definition.

Boundaries are rules for managing physical and psychological distance between family members and for defining the regulation of closeness, distance, hierarchy, and family roles (Minuchin & Fishman, 1981). Although they may sound static, they are organic, living processes. Structural therapists identify three basic types of boundaries:

- Clear boundaries: Clear boundaries are "normal" boundaries that allow for close emotional contact with others while simultaneously allowing each person to maintain a sense of identity and differentiation (Colapinto, 1991). Each culture has a unique style of balancing closeness and distance, with different appropriate outward expressions of this balance. For example, some cultures require more physical space for clear boundaries than do others.
- Enmeshment and diffuse boundaries: Diffuse or weak boundaries lead to relational **enmeshment** (for those who like to be technically correct, boundaries are diffuse and relationships enmeshed). Families with overly **diffuse boundaries** do not make a clear distinction between members, creating a strong sense of mutuality and connection at the expense of individual autonomy (Colapinto, 1991). When talking with an enmeshed family, therapists typically see family members doing the following:

  - Interrupting one another or speaking for one another
  - Mind reading and making assumptions
  - Insisting on high levels of protectiveness and being overly concerned
  - Demanding loyalty at the expense of individual needs
  - Feeling threatened when there is disagreement or difference

How can you tell the difference between clear and close versus diffuse boundaries? Simple. If boundaries are diffuse, the family will report symptoms and problems in one or more individuals and/or complaints about family interactions. Moreover, behaviors that constitute problematic boundaries in one cultural context may be clear in another cultural context (Minuchin & Fishman, 1981). Immigrant and other bicultural families present special problems because there is more than one cultural context at play. Thus, although identifying problem boundaries seems straightforward at first, it quickly becomes murky in actual practice, requiring therapists to proceed mindfully and respectfully and to attend to each family's unique situation.

- Disengagement and rigid boundaries: Rigid boundaries lead to relational **disengagement**. Autonomy and independence are emphasized at the expense of emotional connection, creating isolation that may be more emotional than physical (Colapinto, 1991). These families have excessive tolerance for deviation, often failing to mobilize support and protection for one another. Therapists working with disengaged families notice the following:

  - Lack of reaction and few repercussions, even to problems
  - Significant freedom for most members to do as they please
  - Few demands for or expressions of loyalty and commitment
  - Consistently using parallel interactions (e.g., doing different activities in the same room) as substitutes for reciprocal interactions and engagement

Again, rigid boundaries cannot be accurately assessed without taking cultural and developmental variables into consideration; unless members are experiencing symptoms or problems, there is little ground for identifying boundaries as overly rigid.

Try It Yourself

With a partner or on your own, describe relationships in which you experienced all three types of boundaries: clear, enmeshed, and disengaged.

Juice 2: Enactments

Perhaps the most distinctive of structural interventions, **enactments** are techniques in which the therapist prompts the family to reenact a conflict or other interaction (Colapinto, 1991; Minuchin, 1974; Minuchin & Fishman, 1981). Regardless of the therapy model you choose to use, enactments are one of the most important techniques for therapists to master. Why? Because most couples and families are going to start arguing in your office whether you ask them to or not, so you had better be prepared! Enactments are one of the best ways to handle this.

Minuchin preferred enactments to talking about interactions because often people describe themselves as one way but behave quite differently, not because they are malicious or hypocritical but because it is often difficult to see clearly how our behavior looks from the outside (Minuchin & Fishman, 1981). Enactments are used to both assess and alter the problematic interactional sequences, allowing the therapist to *map, track,* and *modify* the family structure. In the case study at the end of this chapter, the therapist uses enactments to first assess the boundaries between the parents and their sons (the eldest referred for fighting at school) and later uses enactments to strengthen the parental hierarchy and boundaries.

As therapists become more experienced, they require only a few minutes of watching a family interact to know where and how to *restructure* the family. Restructuring may take the form of creating a clearer boundary in enmeshed relationships (e.g., stopping people from interrupting and speaking for one another), increasing engagement by encouraging the expression of empathy or direct eye contact, or improving parental effectiveness by helping the parent successfully manage a child's in-session behavior.

An enactment occurs in three phases, as a "dance in three movements" (Minuchin & Fishman, 1981, p. 81):

1. Observation of spontaneous interactions: Use tracking and mapping. When talking with the family, the therapist closely follows both content and process, listening for the rules and assumptions that coordinate the family's interactions, such as demands for overconnectedness, extreme disconnection, or hierarchical confusion, as well as strengths and resources. The therapist tracks actual transactions more closely than verbal accounts (Colapinto, 1991), while developing a hypothesis that maps the family's boundaries and hierarchy (Minuchin & Fishman, 1981). Once the therapist identifies an area for change, he or she is ready to invite the family into the active phase of enactment.

2. The invitation: **eliciting transactions:** The invitation for an enactment is issued in one of two ways: either the therapist directly asks the family to engage in an enactment or the family spontaneously starts an enactment of at-home behavior, usually in the form of an argument (Colapinto, 1991). Obviously, the therapist does not need to do much when the family spontaneously begins; if the family does not, the therapist must issue an explicit invitation to "show" the problem:

   "Can you reenact what happened last night?" or
   "Please show me what happens at home when he is 'defiant'; can you act out an incident of defiance that happened last week so I have a good idea of what the problem really is?"

3. Redirecting alternative transactions: This is the most important part. It really is not therapeutic to ask a family to start enacting problem behaviors if the therapist does not jump in and help redirect the behavior to clarify boundaries and hierarchies. How therapists redirect the interaction depends on the particular interaction that needs to be changed. Redirection often involves the following:

- Stopping family members from interrupting or speaking for one another
- Directing two people to directly engage each other while asking a third member to allow the other two to communicate
- Encouraging emotional understanding and connection between disengaged parties
- Rearranging chairs physically to increase or decrease emotional closeness
- Requesting parents to actively establish an effective hierarchical position with a child

Enactments are beneficial because they provide live practice with new interactions and family patterns, increasing the likelihood of transitioning in-session gains and insights into everyday family life. They also reduce the illusion that the problem belongs to a single person; when family members demonstrate the problem in front of the therapist, it becomes clear that the reported problem does not belong to a single person but to the larger family unit. Finally, enactments increase the family's sense of competence and strength by helping its members to successfully engage in new preferred behaviors (Minuchin & Fishman, 1981).

Rumor Has It: The People and Their Stories

Salvador Minuchin

Trained as a pediatrician and child psychiatrist, Salvador Minuchin is considered the progenitor of structural family therapy (Colapinto, 1991; Minuchin, 1974). Minuchin lived and worked on three continents; he was born and raised in Argentina and then lived in Israel during two periods of his life before settling in the United States. In 1954, after returning from a two-year period of working with displaced children in Israel, he began his psychiatry training with Harry Stack Sullivan, whose psychoanalytic work emphasized interpersonal relationships. After his training, Minuchin accepted a position at the Wiltwyck School for delinquent boys and suggested to his colleagues—Dick Auerswald, Charlie King, Braulio Montalvo, and Clara Rabinowitz—that they see the entire family. With no formal models to follow, they used a one-way mirror to observe each other and developed a working model as they went along. In 1962, Minuchin visited the Mental Research Institute, where Haley, Watzlawick, Fisch, and others were at the forefront of developing family therapy approaches. There he befriended Jay Haley, who developed the strategic approach to family therapy (see Chapter 4); the mutual influence of this friendship is evident in the work of both men.

From 1965 to 1976, Minuchin served as the director of the Philadelphia Child Guidance Center, and in 1975 he founded the Family Therapy Training Center (later renamed the Philadelphia Child and Family Therapy Training Center). In 1967, Minuchin, Montalvo, Guerney, Rosman, and Schumer published *Families of the Slums*, considered the first book to describe structural therapy and a book that discussed diversity issues before the term *multiculturalism* was coined. Over the years, Minuchin and his colleagues have written numerous books that detail how they have developed and refined this model to address changing cultural contexts and specific diagnoses (Minuchin, Rosman, & Baker, 1978). Minuchin is still an active leader in the field, continuing to teach new generations of therapists (Minuchin, Nichols, & Lee, 2007; Minuchin, Reiter, & Borda, 2014). His influential students and colleagues include Harry Aponte, Jorge Colapinto, Charles Fishman, Marion Lindblad-Goldberg, Jay Lappin, Michael Nichols, Bernice Rossman, and Mary Ann Walters.

Charles Fishman

Also a trained as a child psychiatrist, H. Charles Fishman (1988, 2004, 2012, 2013; Minuchin & Fishman, 1981) served as the director of training at the Philadelphia Child Guidance Center and worked closely with Minuchin in the early years. Since then, much of his work has focused on eating disorders (Fishman, 2004), and most recently, he has developed an intensive structural therapy model, which adds the concept of homeostatic maintainer and includes data-driven methods of measuring client progress (Fishman, Morris, & Fishman, 2016). He currently serves as a clinical professor at the University of Hawaii and clinical director at Reconnect Family Services in New Zealand.

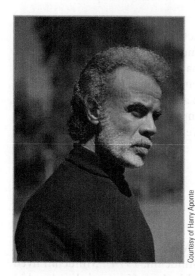

Harry Aponte

Harry Aponte (1994, 1996) attends to issues of spirituality, poverty, and race in the practice of structural family therapy.

Marion Lindblad-Goldberg

Having studied with Minuchin, Marion Lindblad-Goldberg and her colleagues (Lindblad-Goldberg, Dore, & Stern, 1998) developed the empirically supported treatment called "ecosystemic structural family therapy" (ESFT). She directs the Philadelphia Child and Family Therapy Training Center.

Jose Szapocznik

Jose Szapocznik and his colleagues at the Center for Family Studies in Florida developed the empirically supported brief strategic family therapy (BSFT) to address drug abuse problems with Cuban youth in Miami (Szapocznik & Williams, 2000; Szapocznik et al., 2004; Santisteban et al., 1997).

The Big Picture: Overview of Treatment

Three Phases of Therapy

Minuchin (1974) identifies three main *phases* of structural therapy:

1. Join the family and accommodate to its members' style (build an alliance).
2. Map the family structure, boundaries, and hierarchy (evaluate and assess).
3. Intervene to transform the structure to diminish symptoms (address the problems they identified in the assessment).

In general, therapists alternate between phases 2 and 3 many times, revising and refining the map and hypotheses about family functioning until the problems are addressed and resolved. I like to think of it as similar to the golden rule with shampoo: "lather, rinse, repeat" until you achieve the desired effect.

Who Attends Therapy?

To be able to assess the system, structural therapists prefer to begin therapy with the entire family, but they do not insist on it (Colapinto, 1991). However, once the family system has been assessed, the therapist often meets with specific subsystems and individuals to achieve structural goals. For example, often sessions with the couple alone are necessary to strengthen the boundaries between the couple and parental subsystems and to sever cross-generational coalitions.

The Family Therapist's Pouch

In his most recent work, Minuchin (Minuchin et al., 2014) offers the metaphor of the therapist's pouch as a framework for understanding the therapeutic process:

Basic Principles

1. Joining (see "Making Connections," below): Essential for success, joining is first and foremost an attitude of respect, empathy, and curiosity.
2. Assumptions: Families that come to therapy incorrectly assume that there are no alternatives to their problem story: they are too certain in their perspectives.
3. The enemy: The family's strong sense of certainty in their view is ultimately the enemy of therapeutic change.

Techniques

4. Challenging certainty: Challenging the family's sense of certainty about the problem can be done by challenging repetitive patterns or taking a one-down stance, similar to strategic therapists (see Chapter 4).
5. Exploring alternatives: Therapists can help families explore alternatives to their story of certainty, which is frequently done with enactments.
6. Content versus process: To facilitate lasting change, therapists need to use the *content* of family communication to identify the underlying *process* of their dynamics, including the emotional aspect of interactions.
7. Humor and metaphor: Therapists can use humor, stories, and metaphors to facilitate joining as well as challenge certainty.
8. Knowledge: Introducing specific topics at different levels, including knowledge of family structure, future directions, and family ethics.

Working with Subsystems

9. The individual: Exploring the identities of individual members can help identify new alternatives for relating.
10. Subsystems: Therapists can work with individual subsystems—parents together, one parent and child, siblings, etc.—to help shift family structure.
11. Unbalancing: At times, therapists may need to unbalance a system by taking sides with one subsystem.

Self of Therapist

12. Distance: To effectively facilitate, therapists must carefully choose how best to position themselves in relation to each client: close, distant, or somewhere in between.
13. Expertise: Therapists should use their awareness of family dysfunctional patterns as well as facilitating therapeutic conversations.
14. Self: The self of the therapist *is* the primary tool for facilitating change, not the interventions, and therapists need to learn how to challenge families to react to the self of the therapist.

Making Connections: The Therapeutic Relationship

Joining and Accommodating

Structural family therapists have a unique term for the therapeutic relationship: **joining** (Minuchin, 1974; Minuchin & Fishman, 1981; Minuchin & Nichols, 1993). They "join" the system in the sense that they **accommodate** to its style: how people talk, what words they use, how they walk, and so forth. **Mimesis**, a Greek term that means "copy" (as in *mimeograph;* if you're too young to remember that, consider yourself lucky), has also been used to refer to the process of accommodating the family's way of being. In the historical context of psychotherapy, this is a radical concept, because unlike in psychodynamic, cognitive–behavioral, and even experiential therapies, the therapist does not take a superior role.

Minuchin (1974) compared the process of joining a family to an anthropologist studying a new culture, which always begins by sitting back and observing patterns, habits, and behaviors before beginning to address one's own agenda—in this case to alleviate the family's distress. The process of joining can also be likened to falling in rhythm with the family. Do the members of the family talk fast or slow? Do they talk over one another or wait for clear pauses to speak? Do they use teasing and humor, or are their words gentle and soft? A successful structural therapist needs to have a wide repertoire of social skills to successfully join with families, especially when working with diverse populations. In the case study at the end of this chapter, the therapist uses humor and sincerity to balance connecting with the parents with simultaneously gaining the trust of their often-defiant teenage son.

Joining as an Attitude

Colapinto (1991) emphasizes that **joining** is more of an attitude than a technique; it is the glue that holds the therapeutic system together through the often turbulent and challenging journey called therapy (Minuchin & Fishman, 1981). The attitude of joining requires: (a) a strong, clear sense of connection and affiliation (e.g., curiosity, openness, sensitivity, acceptance) and (b) an equally clear sense of distance and differentiation (e.g., questioning, dissenting, promoting change).

Therapeutic Spontaneity

Structural therapists strive to cultivate **therapeutic spontaneity**; this does not mean a do-as-you-please attitude, but rather a relationally and contextually responsive expression of self: "The therapist's spontaneity is constrained by the context of therapy" (Minuchin & Fishman, 1981, p. 3). *Therapeutic spontaneity* refers to the ability to flow naturally and authentically in a variety of contexts and situations. Much in the way riding a bike becomes natural after a painful period of training wheels and falls, therapeutic spontaneity is cultivated and shaped through the training process, which increases therapists' repertoire for "being natural" in a wide range of clinical situations.

Therapist's Use of Self

According to Minuchin, therapists must use themselves to relate to the family, varying from being highly involved to professionally detached (Minuchin & Fishman, 1981). They may be clearly detached from family interactions so that they can clarify boundaries or prescribe a specific intervention, maintain a moderate level of connection to coach the family in new interactions, or assume a fully engaged position by taking sides with one family member to "unbalance" the system (an intervention discussed later in this chapter). The therapist is highly flexible, adapting to each family's needs and cultural norms.

Most recently, Minuchin has described use of self as the therapist's "most significant tool," and states that it appears to be insufficiently addressed in today's training (Minuchin et al., 2014; Wylie & Minuchin, 2013). He encourages new therapists to reflect on aspects of their personal and relational lives that shape their therapeutic style and to recognize how these aspects of the self affect the therapeutic process and client behavior in session. He recommends presenting cases by beginning with an analysis of the therapist's use of self rather than beginning with describing the client. To develop greater awareness of use of self, Minuchin encourages therapists to imagine that a homunculus (an artificially created dwarf; his vocabulary, not mine) sits on the therapist's shoulder during each session and that this little guy observes the therapist's thinking during the session. The homunculus can then engage in imaginary, silent dialogues with the therapist during the session, tracking how the therapist's personal experiences are shaping the action in the room.

Try It Yourself

With a partner or on your own, describe how "who you are" as a therapist is likely to affect therapy with your clients, including your personal strengths, areas for growth, approach to conflict, life experiences, and personality. Describe yourself in at least three different life contexts and how you change in each of these.

"Making It Happen"

The primary injunction from the model to the therapist can be summarized in three words: "Make it happen." —Colapinto, 1991, p. 435

The therapist's job is to find a way to help the family achieve desired change, and he or she must do whatever it takes to make this happen. Therefore, therapists' roles can vary widely: they can be the "producer," who ensures conditions that make therapy possible; the "stage director," who pushes the family toward more functional patterns; the "protagonist," who directly uses himself or herself to alter stuck family interactions'; or the "narrator" or "coauthor," who collaboratively helps the family revise their script. Thus, therapists need to be open to playing whichever role will be most beneficial for a particular family in a given session, rather than being wedded to their own favorite roles.

Recent Adaptation: A Softer Style

In his later work, Minuchin has described a change in approach: "I have moved from being an active challenger—confronting, directing, and controlling—to a softer style, in which I use humor, acceptance, support, suggestion, and seduction on behalf of the same goals" (Minuchin et al., 2007, p. 6). Despite this change, Minuchin has not abandoned the expert role or the goal of achieving change in the present. A recent study that analyzed structural family therapy sessions found that therapist empathy was not only readily evident but appears to be a key ingredient in facilitating change (Hammond & Nichols, 2007).

The Viewing: Case Conceptualization and Assessment

Structural family therapists conceptualize and assess the following factors:

STRUCTURAL ASSESSMENT

- Role of symptom in the family
- Subsystems
- Cross-generational coalitions
- Boundaries
- Hierarchy
- Complementarity
- Family development
- Strengths

Role of the Symptom

Structural therapists identify three possible relationships between the symptom and the family system (Colapinto, 1991):

1. Family as ineffectual challenger of symptom: The family is passive, such as a system that enables an alcoholic. In order to maintain a highly enmeshed or disengaged family structure, it fails to challenge the symptomatic member.
2. Family as "shaper" of individual's symptoms: The family structure shapes the individual's experience and behaviors, such as child who is triangulated into unacknowledged couple conflict.
3. Family as "beneficiary" of the symptom: The symptom performs a regulatory function in maintaining the family structure, such as symptomatic child who gives the parents a reason to unite and/or distracts from marital problems.

As in virtually all forms of family therapy, the *symptom bearer* or *identified patient* is never seen as the sole source of the problem, and instead the family interaction patterns are targeted for intervention.

Subsystems

Minuchin (1974) conceptualized a family as a single system that also had multiple **subsystems**. Some subsystems can be found in almost every family: couple, parent, sibling, and each individual as a separate subsystem. In addition, in some families, other influential subsystems develop along gender lines, hobbies, interests (sports, music), and even personalities (serious vs. fun loving). When assessing a family, in general the most important subsystem issues to consider are: (a) whether there is a clear distinction between the parental and couple subsystems and (b) whether there is a clear boundary between the parental and child/sibling subsystems. Alternatively stated, is there an effective parental hierarchy?

Cross-Generational Coalitions: Problematic Subsystems

One type of subsystem is particularly damaging: **cross-generational coalitions** (Minuchin & Fishman, 1981; Minuchin & Nichols, 1993). A cross-generational coalition is a subsystem that forms between a parent and child *against* the other parent or other key caretaker. This is a common family dynamic; often a mother has grown closer to her children and has unresolved marital or parenting conflicts with her spouse. The inverse, a father in coalition with the children against the mother, is also frequent, as is a family that divides into "teams," with the father and mother heading their team in overt or covert opposition to the other. These coalitions are especially common in divorces, and in fact, both parents typically try to create these coalitions simultaneously against the other; thus, the children become the rope in a tug of war. These coalitions are often *covert,* meaning they are not directly addressed or spoken about in the family but are evident by secrets between the parent and child ("don't tell your mom/dad about this") or comments that compliment the child and disparage the other spouse ("I am so glad you didn't inherit your father's/mother's gene for X"). These coalitions can also involve other caretakers, such as grandparents or parentified children.

Boundary Assessment

This element of case conceptualization is discussed in detail in "The Juice" section, above.

Hierarchy

When working with reported problems in child behavior, therapists must first assess the **parental hierarchy** so that they know how to intervene (Colapinto, 1991; Minuchin, 1974; Minuchin & Fishman, 1981). The three basic forms of parental hierarchy are:

• Effective: When the parental hierarchy is appropriate and effective, parents can set boundaries and limits while still maintaining emotional connection with their children.

- Insufficient: When the parental hierarchy is insufficient, parents are not able to effectively manage the child's behavior and often adapt a permissive parenting style. This style is easy to identify in the therapy office: the parents are not able to keep younger children from tearing up the waiting room and office, or their teens act as though they have the right to set their own curfews and rules. Often the parents hope that the therapist will "teach" their children to listen, but this often requires intervening more with the parents than the children. In general, these parents have enmeshed boundaries with their children, but not always. As with boundaries, the outward expression of effective versus insufficient can be determined only by examining the cultural context, family life stage of development, and symptomatic behavior.
- Excessive: When there is excessive hierarchy, the rules are developmentally too strict and unrealistic and consequences are too severe to be effective. In this situation, there is almost always a rigid boundary between children and parents. These parents need assistance in developing age-appropriate rules and expectations and in developing a stronger emotional bond with their children.

Complementarity

Much like systemic therapists (Chapter 4), structural therapists assess for rigid **complementary patterns** between family members (Colapinto, 1991). Like a jigsaw puzzle, family members develop complementary roles: the overfunctioner/underfunctioner, good/bad child, understanding/strict parent, logical/emotional partner, and so forth. Over time, these systemically generated roles become viewed as inherent personality characteristics that seem unchangeable. The more exaggerated and rigid these roles become, the less adaptable the individuals and family become. Structural therapists recognize the mutually reinforced patterns and target the ones that need to change for members to grow.

Family Development

Rather than a static entity, the family is viewed as continually growing and changing in response to predictable stages of development as well as unexpected life events such as death, a move, or divorce. Minuchin and Fishman (1981) identify four major stages in family development:

1. Couple formation
2. Families with young children
3. Families with school-age or adolescent children
4. Families with grown children

At each stage, the members need to renegotiate boundaries to define the levels of closeness and differentiation that will support individual members' growth needs. Families often get stuck transitioning from one stage to another if they fail to renegotiate boundaries and hierarchy as the family develops.

Strengths

Minuchin feels strongly that therapists should avoid labeling families as dysfunctional and instead recognize their strengths, particularly their cultural and idiosyncratic strengths (Minuchin & Fishman, 1981; Minuchin & Nichols, 1993). He powerfully argues against seeing the family as an enemy of its individual members, as is frequent in the psychological literature, and instead encourages therapists to recognize how the family provides support, protection, and a foundation for its members. Family strengths, such as a strong connection to extended family or community, are identified and used to promote the goals of individual and family growth as well as to reduce symptoms.

Targeting Change: Goal Setting

> *A well-functioning family is not defined by the absence of stress, conflict, and problems, but by how effectively it handles them in the course of fulfilling its function. This, in turn, depends on the structure and adaptability of the family.* —Colapinto, 1991, p. 422

Structural therapists target similar goals for all families (Colapinto, 1991; Minuchin, 1974):

- *Clear boundaries* between all subsystems that allow for connectedness and differentiation congruent with the family's cultural contexts.
- Clear distinction between the *marital/couple subsystem* and the *parental subsystem*.
- *Effective parental hierarchy* and the severing of cross-generational coalitions.
- A family structure that promotes the *development and growth of individuals and the family.*

The Doing: Interventions

Enactments and Modifying Interactions

This intervention is discussed in detail in "The Juice" section, above.

Systemic Reframing

As the family members begin to describe their problems, therapists reflect on their understanding using **systemic reframing** (Colapinto, 1991; Minuchin, 1974; Minuchin & Fishman, 1981). A systemic reframe takes into account that all behavior has reciprocal antecedents: person A affects person B's response, which then affects person A's response, ad infinitum (A → B). Reframes often highlight complementary relationships in the family, such as the pursuer/distancer pattern. Reframing usually involves removing the blame from one person (the identified patient) and "spreading" blame equally by describing how each person's response contributes to the problem dynamic. Once this is done, blame becomes a moot point.

Systemic reframing involves piecing together each member's description of the problem and reframing it to reveal the broader systemic dynamic. Thus, if the wife complains that her husband never listens to her, and he complains that she is always nagging him about something, the therapist can systemically reframe their descriptions to highlight how the more she pushes him to listen and interact, the more he withdraws; and the more he withdraws, the more she feels compelled to pursue him for interaction.

HOW TO GENERATE SYSTEMIC REFRAMES

- Assess broader interactional patterns (complementary relationships, hierarchy, boundaries, etc.)
- Redescribe the problem (use interactional patterns to describe the problem in a larger context)

Try It Yourself

With a partner or on your own, develop a systemic reframe for a current relationship problem in your life.

Boundary Making

Boundary making is a special form of enactment that targets overinvolvement or underinvolvement to help families soften rigid boundaries or strengthen diffuse boundaries (Colapinto, 1991; Minuchin, 1974). Structural therapists use this technique to direct who participates and how. By actively setting boundaries, therapists interrupt the habitual interaction patterns, allowing members to experience underutilized skills and abilities. Boundary making may involve several different directives:

- Asking family members to change seats
- Asking family members to move seats further apart or closer together or turn toward one another
- Having separate sessions with individuals or subsystems to strengthen subsystem boundaries
- Asking one or more members to remain silent during an interaction
- Asking questions that highlight a problem boundary area (e.g., "Do you always answer for your son when he is asked a question?")
- Blocking interruptions or encouraging pauses to enable less dominant persons to speak

Challenging the Family's Certainty and Worldview

Challenging the family's certainty about their worldview and unproductive assumptions can include rigid definitions of the problem, available solutions, and individual member's identity. Therapists challenge these certainties by questioning operational assumptions in the family system, whether overtly spoken or covertly acted upon (Colapinto, 1991; Minuchin, 1974; Minuchin & Fishman, 1981). Common assumptions that create problems for individuals, couples, and families include the following:

- "The only solution to the problem is the one I/we envision."
- "Kids' needs come first."
- "It's better to keep the peace than start conflict."
- "It is easier to sacrifice my needs than ask for what I want."
- "If I give here, you should give there."
- "It's better for the kids for us to stay in this unhappy marriage."

Structural therapists often challenge these assumptions by overtly questioning whether they are actually having the effect family members anticipate. The challenge can be delivered softly or strongly, depending on what will be most effective with a particular family's structure.

Intensity and Crisis Inductions

Intensity and **crisis inductions** are interventions that use affect to create structural shifts in hierarchy and boundaries, especially when the family is having trouble "hearing" the therapist with other interventions (Minuchin, 1974; Minuchin & Fishman, 1981; Minuchin & Nichols, 1993). Because families differ in the degree of loyalty to their reality that they demand, they need different levels and styles of intensity, depending on the issue being discussed. Intensity involves turning up the emotional heat by using tone of voice, pacing, and word choice to break through rigid and stuck interactional patterns. For example, a therapist may say to a couple who claims to have no time for a weekly date because of their children's numerous after-school activities, "Do you think your children would prefer to be in soccer and have divorced parents or to have fewer activities and an intact family?"

Closely related to intensity, *crisis induction* in structural therapy is used with families who chronically avoid a conflict or problem (Colapinto, 1991). For example, in families with anorectic children, the therapist may bring the symptom into the room by staging a meal and having the family deal with it. Similarly, with alcohol or substance abuse issues, the therapist often induces a crisis so that the family will acknowledge and finally address the problem. The therapist can then help the family develop new interactions and patterns.

Unbalancing

Unbalancing is used for more extreme difficulties in hierarchy or when the identified patient is being made a scapegoat. This intervention is used to realign boundaries between subsystems (Minuchin, 1974; Minuchin & Fishman, 1981). Therapists use their expert position to temporarily "join sides" with an individual who is being made a scapegoat or with subsystems that need to develop stronger boundaries by arguing their cause or helping to explain their perspective to others. At first glance, this may seem to go against the general rule of neutrality that characterizes structural therapy specifically and psychotherapy more generally. However, unbalancing is done only briefly and with specific realignment goals in mind, generally only after more direct interventions, such as enactments and challenging assumptions, have failed.

Expanding Family Truths and Realities

Each family develops a unique worldview that defines its realities and truths. When working with a highly rigid family structure, structural therapists directly challenge these beliefs and realities (discussed above in "Challenging the Family's Certainty and Worldview"; Minuchin & Fishman, 1981). However, whenever possible, structural therapists cite these beliefs to *expand* the family's functioning in new directions. For example, they might say, "Because you obviously have such deep concern for your child, you are parents who are likely to understand that the child needs space to grow in order to really flourish." Or "Since you are willing to go to such lengths to be helpful, it seems you are probably able to be helpful in an even more challenging way: allowing him to make his own mistakes." Rather than introduce an entirely foreign concept, the structural therapist takes the family's fundamental premise that has been supporting the problem and redirects its logic to support an alternative set of behaviors and interactions, allowing the family to maintain its core beliefs but to use them in new ways.

Making Compliments and Shaping Competence

Minuchin and Fishman (1981) strongly caution therapists that professional training creates a "search and destroy" (diagnose and treat) approach to psychopathology that often blinds therapists to family strengths and positive interaction patterns. Instead, therapists should augment and reinforce the family's natural positive patterns and strengths. *Compliments* are used to bolster behaviors that support families in moving toward their goals, and **shaping competence** involves noticing small successes along the way to reaching goals. For example, families usually improve after enactments and refrain from interrupting or speaking for each other in later sessions. Therapists can shape competence by noting these changes during the session or as they are reported from week to week.

Shaping competence also involves refusing to function for the family during the session. For example, rather than taking responsibility for having children focus and behave during a session, the therapist asks the parents to do so. If a child is kicking the furniture or gets up to play with a toy during a family session, rather than correct the child, the therapist asks the parents to have the child stop. Similarly, if the therapist is trying to strengthen the parental hierarchy, the therapist asks the parents to answer questions first and recognizes their authority by directing children to ask parents for permission to do such things as go to the bathroom or get some water. In the case study at the end of this chapter, the therapist uses shaping competence with a teen to increase his motivation to pursue his life goals rather than relying entirely on increased parental hierarchy to reduce his fighting at school and improve his grades.

Scope It Out: Cross-Theoretical Comparison

Using Tomm's IPscope described in Chapter 3 (Tomm, St. George, Wulff, & Strong, 2014), this theory approaches the conceptualization of systemic, interpersonal patterns as follows:

Theoretical Conceptualization

Structural case conceptualization maps pathologizing interpersonal patterns (PIPs), primarily by identifying complementary roles. The complementary roles typically correspond directly to the two interlocking dynamics of Tomm's PIPs, such as pursuing/distancing or overfunctioning/underfunctioning. Structural assessment of boundaries, subsystems, hierarchy, coalitions, and role of the symptom often includes elements of the PIP as well.

Goal Setting

Structural family therapists have clearly defined wellness interpersonal patterns (WIPs), which include clear boundaries between all subsystems, clear distinction between the marital and parental subsystems, effective parental hierarchy, and a family structure that promotes the healthy development of individuals and the family.

Facilitating Change

The structural family therapist promotes change by actively using both healing interpersonal patterns (HIPs) and WIPs. Techniques or transforming interpersonal patterns (TIPs) such as unbalancing and crisis inductions are HIPs that are intended create a temporary set of interactions and experiences that will help the client shift to WIPs. In contrast, when therapists use interventions such as enactment and boundary making, they directly facilitate WIPs.

PUTTING IT ALL TOGETHER: STRUCTURAL CASE CONCEPTUALIZATION AND TREATMENT PLAN TEMPLATES

Areas for Theory-Specific Case Conceptualization: Structural

When conceptualizing client *cases,* contemporary structural therapists typically use the following dynamics *to inform their treatment plan.* Go to MindTap® to access a digital version of the theory-specific case conceptualization, along with a variety of digital study tools and resources that complement this text and help you be more successful in your course and career. If your instructor didn't assign MindTap, you can find out more about it at Cengagebrain.com. You can also download the form at masteringcompetencies.com.

Family development

Identify family life-cycle stage and any issues in meeting developmental needs:

- Single adult
- Committed couple
- Families with young children
- Families with school-age or adolescent children
- Divorce
- Blended family
- Launching children
- Later life

Subsystems

Describe who is in each subsystem and the general dynamics of the subsystem and how the subsystem is related to the presenting problem:

- Parental, including grandparents, stepparents, parentified children
- Couple: Is this system distinct from the parental subsystem?
- Sibling, including step-siblings:
- Other:

Hierarchy

Describe parent–child hierarchy and other salient hierarchies in the system:

- Effective (authoritative)
- Insufficient (permissive)
- Excessive (authoritarian)

Boundaries

Describe boundaries in family system between individuals and subsystems:

- Enmeshed
- Clear
- Disengaged

Cross-Generational Coalitions

Describe any cross-generational coalitions within the family or between adult and his/her family of origin.

Complementarity

Describe complementary roles, such as pursuer/distancer, overfunctioner/underfunctioner, logical/emotional, good/bad parent, good/bad child, etc.

Role of Symptom in the Family

Describe relation between the family and symptom:

- Family as ineffectual challenger of the symptom
- Family as "shaper" of the individual's symptom
- Family as "beneficiary" of the symptom

Client/Family Strengths and Diversity

Identify family strengths that may be unique to family or related to diversity factors:

- Identify various forms of strengths:
  - Personal
  - Relational/social
  - Spiritual

- Identify potential resources and limitations available to clients based on their age, gender, sexual orientation, cultural background, socioeconomic status, religion, regional community, language, family background, family configuration, abilities, etc.:
  - Unique resources
  - Potential limitations

TREATMENT PLAN FOR INDIVIDUAL WITH DEPRESSION/ANXIETY: STRUCTURAL

You can download a blank treatment plan (with or without measures) on MindTap at www.cengagebrain.com or www.masteringcompetencies.com.

The following treatment plan template can be used to help you develop individualized treatments for use with individuals with depressive or anxiety symptoms.

Structural Treatment Plan: Client Goals with Interventions

Early-Phase Client Goals

1. Increase *strength of diffuse* [or flexibility, if rigid] *boundaries* with/in [specify person/context] to reduce depressed mood and anxiety.
   a. *Challenge client's worldview* as it relates to maintaining unclear boundaries.
   b. *Shape competence* by helping client transfer strategies for clear boundaries in one area of life to the area where boundaries are a problem.

Working-Phase Client Goals

1. Decrease [specify extreme *complementary roles/behaviors*] to reduce depressed mood and anxiety.
   a. *Intensity and crisis induction* to enable client to see the negative effects of complementary/extreme roles/behaviors.
   b. *Expanding client truths* to use elements of complementary role to reduce its extremity.

2. Increase *strength of diffuse* [or flexibility if rigid] *boundaries* with/in [specify another person/context] to reduce depressed mood and anxiety.
   a. *Enactments* to have client practice setting clearer boundaries.
   b. *Compliments* to shape new behaviors that establish clear boundaries.

3. Increase *clarity and appropriateness of role* in family of origin, partnership, and/or family of procreation to reduce anxiety.
   a. Assign *boundary making* moves for client to use to clarify role out of session.
   b. *Challenge client's worldview* about what "must be done" in specific relationships.

Closing-Phase Client Goals

1. Increase ability to maintain levels of *independence appropriate to current family life stage* of development to reduce depressed mood and increase sense of well-being.
   a. *Challenge client's worldview* to adapt to tasks associated with new stage of development.
   b. *Compliment* behaviors that support stage-appropriate independence.

2. Increase ability to maintain levels of *interdependence and relational connection appropriate to current family life stage* to reduce anxiety and increase sense of well-being.
   a. Use *enactments* to explore new, stage-appropriate ways of relating.
   b. *Shape competence* to enable client to build on current skills to develop new ones.

Treatment Tasks

1. Develop working therapeutic relationship.
   a. *Join* with client, adapting to gender/culture/class norms for relating, expressing emotion, conversational tempo, etc.

2. Assess individual, systemic, and broader cultural dynamics.
   a. Assess structure of family of origin and family of procreation (or current partnership), including *subsystems, coalitions, boundary patterns, hierarchy, complementary relationships, family stage of development,* and *strengths.*
   b. Identify the *role of the symptom* (e.g., depression/anxiety) in the client's family system.

3. Identify needed referrals, crisis issues, collateral contacts, and other client needs.
   a. *Crisis assessment intervention(s):* Address crisis issues such as self-harm, suicidal ideation, substance use, risky sexual behavior, etc.
   b. *Referral(s):* Connect client with *resources* in client's *community* that could be supportive; make collateral contacts as needed.

TREATMENT PLAN TEMPLATE FOR DISTRESSED COUPLE/FAMILY: STRUCTURAL

You can download a blank treatment plan (with or without measures) at www
.cengagebrain.com or www.masteringcompetencies.com.

The following treatment plan template can be used to help you develop individualized
treatments for use with couples and families who report relational distress.

Structural Treatment Plan: Client Goals with Interventions

Early-Phase Client Goals

1. Sever *coalitions* (cross-generational or with external third parties) and reduce conflict.
   a. Use *intensity and crisis induction* to enable clients to see the negative effects of
      coalitions.
   b. Use *boundary making* during the session to expose and realign coalitions.

Working-Phase Client Goals

1. Increase *strength of diffuse* [or flexibility, if rigid] *boundaries* between [person/
   subsystem A] and [person/subsystem B; add more if necessary] to reduce conflict.
   a. *Challenge family's worldview* as it relates to maintaining unclear boundaries.
   b. *Enactments* to enable couple/family experience relating with clear boundaries.

2. Increase [or decrease] *parental hierarchy* and *separate spousal from parental subsystems* to reduce conflict.
   a. Use *enactments* to have couple/family learn how to interact with clear hierarchy
      and subsystem boundaries.
   b. Use *boundary making* to realign hierarchy and subsystems.

3. Decrease *complementary roles* in system and increase *clarity and appropriateness of
   roles* to reduce conflict.
   a. Use *boundary making* to decrease complementary roles.
   b. *Challenge couple/family's worldview* about who is capable of what in system.

Closing-Phase Client Goals

1. Increase ability to maintain levels of *independence appropriate to current family life
   stage* of development to reduce conflict and increase sense of well-being.
   a. *Challenge couple's/family's worldview* to adapt to tasks associated with new stage
      of development to reduce conflict and increase sense of intimacy.
   b. *Compliment* behaviors that support stage-appropriate independence.

2. Increase ability to maintain levels of *interdependence and relational connection appropriate to current family life stage* to reduce conflict and increase intimacy.
   a. Use *enactments* to explore new, stage-appropriate ways of relating.
   b. *Shape competence* to enable couple/family to build on current skills to develop new ones.

Treatment Tasks

1. Develop working therapeutic relationship.
   a. *Join* with system, adapting to gender/culture/class norms for relating, expressing
      emotion, conversational tempo, etc.

2. Assess individual, systemic, and broader cultural dynamics.
   a. Assess structure of system, including *subsystems, coalitions, boundary patterns,
      hierarchy, complementary relationships, family stage of development,* and *strengths.*
   b. Identify the *role of the symptom* (e.g., conflict or identified patient's symptoms) in the system.

3. Identify needed referrals, crisis issues, collateral contacts, and other client needs.
   a. *Crisis assessment intervention(s):* Address crisis issues such as psychological abuse, inti-
      mate partner violence, hidden affair, self-harm, suicidal ideation, substance use, etc.
   b. *Referral(s):* Connect client with *resources* in client's *family and community* that
      could be supportive; make collateral contacts as needed.

Tapestry Weaving: Working with Diverse Populations
Cultural, Ethnic, and Socioeconomic Diversity

Every family has elements in their own culture, which if understood and utilized, can become levers to actualize and expand the family members' behavioral repertory. Unfortunately, we therapists have not assimilated this axiom. Though we pay lip service to the strengths of the family, and talk about the matrix of development and healing, we are trained as psychological sleuths. Our instincts are to "search and destroy": pinpoint the psychological disorder, label it, and eradicate it. —Minuchin & Fishman, 1981, pp. 262–263

Minuchin and his colleagues developed the structural family therapy model to work with poor, ethnically diverse, urban families because they did not find that traditional insight-oriented approaches were effective with these populations (Colapinto, 1991; Minuchin et al., 1967). From its inception, structural family therapy has attended to the dynamics and needs of diverse families, especially those with children who are having difficulties. In addition to Minuchin, structural therapy proponents, such as Harry Aponte (1994, 1996), have been leading voices in the field of family therapy on issues of spirituality, race, and poverty. Because Minuchin and many of the proponents of structural family therapy were themselves from diverse and immigrant backgrounds, they were aware of the strengths of diverse families. Furthermore, several researchers have identified structural family therapy as particularly well suited for diverse families because it does not rigidly define what a healthy family should look like (Epstein et al., 2012; Szapocznik et al., 1997). Structural family therapy employs an active, engaged approach in which the therapist often takes an expert stance in relation to the family, an approach that often fits with the values of traditional cultures.

Hispanic and African American Families

Structural therapy has been widely used and studied with Hispanics, African Americans, and Asian Americans. Most notably, brief strategic family therapy and structural eco-systemic therapy (see "Research and the Evidence Base," below) have been studied and adapted for working with both Hispanic and African American families (Szapocznik & Williams, 2000; Szapocznik, Hervis, & Schwartz, 2000; Szapocznik et al., 1997). In fact, brief strategic family therapy was initially developed specifically for use with Cuban youth with conduct issues; the family focus fits well with Hispanic valuing of family relationships. Current versions of the model, culturally informed and flexible family-based treatment, specifically add content and themes for Hispanic families, specifically acculturation/immigration issues, intrafamilial conflict related to acculturation, and the experience of discrimination in the larger culture (Santisteban & Mena, 2009). Issues of immigration and acculturation are addressed by separating out the cultural "content" of the conflict from the family's structural "processes" to allow them to more effectively engage these difficult topics. Santisteban and Mena (2009) also identify open and honest communication about risky sexual behavior as particularly difficult in Hispanic families because of religious and cultural norms; thus, this is a topic that needs culturally sensitive attention and intervention when working with female and male Hispanic youth and their families.

The careful consideration of culture in brief strategic and structural ecosystemic therapies has also identified different needs of ethnic groups. In one study, researchers compared outcomes of structural ecosystemic therapy with Hispanic versus African American drug-using youth, with Hispanics benefiting differently from the treatment (Robbins et al., 2008). Whereas Hispanic youth experienced a decrease in substance use, African American youth did not, but they did report improved racial socialization and family functioning; the researchers propose that these differences may be related to the relative power of each ethnic group in the Miami community, with African Americans being more disenfranchised. In addition, in another study of HIV-positive African American women, structural ecosystemic therapy was found to be better than person-centered therapy and community controls for reducing psychological distress and family-related hassles but did not significantly improve family support. These sometimes puzzling culture-specific findings remind clinicians to be cautious and attentive when working with diverse families.

Asian American Families

Structural family therapy has also been used with Asian American families (Epstein et al., 2012; Kim, 2003). Kim (2003) describes structural family therapy as ideal for Asian Americans, especially first-generation families: "Its useful concepts, such as hierarchy and its advocacy for a parental executive system, boundaries, and subsystems make it ideal for and compatible with Asian American cultural and family values" (p. 391). Specifically, Kim suggests using the structural concept of parental hierarchy to understand the common Asian value of *filial piety,* the value of high respect for and obedience to parents and elders. In most Asian families, children are expected to sacrifice their own desires for the family, a value that is at odds with many social norms in American society; thus, it is a frequent source of conflict in Asian immigrant families. When working with these families, Kim recommends reframing children's disobedience in terms of children seeking peer approval in the dominant culture rather than a betrayal and devaluing of the family, which is how it appears to many Asian parents. The goal with such families is to help them develop more flexible boundaries to allow members to successfully flow between the two cultural worlds. Yang and Pearson (2002) describe successfully using similar structural practices with families in China to reduce relapses in families with a schizophrenic member.

Epstein and colleagues (2012) caution therapists working with Chinese families about several potential missteps. First, structural therapists should avoid mislabeling the collectivist values of closeness as a form of enmeshment, or, alternatively, misreading their preference for privacy as a form of disengagement. Structural therapists should be sensitive to the Chinese cultural taboos about open conflict; thus, interventions that intensify conflict or require the family to enact their private conflict will likely be met with resistance on the part of Chinese clients who are not acculturated to Western norms. Furthermore, families in China are highly child-focused, and efforts to focus directly on the marital subsystem are likely to be met with resistance. In mainland China, most families have the 4–2–1 structure, with four grandparents and two parents focusing all their attention on one child, who is typically expected to be an "ideal child" who achieves in all areas; structural therapists must account for this unique structure, which may be particularly complex with immigrant families.

Sexual and Gender Identity Diversity

Little specific information has been written on using structural therapy with gay, lesbian, bisexual, and transgender couples or families. However, general research on gay and lesbian families indicates that their basic structure and dynamics are similar to (not statistically different from) those of heterosexual couples (Gottman, 2008); therefore, the same broad family structural considerations are generally the same: having clear boundaries, an effective parental hierarchy, and a separation of the spousal/parental subsystems. Research has also found no difference between children raised by same-sex versus those raised by heterosexual parents on measures of well-being, self-esteem, peer relations, and social adjustment (Biblarz & Savci, 2010). Lesbian families are generally found to have highly egalitarian parenting practices, and they tend to equal or surpass heterosexual couples in time spent with children, parenting skill, warmth, and affection (Biblarz & Savci, 2010). In contrast, gay male couples often must redefine their definitions of masculinity and fatherhood and must acknowledge that the development of their family structures is more complex and unique to each couple; however, like lesbian parents, they are more likely to equally share parenting duties and styles than heterosexual couples (Biblarz & Savci, 2010).

When working with gay/lesbian families, therapists also need to consider the unique experience and pressures on these couples and families. Fitzgerald (2010) identifies common issues that therapists must consider when working with gay/lesbian families: children defending their parents, children needing to determine with whom it is safe to share openly about their family, the process of parents coming out to their children, and parents feeling the need to be "perfect" in society's eyes.

Research and the Evidence Base: Structural

Likely because of its elegant simplicity and clarity, the core components of structural therapy have been used to develop several empirically supported treatments, especially those targeting youth:

- Ecosystemic structural family therapy (Lindblad-Goldberg et al., 1998; see below)
- Functional family therapy (Sexton, 2011; see below)
- Brief strategic family therapy (and two related models: structural ecosystemic therapy and structural ecodevelopmental preventive interventions; Szapocznik & Williams, 2000; see Chapter 4)
- Multisystemic family therapy (Henggeler et al., 1998; see Chapter 4)
- Multidimensional family therapy (Liddle, 2002)
- Emotionally focused therapy (Johnson, 2004; see Chapter 6)

These empirically supported treatments generally target adolescents from diverse families and integrate structural therapy components to assess and restructure the family. The most commonly used elements include the concept of interpersonal boundaries, appropriate family hierarchy, and enactments to facilitate relational change.

Clinical Spotlight: Ecosystemic Structural Family Therapy (ESFT)

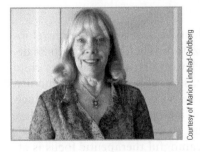

Courtesy of Marion Lindblad-Goldberg

Ecosystemic structural family therapy (ESFT), an empirically supported treatment/supervision/training model was developed by Marion Lindblad-Goldberg initially at the Philadelphia Child Guidance Clinic (1969–1979); it was further elaborated at her Family Therapy Training Center at the University of Cincinnati Medical School (1979–1985), and empirically tested when she returned to Philadelphia to direct the Family Therapy Training Center at the Philadelphia Child Guidance Clinic (1986–1999). The center is now titled The "Philadelphia Child and Family Therapy Training Center" and is its own corporation (1999–present).

ESFT is used to treat a wide range of child, adolescent, and adult clinical or addiction problems across all levels of severity and diverse treatment settings. The empirical support for the ESFT model was conducted in an in-home/community setting and targeted youth who were either at risk of out-of-home placement or who had already spent time in an inpatient or residential setting. The families of these youth tend to be compromised by trauma-induced parental substance abuse, conflictual relationships, emotional disturbance, and the absence of emotional or concrete support (Lindblad-Goldberg et al., 1998; Lindblad-Goldberg & Igle, 2015; Lindblad-Goldberg & Northey, 2013).

The development of ESFT was influenced by Salvador Minuchin (structural family therapy, 1974), Virginia Satir (experiential family therapy, 1964, 1972), John Bowlby (attachment therapy, 1983, 1988), Stanley Greenspan (bio-developmental, 1992), and Bessel van der Kolk (trauma therapy, 1997).

In comparison to structural family therapy, ESFT includes the following;

1. Broader case conceptualization and assessment: Therapists gather more information about the fit of a family in its ecosystem before setting goals, including individual biological, developmental, affective, trauma, relational, and psychological assessment as well as more methodical analysis of larger-system processes (Lindblad-Goldberg et al., 1998).

2. More collaborative therapeutic relationship: In ESFT, therapists have always developed a more collaborative and nonhierarchical relationship with clients, using a strengths-based perspective (Lindblad-Goldberg et al., 1998). In contrast, the position of the therapist in structural family therapy was very hierarchical from its onset in 1974. The development of a more collaborative relationship in structural family therapy has been emphasized since 2007 (Minuchin et al., 2007).

3. Greater emphasis on relational affect, emotion regulation, and the security of attachment: Unlike traditional structural therapists, ESFT therapists focus on affect and emotion regulation both at the family and individual levels as well the quality and patterns of emotional attachment between parents and children (Lindblad-Goldberg & Northey, 2013).

The Big Picture: Overview of Treatment

Ecosystemic structural family therapy (ESFT) has four basic stages:

Stage 1: Constructing a Therapeutic System

In the first phase, therapists identify the relevant parties who need to be part of treatment, including both family and extrafamilial persons. As the "ecosystemic" part of the name implies, the therapist conceptualizes who needs to be part of the process more broadly to include extended family members, caregivers who may not live in the home, school personnel, social workers, clergy, health care providers, etc. ESFT emphasizes the importance of joining on the levels of hierarchy, meaning, and emotional experience at the outset of treatment in order to form a strong therapeutic alliance. This therapeutic alliance will be tested and, if needed, mended throughout the course of treatment.

Stage 2: Establishing a Meaningful Therapeutic Focus

In the second stage, the therapist generates a comprehensive assessment and develops a meaningful focus of treatment from this conceptualization. The therapist gathers descriptions of the child's presenting concerns from all relevant parties and assesses child functioning across all social contexts, including home, school, peers, and community. This assessment process also includes identifying family resources, strengths, and vulnerabilities. Similar to structural therapy, the assessment and intervention processes overlap, often in a cyclical fashion: assess, hypothesize, intervene, and then reassess the family's response (Lindblad-Goldberg & Northey, 2013). A meaningful therapeutic focus is attained when the burden of change is lifted from the shoulders of the symptom-bearer (typically the child) and placed within the context of the symptom-bearer's relationship with the people in his or her life to whom he or she matters the most. The key to generating meaningful therapeutic focus is *reframing* the presenting problem as "something between people" and not "something embedded in the permanent identity of the symptom-bearer."

Stage 3: Creating Key Growth-Promoting Experiences

The focus in stage three is growth, which is facilitated by creating interactional experiences for the family that challenge and dilute the power of the core negative interactional pattern. During this phase, some of the traditional interventions are used, such as directed enactments, boundary making, and continued reframing (Lindblad-Goldberg & Northey, 2013). In addition, ESFT therapists use emotional support and emotional challenge to promote new interactional patterns within the family therapy sessions. These experiments of relational change are aimed at ESFT's essential pillars of healthy family functioning:

1. Increasing parental executive skills
2. Strengthening the caregiver/parental alliance
3. Increasing emotion regulation or distress tolerance individually and as a family
4. Creating age-appropriate secure attachment between parents and children

Stage 4: Solidifying Change and Termination

In the final stage, therapists help families to develop a conceptual understanding of how their new behaviors have enabled them to make their desired changes and help them practice these new behaviors in sessions and between sessions until termination.

The Viewing: Case Conceptualization

ESFT therapists organize their case conceptualization using five interrelated constructs:

Family Structure

Family structure is central to case conceptualization in both traditional structural therapy and ESFT (Lindblad-Goldberg & Northey, 2013). Specifically, they assess for the following:

- Complementary roles
- Mutual expectations with regard to daily operations and routines
- Proximity: affective closeness and distance between family members
- Organization and regulation of the system: boundaries, parameters, etc.
- Power differentials between members and generations (hierarchy)

Core Negative Interactional Patterns

ESFT explores cyclical transactional patterns, called "core negative interactional patterns," that sustain the presenting problem. Therapists assess the family's replication of its core negative interactional patterns in relationships with extrafamilial systems, including schools, community resources, neighborhood, law enforcement, judiciary etc., noting both vulnerabilities and resources available to the family. ESFT therapists use ecomaps, structural maps, genograms, core negative interaction pattern diagrams, and critical life-event time lines as part of this process.

Affective Proximity and Attachment

A significant addition to structural conceptualization, Lindblad-Goldberg has added the language of *affective proximity* and the concept of *attachment* to her theory of relational change (Lindblad-Goldberg & Northey, 2013). Close and securely attached relationships allow family members to feel that they can count on each other and that they are attuned and responsive to one another during times of stress. Secure attachment enhances each family member's ability to regulate emotions and thereby work as a cohesive unit to resolve the presenting problem (Lindblad-Goldberg et al., 1998).

Family and Individual Emotional Regulation and Trauma

Lindblad-Goldberg also adds the concept of trauma and explores the ways that unresolved trauma contributes to family difficulties with emotion regulation in each individual as well as in the family as a whole (Lindblad-Goldberg et al., 1998; Lindblad-Goldberg & Northey, 2013). Patterns of emotion regulation profoundly shape a family's structure and day-to-day interactions by determining how the family handles stress and conflict. Emotional regulation is a major predictor of most childhood and adolescent problems and can clearly predict a child's developmental trajectory. In addition, contemporary neuroscientists have identified untreated trauma as impairing a person's ability to regulate emotions.

Therefore, in ESFT therapy, clinicians assess children and their parents for trauma history, particularly complex histories of trauma and loss (Lindblad-Goldberg & Northey, 2013). People with untreated complex trauma histories tend to have greater difficulty regulating their emotions because of the effects of trauma on the nervous system (Lindblad-Goldberg & Northey, 2013).

Individual Differences and Development

More so than traditional structural therapists, ESFT therapists assess individual differences and needs that include distress tolerance as well as individual developmental, cognitive, biological, historical, learning processes, and temperament and factors associated with race, cultural, socioeconomic status, gender, sexual orientation, and religion (Lindblad-Goldberg & Igle, 2015; Lindblad-Goldberg & Northey, 2013). Seeing, understanding, and responding to these features of the family's ecosystem are considered to be crucial to the clinician's design of a treatment plan that fits the current ecological circumstance of the family (Lindblad-Goldberg & Igle, 2015; Lindblad-Goldberg & Northey, 2013).

Family Development

Similar to traditional structural family therapy, the family life cycle is used to conceptualize client concerns, including normative and nonnormative demands as well as challenges that may come from within or outside the family (Lindblad-Goldberg & Northey, 2013). However, more so than in the past, contemporary ecosystemic work focuses on promoting relationships that enhance the long-term development and maturation of each family member.

Targeting Change: Goals

Lindblad-Goldberg and Northey (2013) identify four overarching goals:

1. Resolve presenting problems and eliminate the core negative interactional pattern that sustains the presenting problems.
2. Shift developmental trajectories of children toward greater capacity for emotional self-regulation and socioemotional intelligence.
3. Recognize patterns of interactions that promote healthy attachment bonds.
4. Enable family to reorganize in such a way as to increase positive and productive engagement with nurturing and growth-promoting community systems.

The Doing: Interventions

The necessary agents of change in ESFT are: (a) the family members in partnership with the therapist and (b) the family–therapist entity in partnership with extrafamilial helpers. ESFT incorporates techniques from many different models of psychotherapy to create relational change. It is the relational objective that determines an intervention's appropriateness. Structural interventions that are used to reorganize or restructure the way family members relate to one another include boundary making, clarifying hierarchy, and enactments. ESFT emphasizes continuing strong therapeutic alliances with all family members.

The most common restructuring interventions used in ESFT are: (1) creating in-session experiments of relational change that flow directly from an interpersonal reframe and (2) validating family members' strengths as they challenge the powerful habits imposed by the core negative interactional pattern. The most common ESFT intervention is *enactment* to help family members practice new ways of relating: adjust the necessary emotional proximity between family members, learn to regulate emotions, and learn to tolerate distress and develop new, positive ways for the family to navigate its ecosystem. Other commonly used techniques address thinking, beliefs, or knowledge in the family; these techniques include reframing, constructing adaptive narratives, psychoeducation, and the use of new rituals to celebrate the family's triumph over the negative interactions that had sustained the presenting problems.

ESFT Supervision/Training Models

The ESFT supervision and training models are isomorphic to the principals of the ESFT treatment model. That is, the supervisor–supervisee relationship and the trainer–trainee relationship are collaborative and nonhierarchical; the supervisee's or trainee's voice is privileged above that of the supervisor or trainer. Relational, experiential activity in both supervision and in training is privileged over lecture just as the best therapy session occurs when the family does all the talking, the best supervision or training occurs when the participant in either context is doing the talking. Emphasis is placed on the use of "raw data" that is, video-recorded sessions in the home or behind a one-way mirror, or having the supervisor live in the in-home session (Lindblad & Igle, 2015).

Clinical Spotlight: Intensive Structural Therapy

Developed by Charles Fishman (2012), intensive structural therapy (IST) was designed to better enable therapists to address interactional processes in a family's broader social context that may impede change, including those in the service delivery network. This approach is brief but concentrated and targets transforming the family's broader context by identifying the specific people or elements that are maintaining the dysfunctional homeostasis. This approach has been used extensively with adolescents diagnosed with anorexia and their families (Fishman, 2006). The four fundamental concepts of this theory are:

1. Social environment: Powerful change is possible by working with key people and forces in the family's social environment, such as extended family, schools, church, and extracurricular activities.
2. Isomorphism: Dysfunctional structural patterns tend to be isomorphically (similar in dynamic) replicated at multiple levels in the family's broader social system. For example, therapists may notice that a family with enmeshed boundaries between the primary caretaker and children may also have an overly involved social worker.
3. Homeostatic maintainer: In dysfunctional systems, some people or social forces serve to maintain the unhealthy family homeostasis through specific interaction patterns. However, this does not imply that one member of the system is blamed for the problematic dynamic. Fishman underscores this fundamental systemic principle, "My rule has always been to confirm [support] the individual and challenge the system—the former at all times, and the latter as needed, and sometimes with intensity" (2012, pp. 79–80).
4. Crisis induction: Similar to traditional structural therapy, crisis induction can be used to create more rapid change.

The Big Picture: Overview of Treatment

Intensive structural therapists use a five-step treatment model to facilitate rapid change (Fishman, 2012):

1. Gathering the members of the system: This step involves first identifying who needs to be involve and, once this is done, identifying who might be missing. Based on the initial contact and description of the problem, the therapist begins to identify who needs to be involved in the treatment system and then motivates them to participate. In some cases, motivating family involvement is challenging. In these situations, the therapist appeals to the family's concerns and their value system as well as underscoring the seriousness of the situation. Once the therapist begins to formulate the case, missing parties may then be identified.

2. Generating goals and planning treatment: Therapists use the four-dimensional assessment described above to identify the goals and plans for treatment. The heart of this step is identifying the homeostatic maintainer and interactional processes.

3. Addressing dysfunctional patterns: In this step, the therapist creates a *therapeutic crisis* to destabilize the system and create discontinuous change, similar to perturbing the system to identify the homeostatic maintainer. Some common methods for creating a therapeutic crisis include:

   ▪ Unbalancing: Therapists can use the structural unbalancing technique (see "The Doing: Interventions," above) in which the therapist temporarily takes sides with the member whose perspective challenges the homeostasis in some way.

   ▪ Amplify present crisis: Similar to crisis induction in traditional structural therapy (see "The Doing," above) and strategic paradoxical directives (see Chapter 4), the therapist can amplify an existing crisis to move the family outside their homeostatic comfort zone.

   ▪ Soft crisis: Therapists can also create a soft crisis, which involves reorganizing the system for "helpful" reasons, such as bringing in help when maintaining the homeostatic pattern requires isolation from others.

4. Establishing and maintaining a new organization: Essential for long-term change, in this step, the therapist targets the family's broader contexts—work, legal, school, hospital, and social service—for change by identifying how these may interfere with the family's new nonsymptomatic structure.

5. Ending therapy: Therapists carefully measure progress using the IST scorecard, which tracks client progress using objective measures determined at the beginning of treatment, such as a achieving a specific weight for an anorexic patient (Fishman et al., 2016). When ending therapy, intensive structural therapists ensure that the family "owns" the change and frame the ending as "unfinished work" to help prepare the family for setbacks and new challenges, which are inevitable in family life.

The Viewing: Case Conceptualization

Assessment in IST involves a four-dimensional model, as discussed below (Fishman, 2012).

Contemporary Developmental Pressures

Intensive structural family therapists begin conceptualization by identifying developmental pressures and challenges on the family using the family life cycle. Each major stage in the cycle—couple union, first child, school-age children, family with adolescents, launching—destabilizes the system and requires it to restructure by shifting the balance of interdependence and independence required in the next stage. In addition, divorce, remarriage, and death necessitate even more complicated structural adaptations for a family. Therapists assess the unique developmental pressures the family is facing to determine the fundamental goals for treatment.

Structure

Similar to traditional structural therapy, IST assesses family structure, focusing on boundaries, hierarchy, complementary patterns, and coalitions. The focus of this assessment is to identify what elements are reinforcing the system's current homeostasis.

History of the System

Next, therapists obtain a history of the system, which includes important family events, births, death, illnesses, major losses, moves, financial strains, career changes, etc. They pay particular attention to any positive or negative destabilizing event that may have increased family stress. The family may have become stuck in shifting their structure to accommodate to the change. As part of this assessment, the therapist takes a careful history of the presenting problem, noting attempted solutions and the various persons involved. In addition, the therapist assesses the symptomatic member to identify any isomorphic processes in their past, such as feeling violated in the current situation and/or a past situation.

Process

Building upon the first three areas of assessment, the therapist then identifies two key structural processes:

- Homeostatic maintainer: The therapist identifies the key person or forces that maintain the dysfunctional structure that keeps the family stuck. In some cases, the *homeostatic maintainer* is readily identifiable, such as parents who do not effectively reinforce problematic child behavior. More often, therapists need to perturb the system to destabilize the current homeostasis (see Chapters 3 and 4) and then observe who or what acts to return the system to status quo. For example, in a family with an underinvolved father, a therapist can perturb the system by staging an enactment that instructs him to be more involved; the therapist then watches to see how others in the system react and how these reactions serve to return the system to its familiar homeostasis.
- Transactional patterns: Once the homeostatic maintainer is identified, the next step is to identify the transactional patterns used to maintain the dysfunctional homeostasis. Therapists look for one or more of these typical patterns:
  - conflict avoidance,
  - schizmogenesis (escalating sequences of complementary or symmetrical behaviors; see Chapter 3)
  - lack of complementarity, which can signal underinvolvement or lack of response on the part of a member
  - enmeshment
  - rigidity
  - overprotectiveness
  - conflict diffusion, when a less-involved family distracts itself from conflict

Measuring Outcomes

In developing the IST model, Charles Fishman was influenced by the words of Peter Drucker: "If you can't measure it, you can't manage it" (Fishman, personal communication). Toward this end, Fishman joined with Friedman (2015), the developer of results-based accountability to develop an effective approach to measuring outcomes in IST. Results-based accountability is a framework utilized by many U.S. states and 30 countries abroad to measure outcomes in multiple disciplines, including health, business, and government. Using this model, treatment begins with all stakeholders agreeing on the treatment goals. Therapists track change over time using a three-part system to measure outcomes in IST:

IST Scorecard

The IST scorecard is designed to enable clinicians to track their outcomes using clear measures and benchmarks (Fishman et al., 2016). Free for download at www.intensivestructuraltherapy.com, the scorecard includes the following elements:

- *Objectives and goals* that are as objectively measured as possible.
- *Plans,* which are the specific interventions that the treatment team will take to achieve the goal.

- *Measures,* which should be as objective as possible, often a relevant psychometric scale and inventory.
- *Targets,* which are the specific score or achievement within a specific timeframe, such as a 10% improvement on a specific inventory.
- *Homeostatic maintainer:* The final element is the identification of the homeostatic maintainer, which is the main barrier to change.

IST Triangulation or IST Single-Parent Scale

Two measures that are specific to intensive structural therapy are often used to measure client progress: the triangulation scale measures the degree to which a child may be triangulated into the couple relationships, and the single-parent scale measures the degree to which there is a sufficient hierarchy in a single-parent family; both forms are available for free download at www.intensivestructuraltherapy.com.

Turning the Curve

Founded on results-based accountability, "turning the curve" refers to aggregating outcome data scores to track a positive direction from baseline, allowing clinicians to measure overall progress and success.

Functional Family Therapy (FFT)

In a Nutshell: The Least You Need to Know

An empirically validated family therapy treatment for working with conduct disorder and delinquency, functional family therapy (FFT) has been studied for over 40 years (Alexander & Parsons, 1982; Alexander & Sexton, 2002; Sexton & Alexander, 2000). Unlike other evidence-based treatments for conduct disorder, FFT has been developed to be used in agency settings as well as by individual practitioners (Sexton, 2011), and that is the reason I highlight it in this book. The approach integrates cognitive theory, systems theory, and learning theory using a combination of structural, strategic, cognitive, and behavioral interventions. In FFT, all behavior is viewed as *adaptive* to serve a particular *function* in the system. Behaviors are viewed as attempts to achieve two basic functions:

- Relational connection: the relative balance of closeness and independence
- Relational hierarchy: defining who has influence and control

The therapist's primary task is to identify the *function* of the problem behaviors—how the behaviors maintain connection and define hierarchy—and then find more effective behaviors that achieve the same basic function (i.e., sense of connection, influence, independence, etc.). Interventions aim to achieve the desired goal or function without the negative consequences that brought the family to therapy. FFT offers therapists a coherent approach for assessing and effectively intervening with families who have children with significant behavioral problems.

The Juice: Significant Contributions to the Field

If you remember one thing from this chapter, it should be the following:

Multisystemic and Family Focus

Similar to other evidence-based treatments for troubled youth, FFT uses a *multisystemic focus,* meaning that the therapy process addresses individual, family, peer, and community system dynamics (Alexander & Parsons, 1982; Sexton, 2011). Furthermore, the evidence is quite clear that the preferred unit of treatment to affect these multiple systems is the *family,* not the individual youth. Research has identified a strong family bond to be one of the most critical protective factors that keep youth out of trouble. Furthermore, current research indicates that group treatment of troubled youth actually augments antisocial behavior rather than reduces it (Lebow, 2006). If you check with your local juvenile justice courts, you may find that teen anger management or adolescent substance abuse classes are mandated for many youth in trouble with the law; it is likely these groups are making the problem worse rather than better. Findings like this underscore the importance of research to help therapists identify when commonsense solutions don't work.

In FFT, the therapist works with the youth's school, probation officer, peers, community, extended family, and immediate family to effect change. This may involve direct interventions with persons in these systems or more indirectly affecting larger systems by helping the youth and family interact with them differently (e.g., increasing parental communication with the school may start to change how teachers, counselors, and/or administrators view and therefore interact with the youth and thereby trigger a cascade of positive changes).

Rumor Has It: People and Places

James Alexander

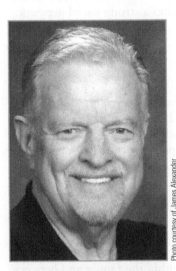

Photo courtesy of James Alexander

James Alexander developed FFT with Bruce Parsons in the 1960s while working at the University of Utah (Sexton, 2011). Alexander had a strong background in systemic theory and used it to build his theory, which was originally developed to help youth in the juvenile justice system.

Bruce Parsons

Beginning as a graduate student in the 1960s, Bruce Parsons has continued to work with James Alexander to develop FFT.

Thomas Sexton

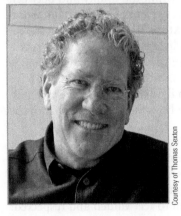

Courtesy of Thomas Sexton

Thomas Sexton (2011) is a well-known practitioner and proponent of FFT, authoring a text that describes how the approach can be used in standard outpatient clinical settings.

The Big Picture: Overview of Treatment

Early Phase: Engagement and Motivation

In the first phase, the therapist aims: (a) to develop a connection with all members of the family and (b) to assess the *function* of the problem behaviors (Alexander & Sexton, 2002; Sexton, 2011). During this phase, the therapist works to reduce anger, blame, and hopelessness. Therapists create a context conducive to change by using cognitive techniques to reduce parents' tendencies to blame the problem on negative characteristics of the child (e.g., laziness or irresponsibility) and to replace these characterizations with descriptions that do not impute negative motives (e.g., experimenting with freedom, exploring identity).

Middle Phase: Behavioral Change

In the middle phase, the therapist aims to modify cognitive sets, attitudes, expectations, labels, and beliefs so that family members see how their actions are interrelated (Alexander & Sexton, 2002). Therapists specifically target parenting skills, negativity, and blaming and intervene by making comments about the impact of a behavior on others; describing the interrelation of feelings, thoughts, and behavior; offering interpretations; stopping negative interactions; relabeling behaviors in nonblaming terms; discussing the implications of symptom removal; changing the context of a symptom; and shifting the focus from one person or problem to another.

Once the family's cognitive set has been changed, the therapist focuses on building interpersonal and practical skills, such as *parent training, problem solving, conflict resolution,* and *communication skills.* Parent training is emphasized with younger children and follows traditional behavioral parenting interventions using operant conditioning principles. Problem solving and conflict resolution are favored when helping parents and older adolescents address their conflict. Communication skills training is based on traditional behavioral techniques that encourage brevity, directness, and active listening.

Late Phase: Generalization

The focus during this phase is to generalize change to the larger social systems in which the family interacts (Alexander & Sexton, 2002). The therapist now works more as a caseworker to encourage families to develop positive relations with community systems, such as mental health and juvenile justice authorities, and to develop a strong social network.

Making a Connection: The Therapeutic Relationship

Alliance: Between Family Members and with Therapist

In FFT, the therapist develops an **alliance** with the family and also helps build up a sense of alliance between family members (Alexander & Sexton, 2002; Sexton, 2011). This alliance is considered a personal connection that includes feeling understood and having trust in the other. What makes the alliance specifically therapeutic is the additional agreement on the goals and tasks of the therapy process. In FFT, a typically family approach, alliance means all members of the family feel safe, heard, and are in agreement about the direction of therapy. The family members feel that they are "on the same page" with each other as well as the therapist.

Motivation and Engagement

If the therapist is successful in creating a sense of alliance within the family and between the therapist and family, this typically results in a subtle yet essential element for therapeutic success: **motivation** (Alexander & Sexton, 2002; Sexton, 2011). Otherwise stated, the purpose of a strong therapeutic alliance is to motivate clients to take the action necessary for change. Although some family members may have some motivation for change upon entering therapy, often the unspoken—or sometimes said aloud—hope is to have the therapist do something to fix another person in the family. Thus, through a strong alliance, the therapist helps inspire all family members to see how they can be a part of the solution and be willing to do so.

Engagement involves having all members of the family actively participating in sessions. Therapists facilitate engagement by using humor, demonstrating respect, sincerely attempting to understand, and bringing therapeutic presence to the room. Moreover, therapists encourage family engagement by bringing a nonblaming and strength-based perspective to the conversation, one that allows each person to feel valued and respected.

Mandated and Reluctant Clients

Because FFT targets delinquent youth, many of the families that come are mandated by an external third party, such as a court or school, or contain at least one member reluctant to be in therapy (sometimes the parent, sometimes the child, sometimes both; Alexander & Sexton, 2002). In addition, most of them have had many painful experiences as well as difficulties and unfair treatment in school, justice, and other systems. Thus, FFT therapists *expect* their clients to come feeling wary, hopeless, blaming, resistant, negative, or otherwise not in a good place (Sexton, 2011).

The FFT therapist's systemic perspective is often experienced as a refreshing reprieve from the family's experiences with other professionals and systems. This systemic perspective refrains from blaming any member of the family and instead encourages them to see the bigger picture and how all members—as well as external systems—contribute to and sustain the problem. This new perspective inspires hope that things can be different and that the family can take action to make meaningful change.

Spirit of Respect and Collaboration

A subtle but particularly important element of FFT is the attitude that the therapist brings to working with youth and families that typically have not been treated well by the system (Sexton, 2011). Often, long before seeing a therapist, delinquent youth have been labeled as failures and outcasts, and their parents are often seen in a similar light. Thus, therapists need to be particularly aware of engaging these families from a place of respect, valuing their experience, and creating space for them to share their side of the story. This requires patience and openness to learning from the client as well as a willingness to engage in a sincere collaborative partnership in the therapeutic process.

Credible Helper

FFT therapists are aware of the importance of having credibility in the eyes of the family. Credibility is not established by promises of future gains but rather by what the therapist says and does in the therapy room, starting with the first session. Therapists need to be able to demonstrate that they understand the family's situation and have effective ways of intervening and assisting the family. This relates closely to the common factor of establishing hope.

The Viewing: Case Conceptualization and Assessment

Relational Functions: The Glue

Like other systemic therapists, when assessing families, FFT therapists identify the **relational functions** of the problem behavior (Sexton, 2011; Sexton & Alexander, 2000). In general, FFT therapists focus on the two essential relational functions of behaviors: (a) relational connection and (b) relational hierarchy.

Relational Connection

Similar to the concept of boundaries in structural therapy, FFT therapists use the concept of **relational connection** to describe how families balance a sense of interdependence (connectedness) and independence (autonomy). In general, there are three ways families can balance these. One is not necessarily better than another; each family's preference is highly influenced by cultural norms:

- High independence: families that value high independence support autonomy and independence but may also risk distance and disengagement
- High interdependence: families that value high interdependence may enjoy closeness and connection but also risk enmeshment and dependency
- Midpointing: these families strive for a balance between the above two

Try It Yourself

> **With a partner or on your own, describe the pattern of relational connection in your family of origin. What were the strengths and limits of this pattern? Describe any ethnic, racial, or religious influences.**

Relational Hierarchy

Relational hierarchy describes relational control and influence in the relationship. There are three general patterns that families can fall into:

- Parent up/adolescent down: The parent–child relationship can have a traditional hierarchy, in which the parent has more power and the child less; of course, this can range from a small power difference to an extreme power difference.
- Adolescent up/parent down: In some families, the power hierarchy is reversed and the adolescent has more influence over outcomes than the parent; this is rarely an appropriate arrangement.
- Symmetrical: Some families have a strong democratic structure in which parents and children have similar levels of power.

Changing the Expression, Not the Function

So, if you have been reading along thinking that the therapist's job is to help families get into some of the categories listed above and out of others, you are in for a surprise. FFT therapists are *not* trying to help all families have the same style or to achieve some "optimal" form of functioning: that would be disrespectful to cultural and individual family differences and needs. Instead, the goal is to help families find better *expressions* of the same function. For example, if parents are using verbally and physically abusive methods to maintain hierarchy, the FFT therapist will help these parents learn new ways to maintain hierarchy that are not abusive. Similarly, FFT therapists would help parents who overfunction for their children to find ways to express their connection and affection that are contingent on the child's appropriate behavior.

RELATIONAL FUNCTION ASSESSMENT

So, the question is this: what function does the symptom serve?

- To create independence or interdependence?
- To establish hierarchy or distribute power?

The next question is this:

- How can the family achieve a similar function with more effective relational interactions?

Answer these questions and you have a plan for success.

Risk and Protective Factors

FFT therapists are quick to identify the various known **risk and protective factors** for troubled youth. Some of these include (Sexton & Alexander, 2000; Sexton, 2011):

Individual Youth and Parent Risk Factors

- History of violence or victimization
- History of early aggressive behavior and general poor behavior control
- Substance, alcohol, and/or tobacco use/abuse
- Diagnosis of an emotional or psychological concern, including attention-deficit/hyperactivity disorder (ADHD), or other deficits in social, cognitive, or information processing
- Low IQ
- Antisocial beliefs or attitudes

Family Risk Factors

- Lack of mutual attachment and nurturing by parents
- Ineffective parenting
- Chaotic home environment
- Lack of a significant relationship with a caring adult
- Caregiver who abuses drugs, commits crimes, or is diagnosed with a mental disorder

Peer/School Risk Factors

- Associates with other troubled youth, including gang involvement
- Frequent social rejection by peers
- Lack of involvement in conventional activities
- Poor academic performance; little commitment to school

Community Risk Factors

- Diminished economic opportunities; high concentration of poor residents
- High level of transience and low levels of community participation
- High levels of family disruption

Protective Factors

- Strong bond between children and family
- Parental involvement in child's life
- Supportive parenting that meets financial, emotional, cognitive, and social needs of child
- Clear limits and consistent enforcement of discipline

Multisystemic Assessment

In FFT, troubled youth are never assessed apart from the multiple systems they inhabit; thus, it is an **ecosystemic approach** (Alexander & Parsons, 1982; Sexton, 2011; Sexton & Alexander, 2000). FFT therapists view people as being made up of internal systems (physiological, cognitive, emotional, behavioral, etc.) that are in constant interaction with multiple external systems, such as the family, neighborhood, school, peers, employment, human service agencies, cultural groups, region, etc. A client's behavior is assessed in terms of the *function* it plays in each of these systems. For example, a youth's or parent's poor choices are not seen as isolated, individual problems but rather as having particular meaning and effects in the multiple systems of which they are a part. Similarly, the interconnection of these systems is also a source of resilience and support, both potential and actualized. Therapists attend to both the untapped resources, potential resources, and negative influences in the multiple systems and use these to inform the direction of therapy. Identifying the effects of multiple systems helps therapists know where and with whom to intervene.

Community and Culture

When assessing families, FFT therapists carefully attend to the family's cultural and community contexts (Sexton & Alexander, 2000). Informed by ethnic and religious norms, "cultural expectations contribute to patterns of interaction within the family, the ways it expresses emotion and organizes around roles, how the roles generally look and feel, and parenting style" (Sexton, 2011, pp. 2–13). Community contexts refer to the family's local community, which is influenced by the cultures that compose them but are a unique expression of them, often combined with regional and other social influences.

When working with delinquent youth, culture and community are of particular importance. Although ethnic minorities make up approximately one-third of the youth population, they account for two-thirds of the population in juvenile detention and correction centers (Sexton, 2011). Furthermore, youth of color are arrested more often, spend more time in detention, and tend to be given longer sentences. Thus, minority and white delinquent youth come to therapy with very different contexts, and the therapy process needs to be responsive to these different experiences.

CULTURAL AND COMMUNITY QUESTIONS TO CONSIDER

- **Cultural Background:** What is the family's cultural background(s)? In which ways do they identify with this background? In which ways do they not?

- **Culture and Family Norms:** What are the norms for family structure, hierarchy, role, and emotional expression in the family's culture? In which ways does the family embrace these? In which ways do they not? How does this compare with norms from their local and regional community?

- **Local Community:** How does the family fit within their local community? Are they connected to meaningful and supportive groups within the community? How are their problems viewed within this community? Are there support persons that can be engaged?

- **Socioeconomic Context:** How does the family's socioeconomic status affect their role in the community and contribute to the problems they experience?

- **Adapting Therapy:** How does the therapy process need to be adapted to be respectful of the family's cultural and community contexts, values, and norms? What type of therapeutic relationship, goals, assessments, and interventions would be most useful?

Strengths and Resiliency

FFT therapists strive to reach a healthy balance between seeing both client problems (glass half empty) and strengths (glass half full) (Sexton, 2011). When working with troubled youth, this balance can be especially challenging because their problems are often in the realm of criminality and are harmful to others, not just themselves. Thus, it is easy to fall into the trap of either labeling the teen as "bad" or "antisocial" or naively viewing everything as a "big mistake." Instead, the therapist is challenged to find a much more uncomfortable position of acknowledging both the bad and the good, even if the good is difficult to see at first.

Commonly Assessed Strengths in Troubled Youth and Their Parents

- A bond of love between one or more family members
- Extended family members or community members who care and are reliable
- At least one prosocial friend
- A meaningful hobby, interest, or ability
- Passing grades
- Holding a job
- A history of doing well socially, in school, or with the family

Targeting Change: Goal Setting

Goals of Initial Phase: Engagement

1. Reduce within-family risk factors
2. Reduce blame and negativity in the family
3. Increase family alliance and family-focused view of problem

Goals of Working Phase: Behavior Change

1. Increase behavioral competencies (e.g., parenting, communication, problem solving) that fit for the family
2. Match these competences to family's relational function

Goals of Closing Phase: Generalization

1. Increase within context protective factors
2. Generalize
3. Support and maintain gains

The Doing: Interventions

Developing a Family-Focused Problem Description

In the initial sessions, FFT therapists help families move from a blame-focused definition of the problem to developing a family-focused definition. This family-focused definition helps build a sense of understanding, alliance, and motivation. The therapist begins by asking each family member to describe the problem, its causes, and how it affects him or her (Sexton, 2011). Based on this, the therapist can identify blaming, problem attributions, and emotions as well as develop a sense of relational patterns and family structure.

Next, the therapist uses reframing to help family members see how their seemingly individual behaviors are part of a larger family interaction pattern: for example, it may be that a teen stays out late to avoid getting pulled into his parents' arguments.

Identifying the Problem Sequence

Similar to strategic and behavioral family therapies (see Chapters 4 and 8), FFT therapists identify the relational sequence or pathologizing interpersonal pattern (PIP) around the presenting problem. This boils down to:

- What behaviors (from all family members) came before the problem?
- What behaviors (from all family members) come after the problem?

Therapists can often assess this indirectly by observing interactions in session as well as from the family's description of the presenting problem. In addition, therapists sometimes directly ask about the problem sequence in order to more carefully assess it.

Relational Reframing

In the initial phases of FFT, therapists help families change the interpretations and meanings about the problem, a process known as *cognitive restructuring*. Therapists move families from blaming another member of the family for the problems to helping them see how the problem is relational: everyone plays a part in maintaining the problem behaviors (Sexton, 2011). Thus, problems are *reframed relationally* to reduce malicious and negative attributions and increase understanding and hope.

FFT therapists use a three-phase process for relational reframing (Alexander & Sexton, 2002; Sexton, 2011):

1. Acknowledgment: Acknowledge each person's initial position, views, understandings, and feelings. Acknowledgment statements—such as "You got really angry"—show that the therapist understands and supports the importance but not necessarily the content of the client's statement. *The therapist avoids generalizations and normalizing comments, and instead focuses on the client's personal experience.*

2. Reattribution: In the next phase, the therapist offers a reattribution for the problem behavior, which generally takes one of three forms:

   - An alternative explanation for the problem behavior (e.g., "perhaps he is getting high to avoid his feelings of being a failure").
   - A metaphor that implies an alternative construction of the problem (e.g., perhaps his drug use is his way of "self-medicating" his ADHD).
   - Humor to imply that not everything is as it seems (e.g., perhaps his drug use is his way of communing with his ancestors and showing respect for a nonconformist family tradition).

   For reframing to be successful, it must include the concept of responsibility: the problem behavior was intended, but the motivation was not as malevolent as it might appear.

3. Assess the impact of the reframe and build on it: Finally, the therapist listens to the family's response to assess the "fit": Is it meaningful and useful to the family? The therapist often works with the client to modify the reframe so that it better fits with each member's worldview. The goal is to find a mutually agreeable—or at least plausible—alternative explanation for the problem behavior. The reframing process is likely to continue across sessions, as the family more finely tunes the possible explanations.

Building Organizational Themes

An outcome of reframing, **organizational themes** are used to describe how the problematic behaviors are motivated by *positive but misguided* intentions (Sexton, 2011). These themes help family members reattribute more positive qualities to one another. Themes are most useful when they are mutually developed by the family and therapist. Common themes are (Sexton, 2011, pp. 4–23):

- Anger implies hurt
- Anger implies loss
- Defensive behavior implies emotional bonds
- Nagging equals importance
- Pain interferes with listening
- Differences can be frightening
- Protection often involves shutting others out

These organizing themes help to describe the origin of the problem without blaming any one person, eliciting greater understanding if not compassion for one another. Ideally, the theme is mutually developed so that it is meaningful to all members of the family while also feeling supportive. Most often, these themes help focus the family on the big picture—such as feeling loved, safe, and valued—rather than getting lost in the details.

Interrupting and Diverting to Structure Sessions

When families begin to escalate or start self-defeating patterns, FFT therapists actively intervene to interrupt or divert the conversation to help structure the session (Sexton, 2011). For example, if a parent begins berating the child, the therapist quickly steps in to stop the unhelpful rant: "I can hear that you are very frustrated by your son's behavior. Can you please describe how it is affecting you?" Such comments stop potentially harmful interactions and keep the therapy on track. In addition, FFT therapists use coaching ("Why don't you try …?), directing (Wait, use the problem-solving steps), or modeling to also help redirect families.

Process Comments

A particular form of diverting, FFT therapists use **process comments** to draw the family's attention to the immediate interactions in the room. These comments serve two functions: (a) they interrupt the problem behavior patterns and (b) they help the family become more consciously aware of the patterns. The process comments can focus on the behavioral sequence patterns or functions of the behaviors. For example, "Did you notice that before he finished making the request, you jumped in with an answer based on your assumption about what he was going to say?" or "Are you noticing how the silence and refusal to look up is how you hold on to your sense of power in the relationship?"

Parent Skill Training

FFT therapists help parents be more effective based on current scientific literature on parenting behaviors that are associated with risk factors and protective factors for youth behavioral problems (Sexton, 2011). For example, supportive yet challenging parenting is predictive of better school performance and social adjustment than authoritarian parenting. In addition, clear expectations with consistent reinforcement has long been associated with fewer emotional and behavioral problems. While parent training may be more effective with younger children, Sexton (2011) and colleagues have found that with adolescents, parenting strategies are best learned by helping families alter their family relational sequences in family therapy.

When working with parents, FFT focuses on three areas:

- Clear expectations and rules: Create mutually agreed-upon and developmentally appropriate behavioral expectations that are concrete and specific. In some cases, *contracts* that specify the rules are written down and signed by all parties, which can help adolescents feel actively involved in the process.
- Active monitoring and supervision: Help parents take an active role in monitoring their children, which is summed up by answering the following: "Who is the teen with? Where is he or she? What is he or she doing? When will he or she be home?" (Sexton, 2011, pp. 5–14)
- Consistent and enforcement of behavioral contingencies: Although most parents of troubled youth hope for a set of consequences that will magically inspire flawless role-model behavior overnight, FFT therapists recognize that consequences are not as effective with teens as with younger children. However, the process of having parents and teens negotiate reasonable terms is more likely to be beneficial (Sexton, 2011). If consequences are to be used, FFT therapists recommend that they be brief, done without anger, and directly linked to the behavior in question (e.g., taking financial responsibility for damages or writing a letter of apology).

Mutual Problem Solving

A subset of parenting skills, problem solving in FFT involves helping parents and children work together to address concerns in a way that strengthens the relationship rather than have the parents dictate how problems will be solved (Sexton, 2011). The typical steps in problem solving include:

- Identify the problem: Defining the problem in relational terms (everyone shares responsibility) and in concrete, behavioral terms (e.g., yelling, drinking and driving, etc.).
- Identify the outcome desired: As simple as it sounds, it is especially important in families with troubled youth to identify the desired outcome in specific, behavioral terms; this discussion alone can help resolve some issues (e.g., having a relatively calm discussion about expectations in which no one curses, raises their voice, or insults another and everyone is seeking a reasonable solution).
- Agree on how to accomplish the goal: Next, the family identifies each person's role in helping to solve the problem; this may involve written contracts or agreements.
- Identify potential obstacles: In most cases, it helps to identify potential obstacles and barriers before trying to act on the plan.
- Reevaluation of outcomes: Finally, the goals are evaluated to establish accountability and determine next steps.

Conflict Management

Some families have painful histories and/or rigid patterns that make it difficult to successfully solve problems In such cases, therapists need to help them move past these past hurts and struggles. Conflict management may not "solve" the painful issue but instead is used by the therapist to help contain difficult interactions. Some commonly used strategies for containing conflict include:

- Remaining focused on a specific issue: The therapist keeps the family focused on a specific current issue rather than bringing up unresolved past issues.
- Adopting a conciliatory mind-set and willingness to talk: The therapist sets an emotional tone that helps reduce conflict.
- Staying oriented to the present: The therapist keeps the focus on reducing the conflict rather than trying to directly solve extremely volatile issues or "rehearsing" them.

If family members get stuck in an issue, the therapist may use the following questions to help move the process forward:

- Exactly what is the issue of concern for you?
- Exactly what would satisfy you?
- How important is that goal to you?
- Have you tried to get what you want through problem solving?
- How much conflict are you willing to risk to get what you want? (Sexton, 2011, pp. 5–18)

Communication Skill Building

In FFT, the family's communication skills are often addressed as part of helping the family resolve their concerns; however, it is not a goal by itself: it is a means to other ends, such as problem solving and parenting. In helping families restructure their interactions, FFT therapists may focus on one or more of the following issues to help improve family communication:

- Responsibility: Each person takes responsibility for his or her words and communications and avoids speaking for others (e.g., not say "in this house" or "kids should …").
- Directness: Families are encouraged to direct their comments to the intended recipient and avoid third-person comments (e.g., "no one in this house" or "she never").
- Brevity: Messages should be kept short to ensure that the recipient understands.
- Concrete and specific: Families are taught to avoid generalizations (e.g., "you never") and broad statements (e.g., "make a good decision") and to make very specific requests for action.
- Congruence: Helping family members have verbal and nonverbal messages that match and are consistent (e.g., not sounding angry when you say everything is okay).
- Active listening: Therapists help family members learn how to be responsive listeners in ways that are natural for them (e.g., a head nod to signal that you have heard the other's message—remember that may be a big step for a teen who hasn't communicated with parents in years).

Matching to Fit the Family

In FFT, therapists maintain realistic goals for their clients. They do not expect their clients to communicate and interact in some idealistic "perfect family" way. Instead, they use ideal forms of communication, parenting, and conflict management to help them develop realistic modifications of the family's current interactions that will help them have better outcomes. For example, many therapists consider yelling "unhealthy" and are quick to target yelling for change. However, in FFT, the therapist first assesses how the yelling functions in the family—how it creates closeness and distance and determines hierarchy—before determining whether and how it needs to change. The key is to introduce new behavioral skills that *fit* for a particular family.

- Matching to the problem sequence: When targeting the sequence of problem interactions, the therapist looks for the easiest (rather than the ideal) place to introduce a new behavior.
- Matching to the relational functions: Rather than trying to change the fundamental quality of relational functions (interdependence, independence, and hierarchy), the therapist helps the family find more effective ways of maintaining the same relational function (e.g., rather than avoid conflict, use a relatively short, structured approach to problem resolution, *or* to express closeness, find mutually enjoyable activities that help the family feel connected rather than having a parent ask a series of endless questions).
- Matching to organization theme: Interventions are linked back to the organization themes identified early in treatment to create a sense of coherency and continuity.

Scope It Out: Cross-Theoretical Comparison

Using Tomm's IPscope described in Chapter 3 (Tomm et al., 2014), this theory approaches the conceptualization of systemic, interpersonal patterns as discussed below.

Case Conceptualization

One of the few approaches that consistently uses all interpersonal patterns, FFT identifies the relational and hierarchy functions of the PIP in their case conceptualizations. In addition, FFT therapists formally assess a broad range of sociocultural interpersonal patterns (SCIPs) as part of their case conceptualization.

Goal Setting

Functional family therapists focus on creating several forms of WIPs:

- Within the family: WIPs that are developmentally appropriate relational bonds and hierarchy
- With the community: WIPs between the adolescent and family with relevant sociocultural systems, including school, peer, extended family, community, neighborhood, etc.

Facilitating Change

FFT therapists use two basic classes of TIPs to facilitate change: systemic and psychoeducational. Systemic interventions include relational reframing, identifying the problem sequence, developing a family-focused problem definition, building organization themes, and interrupting to structure sessions. In addition, they use psychoeducational techniques such as parent training, mutual problem solving, and communication skill training to help the family develop competencies.

Putting It All Together: FFT Case Conceptualization and Treatment Plan Templates

Areas for Theory-Specific Case Conceptualization: FFT

When conceptualizing client cases, functional family therapists typically use the following dynamics to inform their treatment plan. Go to MindTap® **to** access a digital version of the theory-specific case conceptualization, along with a variety of digital study tools and resources that complement this text and help you be more successful in your course and career. If your instructor didn't assign MindTap, you can find out more about it at Cengagebrain.com. You can also download the form at masteringcompetencies.com.

Relational Connection

Describe the family's preferred approach to relational connection:

- High independence
- High interdependence
- Midpointing

Relational Hierarchy

Describe current hierarchy in the family

- Parent up/adolescent down
- Adolescent up/parent down
- Symmetrical

Relational Function of Symptoms

What function does the symptom serve?

- To create independence or interdependence?
- To establish hierarchy or distribute power?

How can the family achieve a similar function with more effective relational interactions?

Risk and Protective Factors

Individual Youth and Parent Risk Factors

- History of violence or victimization
- History of early aggressive behavior and general poor behavior control
- Substance, alcohol and/or tobacco use/abuse
- Diagnosis of an emotional or psychological concern, including ADHD, or other deficits in social, cognitive, or information-processing
- Low IQ
- Antisocial beliefs or attitudes

Family Risk Factors

- Lack of mutual attachment and nurturing by parents
- Ineffective parenting
- Chaotic home environment
- Lack of a significant relationship with a caring adult
- Caregiver who abuses drugs, commits crimes, or is diagnosed with a mental disorder

Peer/School Risk Factors

- Associates with other troubled youth, including gang involvement
- Frequent social rejection by peers
- Lack of involvement in conventional activities
- Poor academic performance; little commitment to school

Community Risk Factors

- Diminished economic opportunities; high concentration of poor residents
- High level of transience and low levels of community participation
- High levels of family disruption

Protective Factors
- Strong bond between children and family
- Parental involvement in child's life
- Supportive parenting that meets financial, emotional, cognitive, and social needs of child
- Clear limits and consistent enforcement of discipline

Multisystem Assessment

Describe the function of symptomatic behavior in other social systems, such as neighborhood, school, peers, employment, human service agencies, cultural groups, region, etc.

Culture and Community

- Cultural background: What is the family's cultural background(s)? In which ways do its members identify with this background? In which ways do they not?
- Culture and family norms: What are the norms for family structure, hierarchy, role, and emotional expression in the family's culture? In which ways does the family embrace these? In which ways do they not? How does this compare with norms from their local and regional community?
- Local community: How does the family fit within their local community? Are they connected to meaningful and supportive groups within the community? How are their problems viewed within this community? Are there support persons who can be engaged?
- Socioeconomic context: How does the family's socioeconomic status affect its role in the community and contribute to their problems?
- Adapting therapy: How does the therapy process need to be adapted to be respectful of the family's cultural and community contexts, values, and norms? What type of therapeutic relationship, goals, assessments, and interventions would be most useful?

Strengths and Resiliency

Describe forms of individual and family strengths and resiliency.

TREATMENT PLAN TEMPLATE FOR FAMILY: FFT

You can download a blank treatment plan (with or without measures) on MindTap at www.cengagebrain.com or www.masteringcompetencies.com. The following treatment plan template can be used to help you develop individualized treatments for use with distressed families.

FFT Treatment Plan: Client Goals with Interventions

Early-Phase Client Goal
1. Decrease *within-family blame* and increase *within-family alliance* to reduce within-family conflict.
   a. *Identify the problem sequence,* including each family member's role in the dynamic, to reduce within-family blame.
   b. *Reframe the problem* and interactions *in relational terms* and identify *organization themes* to reduce within-family blame and increase motivation to change and sense of family alliance.

Working-Phase Goals
1. Increase family's *relational competencies* (e.g., parenting, communication, problem solving) to reduce within-family conflict and improve problem interaction sequence.
   a. *Parent training* and/or *mutual problem solving* matched to the family's problem sequence, relational functioning, and/or organization themes.
   b. *Conflict management* and/or *communication skill training* matched to the family's problem sequence, relational functioning, and/or organization themes.

2. Change *expression of relational functions* to reduce conflict and conduct issues.
   a. *Interrupt self-defeating patterns* and *coach* or *direct* family in more functional interactions.
   b. Use *process comments* to increase family's awareness of their interaction patterns.
   c. *Conflict management, parent training, problem solving,* and/or *communication skill training* matched to the family's problem sequence, relational functioning, and/or organization themes.

3. Increase adolescent's and family's *protective factors* to reduce frequency of conduct issues.
   a. Identify and *engage resources* in other systems: peer, school, social service, community, etc.
   b. Build on *organizational themes* to help teen and family access their own strengths and resources.

Closing-Phase Goals

1. Increase *positive interactions* with [specify *external system:* school, peer, extended family, etc.] to reduce conflict and conduct issues
   a. *Generalize problems solving, conflict management, and communication skills learned* to improve relationships with persons outside the family.
   b. Identify potential *sources of support in the community,* including sources of emotional support, information, and practical assistance.

2. Increasing family's *self-efficacy* and within-family alliance to reduce conflict.
   a. *Coaching* family to successfully respond to new challenges as they arise.

Process comments *to reinforce new, functional patterns.*

Treatment Tasks

1. Build family *engagement* in therapy and their *motivation.*
   a. Demonstrate *respectful* and *collaborative attitude* with each member of the family to create a context of safety.
   b. Develop motivation by establishing self as a *credible helper.*

2. Assess individual, systemic, and broader cultural dynamics. Strategies include:
   a. Assessing *relational function,* including *relational connection* (balance of independence and interdependence) and *relational hierarchy.*
   b. Assessing *risk and protective factors* as well as *strengths and resiliency.*
   c. Assessing how *multiple systems* (school, peer, extended family, community, social service agencies, cultural group, etc.) intersect with family problems and resiliency.
   d. Identifying *organizational themes* that characterize family conflict.

3. Identify needed referrals, crisis issues, collateral contacts, and other client needs. (Note: With troubled teens this often includes probation officers, school counselors, psychiatrists, etc. Also, current research does not support group treatments for conduct-disordered youth; thus, these should not be included.)
   a. *Crisis assessment intervention(s):* Address crisis issues such as psychological abuse, intimate partner violence, hidden affair, self harm, suicidal ideation, substance use, etc.
   b. *Referral(s):* Connect client with *resources* in client's *family and community* that could be supportive; make collateral contacts as needed.

Tapestry Weaving: Diversity Considerations
Ethnic, Racial, and Cultural Diversity

FFT is an approach that has been widely used but not necessarily widely studied with ethnically diverse populations (Hennegler & Sheidow, 2012; Sexton, 2011). In a large

Florida-based study examining the effectiveness of FFT across diverse groups, no significant differences were found in terms of recidivism, posttreatment crime severity, and program completion rates (Dunham, 2010). Embedded within the approach's view of relational function is a respect for a wide variety of family structures, allowing it to be applicable to culturally diverse family forms. The therapist respects culture by acknowledging the relational function of problem exchanges and helping the family to find more effective ways to meet those functions, whether by establishing a more hierarchical or democratic family structure or allowing for more interdependence or independence between family members. Thus, the therapist adapts the goals based on the family's cultural norm, allowing them to honor both collectivist and individualist value systems. Of course, immigrant families are likely to have a significant difference in values between generations, which cannot always be easily bridged, but FFT has many strategies to help create a meaningful common ground.

Research on FFT with diverse populations provides clinically relevant guidance for therapists using FFT with diverse families. For example, one study found that Hispanic adolescents had better outcomes when they worked with a Hispanic therapist; however, in the same study, ethnic match did not affect outcomes for Anglo adolescents (Flicker et al., 2008). This study underscores the importance of cultural competence for Anglo therapists and the need to attend to ethnic match with diverse clients when possible. Future research is likely to refine the implementation recommendations for ethnically diverse families.

Sexual and Gender Identity Diversity

Little has been written specifically about FFT and lesbian, gay, bisexual, transgendered, and questioning (LGBTQ) youth or families. Greenan (2010) describes how he used structural therapy as his main framework and integrated mindfulness and elements of experiential dynamic therapy to successfully work with a gay couple. In addition, one case study has considered using FFT principles when working with a gay male (Datchi-Phillips, 2011). Using FFT and general family systems principles, Datchi-Phillips recommends assessing the multiple systems of which a LGBTQ client is a member, including family of origin, current relationship, LGBTQ community, school, work, neighborhood, religious community, etc. Each system is likely to have a unique response to the client's sexuality. Furthermore, the family's organizing theme may be useful for LGBTQ individuals to make sense of and depersonalize some of their own struggles. Datchi-Phillips also emphasizes that often people who identify as LGBTQ are not fully accepted by their families of origin and therefore must create their own "families." When appropriate these "family members" should also be involved in treatment. Furthermore, an individual's apparent "pathology" should be viewed within the network of family and other social contexts, helping reframe the youth's problem in ways that are less blaming and more hopeful.

Research and the Evidence Base: FFT

With its first efficacy trial over 40 years ago, FFT was one of the first evidence-based treatments (Baldwin et al., 2012; Henggeler & Sheidow, 2012). Used internationally, FFT is one of four widely recognized family treatments for adolescent conduct issues that appears to be moderately superior to other forms of treatment or treatment-as-usual (Baldwin et al., 2012). Over the years, FFT has been on the vanguard with many "firsts" and landmark trials in the research world. For example, the study by Alexander and Parsons (1973) was the one of the first clinical trials to show favorable outcomes in the juvenile justice system. In addition, FFT was the first to have an efficacy study conducted by independent investigators, researchers not directly associated with the theory being studied (and therefore less likely to be biased) (Hennegler & Sheidow, 2012). In addition, they had one of the largest trials to examine the transportability of FFT to real-world settings (Sexton & Turner, 2010). In addition, the rates of adolescent recidivism and relapse have been correlated to the therapist's adherence to the model (Sexton & Turner, 2011). In sum, FFT has a strong evidence base for treating conduct-disordered and substance-abusing youth; future research will hopefully refine applications, especially with diverse families.

QUESTIONS FOR PERSONAL REFLECTION AND CLASS DISCUSSION

1. Describe how the structure of your family of origin reflects its racial, ethnic, religious, gender, and/or socioeconomic backgrounds.

2. Minuchin describes the self-as-the-therapist as the primary tool in therapy, referring to how you use yourself to create relational experiences—including conflict and contradiction—for families to respond to. Provide some examples of how you might do this. What types of relational experiences might be most difficult for you: initiating conflict, confronting beliefs, engaging in emotional intimacy, discussing sex?

3. Enactments are used frequently in structural therapy and in several evidence-based therapies. What benefits do you see to using enactments? What limitations?

4. In FFT, the relational function of the symptom is not challenged, only the means for achieving it. Describe racial, ethnic, religious, and socioeconomic factors that may influence the process of shifting the relational function for a given family.

5. Virtually all evidence approaches for adolescent conduct and substance abuse issues are family-based and rely primarily on structural and systemic–strategic therapy models. What does that tell us about these teen issues?

6. Ecosystemic structural therapy, intensive structural therapy, and FFT all emphasize the broader systems in which families are embedded. How might you go about assessing these systems, which can include school, neighborhood, work, court system, social services, etc.?

7. Describe the potential changes in family structure when an LGBTQ teen or young adult "comes out" and the family is accepting vs. rejecting vs. somewhere in between. What changes in structure are likely if one parent is accepting and the other is not?

ONLINE RESOURCES

The Minuchin Center

www.minuchincenter.org

Philadelphia Child and Family Therapy Training Center

www.philafamily.com

Intensive Structural Therapy

www.intensivestructuraltherapy.com

Brief Strategic Family Therapy Training

www.brief-strategic-family-therapy.com

Functional Family Therapy

www.functionalfamilytherapy.com and www.fftllc.com

National Juvenile Justice Publication on FFT

www.ncjrs.gov/pdffiles1/ojjdp/184743.pdf

Go to MindTap® for an eBook, videos of client sessions, activities, practice quizzes, apps, and more—all in one place. If your instructor didn't assign MindTap, you can find out more information at CengageBrain.com.

REFERENCES

*Asterisk indicates recommended introductory readings.

Alexander, J. F., & Parsons, B. V. (1973). Short-term behavioral intervention with delinquent families: Impact on family process and recidivism. *Journal of Abnormal Psychology, 81*(3), 219–225. doi:10.1037/h0034537

*Alexander, J., & Parsons, B. V. (1982). *Functional family therapy.* Belmont, CA: Brooks/Cole.

Alexander, J., & Sexton, T. L. (2002). Functional family therapy (FFT) as an integrative, mature clinical model for treating high risk, acting out youth. In J. Lebow (Ed.), *Comprehensive handbook of psychotherapy, Vol. IV: Integrative/Eclectic* (pp. 111–132). New York: Wiley.

Aponte, H. J. (1994). *Bread and spirit: Therapy with the new poor: Diversity of race, culture, and values.* New York: Norton.

Aponte, H. J. (1996). Political bias, moral values, and spirituality in the training of psychotherapists. *Bulletin of the Menninger Clinic, 60*(4), 488–502.

Baldwin, S., Christian, S., Berkeljon, A., & Shadish, W. (2012). The effects of family therapies for adolescent delinquency and substance abuse: A meta-analysis. *Journal of Marital and Family Therapy, 38,* 281–304.

Biblarz, T. J., & Savci, E. (2010). Lesbian, gay, bisexual, and transgender families. *Journal of Marriage and Family, 72*(3), 480–497. doi: 10.1111/j.1741-3737.2010.00714.x

Bowlby, J. (1983). *Attachment and loss* (vol.1, 2nd ed.). New York: Basic Books.

Bowlby, J. (1988). *A secure base: Parent-child attachment and healthy human development.* New York: Basic Books.

*Colapinto, J. (1991). Structural family therapy. In A. S. Gurman & D. P. Kniskern (Eds.), *Handbook of family therapy* (vol. 2, pp. 417–443). New York: Brunner/Mazel.

Datchi-Phillips, C. (2011). Family systems (the relational contexts of individual symptoms). In C. Silverstein (Ed.), *The initial psychotherapy interview: A gay man seeks treatment* (pp. 249–264). Amsterdam, the Netherlands: Elsevier. doi:10.1016/B978-0-12-385146-8.00012-2

Dunham, J. (2010). Examining the effectiveness of functional family therapy across diverse client ethnic groups. *Dissertation Abstracts International Section A, 70*(12–A), pp. 45–86.

Epstein, N. B., Berger, A. T., Fang, J. J., Messina, L. A., Smith, J. R., Lloyd, T. D., & ... Liu, Q. X. (2012). Applying western-developed family therapy models in China. *Journal of Family Psychotherapy, 23*(3), 217–237. doi: 10.1080/08975353.2012.705661

Fishman, H. C. (1988). *Treating troubled adolescents: A family therapy approach.* New York: Basic Books.

Fishman, C. (2004). *Enduring change in eating disorders: Interventions with long-term results.* New York: Routledge.

Fishman, C. (2006). Juvenile anorexia nervosa: Family therapy's natural niche. *Journal of Marital and Family Therapy, 32,* 505–514.

Fishman, C. (2012). *Intensive structural therapy: Treating families in their social context.* New York: Basic Books.

Fishman, C. (2013). *You can fix your family.* Seattle, WA: CreateSpace.

Fishman, C., Morris, J., & Fishman, T. (2016). *The IST clinical scorecard: A tool for improving outcomes.* Unpublished manuscript.

Fitzgerald, T. (2010). Queerspawn and their families: Psychotherapy with LGBTQ families. *Journal of Gay & Lesbian Mental Health, 14*(2), 155–162. doi:10.1080/19359700903433276

Flicker, S. M., Waldron, H., Turner, C. W., Brody, J. L., & Hops, H. (2008). Ethnic matching and treatment outcome with Hispanic and Anglo substance-abusing adolescents in family therapy. *Journal of Family Psychology, 22*(3), 439–47. doi:10.1037/0893-3200.22.3.439

Friedman, M. (2015). *Turning curves: An accountability companion reader.* Seattle, WA: CreateSpace.

Greenspan, S. I. (1992). *Infancy and early childhood: The practice of clinical assessment and intervention with emotional and developmental challenges.* Madison, CT: International Universities Press.

Gottman, J. M. (2008, April). *Marriage counseling: Keynote address.* Annual Conference of the American Counseling Association, Honolulu, HI.

Greenan, D. E. (2010). Therapy with a gay male couple: An unlikely multisystemic integration. In A. S. Gurman (Ed.), *Clinical casebook of couple therapy* (pp. 90–111). New York: Guilford.

Hammond, R. T., & Nichols, M. P. (2008). How collaborative is structural family therapy? *Family Journal, 16*(2), 118–124. doi: 10.1177/1066480707313773

Henggeler, S., & Sheidow, A. (2012). Empirically supported family-based treatments for conduct disorder and delinquency in adolescents. *Journal of Marital and Family Therapy, 38,* 30–58.

Henggeler, S. W., Schoenwald, S. K., Borduin, C. M., Rowland, M. D., & Cunningham, P. B. (1998). *Multisystemic treatment of antisocial behavior in children and adolescents.* New York: Guilford.

Johnson, S. M. (2004). *The practice of emotionally focused marital therapy: Creating connection* (2nd ed.). New York: Brunner/Routledge.

Kim, J. M. (2003). Structural family therapy and its implications for the Asian American family. *Family Journal, 11*(4), 388–392. doi: 10.1177/1066480703255387

Lebow, J. (2006). *Research for the psychotherapist: From science to practice.* New York: Routledge.

Liddle, H. A. (2002). *Multidimensional family therapy treatment for adolescent cannabis users.* Rockville, MD: Substance Abuse and Mental Health Services Administration.

Lindblad-Goldberg, M., Dore, M., & Stern, L. (1998). *Creating competence from chaos.* New York: Norton.

Lindblad-Goldberg, M., & Igle, E. A. (2015). Grandparents raising grandchildren: An ecosystemic structural family therapy (ESFT) treatment approach. In S. Browning, K. Pasley, S. Browning, & K. Pasley (Eds.), *Contemporary families: Translating research into practice* (pp. 248–266). New York: Routledge.

Lindblad-Goldberg, M., & Northey, W. F. (2013). Ecosystemic structural family therapy: Theoretical and clinical foundations. *Contemporary Family Therapy, 35*(1), 147–160. http://doi.org/10.1007/s10591-012-9224-4

*Minuchin, S. (1974). *Families and family therapy.* Cambridge, MA: Harvard University Press.

*Minuchin, S., & Fishman, H. C. (1981). *Family therapy techniques.* Cambridge, MA: Harvard University Press.

Minuchin, S., Montalvo, B., Guerney, B. G., Rosman, B., & Schumer, F. (1967). *Families of the slums.* New York: Basic Books.

Minuchin, S., & Nichols, M. P. (1993). *Family healing: Tales of hope and renewal from family therapy.* New York: Free Press.

Minuchin, S., Nichols, M. P., & Lee, W. Y. (2007). *Assessing families and couples: From symptom to system.* New York: Allyn & Bacon.

Minuchin, S., Reiter, M. D., & Borda, C. (2014). *The craft of family therapy.* New York: Routledge.

Minuchin, S., Rosman, B., & Baker, L. (1978). *Psychosomatic families: Anorexia in context.* Cambridge, MA: Harvard University Press.

Robbins, M. S., Szapocznik, J., Dillon, F. R., Turner, C. W., Mitrani, V. B., & Feaster, D. J. (2008). The efficacy of structural ecosystems therapy with drug-abusing/dependent African American and Hispanic American adolescents. *Journal of Family Psychology, 22*(1), 51–61. doi: 10.1037/0893-3200.22.1.51

Santisteban, D. A., Coatsworth, J., Perez-Vidal, A., Mitrani, V., Jean-Gilles, M., & Szapocznik, J. (1997). Brief structural/strategic family therapy with African American and Hispanic high-risk youth. *Journal of Community Psychology, 25*(5), 453–471. doi:10.1002/(SICI)1520-6629(199709)25:5<453::AID-JCOP6>3.0.CO;2-T

Santisteban, D. A., & Mena, M. P. (2009). Culturally informed and flexible family-based treatment for adolescents: A tailored and integrative treatment for Hispanic youth. *Family Process, 48*(2), 253–268. doi: 10.1111/j.1545-5300.2009.01280.x

Satir, V. (1964). *Conjoint family therapy, A guide to theory and technique.* Palo Alto, CA: Science and Behavior Books.

Satir, V. (1972). *Peoplemaking.* Palo Alto, CA: Science and Behavior Books.

Sexton, T. L. (2011). *Functional family therapy in clinical practice: An evidence-based treatment model for working with troubled adolescents.* New York: Routledge.

Sexton, T. L., & Alexander, J. F. (2000, December). Functional family therapy. *Juvenile Justice Bulletin,* U.S. Department of Justice, NCJ 184743.

Sexton, T., & Turner, C. W. (2010). The effectiveness of functional family therapy for youth with behavioral problems in a community practice setting. *Journal of Family Psychology, 24*(3), 339–348. doi:10.1037/a0019406

Sexton, T., & Turner, C. W. (2011). The effectiveness of functional family therapy for youth with behavioral problems in a community practice setting. *Couple and Family Psychology: Research and Practice, 1*(S), 3–15.

Szapocznik, J., Feaster, D. J., Mitrani, V. B., Prado, G., Smith, L., Robinson-Batista, C., & … Robbins, M. S. (2004). Structural ecosystems therapy for HIV-seropositive African American women: Effects on psychological distress, family hassles, and family support. *Journal of Consulting and Clinical Psychology, 72*(2), 288–303. doi:10.1037/0022-006X.72.2.288

Szapocznik, J., Hervis, O. E., & Schwartz, S. (2003). *Brief strategic family therapy for adolescent drug abuse* (NIH publication no. 03-4751). NIDA Therapy Manuals for Drug Addiction. Rockville, MD: National Institute for Drug Abuse.

Szapocznik, J., Kurtines, W., Santisteban, D. A., & Pantín, H. (1997). The evolution of structural ecosystemic theory for working with Latino families. In J. G. García & M. C. Zea. (Eds.), *Psychological interventions and research with Latino populations* (pp. 166–190). Needham Heights, MA: Allyn & Bacon.

Szapocznik, J., & Williams, R. A. (2000). Brief Strategic Family Therapy: Twenty-five years of interplay among theory, research and practice in adolescent behavior problems and drug abuse. *Clinical Child and Family Psychology Review, 3*(2), 117–134.

Tomm, K., St. George, S., Wulff, D., & Strong, T. (2014). *Patterns in interpersonal interactions: Inviting relational understandings for therapeutic change.* New York: Routledge.

Van der Kolk, B. A. (1997). *The psychobiology of posttraumatic stress disorder. Journal of Clinical Psychiatry 58*(9), 16–24.

Wylie, M. S., & Minuchin, S. (2013, September/October). The therapist's most important tool:

Salvador Minuchin on what today's training approaches are missing. *Psychotherapy Networker.* Retrieved from http://www.psychotherapynetworker.org.

Yang, L., & Pearson, V. J. (2002). Understanding families in their own context: Schizophrenia and structural family therapy in Beijing. *Journal of Family Therapy, 24*(3), 233–257. doi: 10.1111/1467-6427.00214

Structural Case Study: Teen Conduct Issues

Bill and Sally bring their son Tom in for therapy after he was suspended a second time for getting into a fight at school. Six months ago, the family moved across town when Bill was transferred, just before Tom was about to start high school. An above-average student in middle school, Tom is now in danger of failing the ninth grade. Bill and Sally have been arguing more since the move, with Bill working longer hours at the new job, leaving Sally to handle the kids. John, Tom's younger brother, is reportedly doing well with the move and tries to stay out of the conflict.

After meeting with the family, a structural family therapist developed the following case conceptualization.

STRUCTURAL CASE CONCEPTUALIZATION

For use with individual, couple, or family clients.

Date: 6/2/16   **Clinician:** Albert Luis, MFT Trainee   **Client/Case #:** 9002

Introduction to Client & Significant Others

Identify significant persons in client's relational/family life who will be mentioned in case conceptualization:

Adults/Parents: Select identifier/abbreviation for use in rest of case conceptualization

AF1:   Female   Age: 40   European American   Married heterosexual   Occupation: pediatric nurse   Other: Italian American

AM1:   Male   Age: 44   European American   Married heterosexual   Occupation: bank executive   Other identifier: Irish American

Children/Adult Children: Select identifier/abbreviation for use in rest of case conceptualization

CM1:   Male   Age: 14   European American   Grade: 9th   School: Alexander High School   Other: track team

CM2:   Male   Age: 12   European American   Grade: 7th   School: Barton Middle School   Other identifier: jazz band

Others: Identify all: _____

Presenting Concerns

Describe each significant person's description of the problem:

AF1:   States that AM44 too harsh on CM14 and that CM14 is just adjusting to HS.

AM1:   States that AF40 too lenient on CM14 and that CM14 is not learning responsibility and is on the road to becoming a failure.

CM1:   States that he is adjusting to HS and move; trying to make friends at a new school and learning how to study.

CM2:   States that his brother and father fight more recently; believes CM14 is rebelling like all teenagers do.

Broader System: Description of problem from extended family, referring party, school, legal system, etc.: Extended Family: AM44's family blames AF40 for being too lenient; AF40s family sees both parents as not being strict enough or effective.

School counselor: States that she believes CM14 is not living up to his potential; has "defiance" issues; difficulty fitting in at school.

Teacher: States that CM14 has difficult time focusing in the classroom.

Background Information

Trauma/Abuse History (recent and past): Both parents report physical punishment as children but deny using it themselves.

Substance Use/Abuse (current and past; self, family of origin, significant others): There is a history of alcohol abuse on both sides of the family.

Precipitating Events (recent life changes, first symptoms, stressors, etc.): After performing above average in middle school, CM14 began high school six months ago after family moved across town because of AM44's job transfer. He was suspended two weeks ago because of fistfight with peer (second incident); he is currently in danger of failing two classes. CM14 reports being motivated to keep his grades up to stay on the track team. He reports experimenting with drinking and pot in the past year. AF40 and AM44 have been arguing more since the move, and CM14 has been having problems in school. CM12 is reportedly doing well. AM44 has been working longer hours with the new job, and AF40 reports he is not helping out like he did before.

Related Historical Background (family history, related issues, previous counseling, medical/mental health history, etc.): Report "normal" family before now: summer vacations, sports and music activities; nightly dinners. AM44 says he went through a "rebellious" period when he was a teen but he never let his grades drop and was never suspended. No reported health concerns.

Family Life Cycle Stage

Check all that apply:

☐ Single Adult
☐ Committed Couple
☐ Family with Young Children
☒ Family with Adolescent Children
☐ Divorce
☐ Blended Family
☐ Launching Children
☐ Later Life

Describe struggles with mastering developmental tasks in one or more of these stages: Family having difficulty adjusting to CM14 adjusting to high school; difficulty helping CM14 take on more freedom and responsibility.

Subsystems

Describe who is in each subsystem and the general dynamics of the subsystem and how the subsystem is related to the presenting problem:

- Parental, including grandparents, stepparents, parentified children: AF40 and AM44

- Couple: Is this system distinct from the parental subsystem? Not really. Since having children the marital relationship has not been well maintained; the couples primary relationship is the coparenting relationship.

(continued)

Subsystems (*continued*)

• Sibling, including step-siblings: <u>CM14 and CM12</u>

• Other: <u>See coalitions below.</u>

Hierarchy

Hierarchy between Parents and Children: ☐ NA

AF1: ☐ Effective ☐ Insufficient (permissive) ☐ Excessive (authoritarian) ☒ Inconsistent/Variable

AM1: ☐ Effective ☐ Insufficient (permissive) ☒ Excessive (authoritarian) ☐ Inconsistent/Variable

Description/Example to illustrate: <u>AF40 inconsistent and lenient; AM44 too harsh in response.</u>

Boundaries

Boundaries with/between:

Primary Couple ☒ Enmeshed ☐ Clear ☐ Disengaged ☐ NA Describe: <u>Each partner wants the other to see situation the way he/she does. Conflict often arises when they have differences of opinion or different emotional responses.</u>

AF1: & Children ☒ Enmeshed ☐ Clear ☐ Disengaged ☐ NA Describe: <u>AF is more</u> emotionally connected to the children than her husband.

AM1: & Children ☒ Enmeshed ☐ Clear ☐ Disengaged ☐ NA Describe: <u>AM is emotionally</u> overinvolved in CM's behavior and sees son's poor choices as sign he is a failure as a father.

Siblings ☐ Enmeshed ☐ Clear ☒ Disengaged ☐ NA Describe: <u>Although close in age,</u> the brothers are fairly disengaged from each other.

Extended Family ☒ Enmeshed ☐ Clear ☐ Disengaged ☐ NA Describe: <u>Extended family can</u> become involved in couple arguments.

Friends/Peers ☐ Enmeshed ☒ Clear ☐ Disengaged ☐ NA Describe: <u>Generally clear</u> boundaries with friends.

Broader Community ☐ Enmeshed ☒ Clear ☐ Disengaged ☐ NA Describe: <u>School counselor</u> appropriately supportive.

Describe patterns of managing closeness and distance, especially when conflict arises: _____

Coalitions

☒ Cross-generational coalitions: Describe: <u>AF40 takes CM14's side in most arguments against AM44.</u>

☒ Coalitions within family of origin: Describe: <u>AM44 agrees with parents that AF40 is not strict</u> enough with the children.

☐ Other coalitions: _____

Complementary Patterns

Complementary Patterns between <u>AF40</u> *and* <u>AM44</u>:

☐ Pursuer/distancer

☐ Overfunctioner/underfuntioner

☐ Emotional/logical

☒ Good/bad parent

☐ Other: _____

Example of pattern: AF40 tends to take the side of CM14 and AM44 is the disciplinarian. The pattern was evident but not as extreme when the kids were younger.

Role of Symptom in the System
Describe relation between the family and symptom:
☐ Family as ineffectual "challenger" of the symptom:
☐ Family as "shaper" of the individual's symptom: _____
☒ Family as "beneficiary" of the symptom: *Couple is able to avoid marital issues by focusing on CM14's behavioral issues.*

Problematic or Contradictory Family Rules and Myths
Describe the family's rules, myths, values, and/or standards that are related to the presenting problem; these often include unspoken rules about achievement, emotional expression, loyalty, valuing of members, etc:

The family seems to be enacting several myths related to gender. First, AF enacts the ideal of "mother as a nurturer," which is strong in her Italian background. The father is also holding strong to his ideas of what it means to be a "man" and how fathers should raise sons.

Client/Family Strengths and Social Location
Strengths and Resources:

Personal: *CM14 is motivated to get his grades up to stay on track team; he and CM12 have made new friends in the neighborhood; AM44 doing well in promotion; both parents motivated to improve situation at home.*

Relational/Social: *CM14 has supportive counselor and good relationship with two teachers; CM14 is close with one uncle, who serves as mentor; has made some friends at new school.*

Spiritual: *AM44 and AF40 are Catholic and use their spiritual tradition to keep them connected; semi-active in local church.*

Based on the client's social location—age, gender race, ethnicity, sexual orientation, gender identity, social class, religion, geographic region, language, family configuration, abilities, etc.—identify potential resources and challenges:

Unique Resources: Strong extended family connections on both Irish and Italian sides; church has been a resource, especially for AF.

Potential Limitations: Parent's move across town to a wealthier neighborhood fulfills a dream for the parents but is creating unexpected stress on the kids who have a more difficult time fitting in; also creating difficulty for whole family to rebuild social network.

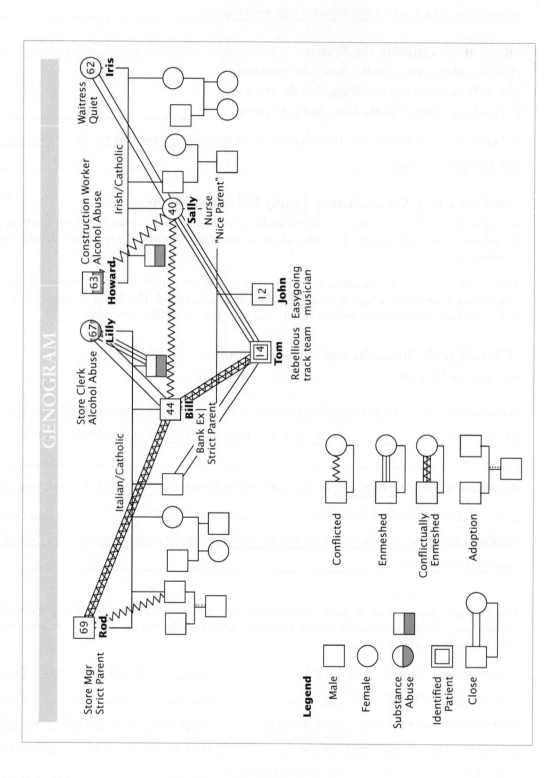

CLINICAL ASSESSMENT

Clinician: Albert Luis, MFT Trainee	Client ID #: 9002	Primary configuration: ☐ Individual ☐ Couple ☒ Family	Primary Language: ☒ English ☐ Spanish ☐ Other: _____

List client and significant others

Adult(s)

Adult Male Age: 44 European American Married heterosexual Occupation: bank executive Other identifier: Irish American

Adult Female Age: 40 European American Married heterosexual Occupation: pediatric nurse Other identifier: Italian American

Child(ren)

Identified Patient: Child Male Age: 14 European American Grade: 9th School: Alexander High School Other identifier: track team

Child Male Age: 12 European American Grade: 7th School: Barton Middle School Other identifier: jazz band

Others: _____

Presenting Problem(s)

Complete for children:

☐ Depression/hopelessness
☐ Anxiety/worry
☒ Anger issues
☐ Loss/grief
☐ Suicidal thoughts/attempts
☐ Sexual abuse/rape
☒ Alcohol/drug use
☐ Eating problems/disorders
☐ Job problems/unemployed

☐ Couple concerns
☒ Parent/child conflict
☐ Partner violence/abuse
☐ Divorce adjustment
☐ Remarriage adjustment
☐ Sexuality/intimacy concerns
☒ Major life changes
☐ Legal issues/probation
☐ Other: _____

☒ School failure/decline performance
☐ Truancy/runaway
☒ Fighting w/peers
☐ Hyperactivity
☐ Wetting/soiling clothing
☐ Child abuse/neglect
☐ Isolation/withdrawal
☐ Other: _____

Mental Status Assessment for Identified Patient

Interpersonal	☐ NA	☒ Conflict ☒ Enmeshment ☐ Isolation/avoidance ☐ Harassment ☐ Other: _____
Mood	☐ NA	☐ Depressed/Sad ☐ Anxious ☐ Dysphoric ☒ Angry ☒ Irritable ☐ Manic ☐ Other: _____
Affect	☐ NA	☒ Constricted ☐ Blunt ☐ Flat ☐ Labile ☐ Incongruent ☐ Other: _____
Sleep	☐ NA	☐ Hypersomnia ☐ Insomnia ☒ Disrupted ☐ Nightmares ☐ Other: _____
Eating	☒ NA	☐ Increase ☐ Decrease ☐ Anorectic restriction ☐ Binging ☐ Purging ☐ Other: _____
Anxiety	☒ NA	☐ Chronic worry ☐ Panic ☐ Phobias ☐ Obsessions ☐ Compulsions ☐ Other: _____
Trauma symptoms	☒ NA	☐ Hypervigilance ☐ Flashbacks/Intrusive memories ☐ Dissociation ☐ Numbing ☐ Avoidance efforts ☐ Other: _____

(continued)

Mental Status Assessment for Identified Patient *(continued)*

Psychotic symptoms	☒ NA	☐ Hallucinations ☐ Delusions ☐ Paranoia ☐ Loose associations ☐ Other:
Motor activity/speech	☐ NA	☐ Low energy ☒ Hyperactive ☐ Agitated ☐ Inattentive ☐ Impulsive ☐ Pressured speech ☐ Slow speech ☐ Other:
Thought	☐ NA	☒ Poor concentration ☐ Denial ☐ Self-blame ☐ Other-blame ☐ Ruminative ☐ Tangential ☐ Concrete ☐ Poor insight ☐ Impaired decision-making ☐ Disoriented ☐ Other:
Sociolegal	☐ NA	☐ Disregards rules ☒ Defiant ☐ Stealing ☐ Lying ☐ Tantrums ☐ Arrest/incarceration ☒ Initiates fights ☐ Other:
Other symptoms	☒ NA	

Diagnosis for Identified Patient

Contextual Factors considered in making diagnosis: ☒ Age ☒ Gender ☒ Family dynamics ☒ Culture ☐ Language ☐ Religion ☐ Economic ☐ Immigration ☐ Sexual/gender orientation ☐ Trauma ☐ Dual diagnosis/comorbid ☐ Addiction ☐ Cognitive ability ☐ Other:

Describe impact of identified factors on diagnosis and assessment process: Norms of teen behavior considered; substance use identified as potential problem and will monitor.

DSM-5 Level 1 Cross-Cutting Symptom Measure (optional): Elevated scores on: (free at psychiatry.org) ☒ I Depression ☒ II Anger ☐ III Mania ☒ IV Anxiety ☐ V Somatic ☐ VI Suicide ☐ VII Psychosis ☐ VIII Sleep ☐ IX Memory ☐ X Repetitive ☐ XI Dissociation ☐ XII Personality ☐ XIII Substance ☐ Not administered

DSM-5 Code	Diagnosis with Specifier *Include Z/T-Codes for Psychosocial Stressors/Issues*
1. F43.24	1. Adjustment Disorder with Disturbance of Conduct, acute
2. Z62.820	2. Parent–child relational problem
3.	3.
4.	4.
5.	5.

List Specific DSM-5 Criterion Met for Diagnosis

1. Stressor: Move to new neighborhood/school; start HS
2. Significant drop in grades
3. Two physical fights at school
4. Increased defiance at home, esp with AM
5. Began experimenting with alcohol and pot use (1–2 times per week)

Medical Considerations

Has patient been referred for psychiatric evaluation? ☐ Yes ☒ No

Has patient agreed with referral? ☐ Yes ☐ No ☒ NA

Psychometric instruments used for assessment: ☒ None ☐ Cross-cutting symptom inventories ☐ Other:

(continued)

Diagnosis for Identified Patient *(continued)*

Client response to diagnosis: ⊠ Agree ☐ Somewhat agree ☐ Disagree ☐ Not informed for following reason: _____

Current Medications (psychiatric & medical) ⊠ NA

1. _____ ; dose _____ mg; start date: _____
2. _____ ; dose _____ mg; start date: _____
3. _____ ; dose _____ mg; start date: _____
4. _____ ; dose _____ mg; start date: _____

Medical Necessity: *Check all that apply*
⊠ Significant impairment ☐ Probability of significant impairment ⊠ Probable developmental arrest

Areas of impairment:
⊠ Daily activities ⊠ Social relationships ⊠ Health ⊠ Work/school ☐ Living arrangement
☐ Other: _____

Risk and Safety Assessment for Identified Patient

Suicidality	**Homicidality**	**Alcohol Abuse**
⊠ No indication/denies	⊠ No indication/denies	☐ No indication/denies
☐ Active ideation	☐ Active ideation	☐ Past abuse
☐ Passive ideation	☐ Passive ideation	⊠ Current; Freq/amt: drunk 1–2x/mo
☐ Intent without plan	☐ Intent without means	**Drug Use/Abuse**
☐ Intent with means	☐ Intent with means	☐ No indication/denies
☐ Ideation in past year	☐ Ideation in past year	☐ Past use
☐ Attempt in past year	⊠ Violence past year	⊠ Current drugs: Marijuana
☐ Family or peer history of completed suicide	⊠ History of assaulting others	Freq/amt: 1–2x/mo
	☐ Cruelty to animals	⊠ Family/sig. other use

Sexual & Physical Abuse and Other Risk Factors
☐ Childhood abuse history: ☐ Sexual ☐ Physical ☐ Emotional ☐ Neglect
☐ Adult with abuse/assault in adulthood: ☐ Sexual ☐ Physical ☐ Current
☐ History of perpetrating abuse: ☐ Sexual ☐ Physical ☐ Emotional
☐ Elder/dependent adult abuse/neglect
☐ History of or current issues with restrictive eating, binging, and/or purging
☐ Cutting or other self harm: ☐ Current ☐ Past: Method: _____
☐ Criminal/legal history: _____
☐ Other trauma history: _____
⊠ None reported

Indicators of Safety

☐ NA
⊠ At least one outside support person
⊠ Able to cite specific reasons to live or not harm
☐ Hopeful
☐ Willing to dispose of dangerous items
⊠ Has future goals

☐ Willingness to reduce contact with people who make situation worse
☐ Willing to implement safety plan, safety interventions
⊠ Developing set of alternatives to self/other harm
☐ Sustained period of safety: _____
☐ Other: _____

(continued)

Elements of Safety Plan

☐ NA
☒ Verbal no harm contract
☐ Written no harm contract
☒ Emergency contact card
☒ Emergency therapist/agency number
☐ Medication management:

☒ Plan for contacting friends/support persons during crisis
☐ Specific plan of where to go during crisis
☐ Specific self-calming tasks to reduce risk before reach crisis level (e.g., journaling, exercising, etc.)
☐ Specific daily/weekly activities to reduce stressors
☐ Other: _____

Legal/Ethical Action Taken: ☒ NA ☐ Action: _____

Case Management

Collateral Contacts

• Has contact been made with treating *physicians or other professionals:* ☐ NA ☒ Yes ☐ In process.
Name/Notes: Called pediatrician to assess and help monitor substance use.

• If client is involved in mental health *treatment elsewhere*, has contact been made? ☐ NA ☒ Yes ☐ In process.

Name/Notes: School counselor
• Has contact been made with *social worker:* ☒ NA ☐ Yes ☐ In process. Name/Notes: _____

Referrals

• Has client been referred for *medical assessment:* ☒ Yes ☐ No evidence for need
• Has client been referred for *social services:* ☒ NA ☐ Job/training ☐ Welfare/Food/Housing ☐ Victim services ☐ Legal aid ☐ Medical ☐ Other: _____

• Has client been referred for *group* or other support services: ☒ Yes: teen group at school ☐ In process ☐ None recommended

• Are there anticipated *forensic/legal processes* related to treatment: ☒ No ☐ Yes; describe: _____

Support Network

• Client social support network includes: ☒ Supportive family ☐ Supportive partner ☐ Friends ☒ Religious/spiritual organization ☐ Supportive work/social group ☐ Other: _____
• Describe anticipated effects treatment will have on others in support system (Children, partner, etc.): Parents involved in treatment; adjust parenting; CM12 also attend.
• Is there anything else client will need to be successful? Parents may need to address couple issues.

Expected Outcome and Prognosis

☒ Return to normal functioning ☐ Anticipate less than normal functioning ☐ Prevent deterioration
Client Sense of Hope: 5 Moderate hope

Evaluation of Assessment/Client Perspective

How were assessment methods adapted to client needs, including age, culture, and other diversity issues?
Used language CM14 and CM12 could understand; respectful of cultural, gender expectations. Using teen-friendly language; allowing family to discuss traditions and values. Considered CM14 behavior in broader system, including parents' conflicting parenting styles and confused parental hierarchy cross-generational coalition.

Describe actual or potential areas of client–clinician agreement/disagreement related to the above assessment:
CM14 does not view situation as "big" problem; AM sees as bigger problem than AF.

_____, _____ _____
Clinician Signature   License/Intern Status   Date

_____, _____ _____
Supervisor   License   Date

TREATMENT PLAN

Date: 06/2/2016   **Case/Client #:** 9002

Clinician Name: Albert Luis, MFT Trainee   **Theory:** Structural

Modalities planned: ☐ Individual Adult ☐ Individual Child ☐ Couple ☒ Family ☐ Group: _____
Recommended session frequency: ☒ Weekly ☐ Every two weeks ☐ Other: _____
Expected length of treatment: 4 months

Treatment Plan with Goals and Interventions
Early-Phase Client Goal

1. Increase clarity of parent–child boundaries by defining parental hierarchy while simultaneously increasing CM14's responsibility for his choices and actions to reduce CM14's need to drink and smoke to distract family from the issues they are avoiding.).

   Measure: Able to sustain pro-social interactions for period of 2 ☐ wk ☒ mo with no more than 0 mild episode of _violence_.

   a. Reframing to increase CM14's internal motivation to choose pursing meaningful life goals over violence.

   b. Separate parenting sessions to strengthen parental coalition by developing an agreed-upon approach to parenting CM14 in regards to fighting at school.

Working-Phase Client Goals

1. Increase clarity of boundaries and mutually satisfying interactions between AF40 and CM14 to reduce enmeshment and clarify parental hierarchy to reduce fights.

   Measure: Able to sustain mutually satisfying exchanges for period of 2 ☐ wk ☒ mo with no more than _1_ mild episode of arguing in a two-week period.

   a. Enactments that reduce aggressive communications, reinforce parental hierarchy, and reduce enmeshment (e.g., direct family to begin reenacting argument from past week and redirect to improve communication and clarify boundaries).

   b. Separate parental sessions to create parental coalition and alliance.

2. Increase and strengthen CM14's personal boundaries by increasing his responsibility for conduct and life direction to reduce parent–child enmeshment to improve grades and motivation.

   Measure: Able to sustain responsibilities at home and school for period of 2 ☐ wk ☒ mo with no more than 1–2 mild episodes of _poor grades, failure to do chores, etc.

   a. Shaping competency by complimenting CM14 and highlighting areas of mature decision making, drawing on motivation to stay on track team (e.g., "Once you made the decision to improve your grades to stay on the team, you knew exactly what to do without your parents telling you").

Treatment Plan with Goals and Interventions (*continued*)

b. Reframe CM14 "rebelling" against father as "wanting to be seen as an adult"; extend metaphor to identify more effective ways of showing father that he is an adult than using drugs and alcohol; draw on cultural, religious, and intergenerational definitions of being a "man."

3. Increase and strengthen parental coalition and marital subsystem boundaries to increase sense of emotional connection to reduce parent–child conflicts.

Measure: Able to sustain effective coalition for period of _2_ ☐ wk ☒ mo with no more than _1_ mild episode of failing to support the other.

a. Reframe each partner's parenting style as a complement to the other and having a place in the successful parenting; draw on religious, intergenerational, and cultural models of good parenting.

b. Clarifying parental subsystem boundaries and strengthen hierarchy by creating agreed-upon roles and limits as well as enable both parents to have a strong emotional connection with children; develop plan for addressing alcohol and substance issue if CM14 continues to make poor decisions related to use.

c. Enactments to increase emotional intimacy and help couple reconnect as couple, not just coparents.

Closing-Phase Client Goals

1. Increase ability to maintain levels of independence appropriate to current family with adolescents to reduce reduce conflict and increase sense of well-being.

Measure: Able to sustain age-appropriate levels of independence for period of _2_ ☐ wk ☒ mo with no more than _1_ mild episode(s) of failing to make responsible choices.

a. Challenge couple's/family's worldview to adapt to tasks associated with new stage of development to reduce conflict and increase sense of intimacy.

b. Compliment behaviors that support stage-appropriate independence

2. Increase ability to maintain levels of interdependence and relational connection appropriate for families with adolescents to reduce conflict and increase intimacy.

a. Enactments to explore new, stage-appropriate ways of relating.

b. Shaping competence to enable couple/family to develop rituals for connecting at home.

Treatment Tasks

1. Develop working therapeutic relationship using theory of choice.

Relationship-building approach/intervention:

a. Mimesis to join, carefully gaining CM14's trust while ensuring AM44 feels respected using cultural/religious norms; using humor with CM14.

(continued)

2. Assess individual, relational, community, and broader cultural dynamics using theory of choice.

Assessment strategies:

   a. Enactments to map structure to identify potential cross-generational coalitions, effectiveness of parental hierarchy, quality of parent/couple relationships.

   b. Assess boundaries at home, school, and with extended family system.

3. Identify needed referrals, crisis issues, collateral contacts, and other client needs.

   a. *Crisis assessment intervention(s):* Continue to assess for potential for future violence and substance misuse. Connect with school counselor and teachers to provide support on campus for prosocial activities.

   b. *Referral(s):* Rule out medical causes, substance abuse, danger to others (potential gang involvement).

Diversity Considerations

Describe specifically how treatment plan, goals, and interventions were adapted to address each area of diversity (note: identify specific ethnicity, e.g., Italian American rather than white):

Age: Use humor to join with CM14 and CM12. Attend to transition in family life cycle from school-aged to adolescent children by increasing youth's independence and responsibility and reducing reliance on parents to make good decisions.

Gender/Sexual Orientation: Address differences in cross-generational gender expectations between father and son; also gender polarity between father and mother.

Race/Ethnicity Religion/Class/Region: Assess roles of Itialian American and Irish American extended families; how couple experiences/handles ethnic differences; also address socioeconomic status issues with family moving to wealtahier neighbhorhood and how this may related to CM's difficulty adjusting to his new school.

Other factors: Help family develop connections in new community, perhaps around religion. Identify peer and school resources to engage CM14 in prosocial activities.

Evidence-Based Practice (Optional)

Summarize evidence for using this approach for this presenting concern and/or population: All evidence-based treatments for adolescent substance abuse and conduct disorder include elements of structural therapy. Engaging the entire family is considered to be the ideal form of therapy for such teens.

Client Perspective (Optional)

Has treatment plan been reviewed with client: ☒ Yes ☐ No; If no, explain: _____

Describe areas of Client Agreement and Concern: Family willing to meet as family to work on issues outlined in plan; general agreement with identified areas of intervention.

_____, _____ _____   _____, _____   _____
Therapist's Signature   Intern Status   Date   Supervisor's Signature   License   Date

PROGRESS NOTE

Date: 06/9/16 **Time:** 6:30 ☐ am/☒ pm **Session Length:** ☐ 45 min. ☐ 60 min.

☒ Other: 50 minutes

Present: ☒ Adult Male ☒ Adult Female ☒ Child Male ☐ Child Female ☐ Other: _____

Billing Code: ☐ 90791 (eval) ☐ 90834 (45 min. therapy) ☐ 90837 (60 min. therapy)
☒ 90847 (family) ☐ Other: _____

Symptom(s)	Duration and Frequency since Last Visit	Progress
1: Conflict w AM	2 moderate arguments w AM/ past wk	No Progress
2: Fights with peers	No new incidents this week	Maintained
3: Grades drop	Report increase in completing HW/5 days	Progressing

Explanatory Notes on Symptoms: Denies drinking this week; reports less defiance/arguing with AM; AF reports being more supportive of AM; report family had "fun" movie night on Saturday. CM14 reports meeting a new group of friends who are less "trouble-prone" than those he had met previously.

In-Session Interventions and Assigned Homework

Enactments in session to encourage CM14 to take greater responsibility for choices, clarify boundaries between AF, AM, and CM14, and interrupt cross-generational coalition. Identified rules for going out and how greater freedom can be earned. Met with AM and AF alone briefly to discuss parental coalition issues: agreeing on rules and limits. HW: continue with one fun weekend activity.

Client Response/Feedback

CM14 receptive to viewing self as taking responsibility for his life direction. Family receptive to redirection in enactments and open to working with parents alone. Enthusiastic about HW.

Plan

☒ Continue with treatment plan: plan for next session: Parents only to discuss parenting next week; CM14 only following.
☐ Modify plan: _____

Next session: Date: 6/16 Time: 6:30 ☐ am/☒ pm

Crisis Issues: ☒ No indication of crisis/client denies ☐ Crisis assessed/addressed: describe below

CM14 denies current alcohol and substance use; no reported fighting or plans for fighting

_____, _____ _____
Clinician's Signature   License/Intern Status   Date

(continued)

◇◇

Case Consultation/Supervision ☐ Not Applicable
Notes: Supervisor recommended individual session with parents to address parenting and one alone with CM14 to increase his motivation.

Collateral Contact ☐ Not Applicable

Name: <u>Courtney Markowitz</u>   Date of Contact: <u>5/23</u> Time: <u>2:00</u> ☐ am/☒ pm
☒ Written release on file: ☒ Sent/☐ Received ☐ In court docs ☐ Other: _____
Notes: School counselor reports working on plan to make up work to ensure passes 9th grade; will have to take summer school; report CM14 participating well in teen group; report no new fights at school.

_____,   _____   _____
Clinician's Signature   License/Intern Status   Date

_____,   _____   _____
Supervisor's Signature   License   Date

CHAPTER

6

Experiential Family Therapies

Learning Objectives

After reading this chapter and a few hours of focused studying, you should be able to:

- **Theory:** Describe the following elements of the Satir model and emotionally focused therapy:

    - Process of therapy
    - Therapeutic relationship
    - Case conceptualization
    - Goal setting
    - Interventions

- **Case conceptualization and treatment plan:** Complete a theory-specific case conceptualizations and treatment plans for Satir family therapy and emotionally focused couples therapy using templates that are provided.

- **Research:** Provide an overview of significant research findings for Satir family therapy and emotionally focused couples therapy.

- **Diversity:** Analyze strengths, limitations, and appropriate applications for using experiential approaches with clients in relation to their social location/diverse identities, including but not limited to ethnic, racial, and/or sexual/gender identity diversity.

- **Cross-theoretical comparison:** Compare how experiential therapies utilize interpersonal patterns (IPs) with other approaches described in this book.

Life is not the way it's supposed to be. It's the way it is. The way you cope with it is what
makes the difference.
—Virginia Satir

Lay of the Land

If you have been hoping an approach with a softer style, you may have found your chapter. Integrating systemic theory with humanism, experiential family therapists are noted for their warmth and direct emotional engagement with clients. These approaches include:

- The Satir model: Considered one of the top five most influential therapists in America (Banmen & Maki-Banmen, 2014), Satir was a vibrant pioneer in the field of family therapy. Arguably the field's most influential woman, her approach focuses on teaching families how to communicate effectively and reach their full human potential.
- Emotionally focused therapy (EFT): One of two leading evidence-based approaches for couples therapy, EFT integrates experiential, systemic, and attachment theories to help couples and families create emotional safety to foster wellness interaction patterns.
- Symbolic–experiential therapy: A vivacious pioneer in the field of family therapy, Carl Whitaker developed symbolic–experiential therapy, which focuses on symbolic meanings and emotional exchanges within the family using a balance of warmth and confrontation to promote change. As few contemporary clinicians practice this approach in its original form, and this text provides a brief overview of his original theoretical contributions; those interested in reading can consult Gehart (2015), which has an extended section that is also available as an eChapter directly from Cengage.

Shared Assumptions and Practices in Experiential Approaches

Targeting Emotional Transactions

Whereas systemic, strategic, structural, and cognitive–behavioral family therapists primarily track *behavioral* interaction sequences, experiential family therapists focus more on the *affective* or *emotional* layer of those same interactions—while still attending to behavior and cognition (Johnson, 2004; Satir et al., 1991; Whitaker & Bumberry, 1988). Assessment and intervention target the emotional exchanges between family members and significant others in relation to the presenting problem.

Warmth, Empathy, and the Therapist's Use of Self

More so than strategic, structural, and intergenerational family therapists, experiential family therapists use warmth and empathy in building relationships with clients (Johnson, 2004; Satir, 1988; Satir et al., 1991; Schwartz, 1995; Whitaker & Bumberry, 1988). Therapists use themselves—their personhood—to make this strong affective connection with clients. This approach creates a sense of safety that allows clients to explore areas of emotional vulnerability.

Individual and Family Focus

Experiential family therapies address individual and family concerns as distinct sets of problems (Johnson, 2004; Satir et al., 1991; Schwartz, 1995; Whitaker & Bumberry, 1988). In contrast, systemic, structural, and intergenerational therapies conceptualize individual systems as part of the family system; they assume that individual symptoms will resolve if the family system is treated. Experiential therapists may not entirely disagree with this perspective but are much more deliberate in treating problems at the individual level.

The Satir Model

In a Nutshell: The Least You Need to Know

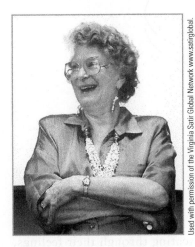

Virginia Satir

One of the first prominent women in the field, Virginia Satir began her career in family therapy at the Mental Research Institute (MRI; see Chapter 4) working alongside Jay Haley, Paul Watzlawick, Richard Fisch, and the other leading family therapists in Palo Alto (Satir, 1967/1983, 1972). She eventually left the MRI to develop her own ideas, which can be described broadly as infusing humanistic values into a systemic approach. She brought a warmth and enthusiasm for human potential that is unparalleled in the field of family therapy. Her therapy focused on fostering individual growth as well as improving family interactions. She used experiential exercises (e.g., family sculpting; see section on "Sculpting, or Spatial Metaphor," below), metaphors, coaching, and the self-of-the-therapist to facilitate change (Satir & Baldwin, 1983; Satir et al., 1991). Her work is practiced extensively internationally, with Satir practitioners connecting through the Satir Global Network.

The Juice: Significant Contributions to the Field

If you remember one thing from this chapter, it should be the following:

Communication Stances

The **communication stances** in the Satir model offer a clinician of any theoretical orientation an efficient and effective means of conceptualizing how best to communicate and interact with a client (Satir, 1967/1983, 1988; Satir et al., 1991). Satir describes four communication survival or coping stances: placator, blamer, superreasonable, and irrelevant (Banmen & Maki-Banmen, 2014). These stances develop in childhood and reveal how a person communicates under stress, especially when he or she does not feel emotionally safe in intimate relationships. And, yes, a person can use more than one, but typically a person uses one style predominantly. Each stance acknowledges or minimizes three basic realities: self, other, and context. Survival stances often fit together like puzzle pieces within a family, with people assuming complementary stances to create balance, such as placating and blaming.

In all cases, the goal is to move people toward *congruent communication,* in which they respectfully balance the needs of *self* and *others* while responding appropriately within and acknowledging the *context.* Most of us use congruent communication when we feel secure. The challenge is use congruent communication during stressful times, such as moments of conflict or strong emotion.

At first glance, these stances appear too simplistic to be of much clinical relevance. I believed this myself until I started teaching case conceptualization (see Chapter 11). Over time, however, I began to appreciate their remarkable sophistication and the insights they offer. Identifying a client's communication stance can help therapists design interventions more effectively and use almost every utterance to move clients toward their goals, whether working solely from a Satir approach or from an entirely different approach. Therapists can also communicate with a wide range of clients, adjusting their comments and interventions to accommodate the client and using consistent and focused language to reinforce therapeutic movement with every communication, from scheduling an appointment to wording interventions from any model.

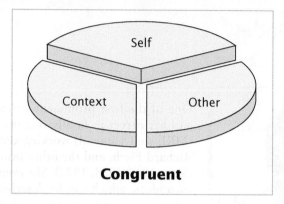

Congruent

Survival Stances

Unlike the congruent stance, each survival stance minimizes one or more essential parts of the total picture, as illustrated by the dark shading in the following diagrams.

Placating Stance

Therapists can make connection with those using placating through their feelings, to which they are closely attuned (Banmen, 2002). Because placatory have people-pleasing tendencies, therapists use less directive therapy methods, such as multiple-choice questions and open-ended reflections, to require them to voice their opinion and take a stand. Often this is quite painful and scary for **placators**. With clients who tend toward placating, therapists should carefully avoid giving opinions, making it seem that they have an opinion, or offering too much personal information. Clients will use this type of information to know what parts of themselves to hide and what parts to foreground to gain therapist approval. Never underestimate placators; they are skilled in the art of people pleasing. Research indicates that some clients make up things to give the impression that therapy is progressing (Gehart & Lyle, 2001). Not until the placator regularly and openly *disagrees* with the therapist has rapport been established.

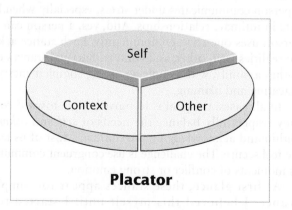

Placator

Blaming Stance

Therapists can best connect with those who blame through by addressing their expectations (Banmen & Maki-Banmen, 2014). The goal often is to increase blamers' awareness of others' thoughts and feelings and help them learn how to communicate their personal perspectives in ways that are respectful of others. Counter to what one might expect, with these clients, direct confrontation often strengthens the therapeutic relationship. Most blamers lose respect for "wimpy" (think "placating") therapists who do not speak their minds honestly and directly, a skill that blamers have mastered. Blamers generally prefer more upfront and direct communication than is generally tolerated in polite society.

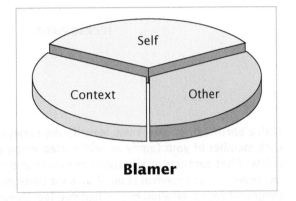

Blamer

Superreasonable Stance

When working with those who use a superreasonable stance, logic and rules reign supreme. Since these client tend to avoid all emotions, therapists might best engage them by starting with their bodily reactions and expectations before moving onto feelings (Banmen & Maki-Banmen, 2014). The goal with this stance is to help clients value the internal, subjective realities of themselves and others.

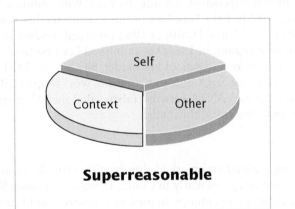

Superreasonable

Irrelevant Stance

A client with the irrelevant stance creates a unique challenge for therapists because there is no consistent grounding in self, other, or context for the therapist to use in understanding and communicating with the client. Instead, the therapist must spend time "floating" along with the client's distractions to identify the unique "anchors" of the client's reality that the therapist can tap into. Often the first step is to make the therapeutic relationship a place of utmost safety so that there is less need for distracting communication. Toward that end, bodily sensations, touch, and physical activities often work best with this client stance. As treatment progresses, the therapist works with these clients to increase their ability to recognize the thoughts and feelings of self and others and to acknowledge the demands of context. Progress is typically slower with those who use this stance frequently.

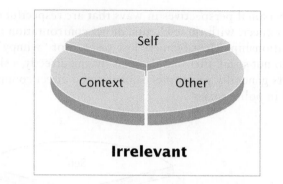

Irrelevant

Try It Yourself

With a partner or on your own, identify the survival communication stances that each member of your family of origin used when there was a loss of relational safety. What contexts or situations are most likely to trigger you to feel unsafe and revert to your survival stance? In what contexts have you learned to maintain congruent communication even when you feel threatened?

Rumor Has It: The People and Their Stories

Virginia Satir

A true pioneer, Virginia Satir was one of the first therapists to work with entire families. She began her private practice in 1951, and by 1955, she was training therapists at the Illinois Psychiatric Institute to work with families. She then joined the newly established MRI in Palo Alto, California, to continue her research. A grant from the National Institute of Mental Health in 1962 provided funding to establish the first family therapy training program. In 1964, she published her first book, *Conjoint Family Therapy*, which outlines the key aspects of her model. She left the MRI to become the director of Esalen Institute in Big Sur, California, offering workshops facilitating personal growth. She also founded the AVANTA network (also called the "Virginia Satir Global Network") to connect practitioners of the model.

John Banmen

Having trained and worked closely with Satir, Banmen now teaches the Satir model internationally, particularly in China, Taiwan, and Hong Kong, where Satir's work is highly influential, and continues to publish on current applications of her work (Banmen, 2002, 2003). He has continued to develop the theory, integrating more spiritual and wellness elements (Banmen & Maki-Banmen, 2014).

The Big Picture: Overview of Treatment

Satir et al. (1991) use a six-stage model of change that is based on research on cybernetic systems conducted by Satir while at the MRI and that draws from humanistic principles, including the assumption that people naturally strive toward growth. Her six-stage model describes how the therapy process helps families move toward a *second-order change* in the family structure (see Chapter 3). The model also emphasizes that the therapist perturbs the system—shakes it up and respects its ability to naturally reorganize itself in a more useful way—rather than attempting to direct and control the system from the outside. Thus, even though Satir uses education and coaches clients on how to better communicate, the aim is not for clients to follow her instructions literally but rather to adapt and respond to the instructions in a way that works for their system. The six stages are as follows:

1. Status quo: This is a state of homeostasis that includes at least one symptomatic member.
2. Introduction of foreign element: A *foreign element*, which may be a life crisis, tragedy, or therapeutic intervention, gets the system off balance.
3. Chaos: The new perspective creates a *positive feedback* loop that throws the system into a state of chaos; at this point the "natural" response is to feel uncomfortable, and in almost all cases the family tries to regain the status quo (stage 1), which may or may not be possible.
4. Integration of new possibilities: Eventually, the family system interprets the new information in a meaningful way; the therapist needs to be respectful of how the system uses the information and responds to therapist–client interactions, honoring and trusting the system's autonomy.
5. Practice: The system develops a new set of interaction patterns based on the new information. This may or may not look like what the therapist expects, but the therapist asks two key evaluative questions: Are the symptoms improving? and Is each person able to self-actualize and grow?
6. New status quo: This is a state of new homeostasis that does not include a symptomatic member and that allows all members to grow and flourish.

In most cases, therapy involves going through these six stages several times, with the discomfort and relative sense of chaos diminishing each time the client cycles through, becoming increasingly comfortable with change.

Making Connections: The Therapeutic Relationship

Humanistic and Systemic Foundations

Satir et al. (1991, pp. 14–15) state four primary assumptions about people and therapy; the first two reflect *humanistic* assumptions and the latter two a *systemic* view.

ASSUMPTIONS OF SATIR'S MODEL

1. People naturally tend toward positive growth (humanistic principle).
2. All people possess the resources for positive growth (humanistic principle).
3. Every person and every thing or situation impacts and is impacted by everyone and everything else (systemic principle).
4. Therapy is a process that involves interaction between a therapist and a client; in this relationship, each person is responsible for himself/herself (systemic and humanistic principle).

These assumptions clarify the therapist's role in the process (the therapist is "responsible for him/herself"), but also how the therapist believes the therapeutic process works: clients already possess the natural inclination toward growth and the resources for it, and it is the therapist's job to activate these tendencies. These assumptions inform the role of the therapist as a *guide* to the process of becoming more fully human.

Therapeutic Presence: Warmth and Humanity

Carl Rogers (1961, 1981), a leader in humanistic, experiential therapies, based his client-centered approach on three therapist qualities: (a) congruence or genuineness,

(b) accurate empathy, and (c) unconditional positive regard. These conditions are the theoretical foundation of the warmth and humanity for which Satir is legendary (Satir et al., 1991). Her way of being in the world radiated an unshakable hope and deep-felt respect for her clients. Her presence in the room put people at ease and allowed them to feel secure enough to relate to one another nondefensively. She created a safe haven that made it easy for her clients to address the issues in their lives. How she did this is a difficult question to answer. This quality of being, or *therapeutic presence,* is difficult to define, and there are few methods for systematically developing it (Gehart & McCollum, 2008). The more that therapists are *congruent*—that is, able to communicate authentically while responding to the needs of both self and others—the better they can create the therapeutic warmth and humanity that characterized the work of Satir.

Making Contact

Satir et al. (1991) describe establishing a therapeutic relationship as "**making contact**," which refers to a series of connections both within the therapist and between the therapist and the client. Making contact begins with the therapist being in contact with himself or herself, including all resources of the self as defined in the *self-mandala:* physical, intellectual, emotional, sensual, interactional, nutritional, contextual, and spiritual. In addition, the therapist prepares to meet another "miracle," a fellow human being. Then, the therapist works to make contact with each client in the room, engaging them on "all channels": mind, body, and spirit. Thus open body positioning and congruent communication are critical. Once the therapist has made contact with each person, the therapist works to help family members make contact with each other and ultimately with others in their broader social system. The therapy process cannot move forward until the therapist has made contact with the client. When contact is made, clients feel valued for who they are, regardless of their problem, and they feel free to make mistakes in the therapist's presence. Making contact involves the following:

- Making direct eye contact with clients
- Touching clients (e.g., shaking hands)
- Sitting or standing at the same physical level so that eye contact is easy (i.e., leaning down to talk with children)
- Asking each person's name and how he or she prefers to be called (Satir et al., 1991)

Try It Yourself

When are you able to make authentic contact as Satir describes? Describe relationships in which you feel most authentic and able to fully connect with another. Why does this connection matter? What helps you to "make contact" with others?

Empathy

Satir practitioners convey their understanding of clients' subjective, inner realities by expressing *empathy,* an accurate understanding of another's emotional reality. Having empathy does not mean that a therapist takes the client's side, avoids confronting inconsistencies, or ignores the client's responsibility. Don't get me wrong; clients *like* therapists who take their side, don't confront them, and ignore their responsibility in the problem situation. It feels good to be validated in this way, but this type of validation is detrimental to therapeutic progress. Similarly, comments that imply a client has a right to feel a certain way can also shut down the process of reflecting on the client's responsibility for his or her half of an interaction. On the other hand, expressing empathy emphasizes that it is not wrong or right, normal or abnormal, to feel a certain way—it is simply how the client feels and means that this is his or her "truth," at least for the moment (e.g., "It sounds as though you felt betrayed"). Honoring the client's unique experience without validating it as right or normal makes it much easier to move the client toward seeing that the other person has his or her unique experience that is also "true" for that person, creating a context from which to understand how these two (or more) realities may collide and create problematic interactions.

Conveying Hope

In joining with clients, therapists instill hope that they can change and that the situation can be better, even if it seems hopeless at the moment. Satir et al. (1991) emphasize that clients must have faith that change is possible before they can move forward with treatment.

Establishing Credibility

Clients also need to believe that therapy and their particular therapist can help them resolve their problems. Therapists establish credibility by making a personal connection (making contact) and by being confident and competent (modeling high self-esteem; Satir et al., 1991).

The Viewing: Case Conceptualization and Assessment

In the Satir model, both family functioning and individual functioning are assessed.

ASSESSMENT OF FAMILY FUNCTIONING

- *Role of the symptom in the system:* Describe how the symptom maintains the family's homoeostasis at an emotional level, often regulating closeness and distance.
- *Family dynamics:* Identify salient dynamics:
  - Power struggles
  - Parental conflicts
  - Lack of validation
  - Lack of intimacy
- *Family roles:* Identify possible family roles:
  - The martyr
  - The victim or helpless one
  - The rescuer
  - The good child or parent
  - The bad child or parent
- *Family life chronology:* Describe key historical events, deaths, births, divorces, major life changes.
- *Survival triad:* Describe the emotional and nurturing relationships between each child and parents.

ASSESSMENT OF INDIVIDUAL FUNCTIONING

- *Survival stances:* Identify the survival stance of each person in the system:
  - Placator
  - Blamer
  - Superreasonable
  - Irrelevant
  - Congruent
- *Six levels of experience: The iceberg:* For symptomatic behavior, describe:
  - Behavior
  - Coping
  - Feelings
  - Perceptions
  - Expectations
  - Yearnings
- *Self-worth and self-esteem:* Describe each person's level of self-worth.
- *Mind–body connection:* Describe any salient mind–body connections.

Role of the Symptom in the System

Much like other systemic therapists, Satir (1972) viewed the symptom as having a role in the family system. For example, a child's exaggerated acting out, such as with drug use or sexual activity, may serve to reduce tension in the marriage by getting the parents on the same page about the child's issue. Similarly, a person's depression may be a means of avoiding an unpleasant confrontation with a spouse or boss. Basically, symptoms always have an emotional function in the family system, even if they are consciously and logically unwanted. The question is, Why is this particular symptom manifesting in this particular family (or relationship)? If the therapist can understand how the symptom makes emotional sense in the family dance, it will be easier to help the family find ways to interact successfully without the need for the symptom.

Family Dynamics

Along with assessing family roles, Satir et al. (1991) identify problematic family dynamics:

- Power struggles: These can be within the family and couple or with extended family members.
- Parental conflicts: These can involve parents disagreeing about how to parent and care for children.
- Lack of validation: The family openly expresses little emotional support or validation.
- Lack of intimacy: There is minimal sharing of significant personal information and one's emotional life.

Family Roles

Satir (1972, 1988) assessed each person's role in the family system to understand the function of the problem. Possible roles include the following:

- The martyr
- The victim or helpless one
- The rescuer

- The good child or parent
- The bad child or parent

Family Life Chronology

The **family life chronology** (Satir, 1967/1983; Satir et al., 1991) is a timeline that includes the major events in an individual's or family's life:

- Births and deaths
- Important family events: marriages, moves, tragedies, major illnesses, job loss
- Important historical events: wars, natural disasters, economic downturns

This chronology gives both the therapist and the client a "big picture" view of the context for the potential problem and provides clues as to what old wounds may be fueling the current problems, as well as what potential strengths and resources might exist.

Survival Triad

Another area for assessment is the **survival triad** (Satir, 1988)—the child, mother, and father—and the quality of the relationship between all three. Satir asserted that it was in this primary triad that a child learns how to be human (Azpeitia, 1991). Is there an emotional bond between each parent and the child, or do the parents have significantly different levels of connection with the child? Because the survival triad should serve as a nurturing system for the child, when the child is experiencing difficulty, the therapist considers how the nurturing function of these relationships can be improved.

Survival Stances

This element of case conceptualization is discussed in detail in "The Juice" section, above.

Six Levels of Experience: The Iceberg

One of Satir's last theoretical developments and central focus of contemporary work was the **six levels of experience**. Satir practitioners use these to help clients *transform* their feelings about feelings to make lasting change (Satir et al., 1991). These levels are likened to an *iceberg*, with the behavior the only visible layer and the other five layers unseen beneath the surface. At any moment, all six aspects are in play, but often we are not conscious of most of them. The iceberg model is used to help individuals better understand their intrapsychic experience and for couples to understand how the levels of each person's experience resonates with the other (Banmen & Maki-Banmen, 2014). Contemporary Satir practitioners help clients achieve *intrapsychic congruence* by identifying contradictions between these layers, such as taking actions one does not ultimately believe in (Lee, 2002). The six layers of the iceberg are as follows:

- Behavior: The behavior on the surface; the external manifestation of the person's inner world
- Coping: Defenses and survival stances: placating, blaming, superreasonable, and irrelevant; these come out in times of stress, and a person may use different stances in different relational contexts
- Feelings: Present feelings that are strongly past-based, using past events to interpret the present. Contemporary practitioners also ask about a person's feelings about his or her feelings, which invites clients to relate to their feelings differently.
- Perceptions: Beliefs, attitudes, and values that inform one's sense of self; most people form their perceptions when very young, and they are based on a limited view of reality.
- Expectations: A strong belief about how life should go, how people should behave, and how one should perform; most people form their expectations when young, and they are often unrealistic and/or may not apply to a particular situation.
- Yearnings: Universal longings to be loved, accepted, validated, and confirmed; this level closely parallels the emphasis on secure attachment emotionally focused therapy (see below).

In therapy, Satir practitioners use the six levels of experience to assess the motivation behind problematic behaviors and interactions. By understanding the *yearnings* as well as *perceptions* and *expectations* that fuel problematic behavior, coping, and feelings, therapists are able to help clients transform their feelings about their feelings (for example, being embarrassed about feeling angry) to more effectively meet the underlying longing for love and acceptance.

Try It Yourself

With a partner or on your own, identify a recent stressful event that made you feel strong negative emotion of some kind. Use the iceberg to describe the multiple layers of experience related to the one event. Are some levels incongruent with other layers? Does identifying the different layers of experience help you understand the situation differently? Do you see any new options?

Self-Worth and Self-Esteem

Satir was one of the first to recognize the importance of **self-worth** and **self-esteem**, and she always assessed a person's level of self-esteem (Satir, 1972). Clinically, it is generally unhelpful to assess self-esteem in an all-or-none fashion (i.e., high versus low), as is frequently done by teachers, parents, and concerned others who believe they have identified the secret cause behind a child's poor behavior. Instead, it is more useful to consider the specific *aspects of the self* that a client *values* and the aspects of which he or she is ashamed. For example, a child may value and have confidence in her ability to make friends but have less confidence in her scholastic abilities.

More recent research on self-esteem indicates that *self-compassion*, or acceptance of one's strengths and weaknesses, is a better indicator of happiness than self-esteem, which can be artificially high (Neff, 2003). People who overestimate their abilities and worth often have high self-esteem but significant problems in their interpersonal and work or school relationships because they have unrealistic expectations of "what is due to them." The best indicator of health, self-compassion is one's ability to accept strengths and weaknesses in oneself and others. People who are judgmental, impatient, or intolerant of others' weaknesses are almost always equally harsh on themselves; conversely, those who are hard on themselves are almost always equally harsh on others, even if it is not verbalized. As self-compassion and self-worth rise, people become more realistic and tolerant of their own and others' weaknesses while realistically assigning and assuming responsibility for their actions.

Mind–Body Connection

Satir et al. (1991) also consider the mind–body connection: how emotional issues may manifest in the body, either *symbolically* or *functionally*. For example, if a person is feeling burdened, this emotional feeling may manifest symbolically as stooped shoulders ("shoulders") or as a "burdened" posture. Similarly, if a person is feeling overwhelmed, this may manifest functionally in often being ill or exhausted. In addition, the role of nutrition and exercise is assessed. Finally, Satir maintained that the way the body is used indicates the person's communication stance:

- Congruent communication and self-esteem: Open and relaxed body postures
- Placating: Timid and reserved postures
- Blaming: Pointing, angry, and stiff postures
- Superreasonable: Cold and distant postures
- Irrelevant: Hyper and distracted

Targeting Change: Goal Setting

At the most general level, the goal of Satir's model is transformation: to achieve optimal realization of a person's full potential (Azpeitia, 1991). This goal translates into two broad sets of practical goals for treatment planning:

1. Relational, family, or systemic goals
2. Individual goals

Satir therapists' attention to individual goals reflects their humanistic foundations and is unique among systemically based therapists; symbolic–experiential therapists, who share this humanistic foundation, also have systemic and individual goals (see "Clinical Spotlight: Symbolic–Experiential Therapy" later in the chapter).

Relationally Focused Goals: Congruent Communication

The heart of relational goals in Satir's approach is **congruent communication**: the ability to communicate authentically while responding to the needs of both self and others. Specifically, the goal is to help the family develop ways for all members to communicate so that the system's homeostasis no longer needs the initial symptoms (problems) to maintain balance. The following are examples of specific goals (Satir, 1967/1983; Satir et al., 1991).

EXAMPLES OF RELATIONALLY FOCUSED GOALS

- Increase congruent communication in relationships with spouse, parent, child, etc.
- Change family rules and *shoulds* to general guidelines.

Individually Focused Goals: Self-Actualization

The overarching individual goal is consistent with other humanistic approaches: to promote the self-actualization of all members of the system. Self-actualization means fulfilling one's potential and living an authentic and meaningful life. The more a person self-actualizes, the greater his/her sense of self-worth and self-esteem. Examples of specific goals (Satir et al., 1991) are as follows:

EXAMPLES OF INDIVIDUALLY FOCUSED GOALS

- Increase sense of self-worth and self-compassion.
- Reduce defensiveness and use of survival stances.

In the case study at the end of this chapter, the goals focus on: (a) helping a teen who has been sexually abused regain her sense of self-worth (especially after the abuse) and autonomy (developmental task), and (b) helping the couple and family develop congruent communication regarding the abuse as well as resolve couple concerns that were there prior to the abuse.

The Doing: Interventions

Therapist's Self

Therapists' use of self—being authentically who they are—is one of the most essential interventions in Satir's approach (1988). By being authentic, therapists provide a role model for how to communicate congruently and also show the effects of increased self-actualization. Furthermore, the use of the therapist's self in therapy, which may include self-disclosure, creates a safe relationship in which clients can practice communicating congruently without negative consequences and learn to tap into more authentic modes of expression.

Ingredients of an Interaction

The foundation for all other interventions (Azpeitia, 1991), the **ingredients of an interaction** details the internal communication process and can be used to teach clients about internal and relational processes (Satir et al., 1991). The ingredient questions are used to help people better understand their interactions with others and can be used with individuals, couples, or families. When a client shares a troubling interaction with another, the therapist uses the following seven questions to walk the client through the "ingredients of an interaction" (Azpeitia, 1991; Satir et al., 1991):

1. What do I HEAR AND SEE? The therapist prompts clients to describe behaviorally what happened without adding interpretations; this is similar to "videotalk" in solution-based therapies (Chapter 9) (e.g., "My child did not take out the trash immediately upon my asking her to do so").

2. What MEANINGS do I make of what I hear and see? After obtaining a clear, behavioral description, the therapist facilitates a discussion of how the clients interpreted these behaviors; meanings often connect back to past experiences (e.g., "My child does not respect me; I would never have spoken to my parents that way").

3. What FEELINGS do I have about the meanings I make? Next, the therapist helps clients identify specific feelings about the meanings and interpretations (e.g., "This makes me angry and hurt"). Therapists use "facilitation of emotional expression" techniques, described in detail in next section.

4. What FEELINGS do I have *ABOUT* THESE FEELINGS? Then the therapist asks clients about whether they can accept and tolerate the feelings; the more congruent a person is, the more accepting he or she is of various feelings. If a person is not accepting, survival stances will be triggered (e.g., *congruent:* "I don't like these feelings, but I know that they are natural"; *incongruent:* "I don't like these feelings and need my child to do what I say so that I don't have such feelings anymore"). Subsequent interventions target this level of feeling, not the emotions attached to the interpretation.

5. What DEFENSES do I use? When people use incongruent communication, they respond in the interaction using defense mechanisms such as projection, denial, ignoring, or one of the communication stances (e.g., "I get angry and yell at my child for not following my request"; "I blame my spouse for spoiling the child").

6. What RULES FOR COMMENTING do I use? Each person's family of origin and early significant others impart rules for commenting on interpersonal interactions that may limit self-worth, restrict choices, and determine what actions are "allowed" and "appropriate"; most of these rules are unspoken and brought into future relationships without reflection on whether they are appropriate or useful (e.g., "It is not okay for a parent to be vulnerable with a child"; "Parents should always be in charge"). These rules are transformed using "softening" techniques (described in "Softening Family Rules," below).

7. What is my RESPONSE in the situation? How does the client respond behaviorally and verbally (e.g., "I tell my child 'You don't respect me.' in an angry, hostile tone and stay angry even after the child does the chore"; "I also get angry at my spouse for not being stricter with the children")? Incongruent and problematic responses are targeted for change.

Facilitating Emotional Expression

Satir therapists work with clients to help them express difficult-to-articulate emotions related to the presenting problem (Satir et al., 1991). If clients complain about family members or a difficult life situation, experiential therapists listen closely for the emotions, expressed or unexpressed, that are related to the problem circumstance. They listen not just for the surface emotions (e.g., "I am angry that my partner was late") but also for deeper levels of emotion (e.g., "My partner does not care about me") and use questions and empathetic reflections to focus clients on those deeper emotions.

Examples:

- If a client tells a story without identifying their emotions directly:
  - "As I listen to you explain what happened to you during that argument, I am getting a sense that you were feeling [name the emotion]. Does that sound right?"
  - "That sounds like a very difficult situation. Can you share some of the emotions you have been experiencing as you go through this?"
- If a client does identify emotions, the therapy can help explore them with questions such as:
  - "You say you were feeling [emotion]. I am wondering if part of you is also feeling [name another emotion that client seems to be experiencing]."
  - "Can you say more about what feeling [name emotion] feels like for you."

Softening Family Rules

Satir et al. (1991) coached families in softening rigid family rules by changing them to *guidelines*. For example, rather than saying "I should not get angry," a client or family was encouraged to revise the limiting rule to "When I am angry, I will express this anger in a way that is respectful to the others and myself." In addition, Satir encouraged families to have as few rules as possible and to be flexible, adapting them for each context and as children's developmental needs change.

Communication Enhancement: Coaching, Role Play, and Enactment

A hallmark of Satir's approach, coaching clients in how to have authentic, congruent communication in session, involves the "ingredients of an interaction" (previously discussed) combined with specific communication coaching strategies (Satir, 1988; Satir et al., 1991). When coaching communication, Satir had clients turn their chairs toward one another and gave the clients prompts, such as "Tell your partner how you feel about what happened on Saturday night." If the client was able to congruently address his or her partner about this, she then prompted the partner to respond in kind, continuing this process until the problem was resolved. When a person had trouble communicating congruently and reverted to a survival stance, Satir interrupted the conversation and suggested how to rephrase the statement or how to make the client's nonverbal communications more congruent (e.g., "Now, can you say that starting the statement with 'I' instead of 'you'?" or "Can you show the emotion you say you are feeling when you speak to your wife?").

COMMON AREAS OF COMMUNICATION COACHING

- Ask clients to start statements using "I" rather than "You."
- Ask clients to take full responsibility for their feelings rather than blaming others (e.g., "Instead of 'You made me feel . . .,' try 'When X happened, I felt . . .'").
- Encourage clients to be direct and honest rather than expecting the other to read between the lines.
- Identify double binds (e.g., "You asked your husband to show more affection, but when he does, you are upset and say he only did so because you asked").

In addition, the "ingredients of an interaction" technique (see previous discussion) was used to help coach clients through what they heard and saw, how they interpreted and felt about it, and the feelings about feelings and family-of-origin rules for communicating about what happened. In the case study at the end of this chapter, the therapist plans to use role-play to help a teen who has been sexually abused regain her sense of safety, ability to set boundaries, and confidence in her ability to say "no."

Sculpting, or Spatial Metaphor

Satir's most distinctive intervention is **family sculpting**, which is done either with the family or in a group setting (Satir, 1988; Satir et al., 1991). Sculpting involves putting family members in physical positions that represent how the "sculptor" sees each person's role in the family. For example, if a child sees a parent as blaming or harshly punitive, he may sculpt that parent with a harsh look and angry pointing finger and perhaps himself as the child cowering or hiding. Typically, either the therapist or the client may direct the sculpting. If family members are directing the sculpting, each person in the family is given an opportunity to sculpt the family as he or she sees it. Sometimes the sculptor assigns each family member to say a line that represents how he or she might be feeling, thinking, or viewing the situation. Usually, however, the essence of this intervention is to give a nonverbal, symbolic depiction of the family process from each person's perspective.

In most cases, sculpting is a highly effective nonverbal confrontation that bypasses cognitive defenses. Through the sculpting process, a person is able to literally *see* how he or she is contributing to the problematic family process far more quickly than when the same information is provided with words. For example, if a person places herself far away from the rest of the family because she feels as though she is being made a scapegoat or is being ostracized, this often communicates the emotional reality of her situation far more effectively than if she were to use words, which would usually generate a verbal rationalization. When all family members are sculpting, it is generally best to let all family members sculpt how they see the family before allowing discussion of one another's sculpting. Therapists encourage family members to respect each person's subjective experience as illustrated in the sculpting and to use the experience to deepen their understanding of one another.

In the case study at the end of this chapter, the therapist uses sculpting with a teen who has been sexually abused at a time when her mother is significantly increasing her business travel; to assess the emotional impact of these changes, the therapist has the family sculpt what the family was like prior to the abuse and after.

Touch

Satir (1988) used touch in therapy to initially connect with clients and to encourage and reassure them when they were practicing new ways of communicating. In this way, she underscored emotional content and provided palpable support. She also used touch with children to help teach alternatives to violent behavior and to model for parents how to manage difficult children. The fact that she was an extremely nurturing female figure contributed significantly to how clients experienced her touch. In today's practice environments, touching is generally discouraged because it can easily be misinterpreted as sexual harassment or may make a client feel uncomfortable. Thus, therapists need to carefully consider the legal and ethical issues of using touch. That said, touch may be appropriate in certain practice and cultural contexts. At a minimum, therapists can learn from Satir the importance of coaching clients in touching *each other*—their children and spouses—in more loving and helpful ways. For example, rather than using a demonstration, therapists can guide a parent on how to hold children who are having a tantrum.

Interventions for Special Populations

Family Reconstruction: Group Intervention

A form of group psychodrama, the **family reconstruction** is used to allow clients to explore unresolved family issues and life events in the safety of the group setting (Satir et al., 1991). The client, who is called the "star," first identifies key events in his or her life chronology and significant sources of influence. The star then picks people from the group to reenact pivotal life experiences and relationships. The therapist facilitates the reenactment with the following three goals in mind:

• Identifying the roots of old learning and their role in the present
• Developing a more realistic picture of the client's parents
• Discovering unique strengths and potentials

Parts Party

A group activity similar to the family reconstruction, the **parts party** involves the client identifying group members to represent aspects of the self (Satir et al., 1991). The person may have members enact generic characteristics (martyr, victim, savior) or use famous figures to represent different aspects of the self. In this way, the therapist facilitates a process in which the client is better able to accept different aspects of the self and to identify the contexts in which these aspects have been and continue to be useful. The language of "parts" can also be used to facilitate similar discussions and insights in individual, couples, and family therapy.

Scope It Out: Cross-Theoretical Comparison

Using Tomm's IPscope described in Chapter 3 (Tomm, St. George, Wulff, & Strong, 2014), this theory approaches the conceptualization of systemic, interpersonal patterns as follows:

Theoretical Conceptualization

Satir's approach tracks pathologizing interpersonal patterns (PIPs) with a specific focus on the emotional level of the interaction and adds to it an understanding of the intrapsychic experiences within each person. The "iceberg" (six levels of experience) helps therapists assess the internal PIPs that are part of the external PIP with others. In addition, survival stances often can be at the heart of a PIP, such as placating/blaming or blaming/distracting.

Goal Setting

In the Satir model, wellness interpersonal patterns (WIPs) are conceptualized in terms of congruent communication (relationally) and self-worth (intrapersonally). These can take the form of listening compassionately/sharing vulnerably or acknowledging self/appreciating self.

Facilitating Change

When facilitating change, the therapist uses several forms of transformational interaction patterns (TIPs). Often, family sculpting takes the form of having everyone first sculpt the PIP and then having each person sculpt their desired WIPs. When working more intrapsychically, the iceberg is used to identify both PIPs and WIPs as well, first identifying the negative inner dialogue patterns (disapproving of self/disapproving of others) and then identifying alternatives (approving of self/approving of others). In addition, much of the family-of-origin work that characterize this approach involve healing interpersonal patterns (HIPs), especially the family reconstruction and parts party; this is typically done by having another group member say what she always wished her parents would have said.

Putting It All Together: Satir Case Conceptualization and Treatment Plan Templates

Areas for Theory-Specific Case Conceptualization: Satir

When conceptualizing client **cases**, contemporary Satir family therapists typically use the following dynamics **to inform their treatment plan.** Go to MindTap® to access a digital version of the theory-specific case conceptualization, along with a variety of digital study tools and resources that complement this text and help you be more successful in your course and career. If your instructor didn't assign MindTap, you can find out more about it at Cengagebrain.com. You can also download the form at masteringcompetencies .com

Communication and Validation Patterns

Describe the communication and validation patterns for all significant persons related to client. For each person describe the:

- Survival stance used when person feels invalidated: placating, blaming, superreasonable, or irrelevant.

Self-Worth and Self-Esteem

- Describe the dynamics of each person's sense of self-worth and self-esteem, including contexts in which each has a greater or lesser sense of worth.
- Describe dynamics of social location, such as cultural, gender, social class, or other diversity factors, that inform the evaluation of self.

Relational Life Chronology

Describe significant events, specifically those that may relate to sense of validation and worth, in family and/or relational life; list in chronological order.

Relational and Family Dynamics

Describe the following:

- Power struggles and collations
- Parental conflicts
- Expression of intimacy/warmth between members
- Salient family roles, including: martyr, victim, rescuer, good/bad parent or child, etc.
- How the client or family's social location affects these dynamics, such as gender, ethnicity, socioeconomic class, sexual/gender orientation, etc.

Role of the Symptom in the System

Hypothesize homeostatic function of presenting problem: How might the symptom serve to maintain connection, create independence/distance, establish influence, reestablish connection, or otherwise help create a sense of balance in the family?

TREATMENT PLAN TEMPLATE FOR INDIVIDUAL WITH DEPRESSION/ANXIETY: SATIR

The following treatment plan template can be used to help you develop individualized treatments for use with individuals with depressive or anxiety symptoms. You can download a blank treatment plan (with or without measures) on MindTap at www.cengagebrain .com or www.masteringcompetencies.com.

Satir Treatment Plan: Client Goals with Interventions

Early-Phase Client Goal

1. Decrease use of *survival stance* in [key context where symptoms occur] to reduce depressed mood and anxiety.
   a. Use *ingredients-of-interaction* technique to identify meanings, feelings, defenses, and rules for commenting in problem interactions.
   b. **Facilitate emotional expression** related to depression and anxiety feelings.

Working-Phase Client Goals

1. Reduce *shoulds* and alter *expectations* for [specify area of life] to reduce sense of depression, hopelessness, and anxiety.
   a. Use *ingredients-of-interaction* technique to identify and alter *shoulds* and expectations related to depressive and anxious feelings.
   b. *Sculpt* shoulds and expectations to increase awareness of emotions and history related to expectations.

2. Increase realistic *perceptions, attitudes, and beliefs* that inform the *sense of self* to reduce depression, hopelessness, and anxiety.
   a. *Soften family rules* to reduce rigidity of beliefs and attitudes learned in family of origin.
   b. *Coach* how to act from more realistic perceptions and attitudes.

3. Increase behaviors that more effectively fulfill client's *yearnings for love and acceptance* to reduce sense of depression and anxiety.
   a. Use *ingredients-of-interactions* intervention to identify underlying yearnings.
   b. *Role-play* new behaviors and forms of communication that help client fulfill yearnings for love and acceptance.

Closing-Phase Client Goals

1. Increase daily experience of *self-worth* and ability to express and relate from **authentic self** in all areas of life to reduce depression and increase sense of wellness.
   a. *Sculpt* from old versus new self to experientially understand the difference.
   b. *Coach* to practice making decisions from authentic self.

2. Increase *congruent communication in couple/family relations* to reduce depression and anxiety.
   a. *Sculpt* key relationships from survival stance versus congruent stance to experience the difference.
   b. *Role-play* to practice communicating with others from congruent position.

Treatment Tasks

1. Develop working therapeutic relationship.
   a. *Make contact* with client's authentic self using *empathy* and *therapeutic presence*.

2. Assess individual, systemic, and broader cultural dynamics.
   a. Assess individual functioning by noting *survival stance, six levels of experience* related to problem areas, and sense of *self-worth*.
   b. Assess relational functioning by identifying *relational dynamics, family roles, survival triad,* and *family life chronology.*

3. Identify referrals, crisis issues, collateral contacts, and other client needs.
   a. Crisis assessment intervention(s): Address crisis issues such as self-harm, suicidal ideation, substance use, risky sexual behavior, etc.
   b. Referral(s): Connect client with *resources* in client's *community* that could be supportive; make collateral contacts as needed.

TREATMENT PLAN TEMPLATE FOR DISTRESSED COUPLE/FAMILY: SATIR

You can download a blank treatment plan (with or without measures) on MindTap at www.cengagebrain.com or www.masteringcompetencies.com.

The following treatment plan template can be used to help you develop individualized treatments for use with couples and families who report relational distress.

Satir Treatment Plan: Client Goals with Interventions

Early-Phase Client Goal

1. Decrease use of *survival stances* in couple/family relating to reduce conflict.
   a. Have *family sculpt* each person's perception of others and their roles in family system.
   b. *Coach* family in *direct communication of emotions*.

Working-Phase Client Goals

1. Reduce and alter *expectations* of others in system and increase acceptance to reduce conflict.
   a. Use *ingredients-of-interaction* technique to identify and alter should and expectations of others.
   b. *Sculpt* shoulds and expectations to increase awareness of emotions and history related to expectations.

2. Increase realistic *perceptions, attitudes,* and *beliefs* that inform incongruent communication reduce conflict.
   a. *Soften family rules* to reduce rigidity of beliefs and attitudes learned in family of origins.
   b. *Coach* how to interact with more realistic perceptions and attitudes.

3. Increase behaviors that more effectively fulfill clients' *yearnings for love and acceptance* to reduce conflict.
   a. Use *ingredients-of-interactions* intervention to identify and express underlying yearnings.
   b. *Role-play* new behaviors and forms of communication that help client fulfill yearnings for love and acceptance.

Closing-Phase Client Goals

1. Increase each person's daily experience of *self-worth* and ability to express and relate from *authentic self* to reduce conflict and increase sense of wellness.
   a. *Sculpt* from old versus new selves to experientially understand the difference.
   b. Coach to practice making decisions from authentic self.

2. Increase *congruent communication* in work/school/extended family relations to reduce conflict and increase sense of wellness.
   a. *Sculpt* key relationships from survival stance versus congruent stance to experience the difference.
   b. *Role-play* to practice communicating with others from congruent position.

Treatment Tasks

1. Develop working therapeutic relationship.
   a. *Make contact* with each client's authentic self using *empathy* and *therapeutic presence*.

2. Assess individual, systemic, and broader cultural dynamics.
   a. Assess each individual's level of functioning by noting *survival stance, six levels of experience* related to problem areas, and sense of *self-worth*.
   b. Assess relational functioning by identifying *relational dynamics, family roles, survival triad,* and *family life chronology*.

3. Identify referrals, crisis issues, collateral contacts, and other client needs.
    a. Crisis assessment intervention(s): Address crisis issues such as psychological abuse, intimate partner violence, hidden affair, self-harm, suicidal ideation, substance use, etc.
    b. Referral(s): Connect client with *resources* in client's *family and community* that could be supportive; make collateral contacts as needed.

Tapestry Weaving: Working with Diverse Populations
Cultural, Ethnic, and Gender Diversity

Used with a wide range of clients, experiential approaches value clear, congruent emotional expression and the willingness to be vulnerable. Therefore, when working with populations that have different attitudes toward emotional expression and/or are in a treatment context where such vulnerability feels unsafe, therapists need to proceed thoughtfully. For example, the emotional expression often promoted in Satir's communication approach may not be comfortable for some men or East Asian–Americans (Wang, 1994), populations that generally value less dramatic and more indirect emotional expression; thus, they should be used with caution. In addition, an experiential approach may initially be too threatening for clients who have been mandated to receive treatment; they often feel that they might be in a worse position with the courts or social agencies that mandated their treatment if they express too much or certain emotions. Given the fact that a report will be sent to an outside party, these clients are less trusting of the therapeutic relationship.

Experiential therapists also need to monitor their expectations for the level and style of women's emotional expression; nontraditional female clients report feeling that their therapists expect that they express their emotions in a certain way and report feeling judged and misunderstood because they do not subscribe to stereotyped modes of female emotional expression (Gehart & Lyle, 2001). Therapists working with such clients must be very careful to: (a) avoid inaccurate assessment caused by different cultural and gender standards and values concerning emotional expression, (b) adjust the level of intimacy in the therapeutic alliance to fit with the client's level of comfort, and (c) choose interventions that actively engage clients at their comfort level. The case study at the end of this chapter details how an experiential therapy would design treatment for a Greek Armenian family whose teenage daughter has been sexually molested.

Asian Families

Although there are some cautions for using Satir's approach with collectivist cultures, her model is more popular internationally, particularly in Asia, than in the United States (Banmen & Maki-Banmen, 2014). This preference seems to hold true for Asian Americans; in one study, Asian American college students rated experiential therapy approaches more positively than cognitive–behavioral or psychodynamic approaches (Yu, 1998). Epstein and colleagues (2014) note that Satir's focus on the mind–body–spirit connection aligns closely with both traditional Taoist and Confucian traditions in China and East Asia (Epstein et al., 2014). However, the emphasis on self-esteem and the individual contrasts sharply with Chinese values of collectivism, hierarchy, and filial piety. In addition, the direct communication encouraged in this approach goes against traditional Chinese norms, but sculpting, which is largely nonverbal, may be a particularly useful way of helping Chinese families address problematic family dynamics using metaphor and more indirect communications (Epstein et al., 2014). Along similar lines, researchers have found that expressive writing—again, a less direct form of communication—was found to be beneficial for most people but especially for those of Asian origin (Lu & Stanton, 2010).

In summary, there are cautions for some things but there also seems to be a cultural fit in other ways; therapists should take care to adapt the approach based on a client's level of acculturation.

Hispanic Families

Bermudez (2008) describes several considerations for using the Satir approach with Hispanic families, who embrace collectivist values.

- Acknowledging cultural differences: Because the theory relies heavily on self-of-the-therapist, therapists should address cultural differences with clients directly to ensure transparency.
- Metaphors: Most Hispanic cultures are rich with metaphor, stories, and symbolism, which Satir also used. However, metaphors such as iceberg may have little meaning for Hispanic families, and therefore the therapist should find an appropriate metaphor, such as "molas," which are multilayered decorative textiles.
- Values: Therapists should familiarize themselves with cultural values, such as
    - Familism: valuing family closeness, which is not necessarily enmeshment
    - Respect: honoring hierarchical position of parents and authority
    - *Simpatia:* treasuring the value of friendliness and avoiding confrontation.
- Goal setting: Goals should be set in collaboration with clients to ensure that they are congruent with the client's values, specifically that individual goals of self-actualization do not create new stressors for the family.
- Contextual issues: Satir's approach does not directly address issues of immigration, acculturation, social support, and marginalization, and therefore, therapists working with Hispanic families should make a conscious effort to address these critical issues.

Sexual and Gender Identity Diversity

Grounded in their values of authentic self-expression, experiential therapists avoid conceptualizations of sexuality that are based on norms and performance (Kleinplatz, 1996). Thus, experiential therapies have been widely used with lesbian, gay, bisexual, transgendered, and questioning (LGBTQ) clients (Davies, 2000). When considering the experience of LGBTQ clients, experiential therapists focus on the burden of societal rejection of the client's authentic self and help clients move toward finding safe ways and contexts in which to express their authentic selves (Pachankis & Bernstein, 2012). Experiential therapists should also consider how their social contexts may more seriously constrain communication styles, both in their intimate relationships, with supportive versus nonsupportive family members, as well as with colleagues and strangers. Experiential practices, such as Satir's parts party and family reconstruction, have been used in gay and lesbian group programs to allow them to reexperience support and their family-of-origin relationships in new and more empowering ways (Picucci, 1992).

Research and the Evidence Base: Satir Model

With the notable exception of emotionally focused couples therapy (Johnson, 2004), an empirically supported treatment (see below), there has been little outcomes research on the effectiveness of specific experiential family therapies. Some initial research on Satir's approach has begun with the development of a scale that can be used to measure a person's level of congruence (Lee, 2002). However, what has received attention is the effectiveness of the therapeutic relationship as defined by experiential and humanistic therapies. Both streams of common factors research (see Chapter 2) identify the quality of the therapeutic relationship as highly correlated with therapeutic outcome, with Lambert (1992) estimating that 30% of therapeutic outcome in any form of therapy can be attributed to the therapeutic relationship as defined in the humanistic tradition: non-judgmental, empathetic, and engaged (Miller, Duncan, & Hubble, 1997). Furthermore, the vast majority of studies over the past four decades have found that the *client's* perception of the therapeutic relationship—more so than that of the therapist or a neutral third party—is correlated with positive outcome; thus, it is key to use the client's perception to measure the quality of the therapeutic relationship (Kirschenbaum & Jourdan, 2005). To support this claim, Duncan et al. (2003) have found that they can predict therapy outcome by measuring the quality of the therapeutic alliance in the first three sessions, suggesting that clients must experience the relationship with the therapist as safe and effective early in treatment.

A significant stream of research provides additional evidence for experiential approaches, supporting experiential therapists' claims that emotional expression promotes well-being (Stanton & Low, 2012). In particular, writing to express emotions has been found to transform meaning and increase positive emotion related to the event (Langens & Schüler, 2007). Of particular interest to family therapists, constructive expression of emotion characterizes more satisfying intimate relationships (Yoshida, 2011). In addition, young families with a positive attitude toward emotional expression also reported a greater sense of social support, suggesting that such an attitude may strengthen relationships on multiple levels (Castle et al., 2008). In summary, although the specific interventions and overall outcomes have not received significant research support, the principles and practices behind the humanistic approach to therapeutic relationships and to facilitating emotional expression have strong, consistent support.

Emotionally Focused Therapy (EFT)

In a Nutshell: The Least You Need to Know

Emotionally focused therapy (EFT) is one of the most thoroughly researched approaches in the field and is an empirically validated treatment for treating couples and families (Johnson, 2004). It more than qualifies as an evidence-based treatment, and it is an efficacious treatment, one that has been clinically tested in independent trials (see Chapter 2 for a painfully detailed definition; Furrow & Bradley, 2011; Lebow et al., 2012). Sue Johnson and Les Greenberg (1985, 1994) developed the model by integrating individual and systemic theories and by carefully observing what works in effective couples therapy. EFT uses an integration of: (a) attachment theory, (b) experiential theory (specifically, Carl Rogers's person-centered therapy), and (c) systems theory (specifically, systemic–structural therapies; see Chapters 4 and 5; Johnson, 2004). Emotionally focused therapists focus on the emotional system, which includes both interpersonal (i.e., couple and family) and intrapsychic (i.e., individual) systemic processes. In the first stage of therapy, the therapist identifies the couple's behavioral interactional patterns (just like most other systemic therapists) but also identifies the perceptions, emotions, and underlying attachment needs (need for safe connection) that fuel the problematic behavioral interactions. In the middle stage of therapy, the therapist helps couples fundamentally restructure their interactions so that each partner is able to experience a sense of safety and connection with the other (i.e., attachment needs are met). In the last phase of therapy, the therapist helps the couple solidify the new patterns. The approach is generally brief (approximately 8 to 12 sessions) with 70 to 73% of couples resolving issues and recovering from distress and 86% showing significant improvement within 12 sessions with a formally trained EFT therapist (Johnson et al., 1999). Although most of the research has been conducted with couples, the same principles and techniques can also be used for family therapy (Johnson, 2004).

The Juice: Significant Contributions to the Field

If you remember one thing from this chapter, it should be the following:

Attachment and Adult Love

Sue Johnson's (2004, 2008) emotionally focused couples therapy is based on a new paradigm for understanding adult love relationships. The premise is basically this: *humans need* **secure attachment** *relationships across the life span, not just in infancy and early childhood.* This claim was not widely accepted a few decades ago, but it is now enjoying a strong evidence base, which is likely to radically reshape the direction of couple and family therapy in the 21st century (Furrow & Bradley, 2011). This, dear reader, is big news. So you may want to pull out a highlighter for this section.

Bowlby's (1988) attachment research with human and primate infants established the physiological, emotional, and survival need for a safe, nurturing relationship between caregiver and child and has long been accepted in the human sciences. However, it was commonly believed that this need dissipated with time and that adults could theoretically be psychological and physically healthy without such a secure relationship. Current medical research not only supports the claim that secure attachment affects physical health, but specific correlations have also been identified: avoidant attachment styles are correlated with pain-related complaints and anxious attachment styles with cardiovascular conditions, yet secure attachment was not correlated with any specific health condition (McWilliams & Bailey, 2010). Insecure attachment has long been correlated with higher rates of psychopathology (Mason, Platts, & Tyson, 2005). Additional research has shown that securely attached adults are better able to withstand physical pain than those with insecure attachment styles (Meredith, Strong, & Feeney, 2006). Neurological research suggests that humans need secure relationships in order to emotionally self-regulate (Siegel, 2010).

Sue Johnson's work has been on the vanguard of the application of adult attachment theory to therapy, offering the most comprehensive approach for helping couples develop secure attachments in their intimate relationships. The theory of adult attachment helps explain much of the puzzling behavior related to intimate couple and family relationships: Why do humans so often treat poorly those they claim to love the most? The problem is that humans are trapped in a paradox when tension arises in attachment relationships: the other person is both the primary source of comfort and safety and—during conflict—the most threatening danger (Johnson, 2008). This paradox goes a long way in explaining much of the extreme behavior that therapists often see in couple and family relationships.

Using Bowlby's (1988) theory of attachment to conceptualize adult love, Johnson (2004, pp. 25–32) identifies 10 tenets of this theory, which I paraphrase below.

1. **Attachment is an innate motivating force.** The desire to be connected to others is an intrinsic physiological need of all humans. This implies that a therapist's work is not done until the client has at least one secure relationship in his or her life.

2. **Secure dependence complements autonomy.** Neither complete independence nor overdependence is possible, only effective or ineffective dependency. Thus, in therapy, the therapist's goal is to help clients develop an effective dependency (or interdependency, if you prefer) with significant persons in their lives.

3. **Attachment offers an essential safe haven.** Secure attachment provides a buffer against the stresses of life and measurably reduces their psychological and physiological effects.

4. **Attachment offers a secure base.** Just like young children, adults also need a secure base to enable them to feel free to experience exploration, innovation, and openness, which are all correlated with positive psychological health and growth.

5. **Emotional accessibility and responsiveness build bonds.** Secure attachment is established by being emotionally accessible and responsive; thus, this is the focus of the working phase of EFT.

6. *Fear and uncertainty activate attachment needs.* When threatened, a person experiences an unusually strong emotional need for comfort and connection; it is this need that fuels the destructive patterns too often observed in couples and families.
7. *The process of separation distress is predictable.* If attachment needs are not met, the person experiences predictable responses of anger, clinging, depression, and despair. *This distress is experienced as a primal survival need, thus helping to explain—but not justify—the often extreme and cruel acts committed in the name of love.*
8. *There are a finite number of insecure attachment styles.* When a secure relationship no longer feels secure, a person will use one of these three typical patterns to defend himself or herself against the trauma of having a secure relationship threatened.
   - *Anxious and hyperactivated:* When needs are not met, the person becomes anxious, relentlessly pursues connection, and may become clingy, aggressive, blaming, and/or critical.
   - *Avoidance:* When needs are not met, the person suppresses attachment needs and instead emotionally and physically withdraws, often focusing on unrelated tasks or other distractions.
   - *Combination anxious and avoidant:* In this style, the person pursues closeness and then avoids it once offered.
9. *Attachment involves working models of self and other.* People use the quality of attachments to define themselves and others as lovable, worthy, and competent and develop internal models about what can be expected and how to engage in attachment relationships.
10. *Isolation and loss are inherently traumatizing.* Isolation and loss of connection are inherently traumatic experiences that can trigger a panicked survival responses. Solitary confinement is a universal form of torture.

Rumor Has It: The People and Their Stories

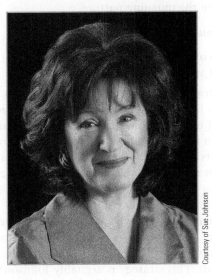

Courtesy of Sue Johnson

Susan Johnson

Sue Johnson, with Les Greenberg, began developing emotionally focused therapy in the 1980s. They developed this approach by refining their methods based on the outcomes of their research and their observations of what worked and what did not work. Johnson has continued research and development of the model, particularly as it applies to couples and families and also teaches internationally throughout the world. She has applied emotionally focused therapy to the treatment of a host of issues, including couples therapy with trauma survivors (Johnson, 2005), depression, and couples with chronically ill children (Johnson, 2004). She has also created, with her colleagues, a detailed workbook for people learning EFT (Johnson et al., 2005) as well as a self-help book for couples (Johnson, 2008).

Les Greenberg

Les Greenberg codeveloped EFT with Sue Johnson while serving as a professor at York University in Toronto and the director of the York University Psychotherapy Research Clinic. He teaches internationally and continues to research and refine a version of the model he calls emotion-focused therapy. He has focused primarily on its application to individuals, although he has recently written a book called *Emotion-Focused Couple Therapy: The Dynamics of Emotion, Love, and Power* (Greenberg & Goldman, 2008).

The Big Picture: Overview of Treatment

The EFT therapy process is clearly structured (this is where the manualized treatment part comes in) in three stages with nine steps that describe the progression of therapy (Johnson, 2004). But before you have pie-in-the-sky fantasies of a step-by-step recipe for success, let me bring you down to Earth and say that these steps are not perfectly linear, and most clients cycle back and forth. Alas, not even in evidence-based treatment does therapy go perfectly according to plan. Thus, the steps are mainly instructive for helping the therapist guide the process of therapy and track progress and setbacks as well as have a very clear treatment plan (note to self: therefore, these are some of the easiest treatment plans to write).

Stage 1: De-Escalation of Negative Cycles

Step 1: Create an alliance and delineate conflict in the attachment struggle.
Step 2: Identify the negative interaction cycle.
Step 3: Access unacknowledged emotions and underlying interactional positions.
Step 4: Reframe the problem in terms of the negative cycle and attachment needs, with the cycle being the common enemy.

Stage 2: Change Interactional Patterns and Creating Engagement

Step 5: Promote identification of disowned attachment needs and aspects of self, integrating these into relational interactions.
Step 6: Promote acceptance of the partner's experience along with new interaction sequences.
Step 7: Encourage direct expression of needs and wants while strengthening emotional engagement and attachment bonds.

Note: Steps 5 to 7 are generally first done focusing on the withdrawing partner, and then the same steps are repeated focusing on the pursuing partner.

Stage 3: Consolidation and Integration

Step 8: Facilitate new solutions to old problems.
Step 9: Consolidate new positions and new cycles of attachment.

Just in case your eyes glazed over reading that list, let me break it down a bit. The first stage of therapy is about two things: (a) establishing a strong therapeutic relationship needed for the exploration of difficult emotions, and (b) developing a clear case conceptualization using attachment theory. In the final step of this phase, the therapist will help the couple both reframe (see Chapters 4 and 5) and externalize (see Chapter 10) their negative interaction cycle in such a way that the couple/family conflict can be seen as failed attempts to connect (rather than believing that the partner has become a horrible, terrible person, which is where many start the conversation).

The second stage of therapy is where the therapy gets intense, and where EFT therapists earn their keep. In this stage, the therapist starts with the most emotionally *withdrawn* partner and helps this person identify, own, and directly express to the other partner his/her unmet attachment needs. This strategy is arguably Johnson's second most brilliant contribution—second, of course, to her theory of adult attachment, described in "The Juice" above. This move is radical because the withdrawer is generally the partner with the fewest complaints, so most therapists end up focusing on the *pursuer,* the one who is pursuing connection, which often takes the form of complaining (here's a hint for case conceptualization: the pursuer is generally the partner who makes the call to the therapist, unless the withdrawer has just been threatened with divorce). However, once the couple is deescalated (Stage 1), Johnson starts with the withdrawer; she does this because once the withdrawer reconnects, it becomes easier for the pursuer to vulnerably ask for needs to be met rather than criticize because now he or she is getting the connection he or she has been pursing in some form. So, in this phase, the therapist first works with the withdrawer to identify and express unmet attachment needs and then does the same with the pursuer. In both cases, the therapist helps the partner learn how to respond effectively to bids for connection. Interestingly, it is often more difficult to get the complaining pursuer to soften because there is a painful history of reaching out and being rejected by the withdrawer (Furrow, Ruderman, & Wooley, 2011).

The third phase is a more hopeful one, as couples learn how to work through old issues using their new safely connected relational patterns (generally with far better results). Since this is real life, not a fairy tale, there are typically quite a few bumps along the way as couples learn to relate to each other differently. EFT therapists are not surprised when old patterns reemerge; the therapist helps the couple identify what is going on and reconnect; this creates a sense of safety.

In addition to the stages and steps, Johnson (2004) identifies three primary therapeutic tasks:

> **Task 1:** Creating and maintaining alliance
> **Task 2:** Assessing and formulating emotion (most critically attachment emotions)
> **Task 3:** Restructuring interactions

If you were conscious while reading the last couple chapters, the first therapeutic task probably should look familiar (see, you are almost an expert). But the second is unique to EFT in that the couple's or family's interaction cycle is conceptualized in terms of attachment needs. Finally, the last task (which is where most of the action happens) involves helping couples learn to change—primarily through experiential means—how they relate with one another so that they can reliably create a strong sense of safety and love.

Making Connection: The Therapeutic Relationship

Empathetic Attunement

As the name suggests, *emotionally* focused therapy focuses on emotions; thus, the therapist's ability to deeply empathize and attune is essential—without it, the therapy will not work. In EFT, the therapist attunes to each partner's emotions with the intent to make contact with the emotional worlds of each (Johnson, 2004). *Empathetic attunement* requires listening to clients, connecting what they say with the therapist's personal experience, and then staying within the client's subjective perspective. Such attunement typically happens more at the nonverbal level, both in perceiving the client's emotional state and in reflecting it back through nonverbal communication (e.g., by softening the voice, nodding the head). The key here is for *the client* to feel deeply heard and understood—by whatever means the therapist does it—and to experience a sense of emotional safety in the therapy room. The therapist's empathic attunement with each partner serves as a model for them to relate to one another.

Expression of Empathy: RISSSC

If you get a chance to watch Sue Johnson doing therapy, you will note that she talks a bit differently than many others. At critical points, she will slow down significantly, repeat herself, and clearly highlight words or images. As you might imagine, this is done on purpose. Johnson (2004) summaries her unique approach to empathy in the following techniques (**RISSSC**) to express understanding of the client's affective reality:

- Repeat: Repeat key words and phrases that the client says.
- Images: Use images to capture emotion in a way that abstract words cannot.
- Simple: Use simple words and phrases.
- Slow: Maintain a slow pace that enables an emotional experience to unfold.
- Soft: Use a soft voice to soothe and encourage deeper experiencing and risk taking.
- Clients' words: Adopt clients' words and phrases in a validating way.

Examples of RISSC from the EFT training manual (Johnson et al., 2005) include:

- "Livid and disappointed, yes? So how did that go between you?" (p. 166)
- "Sounds like that was a pivotal time for you … that you needed him" (p. 167)
- "All your life it's been like that. Never getting the message that you're precious and [that] you count, wondering if there's something wrong with you." (p. 168)

Genuineness

Genuineness requires that the therapist be real and emotionally present with clients without being impulsive or constantly disclosing personal information (Johnson, 2004). Therapists are humble and able to admit mistakes and misunderstandings. As a result, clients experience the relationship between them and the therapist as an authentic human encounter.

Acceptance

Therapists maintain a nonjudgmental stance that is grounded in a positive view of human nature, an acceptance of human struggles, and a humble recognition of how hard it can be to create secure relationships with those we love (Johnson, 2004). Acceptance involves honoring and prizing clients *as they are* and acknowledging the fullness of their humanity. If you are nodding your head at this point, I should perhaps point out that this is far more challenging in practice than it sounds in theory (just remember, you heard it here first).

Self-Disclosure

Used infrequently, self-disclosure can build rapport or intensify validation of client responses (Johnson, 2004). However, the therapist keeps self-disclosure to a minimum to maintain a focus on the emotional process of the couple.

Continuous Monitoring of the Alliance

The therapist continually monitors the therapeutic alliance with each partner to ensure that a strong affective connection and sense of safety continue through all stages of therapy (Johnson et al., 2005). When expressing empathy in couples therapy, it is particularly easy for the alliance with one partner to weaken as the therapist expresses an understanding of the other partner, because for a moment, the therapist may appear to be taking sides in the attempt to understand. Thus, therapists need to constantly balance their focus between the two partners. Therapists monitor the alliance both verbally (directly asking about their experience of therapy) and nonverbally (identifying signs of defensiveness, checking out, etc.).

Joining the System

The therapist must build an alliance not only with each individual but also with the relationship as a system, accepting it as it is, just as each individual is accepted. Joining the system involves not only identifying relational patterns (e.g., nag/withdraw, pursue/distance, criticize/defend) but also reflecting these back to the couple so that they can better understand their relationship.

The Therapist's Role

According to Johnson (2004), the therapist is the following:

- A process consultant who helps the couple reprocess their emotional experiences
- A choreographer who helps the couple restructure their relationship dance
- A collaborator who follows and leads the therapeutic alliance

The therapist is *not* the following:

- A coach teaching communication skills
- A "wise creator of insight" into the past and/or future
- A strategist employing paradox or problem prescription

The Viewing: Case Conceptualization and Assessment

Intrapsychic and Interpersonal Issues

Much like other experiential family therapists the EFT therapist attends to both intrapsychic and interpersonal issues.

- Intrapsychic: How individuals process their experiences, particularly their key attachment-oriented emotional responses
- Interpersonal: How partners organize their interactions into patterns and cycles

Primary and Secondary Emotions

How does an emotionally focused therapist know which emotions to focus on? Is any emotion that a client expresses worthy of focus? The answers to these questions are multilayered. First, emotionally focused therapists distinguish between primary emotions and secondary emotions:

- Primary emotions: **Primary emotions** are the initial reactions to a given situation; these typically represent attachment fears and needs (usually softer, more vulnerable emotions, such as feeling abandoned, alone, helpless, unloved, unwanted, inadequate, etc.)
- Secondary emotions: **Secondary emotions** are emotions *about the primary emotions,* not about the actual situation. For example, if the given situation is a critical remark, the primary emotion may be feeling inadequate, but the secondary emotion is likely to be anger about feeling inadequate. Secondary emotions often take the form of anger, frustration, or withdrawal; these emotions often allow the person to avoid the sense of vulnerability associated with primary emotions. They must be explored so that the underlying primary emotion can be identified.

In the early phases of therapy, the therapist focuses on the salient secondary emotions because these are typically what couples initially present and are the only emotions of which many are conscious. As therapy progresses, the therapist begins to raise each partner's awareness of the primary emotion underlying the secondary emotion, such as the hurt that is beneath the anger of having one's partner no longer express sexual interest. By the working stage of therapy, the focus is mainly on the primary emotions.

Negative Interaction Cycle: Pursue/Withdraw

Similar to other systemic therapists (see Chapter 4 for a refresher), one of the therapist's first tasks is to identify the couple's or family's **negative interaction cycle,** which is typically conceptualized in EFT as a pursue/withdraw pattern (Johnson et al., 2005). The *pursuer* is protesting the separation and distance he or she is experiencing in the relationship; this is indicative of an anxious attachment style. In contrast, the *withdrawer* creates distance to protect himself or herself from the perceived lack of safety in the relationship, often in the form of criticism or rejection; this is typical of an avoidant attachment style. Of course, the more the pursuer tries to connect (often through nagging, criticizing, and demanding closeness), the more the withdrawer feels a need to distance himself or herself in order to create safety. Pursuers typically express emotions such as feeling hurt, alone, and unwanted, whereas withdrawers typically report feeling rejected, inadequate, or judged.

Couples typically present with one of four basic pursue/withdraw patterns (Johnson et al., 2005):

- Pursue/withdraw: The most common cycle, this cycle involves a readily identifiable partner who pursues connection and one who withdraws. In most cases, the female is the pursuer, and the male is the withdrawer. In some cases, the distancing male pursues for sex but otherwise distances from other forms of connection; this is still considered a pursue/withdraw pattern.

- Withdraw/withdraw: Some couples present with what appears to be two withdrawers; however, in these cases there is typically a *burned-out pursuer,* a pursuer who has given up trying to connect because of repeated failures to do so (Furrow et al., 2011). Generally, the prognosis for these couples is less optimistic because typically more damage has been done to the relationship. These couples often describe feelings of numb distancing and refusals to engage.

- Attack/attack: This pattern typically involves a withdrawer who sometimes turns, erupts into anger, and fights when provoked by his/her partner's pursuit (often in the form of criticism). However, after the fight, the withdrawer typically reverts back to the withdrawn position.

- Complex cycles: Trauma survivor couples often present with a complex, multiple-move cycle that involves both high levels of anxiety and avoidance.

In session, the pursue/withdraw pattern is initially traced in the first phase of therapy by asking couples to describe the behaviors and secondary emotions that characterize a typical negative interaction cycle. The therapist slows down the process, inquiring about each partner's inner emotional experience in the cycle and connecting each partner's description to the context of the other's experience. In this process, the therapist tries to move the couple to identify and acknowledge more primary attachment emotions.

Try It Yourself

> With a partner or on your own, identify the negative interaction pattern in your current or a past relationship. Which of the four basic patterns best describes the pattern? Identify each person's observable behavior in the interaction and each person's primary and secondary emotions. Which attachment style best describes each person's behavior during the negative interaction?

Attachment History

EFT therapists assess clients' attachment history, both with their primary caregivers and in adolescent and adult intimate relationships. Therapists do this by asking questions about the qualities of these relationships. To assess the quality of attachment bonds, EFT therapists use the acronym ARE: Are you there for me? Accessible, Responsive, and Engaged (Johnson, 2008).

QUESTIONS FOR ASSESSING ATTACHMENT HISTORY

- Describe your parents' relationship? Were they close? Did they regularly express affection for one another? Did they fight and if so how? Were they generally able to resolve their conflicts in a way that restored harmony and safety in the family?

- When you were young, to whom did you turn to for comfort and nurturing? Was this source of comfort reliable?

> - Describe your relationship with your parents and significant childhood caregivers? How did you know you were loved? Did you feel safe, physically and emotionally? How was conflict or disappointment handled? How was it resolved? Was there abuse or trauma?
> - Describe significant love relationships in your adulthood. Did you feel safe, cared for, and nurtured? Were there significant betrayals or other trauma?
> - Describe the early phases of your relationship when you felt more connected to your partner. How accessible were each of you? How did you show responsiveness? How did you engage one another? (Furrow et al., 2011)

Attachment Injury

In addition to an attachment history, the therapist also assesses for **attachment injuries** that may have occurred in the couple's relationship. An attachment injury is a specific type of betrayal, abandonment, or violation of trust in a couple's relationship (Furrow et al., 2011). Attachment injury occurs when one partner is in a moment of high need and vulnerability (e.g., pregnancy, loss, crisis, affairs, etc.) and the other partner fails to offer the needed support and nurturance. This injury fundamentally redefines the relationship for the injured party as being unsafe. The person may still remain in the relationship, but the quality of his or her participation is different in order to protect himself or herself.

Therapists must identify and directly address attachment injuries for the EFT process to work. Thus, the therapist needs to assess for attachment injuries and repair them (using steps 5 to 7). Identifying attachment injuries can sometimes be done directly, especially in the individual assessment sessions (see section on "Initial Assessment Sessions"): "Is there any event in your relationship that was so painful, possibly felt traumatic, that you feel it has left you feeling fundamentally unsafe in your relationship?" But most often you will blindly stumble upon these because therapy gets stuck: you hit an impasse. And often, when you probe deeper, you learn about the attachment injury, which may even have been discussed earlier but in a way that glossed over its significance.

Initial Assessment Sessions

EFT therapists have a somewhat structured series of initial sessions to determine if the couple is appropriate for EFT (Furrow et al., 2011). Typically, the assessment sessions are scheduled as follows: a joint couple session, followed by individual sessions with each partner, and then a return to regular conjoint sessions. In the conjoint session, the therapist assesses for:

- Perceptions of problems and strengths
- Negative and positive interaction cycles
- Relationship history and key events
- Brief attachment history of each
- Interactions observed in session
- Violence, abuse, or other contraindications
- Prognostic indicators: degree of reactivity, strength of attachment, and openness (response to therapist)

In the individual sessions, the therapist assesses for each partner's:

- Commitment to the relationship
- Sense of physical and emotional safety
- Potential, current, and past affairs
- Trauma history
- Detailed attachment history

Contraindications to EFT

Not all couples or families are appropriate for EFT, and the initial case conceptualization process involves identifying whether this is an appropriate approach. Common contraindications for EFT (reasons for not using EFT) include (Johnson et al., 2005):

- Different agendas for the relationship and therapy: Such as one wanting to marry and the other to remain single, or one partner having an outside romantic relationship.
- Separating couples: When it is clear that one partner has emotionally left the relationship.
- Abusive relationships: Couples in which there is physical, sexual, and/or emotional abuse are not appropriate for EFT. More subtle forms of abuse are often identified by one partner being afraid of the other.
- Untreated addiction: Alcohol and substance abuse do not preclude EFT, but it must be determined whether both parties can participate in therapy while sober. If one or both parties have substance abuse issues, an EFT therapist refers the person out for substance abuse treatment while focusing the EFT process on how substances affect the interaction cycle.

Targeting Change: Goal Setting

The overarching goals of EFT are straightforward and focused, providing couple therapists with consistent direction during what is often a tumultuous adventure (Furrow et al., 2011):

- Creating secure attachment for both partners
- Developing new interaction patterns that nurture and support each partner
- Increasing direct expression of emotions, especially those related to attachment needs

The Doing: Interventions

Interventions by Stage of Therapy

EFT therapists have several interventions they use, with certain ones being more common during particular phases of therapy. They tend to be divided as follows:

Early-Phase Interventions for Deescalating and Identifying the Cycle

- Validation
- Reflecting emotions
- Tracking the cycle (see section on "Case Conceptualization")
- Evocative responding
- Empathic conjecture

Working-Phase Interventions for Restructuring Interactions

- Evocative responding
- Empathic conjecture
- Heightening
- Reframing
- Restructuring Interactions (enactments)

Closing-Phase Interventions

- Validation
- Evocative responding
- Reframing
- Restructuring interactions (enactments)

Validation

Rather than implying some kind of godlike approval, therapists use **validation** to communicate to clients that their emotional experiences are understandable and understood by the therapist, rather than that their emotions are "correct" and "only to be expected" (such implications can weaken the therapist's alliance with the other partner). Therapists use validation to convey that each partner is entitled to his or her experience and emotional responses, helping articulate the underlying logic and emotions of each person's behaviors: "At first, you feel very sad that he does not seem to want to spend time with you, but after a while, you become angry and then try to force him to spend time with you."

Reflecting Primary and Secondary Emotions

The EFT therapist attends to poignant emotions and *reflects* back to the client a deep understanding and acceptance of these emotions (Johnson, 2004; Johnson et al., 2005). The goal of reflection is to help clients more fully experience their emotions, both primary (attachment-based) and secondary. Reflecting secondary emotions involves helping clients identify what they are feeling in the negative interaction cycle: "So when you shut down and pull away, it's when you see her disappointment and anger. It is too much to handle." As therapy progresses, reflections should highlight primary emotions related to unmet attachment needs: "What I hear you saying is not only that you feel like you need to hide when she gets angry, but that you begin to fear she does not love or respect you anymore."

Tracking Interaction Patterns and Cycles

Using methods similar to those of other systemic therapists, EFT therapists track patterns and cycles of interactions and then reflect on these patterns to help couples better understand the nature of their relationship (Johnson, 2004). For example, they look for common pursue/withdrawal and blame/defend patterns and attend to the unique sequences of each couple's interactions. In addition, as therapy progresses, therapists track positive interaction cycles in a similar way, helping reinforce the new interaction cycle.

Evocative Responding: Reflections and Questions

Whether phrased as reflections or questions, therapists use **evocative responding** to bypass superficial issues and identify unexpressed emotions and needs (Johnson, 2004). Because evocative responses are based on conjecture, the therapist offers these *tentatively*, allowing the client to correct or rephrase: "I think that part of the reason you may be pulling away is that you want closeness and connection so badly; if you were to be rejected, you would be devastated."

Empathetic Conjecture and Interpretation

At times, the EFT therapist will offer an **empathetic conjecture** or interpretation, typically addressing defensive strategies, attachment longings, and attachment fears (Johnson, 2004). This process is similar to evocative responding in that the therapist aims to deepen emotional experiencing, but empathic conjecture and interpretation more critically involve generating new meanings, not only touching on the emotion just below the surface. Often the therapist is making a link between the secondary and primary emotions: "So, on the surface you look angry and sure of yourself when you are arguing with him. But inside, something very different seems like it might be going on. Inside, it seems you feel more like a sad and lonely little girl who isn't too sure of herself ... sure if she is good enough or worthy of his love. Is that what is going on here?" In the later phases of therapy, conjecture is used to *seed attachment* by highlighting the desire for attachment that is blocked by fear or anger.

Heightening

Heightening involves using repetition, metaphors, images, and enactments to "heighten" key emotions and interactions that play a crucial role in maintaining the couple's negative cycle (Johnson, 2004). For example, the therapist can heighten by repeating a high-impact phrase (e.g., "feeling betrayed"), using nonverbal gestures like leaning forward or lowering the voice, using images and metaphors, or directing clients to enact responses. The therapist may also ask the client to repeat poignant moments: "Can you say that again—that you need her? Can you look at her and say that again?" Let's be honest: out-of-context these can seem phony and fake. But in the right context and at the right moment, these can be exactly what a person needs to explore complex and often painful feelings that arise in couples therapy.

Attending to Nonverbal Communication

Nonverbal communications often provide clues to primary emotions. EFT therapists closely monitor for nonverbal signs of unexpressed primary emotions. These may include (Furrow et al., 2011):

- Changes in tone of voice
- Bodily reactions
- Looks and glances
- Giggles, jokes, and laughter
- Sighs
- Silence
- Deep breath
- Tight lips

Reframing in Context of Cycle and Attachment Needs

EFT therapists regularly use two types of reframing of each partner's behavior: in the context of the negative cycle and in the context of attachment needs. Consistent with Johnson's systemic perspective, problems are reframed in the broader context of the relationship to help the couple see the cycle as the common enemy and to help each see how he or she contributes to the negative cycle (Johnson, 2004). For example, one partner's anger and the other's silence can be reframed to see how each response serves as a protective mechanism but that each contributes to maintaining the negative cycle. To increase solidarity, the negative interaction cycle is always framed as the couple's common enemy.

Similarly, reframing is used to help move clients from secondary to primary emotions. For example, "your stone-cold silence and distance is all that is showing on the outside. But inside, you are panicking; you're running scared. Because it seems that you have failed her again, and you just can't bear the thought. You can't bear the thought of having failed again."

Try It Yourself

With a partner or on your own, practice reframing the negative interaction cycle in the last "try it yourself" activity as the "problem" as if you were doing it for a client to help them see the cycle, not each other, as the problem.

Enactments, Restructuring, and Choreography

As in structural therapy, couples are asked to enact their present positions so that the therapist can help them more fully experience their underlying emotions (Johnson, 2004). The therapist then redirects or "choreographs" the couple's interaction to be less constricting and more accepting, perhaps by asking a partner to share a new affective insight directly with the other or by physically repositioning the couple to increase emotional intensity. In the later stages of therapy, the therapist usually uses enactments to choreograph partners' requests of each other and to create new positive responses that will lead to new bonding experiences that redefine the relationship as safe and secure.

Common Prompts for Choreographing New Interactions

- "What just happened here? Let's go back and see what was going inside for each of you?"
- "Can you turn to her (him) and tell him that right now?"
- "Can you turn to him (her) and ask for what you are saying you need right now?"

Blamer Softening

A hallmark EFT technique—the change event most associated with treatment success—softening of emotions is used to create emotional bonding, change interactional positions, and redefine the relationship as safe and connected. A softening occurs when a previously blaming, critical partner asks, from a position of emotional vulnerability, a newly accessible partner to meet his or her attachment needs and longings (Bradley & Furrow, 2004; Furrow et al., 2012; Johnson, 2004). The more critical partner softens his or her stance and words, allowing the more vulnerable or anxious partner to reduce emotional reactivity and defensiveness. Therapists can facilitate softening by encouraging partners to express their underlying attachment-based fears, including hurt and disappointment, when discussing conflict areas. Typically, this is done by underscoring the attachment issues, such as fear of rejection, in a particular area of tension. For example, if the wife is complaining that the husband does not spend enough time with her and the children, the emotionally focused therapist helps her articulate the fear of abandonment and/or feelings of rejection that underlie the complaint, thus revealing the wife's vulnerability and fears rather than her anger and frustration. When she expresses these softer emotions of vulnerability and asks her husband directly for comfort and connection, a more productive and healing conversation generally occurs, and this creates new bonding events. Process research on blamer softening identifies two factors that best predict heightened levels of client emotion and a successful softening event: (a) the therapist's emotional presence, and (b) the therapist's corresponding evocative vocal quality.

Bradley and Furrow (2004, 2007) have developed an extensive mini-theory about blamer softening to help guide therapists step-by-step through this often challenging process.

MINI-THEORY OF BLAMER SOFTENING EVENTS

Six key therapist content themes:

1. **Possible blamer reaching:** Therapist invites blaming partner to reach toward withdrawing partner after having blaming partner experience more vulnerable attachment needs.

2. **Processing fears of reaching:** This is the most critical theme in the softening event. The therapist helps process the blaming partner's fears of reaching out to his or her partner and being rejected yet again. During this process, therapists specifically explore fears related to a negative view of self and others that have developed from prior failed bids for affection. Therapists use the most heightening, evocative responses and empathetic conjectures in this theme, with clients typically needing to reach an emotional processing "boiling point" before successfully moving on to the enactment of the softening reach. Then, the therapist reissues the invitation to make the softening reach, this time highlighting both the attachment need and the newly processed fears related to reaching.

3. **Actual blamer reaching:** The therapist makes a directive statement to the blaming partner to reach for the other using a very simple request: "Can you turn to your partner and tell him how scary this is for you and let him know what you need right now?"

4. **Supporting the softening blamer:** The therapist stays active in the enactment and then affirms the clients sense of vulnerability and the new position.

5. **Processing with engaged withdrawer:** Continuing to be actively involved in the enactment, the therapist shifts to the withdrawer, again, validating the softened blamer in third person—"your partner just took a huge risk just now"—and helps "set the stage" for the withdrawer by focusing on the attachment significance of the blamer's reaching out.

6. **Engaged withdrawer reaches back with support:** Finally, after heightening the withdrawer's emotional response, the withdrawer is able to respond with support to his partner's request.

Bradley and Furrow (2007) identified five common obstacles to successful blamer softening:

1. Absence of attachment base in emotional reflections: Therapists simply reflect back emotions without contextualizing them within the larger frame of yearning for safe connection (e.g., "you feel sad" vs. "when you reach for your partner and she does not respond, you feel hurt and alone.").

2. Attachment-related affect distance: Insufficient emotional intensity is used in the softening event; therapists and clients are talking "about" softening rather than experiencing it.

3. Overlooking attachment-related fears: The therapist overlooks the importance of fully exploring attachment-related fears in step 2, either because of the therapist's own fears or rushing to the next step.

4. Internal views of self and other unacknowledged: When exploring fears of reaching out, the therapist needs to separate the fear of reaching from fears related to negative views of self and other that have developed from prior failed bids. EFT therapists typically do this by using "parts" language: "There is a part of you that fears he does not really care because he has not been there in the past when you reached out…. But there is another part of you that sees signs that he might have changed. This gives you hope that he will be there this time."

5. Interpersonal enactment failure: no softening reach: And sometimes, the therapist simply forgets to give a clear direction to have the blaming partner make the softening reach (step 3).

Attachment Injury Resolution Model

EFT therapists use the Attachment Injury Resolution Model (AIRM) with couples who have experienced an attachment injury (Zuccarini et al., 2013). Typically, couples need to resolve attachment injuries before they can effectively move to the second phase of EFT. In one study, 63% of couples were able to resolve the attachment injury using this model (Makinen & Johnson, 2006). The AIRM (a model within a model) has three phases and eight steps.

ATTACHMENT INJURY RESOLUTION MODEL

Phase 1: Steps 1–4: Cycle Deescalation Related to Injury

1. Injured partner provides account of incident, including description of secondary emotions.

2. Offending partner provides account of the same incident with his or her description of secondary protective responses.

3. Injured partner, with the help of the therapist, unpacks the negative models of self and partner and the attachment significant of the event.

4. Offending partner, with the help of the therapist, unpacks secondary emotions, negative models of self and partner, and attachment significance of event.

Phase 2: Steps 5–6: New Cycles of Emotional Engagement

5. Injured partner shares primary vulnerable attachment related emotional expression; this process includes an injury-specific blamer-softening process.

6. Offending partner is emotionally accessible and provides vulnerable expressions of responsibility, apology, and own desire for attachment.

Phase 3: Steps 7–8: Reconsolidation of Frayed Bond

7. Injured party accepts apology and is receptive to the offending partner's accessibility and expression of partner's attachment needs.

8. Offending partner provides responsiveness to the injured partner's expression of attachment needs. However, even if there is forgiveness at this point, reconciliation often requires the injured party to witness behaviors that show the intention to restore trust and maintain the relationship.

Research on the process of AIRM identifies steps 5 and 8 as the critical elements of the model, namely injury-specific softening processes (Zuccarini et al., 2013). Couples who are unable to resolve attachment injuries tend to not process the primary emotions in a highly emotional, differentiating and affiliative manner, and even if they deescalate in phase 1 are unable to move through stage 5.

Turning the New Emotional Experience into a New Response

After helping one partner explore an emotional experience, the therapist uses this experience to allow the other partner to respond in new ways, creating a positive interaction cycle in which each partner is better able to understand himself or herself and the other: "What is happening for you when you hear him say that his avoidance is not motivated by disinterest but by fear of rejection?" (Johnson, 2004).

Scope It Out: Cross-Theoretical Comparison

Using Tomm's IPscope described in Chapter 3 (Tomm et al., 2014), this theory approaches the conceptualization of systemic, interpersonal patterns as follows:

Theoretical Conceptualization

EFT clearly aligns with the various interpersonal patterns (IPs). The primary focus of stage 1 is to identify the pathologizing IP (PIP). EFT therapists do this by first tracking behavioral interactions, then secondary emotions, and then primary emotions. Once the PIP is identified at the end of stage 1, the therapist uses it to externalize the problem and reduce partner blame and unify the couple against the PIP: the PIP is the problem, not one's partner. Stage 2 is then about healing IPs (HIPs) and stage 3 about wellness IPs (WIPs).

Goal Setting

In EFT, WIPs are defined as interactions in which the couple and family are still able to maintain or quickly repair a secure connection even when their sense of secure attachment is threatened. The third stage of EFT is dedicated to helping couples learn how to stabilize these patterns so that they are the default interactions for the couple.

Facilitating Change

The facilitation of change in EFT follows a clear progression from PIP to HIP to WIP. After identifying the PIP in stage 1, the therapist moves on to facilitating HIPs in stage 2. The HIPs in EFT are clearly conceptualized as healing—repairing the loss of secure attachment and loss of emotional safety. During this phase, attachment injuries are attended to first, because they have done the most damage and must be repaired before any other healing can occur. After that, EFT therapists continue healing by first reengaging the withdrawn partner and having this partner begin the process of reconnecting with the pursuer. The last component of healing is having the pursuer reengage. This process can be particularly difficult because the pursuer has typically been actively shut out for a long time; in such situations, the therapists may use the mini-theory of blamer softening to facilitate the reconnection and healing.

Putting It All Together: EFT Case Conceptualization and Treatment Plan Templates

Areas for Theory-Specific Case Conceptualization: EFT

When conceptualizing client cases, EFT therapists typically use the following dynamics to inform their treatment plan. Go to MindTap® to access a digital version of the theory-specific case conceptualization, along with a variety of digital study tools and resources that complement this text and help you be more successful in your course and career. If your instructor didn't assign MindTap, you can find out more about it at Cengagebrain.com. You can also download the form at masteringcompetencies.com.

Negative Interaction Cycle

Describe the cycle and who does what using one of the four types below:

- Pursue/withdraw
- Withdraw/withdraw
- Attack/attack
- Complex cycles

Primary and Secondary Emotions

For each person describe:

- Behavior in the cycle
- Secondary emotions
- Primary emotions
- Attributions of the other

Sociocultural Factors

Describe how each party's social location relates to the problem interaction cycle, including gender, race, ethnicity, immigration status, socioeconomic class, sexual/gender orientation, religion, and ability

Attachment History

Describe key events in each person's attachment history, including current attachment patterns.

Attachment Injuries

- Describe any known attachment injuries in the current relationship.

Attachment Patterns

Describe when (if at all), client(s) feel securely connected in their current attached relationship(s), including:

- Relationships and conditions for secure attachment
- Regularity of secure attachment

Describe typical attachment behavior when person does not feel secure in relationships; specify with anxious, avoidant or anxious/avoidant:

- Frequency of insecure attachment
- Describe specific behavior

Potential Contraindications to EFT

- Different agendas for the relationship and therapy
- Separating couples
- Abusive relationships
- Untreated addiction

TREATMENT PLAN TEMPLATE FOR DISTRESSED COUPLE/FAMILY: EFT

The following treatment plan template can be used to help you develop individualized treatments for use with couples and families who report relational distress. You can download a blank treatment plan (with or without measures) on MindTap at www.cengagebrain.com or www.masteringcompetencies.com.

EFT Treatment Plan: Client Goals with Interventions

Initial Phase

1. Increase couple/family's awareness of *negative interaction cycle* and the *primary emotions* that fuel it to reduce conflict and hopelessness.
   a. Use *validation, reflecting emotions, evocative responding,* and *empathic conjecture* to identify secondary and primary emotions.
   b. *Track the negative interaction cycle,* first with secondary emotions and later identifying primary emotions.
   c. *Reframe* in the context of the negative interaction cycle and attachment needs.

Working Phase

1. *Increase engagement and emotional expression* of withdrawn party to reduce conflict/avoidance.
   a. Use *empathy, validation,* and *conjecture* to facilitate identification and expression of *attachment needs.*
   b. Use *enactments* to allow for direct communication of needs, the *acceptance* of other(s), and *new interaction sequences.*

2. *Decrease criticism* from pursuing party's and increase pursuer's expression of *attachment emotions* to reduce conflict.
   a. *Heighten* pursuer's primary emotions to facilitate *softening* of blaming position.
   b. Use *enactments* to promote *acceptance* by other(s) and to facilitate *new interaction sequences.*

3. Increase the ability of both/all to respond to the other(s) in ways that *create a sense of relational safety and bonding* even in moments of tension to reduce conflict, depressed mood, and/or anxiety.
   a. *Track the interaction cycle* and *empathetic conjecture* to help each person's see how his or her response affects others.
   b. Use *enactments* that help directly express primary emotional needs as well as respond in supportive ways when the other reaches out.

Closing Phase

1. Increase couple/family's ability to *respond effectively* to new stressors to reduce conflict and hopelessness.
   a. *Track positive interaction cycles* to reinforce positive changes.
   b. *Reframe* both positive and negative interaction cycles in terms of *attachment needs.*

2. Increase couple/family's ability to consistently respond to one another in ways that *solidify a secure bond* to reduce conflict, depression, and anxiety.
   a. Use enactments to facilitate *direct expression of emotional needs.*
   b. Facilitate turning the *new emotional experience* into a new response.

Treatment Tasks

1. Create a working alliance with both partners/family.
   a. Use *empathic attunement, RISSSC,* and *genuineness* to develop a safe emotional context for the therapy process.

2. Assess individual, systemic, and broader cultural dynamics.
   a. Identify the *negative interaction cycle,* including *pursuer/distancer roles.*
   b. Identify *secondary and primary (attachment) emotions* that characterize cycle.
   c. Assess *attachment history,* including *attachment injuries,* as well as history of *trauma.*

3. Identify needed referrals, crisis issues, collateral contacts, and other client needs.
   a. Assess for *appropriateness of EFT,* ruling out substance abuse, trauma, abuse/neglect, violence, conflicting agendas, or other contraindications.

  b. *Crisis assessment intervention(s):* Address crisis issues such as psychological abuse, intimate partner violence, hidden affair, self-harm, suicidal ideation, substance use, etc.
  c. *Referral(s):* Connect client with *resources* in client's *family and community* that could be supportive; make collateral contacts as needed.

Tapestry Weaving: Diversity Considerations

Ethnic, Racial, and Cultural Diversity

EFT has been studied on a range of ethnically diverse couples (Liu & Wittenborn, 2011) and has been specifically adapted for work with Latino clients (Parra-Cardona et al., 2009). In addition, attachment has been studied cross-culturally since 1967, and the general consensus is that attachment needs are normative and universal across theory; thus, this theory has elements that should be applicable with diverse clients. Liu and Wittenborn (2011) highlight that EFT therapists need to adapt and to tailor their interventions to work effectively with diverse clients. Many of the signature nonverbal interventions, such as heightening emotion by leaning forward, may be interpreted as inappropriate or invasive depending on the client's cultural background. Furthermore, cultural norms generally have highly specific rules for emotional expression, which is a key focus of EFT; thus, EFT therapists need to understand these norms to be effective. When working with diverse clients, EFT therapists need to identify the specific cultural meanings and functions associated with the expression of emotion and attachment behaviors as well as recognize the socially constructed meaning of emotion. Finally, EFT therapists need to be mindful of these cultural meanings when they choose the words and metaphors to reflect feeling to ensure that they clearly convey their intended meaning with diverse clients.

Gender Identity Diversity

Working with lesbian, gay, bisexual, or transsexual (LGBT) couples using EFT requires attention to their unique stresses and circumstances that often make forming a secure attachment more difficult for these couples. Zuccarini and Karos (2011) describe how EFT can be adapted to be sensitive to the needs of gay and lesbian (GL) couples. Although the general process remains the same, there are many predictable issues to which therapists must attend. In the first stage, therapists need to consider the impact on sexual identity–related stress on the formation of the couple and their generally complex interaction cycle: "negative emotional experiences and attachment related to the GL identity block the acceptance of sexual orientation and seriously undermine any kind of safe emotional engagement in GL relationships" (p. 320). In addition, the coming out process as well as the effects of living in a heterosexist society frequently involve significant trauma and betrayals in significant relationships; the effect of these traumatic betrayals and attachment injuries frequently affect a person's ability to develop secure relationships. Furthermore, when assessing the couple's negative interaction cycle, the therapist needs to consider the stresses of living in a heterosexist context and how rejection in the relationship is compounded by ongoing rejection in society.

Stage 2 involves the standard process of withdrawer reengagement and pursuer softening, but with GL couples therapists must explore the multiple and complex traumas they have experienced because of their sexual orientation; these traumas make it particularly difficult to risk being vulnerable enough to form a secure attachment bond. Exploring these past traumas can help partners feel compassion for one another and safe enough to trust one another. In stage 3, therapists should help each partner to address lingering identity issues and address the chronic stress related to being a sexual minority.

EFT has also been used with couples in which one partner identifies as transgender (identifying with opposite gender and wanting to change their public gender identification) or transsexual (one partner wants to modify their body to match their gender identification) (Chapman & Caldwell, 2012). Coming out to one's partner as trans-identified (TI) typically results in attachment injury for the non-trans partner because of the significant and often sudden role and identity change. Depending on the response, the TI partner is also likely to experience an attachment injury. For most, the revelation ends their sense of emotional security in the relationship and puts the partnership or marriage at immediate risk for dissolution. The double-bind that the non-trans partner experiences is that the trans partner is both the source of the injury and the source of security, creating major crisis in the attachment system. Chapman and Caldwell (2012) propose the following adaptation of the EFT attachment resolution model to help TI couples work through attachment injuries (see "The Viewing," above), specifically for the non-TI partner:

1. Reestablish a safe connection: If the TI partner is emotionally available, the therapist facilitates the injured party (non-TI partner) to reconnect by having him or her express secondary and primary emotions without blaming the TI partner.
2. Differentiate the injured party's primary emotions: Next, therapists help the TI partner to hear that the injured party's response is about attachment needs and the personal meaning of event in his or her life and that it is not ultimately a reflection on the worth of the TI partner. As TI processing often involves a significant degree of self-centeredness because of highly oppressive societal forces, it can be challenging to facilitate the TI partner's understanding (Chapman & Caldwell, 2012). The therapist facilitates the injured party's direct expression of his or her sense of loss and grief, and the TI partner is allowed see the other's vulnerability and to respond appropriately.
3. Reengagement: As the injured party becomes more engaged and owns his or her part in creating additional injury to the TI party (such as expressing hatred, blame, or rejection in response to his or her coming out), the injured party may be able to reach out to the TI partner for caring and possibly comfort.
4. Forgiveness and reconciliation: Finally, the TI partner can respond in a caring manner, which is the antidote to the traumatic experience. At this point, the couple can develop together a new narrative of the attachment injury event (coming out) and ultimately of the relationship. The therapist helps to foster trust and positive interaction patterns (WIPs) for the couple in their newly defined relationship, which may be as co-parents or friends.

Research and the Evidence Base: EFT

Researched for over 25 years, EFT is currently one of two empirically validated couples therapies (the other being integrative behavioral couples therapy; Lebow et al., 2012). EFT has an overall 70 to 73% recovery rate in 10 to 12 sessions, with 90% of all couples showing significant improvement (Johnson et al., 1999). However, often a course of treatment of more than 12 sessions is needed to alleviate couple distress (Johnson & Wittenborn, 2012). Follow-up studies show that the results tend to be stable, even with difficult-to-treat couples, such as trauma survivors and parents of chronically ill children (Clotheir et al., 2002). In addition, four studies, including one randomized clinical trial has examined EFT with female sexual abuse survivors and their partners, which is a population with very high risk of divorce and marital dissatisfaction. Researchers in these studies found clinically significant improvement in marital adjustment in almost all cases and in trauma symptoms in at least half of the participants (Dalton et al., 2013; Johnson & Wittenborn, 2012).

Since 1988, researchers have also studied the active ingredients of the change process in EFT, and they have identified three key process variables:

1. the depth of emotion in key sessions in stage 2
2. facilitating new interactions in which couples are able to express their attachment needs and be responsive to the other
3. the quality of the therapeutic relationship, especially the perceived relevance of the focus and tasks of therapy by clients (Greenman & Johnson, 2013; Johnson & Wittenborn, 2012; Lebow et al., 2012)

In addition, researchers have identified factors that moderate the impact of EFT. Surprisingly, a couple's initial level of distress does not seem to matter as much as their level of engagement in session or the male partner's level of trust in heterosexual couples. In one study, couples who made the most gains were those with high levels of attachment anxiety (e.g., worrying about the quality of connection) and emotional control (e.g., over-control of affect) (Dalgleish et al., 2015). Regarding gender differences, researchers found that therapists' warmth toward husbands was significantly correlated with husbands' warmth toward their wives, but the same was not true for wives; this finding suggests that therapists can potentially shift the trajectory of therapy by attending to warmth, especially as therapy progresses and husbands' warmth tends to wane (Schade et al., 2015). One study also considered treating attachment injuries within the relationship using EFT, with nearly two-thirds of couples resolving such injuries with a brief intervention; these results were stable at a three-year follow up (Johnson & Wittenborn, 2012). To meet the highest level of validation, EFT has also been studied by independent researchers, those not affiliated with the originator of the theory; two such studies have been conducted and have shown that even novice therapists with limited supervision can learn to conduct successful EFT sessions (Johnson & Wittenborn, 2012).

Clinical Spotlight: Symbolic–Experiential Therapy

In a Nutshell: The Least You Need to Know

Symbolic–experiential therapy is an experiential family therapy model developed by Carl Whitaker. Whitaker referred to his work as "therapy of the absurd," highlighting the unconventional and playful wisdom he used to help transform families (Whitaker, 1975). Relying almost entirely on emotional logic rather than cognitive logic, his work is often misunderstood as nonsense, but it is more accurate to say that he worked with "heart sense." Rather than intervene in behavioral sequences like strategic–systemic therapists, Whitaker focused on the emotional process and family structure (Roberto, 1991). He intervened directly at the emotional level of the system, relying heavily on symbolism and real-life experiences as well as humor, play, and affective confrontation.

For the astute observer, Whitaker's work embodied a deep and profound understanding of families' emotional lives; to the casual observer, he often seemed rude or inappropriate. When he was "inappropriate," it was always for the purpose of confronting or otherwise intervening in emotional dynamics that he wanted to expose, challenge, and transform. He was adamant about balancing strong emotional confrontation with warmth and support from the therapist (Napier & Whitaker, 1978). In many ways, he encouraged therapists to move beyond the rules of polite society and invite themselves and clients to be genuine and real enough to speak the whole truth. Although few contemporary practitioners practice purely in this style, Whitaker's approach has several unique elements that are still relevant today.

The Juice: Significant Contributions to the Field

If you remember one thing from this chapter, it should be the following:

The Battle for Structure and the Battle for Initiative

Whitaker referred to two "battles" in therapy: the **battle for structure** and the **battle for initiative**. Even if you are turned off by the war metaphor, every competent therapist should consider the principles he or she is describing. The battle for structure should be won by the *therapist,* who sets the boundaries and limits for therapy (Whitaker & Bumberry, 1988). Therapists need to win this battle because they are responsible for setting up a program for change. They, therefore, need to ensure that the following necessary structure for change is in place:

- The necessary people attend therapy
- Therapy occurs frequently enough to produce progress
- The session content and process will produce change

The "battle" occurs when the therapist must insist on these key pieces. Whitaker was quite clear that if clients were not able to meet the minimal structure requirements, he would not do therapy with them. He saw the therapist's personal integrity to be the heart of this battle:

> The key point here is for the therapist to face the need to act with personal and professional integrity. You must act on what you believe. Betrayals help no one. The Battle for Structure is really you coming to grips with yourself and then presenting this to them. It's not a technique or power play. It's a setting of the minimum conditions you require before beginning.—Whitaker & Bumberry, 1988, p. 54

Although it is unethical to do therapy if you do not believe that you can render successful treatment, frequently therapists "settle" for trying to do marital or family therapy without the key players attending sessions or do not direct the content or process to the areas they believe need to be addressed. Losing this battle results in stagnant therapy.

Conversely, the battle for *initiative* needs to be won by the client. It is the client who must have the most investment and initiative to pursue change. This insight is often summarized as: *therapists should never work harder than their clients.* This is a particularly challenging battle for new therapists, who can be overly helpful and often want to move faster than their clients are able. The therapist wanting change more than the client does creates a problematic dynamic and, paradoxically, often stalls change. The therapist needs to wait and sometimes let the tension and crisis build until the client develops the incentive and motivation to make changes. If the therapist has more initiative toward change, clients feel they are being dragged or forced and then start to dig in their heels or find little ways to sabotage the therapist's efforts at change. When the client has the greater motivation for change, the process flows more smoothly. Thus, therapists must be ready to follow clients' lead on how hard to work, following their flow of energy and enthusiasm.

The battle for initiative can be interpersonally uncomfortable, involving awkward silences, "I don't know" answers, or tension. Clients may feel frustrated that the therapist is not taking the lead in choosing topics of discussion and providing ready solutions. Whitaker and Bumberry (1988) explain the purpose of allowing this tension to build: "It's an issue of the family becoming somebody. They need to grapple with each other. It's an invitation to them to come alive and stop play-acting" (p. 66).

The Big Picture: Overview of Treatment

Therapy of the Absurd

Symbolic–experiential therapy is often referred to as the "therapy of the absurd" (Whitaker, 1975). However, in this case it is not absurdity for absurdity's sake (whatever that might be); instead, symbolic–experiential therapists employ a specific form of absurdity for a specific purpose. Absurdity is used to *perturb* (shake or wake up) the system in a compassionate and caring way. Sometimes the "caring" takes the form of speaking a truth no one else has been willing to speak, but the therapist is always careful to convey the spirit of caring behind such brutally honest comments (Whitaker & Bumberry, 1988). Usually, however, therapy of the absurd involves humor, playfulness, and silliness. By being able to play with otherwise "serious matters," therapists invite themselves as well as their clients into a more resourceful position in relation to the problem. A new attitude of lightness and hope emerges from this playfulness. Therapy of the absurd also uses paradoxical techniques that take the symptom and exaggerate it 10% so that clients can see the folly of their fears and habits. Symbolic–experiential therapists almost always employ paradox in a playful way.

Making Connections: The Therapeutic Relationship

Families do not fail, therapists do.—Whitaker and Ryan, 1989, p. 56

Therapist's Authentic Use of Self

Symbolic–experiential therapists strive to be authentic and genuine and, arguably, are the most authentic of family therapists. This is because they do not follow many of the pretenses that many would consider professional or appropriate boundaries; they are the first to point out that the emperor has no clothes (Connell, Mitten, & Bumberry, 1999; Napier & Whitaker, 1978; Whitaker & Bumberry, 1988). They are fully themselves and do not hide this from their clients. If they are bored, they show it; if they are annoyed, they express it. If they see an elephant in the middle of the room, they say something. This level of authenticity requires extensive supervision and training to ensure that therapists are able to maintain exceptionally clear boundaries between their personal issues and their clients' issues. Therapists who do not work this way are often baffled when watching symbolic–experiential therapists in action because they use a different set of relational rules for being "professional." In the end, being authentic at this level is primarily for the benefit of the client: to model the type of authenticity the therapist wants the client to develop and to create an environment in which the client can do this. If the therapist is hiding behind professional boundaries and the "role," the client has little chance of fully developing this type of authenticity.

Personal Integrity

Whitaker insisted that the therapist maintain a clear and unwavering integrity as a person (Whitaker & Bumberry, 1988). This integrity requires a fierce adherence to personal beliefs and a willingness to stand up for them, even when they are unpopular and may make people upset. Integrity is required to push families to address the painful issues they have been avoiding.

Therapists' Responsibility

Symbolic–experiential therapists strive "to be responsive *to* the family without being responsible *for* them" (Whitaker & Bumberry, 1988, p. 44). They are careful not to take on responsibility for clients' lives, but instead are responsible for pushing clients to accept full responsibility for their own lives. The therapist's greatest responsibility is to ensure that the therapeutic process promotes change: to win the battle for structure. The therapist is *active* but not directive.

Stimulating Mutual Growth

The therapeutic process in symbolic–experiential therapy stimulates mutual growth: the therapist and the client grow together through their authentic encounter with each other (Connell et al., 1999; Napier & Whitaker, 1978). Because therapists are fully authentic—the same people they are in other relationships—they learn about their own limitations, blind spots, and weaknesses and use the encounters with clients to also grow and become more fully authentic people themselves. The encounter touches each participant—client and therapist—at a deeply profound level, leaving both transformed.

Spontaneity, Play, and "Craziness"

Experiential therapists use spontaneity and fun toward several ends (Mitten & Connell, 2004; Roberto, 1991; Whitaker & Bumberry, 1988). First, by being playful, therapists build a strong therapeutic relationship that allows them to directly and honestly confront clients without encountering resistance. When working alone, they position themselves to be the type of person whom the client trusts enough to listen to the raw truth; when working as cotherapists, one therapist tends to be nurturing and the other confrontational. Playfulness also helps reframe problems that have been unrealistically magnified, as is often the case with parents or spouses who magnify a single flaw in the other and deemphasize the balance of good qualities. As folk wisdom teaches, laughter is often the best medicine, and symbolic–experiential therapists are skilled in using laughter to help their clients heal. The use of humor and play often goes against common stereotypes about therapists and therapy, which are based primarily on psychodynamic therapies, but most clients find laughter helpful, or at least enjoyable. Thus, if you observe symbolic–experiential therapists in action, you may see them tossing a Frisbee, singing a silly song, telling a well-chosen joke, or playing musical chairs.

Use of Cotherapists

Whitaker encouraged the use of a cotherapist, recommending that one therapist be nurturing and the other more confrontational so that the family has a strong base of support as well as a process for raising and addressing difficult issues (Napier & Whitaker, 1978). In providing a balance of support and challenge, the cotherapy team models a coparenting relationship.

The Viewing: Case Conceptualization and Assessment

Authentic Encounters and the Affective System

Case conceptualization in symbolic–experiential therapy is one of the most difficult to fully capture in words. In one sense, the therapist relies primarily on the in-the-moment *authentic encounters* with the client to directly experience who the other is in a holistic way (Connell et al., 1999; Whitaker & Bumberry, 1988). To anyone new to the practice, that statement is a bit too vague to be helpful. It is much like riding a bike: beginners need each step broken down, whereas those who are experienced say, "it's easy; just pedal," forgetting how difficult it was to get started (and how long dad pushed from behind). The little steps that allow symbolic–experiential therapists to effortlessly "roll" along and "intuit" their case conceptualization are grounded in a systemic understanding of the family: boundaries, homeostasis, triangles, and other factors. However, symbolic–experiential therapists focus primarily on the family's *emotional system* rather than their behavioral interactions. When they get a sense of boundaries or triangles, they focus on the emotional exchange between parties rather than on their actions. Therapists "feel" their way through the system.

Trial of Labor

The assessment of the family is accomplished through a ***trial of labor***—observing how the family responds to the therapist's interventions and interactions (Whitaker & Keith, 1981). During the trial of labor, the therapist tries to understand each person's preferred family roles, beliefs about life, values within relationships, developmental and family histories, and interactional patterns. More specifically, the therapist attends to two broad patterns: (a) the structural organization of the family and (b) the emotional processes and exchanges within the family (Roberto, 1991). In assessing structure, Whitaker used many of the same criteria as structural therapists.

Assessing Structural Organization

- Permeable boundaries within the family: Interpersonal boundaries should be permeable, not overly rigid or diffuse.
- Clear boundaries with extended family and larger systems: Boundaries with larger systems should allow for the autonomy of the nuclear family as well as connection with broader systems.
- Role flexibility: Family roles, including the scapegoat or good/bad child, should rotate frequently.
- Flexible alliances and coalitions: Alliances and coalitions are inevitable but should be flexible, changing with each new situation or challenge rather than always involving the same people on the same team.
- Generation gap: Generations should have clear boundaries, resulting in strong marital and sibling subsystems.
- Gender-role flexibility: Gender roles should be negotiable, resisting stereotyped gender norms in favor of the ability of each parent or partner to assume a wide range of roles as necessary.
- Transgenerational mandates: Transgenerational behavioral expectations and values are assessed across three to four generations; in healthy families, these are open to renegotiation.
- "Ghosts": Therapy identifies deceased or living extended family members who are creating cross-generational stress.

Assessing Emotional Process

- Differentiation and individuation: Each family member should be able to hold unique opinions and speak for himself or herself.
- Tolerance of conflict: Healthy families are able to tolerate the overt and explicit expression of differences and conflict.
- Conflict resolution and problem solving: Healthy families are able to engage in overt conflict and successfully resolve conflicts and solve problems, which may involve win–win scenarios, compromises, or acceptance of differences.
- Sexuality: In healthy families, couples share sexual intimacy, and sexuality is contained within generational lines.
- Loyalty and commitment: Members experience a clear sense of loyalty and commitment while allowing for individual autonomy.
- Parental empathy: Parents should demonstrate empathy for children's experience while still maintaining boundaries and structure; parents who were abused as children often fail to have sufficient empathy or are overly empathetic and do not set healthy boundaries.
- Playfulness, creativity, and humor: Fun and laughter are signs of healthy family functioning.
- Cultural adaptations: Immigrant families are able to balance the needs of their culture of origin and their current cultural context.
- Symbolic process: Each family has particular symbols and images that are "affectively loaded" and thus helpful in facilitating change.

QUESTIONS FOR PERSONAL REFLECTION AND CLASS DISCUSSION

1. Satir's family sculpting is particularly effective in bypassing client's rational defenses because it involves minimal language and instead uses the visual representation of each person's emotional experiences. In what types of situations and clients might this be especially appropriate or useful?

2. The two leading experiential approaches to family therapy were developed primarily by women. Why do you think this is? On what do you base your opinion?

3. What considerations should a therapist focus on when using the Satir approach or EFT with men? Women? Children? Persons from collectivist cultures? Persons from individualist cultures?

4. Describe the similarities and differences between Satir's survival stances and attachment theory.

5. In Phase 2 of EFT, therapists begin by reengaging the withdrawn partner rather than the pursuer because research has found this to be most effective. Why do you think that is? How is this similar to or different from the socioemotional relational therapy described in Chapter 3?

6. A highly effective and efficient evidence-based treatment, EFT guides therapists to focus primarily on the quality of attachment and repair the sense of trust in the relationship. Why do you think this focus on trust may be superior to other approaches?

7. Satir was recently named the fifth most influential psychotherapist by American therapists yet there is little formal research on her specific approach. Why do you think this is? Conversely, EFT is one of the best-researched approaches in the field. What might explain these differences?

8. Have you ever experienced an attachment injury or potentially caused one for someone else? At the time, did involved parties sense the event was creating significant damage, or was it not clear? Describe how it shifted the relationship, identifying different behaviors, interactions, and emotions. Was it ever resolved?

ONLINE RESOURCES

Satir Global Network (formerly AVANTA): Includes links to training institutes in Asia, Europe, South America

www.avanta.net

Satir Institute of the Pacific: John Banmen

http://www.satirpacific.org

Satir Institute of the Rockies

http://www.satirtraining.org

Satir Institute of the Southeast

http://www.satirinstitute.org

Emotionally Focused Therapy: Sue Johnson, Canada

www.eft.ca

Emotionally Focused Therapy: Los Angeles and Houston

www.theeftzone.com

Emotion-Focused Therapy: Les Greenberg, Canada

www.emotionfocusedtherapy.org

Go to MindTap® for an eBook, videos of client sessions, activities, practice quizzes, apps, and more—all in one place. If your instructor didn't assign MindTap, you can find out more information at CengageBrain.com.

REFERENCES

*Asterisks indicate recommended introductory readings.

Azpeitia, L. M. (1991). The Satir model in action [course reader]. Encino, CA: California Family Study Center.

Banmen, J. (2002). The Satir model: yesterday and today. *Contemporary Family Therapy, 24*, 7–22.

Banmen, J. (2003). *Meditations of Virginia Satir.* Palo Alto, CA: Science and Behavioral Books.

Banmen, J., & Maki-Banmen, K. (2014). What has become of Virginia Satir's therapy model since she left us in 1988? *Journal of Family Psychotherapy, 25,* 117–131. doi:10.1080/08975353.2014 .909706

Bermudez, D. (2008). Adapting Virginia Satir techniques to Hispanic families. *Family Journal, 16*(1), 51–57. doi: 10.1177/1066480707309543

Bowlby, J. (1988). *A secure base: Parent-child attachment and healthy human development.* London: Routledge.

Bradley, B. & Furrow, J. L. (2004). Toward a mini-theory of the blamer softening event: Tracking the moment-by-moment process. *Journal of Marital and Family Therapy, 30,* 233–246.

Bradley, B., & Furrow, J. (2007). Inside Blamer softening: Maps and missteps. *Journal of Systemic Therapies, 26*(4), 25–43. doi:10.1521/jsyt.2007.26.4.25

Castle, H., Slade, P., Barranco-Wadlow, M., & Rogers, M. (2008). Attitudes to emotional expression, social support and postnatal adjustment in new parents. *Journal of Reproductive and Infant Psychology, 26*(3), 180–194.

Chapman, D. M., & Caldwell, B. E. (2012). Attachment injury resolution in couples when one partner in trans-identified. *Journal of Systemic Therapies, 31*(2), 36–53. doi:10.1521/jsyt.2012.31.2.36

Clotheir, P., Manion, I., Gordon-Walker, J., & Johnson, S. M. (2002). Emotionally focused interventions for couples with chronically ill children: A two-year follow-up. *Journal of Marital and Family Therapy, 28*, 391–399.

Connell, G., Mitten, T., & Bumberry, W. (1999). *Reshaping family relationships: The symbolic-experiential therapy of Carl Whitaker*. Philadelphia, PA: Brunner/Mazel.

Dalgleish, T. L., Johnson, S. M., Burgess Moser, M., Lafontaine, M., Wiebe, S. A., & Tasca, G. A. (2015). Predicting change in marital satisfaction throughout emotionally focused couple therapy. *Journal of Marital and Family Therapy, 41*(3), 276–291. doi:10.1111/jmft.12077

Dalton, E. J., Greenman, P. S., Classen, C. C., & Johnson, S. M. (2013). Nurturing connections in the aftermath of childhood trauma: A randomized controlled trial of emotionally focused couple therapy for female survivors of childhood abuse. *Couple And Family Psychology: Research And Practice, 2*(3), 209–221. doi:10.1037/a0032772

Davies, D. (2000). Person-centered therapy. In D. Davies, C. Neal (Eds.), *Therapeutic perspectives on working with lesbian, gay and bisexual clients* (pp. 91–105). Maidenhead, England: Open University Press.

Duncan, B. L., Miller, S. D., Sparks, J. A., Claud, D. A., Reynolds, L. R., Brown, J., & Johnson, L. D. (2003). The Session Rating Scale: Preliminary psychometric properties of a "working" alliance measure. *Journal of Brief Therapy, 3*, 3–12.

Epstein, N. B., Curtis, D. S., Edwards, E., Young, J. L., & Zheng, L. (2014). Therapy with families in China: Cultural factors influencing the therapeutic alliance and therapy goals. *Contemporary Family Therapy: An International Journal, 36*(2), 201–212. doi:10.1007/s10591-014-9302-x

Furrow, J. L., & Bradley, B. (2011). Emotionally focused couple therapy: Making the case for effective couple therapy. In J. L. Furrow, S. M. Johnson, B. A. Bradley (Eds.), *The emotionally focused casebook: New directions in treating couples* (pp. 3–29). New York: Routledge/Taylor & Francis.

Furrow, J. L., Edwards, S. A., Choi, Y., & Bradley, B. (2012). Therapist presence in emotionally focused couple therapy blamer softening events: Promoting change through emotional experience. *Journal of Marital And Family Therapy, 38*(Suppl 1), 39–49. doi:10.1111/j.1752-0606.2012.00293.x

Furrow, J., Ruderman, L., & Woolley, S. (2011). Emotionally focused therapy four-day externship. Santa Barbara, CA, September 7–10.

Gehart, D. (2015). *Theory and treatment planning in family therapy*. Pacific Grove, CA: Brooks/Cole.

Gehart, D. R., & Lyle, R. R. (2001). Client experience of gender in therapeutic relationships: An interpretive ethnography. *Family Process, 40*, 443–458.

Gehart, D., & McCollum, E. (2008). Teaching therapeutic presence: A mindfulness-based approach. In S. Hicks (Ed.), *Mindfulness and the healing relationship*. New York: Guilford.

Greenberg, L. S., & Goldman, R. N. (2008). *Emotion-focused couple therapy: The dynamics of emotion, love, and power*. Washington, DC: American Psychological Association.

Greenman, P. S., & Johnson, S. M. (2013). Process research on emotionally focused therapy (EFT) for couples: Linking theory to practice. *Family Process, 52*(1), 46–61. doi:10.1111/famp.12015

*Johnson, S. M. (2004). *The practice of emotionally focused marital therapy:*

Creating connection (2nd ed.). New York: Brunner/Routledge.

Johnson, S. M. (2005). *Emotionally focused couple therapy with trauma survivors: Strengthening attachment bonds.* New York: Guilford.

Johnson, S. (2008). *Hold me tight: Seven conversations for a lifetime of love.* New York: Little, Brown.

Johnson, S. M., Bradley, B., Furrow, J., Lee, A., Palmer, G., Tilley, D., & Woolley, S. (2005). *Becoming an emotionally focused couples therapist: A workbook.* New York: Brunner/Routledge.

Johnson, S. M., & Greenberg, L. S. (1985). The differential effects of experiential and problem solving interventions in resolving marital conflicts. *Journal of Consulting and Clinical Psychology, 53,* 175–184.

Johnson, S. M., & Greenberg, L. S. (Eds.). (1994). *The heart of the matter: Perspectives on emotion in marital therapy.* New York: Brunner/Mazel.

Johnson, S. M., Hunsley, J., Greenberg, L. S., & Schindler, D. (1999). Emotionally focused couples therapy: Status and challenges. *Clinical Psychology: Science and Practice, 6,* 67–79.

Johnson, S. M., & Wittenborn, A. K. (2012). New research findings on emotionally focused therapy: Introduction to special section. *Journal of Marital and Family Therapy, 38*(Suppl 1), 18-22. doi:10.1111/j.1752-0606.2012.00292.x

Kirschenbaum, H., & Jourdan, A. (2005). The current status of Carl Rogers and the Person-Centered Approach. *Psychotherapy: Theory, Research, Practice, Training, 42,* 37–51.

Kleinplatz, P. J. (1996). Transforming sex therapy: Integrating erotic potential. *Humanistic Psychologist, 24*(2), 190–202. doi:10.1080/08873267.1996.9986850

Lambert, M. (1992). Psychotherapy outcome research: Implications for integrative and eclectic therapists. In J. C. Norcross & M. R. Goldfried (Eds.), *Handbook of psychotherapy integration* (pp. 94–129). New York: Wiley.

Langens, T. A., & Schüler, J. (2007). Effects of written emotional expression: The role of positive expectancies. *Health Psychology, 26*(2), 174–182. doi:10.1037/0278-6133.26.2.174

Lebow, J., Chambers, A., Christensen, A., & Johnson, S. (2012). Research on the treatment of couple distress. *Journal of Marital and Family Therapy, 38,* 145–168.

Lee, B. K. (2002). Development of a congruence scale based on the Satir model. *Contemporary Family Therapy: An International Journal, 24*(1), 217–239. doi:10.1023/A:1014390009534

Liu, T., & Wittenborn, A. (2011). Emotionally focused therapy with culturally diverse couples. In J. L. Furrow, S. M. Johnson, B. A. Bradley (Eds.), *The emotionally focused casebook: New directions in treating couples* (pp. 295–316). New York: Routledge/Taylor & Francis.

Lu, Q., & Stanton, A. L. (2010). How benefits of expressive writing vary as a function of writing instructions, ethnicity and ambivalence over emotional expression. *Psychology & Health, 25*(6), 669–684.

Makinen, J. D., & Johnson, S. M. (2006). Resolving attachment injuries in couples using emotionally focused therapy: Steps toward forgiveness and reconciliation. *Journal of Consulting and Clinical Psychology, 74,* 1055–1064.

Mason, O., Platts, H., & Tyson, M. (2005). Early maladaptive schemas and adult attachment in a UK clinical population. *Psychology and Psychotherapy: Theory, Research and Practice, 78*(4), 549–564.

McWilliams, L. A., & Bailey, S. (2010). Associations between adult attachment ratings and health conditions: Evidence from the National Comorbidity Survey Replication. *Health Psychology, 29*(4), 446–453. doi:10.1037/a0020061

Meredith, P. J., Strong, J., & Feeney, J. A. (2006). The relationship of adult attachment to emotion, catastrophizing, control, threshold and tolerance, in experimentally-induced pain. *Pain, 120*(1–2), 44–52. doi:10.1016/j.pain.2005.10.008

Miller, S. D., Duncan, B. L., & Hubble, M. (1997). *Escape from Babel: Toward a unifying language for psychotherapy practice.* New York: Norton.

Mitten, T. J., & Connell, G. M. (2004). The core variables of symbolic-experiential therapy: A qualitative study. *Journal of Marital and Family Therapy, 30,* 467–478.

*Napier, A. Y., & Whitaker, C. (1978). *The family crucible: The intense experience of family therapy.* New York: Harper.

Neff, K. (2003). Self-compassion: An alternative conceptualization of a healthy attitude toward oneself. *Self and Identity, 2,* 85–101.

Pachankis, J. E., & Bernstein, L. B. (2012). An etiological model of anxiety in young gay men: From early stress to public self-consciousness. *Psychology of Men & Masculinity, 13*(2), 107–122. doi:10.1037/a0024594

Parra-Cardona, J., Córdova, D. R., Holtrop, K., Escobar-Chew, A., & Horsford, S. (2009). Culturally informed emotionally focused therapy with Latino/a immigrant couples. In M. Rastogi & V. Thomas (Eds.), *Multicultural Couple Therapy* (pp. 345–368). Thousand Oaks, CA: Sage.

Picucci, M. (1992). Planning an experiential weekend workshop for lesbians and gay males in recovery. *Journal of Chemical Dependency Treatment, 5*(1), 119–139. doi:10.1300/J034v05n01_10

*Roberto, L. G. (1991). Symbolic-experiential family therapy. In A. S. Gurman & D. P. Kniskern (Eds.), *Handbook of family therapy* (vol. 2, pp. 444–476). New York: Brunner/Mazel.

Rogers, Carl. (1961). *On becoming a person: A therapist's view of psychotherapy.* London: Constable.

Rogers, C. (1981). *Way of being.* Boston, MA: Houghton Mifflin.

Satir, V. (1967/1983). *Conjoint family therapy* (3rd ed.). Palo Alto, CA: Science and Behavior Books.

Satir, V. (1972). *Peoplemaking.* Palo Alto, CA: Science and Behavior Books.

Satir, V. (1988). *The new peoplemaking.* Palo Alto, CA: Science and Behavior Books.

Satir, V., & Baldwin, M. (1983). *Satir step by step: A guide to creating change in families.* Palo Alto, CA: Science and Behavior Books.

*Satir, V., Banmen, J., Gerber, J., & Gomori, M. (1991). *The Satir model: Family therapy and beyond.* Palo Alto, CA: Science and Behavior Books.

Schade, L. C., Sandberg, J. G., Bradford, A., Harper, J. M., Holt-Lunstad, J., & Miller, R. B. (2015). A longitudinal view of the association between therapist warmth and couples' in-session process: An observational pilot study of emotionally focused couples therapy. *Journal of Marital and Family Therapy, 41*(3), 292–307. doi:10.1111/jmft.12076

Schwartz, R. C. (1995). *Internal family systems therapy.* New York: Guilford.

Siegel, D. J. (2010). *The mindful therapist: A clinician's guide to mindsight and neural integration.* New York: Norton.

Stanton, A. L., & Low, C. A. (2012). Expressing emotions in stressful contexts: Benefits, moderators, and mechanisms. *Current Directions in Psychological Science, 21*(2), 124–128. doi:10.1177/0963721411434978

Tomm, K., St. George, S., Wulff, D., & Strong, T. (2014). Patterns in interpersonal interactions: Inviting relational understandings for therapeutic change. New York: Routledge.

Wang, L. (1994). Marriage and family therapy with people from China. *Contemporary Family Therapy: An International Journal, 16*(1), 25–37. doi:10.1007/BF02197600

Whitaker, C. A. (1975). Psychotherapy of the absurd: With a special emphasis on the psychotherapy of aggression. *Family Process, 14,* 1–15.

*Whitaker, C. A., & Bumberry, W. M. (1988). *Dancing with the family.* New York: Brunner/Mazel.

*Whitaker, C. A., & Keith, D. V. (1981). Symbolic-experiential family therapy. In A. S. Gurman & D. P. Kniskern (Eds.), *Handbook of family therapy* (pp. 187–224). New York: Brunner/Mazel.

Whitaker, C. A., & Ryan, M. C. (1989). *Midnight musings of a family therapist.* New York: Norton.

Yoshida, T. (2011). Effects of attitudes toward emotional expression on anger regulation tactics and intimacy in close and equal relationships. *Japanese Journal of Social Psychology, 26*(3), 211–218.

Yu, J. (1998, November). Asian students' preferences for psychotherapeutic approaches: Cognitive-behavioral, process-experiential and short-term dynamic therapies. *Dissertation Abstracts International, 59,* 2444.

Zuccarini, D., & Karos, L. (2011). Emotionally focused therapy for gay and lesbian couples: Strong identities, strong bonds. In J. L. Furrow, S. M. Johnson, & B. A. Bradley, (Eds.), *The emotionally focused casebook: New directions in treating couples* (pp. 317–342). New York: Routledge/Taylor & Francis.

Zuccarini, D., Johnson, S. M., Dalgleish, T. L., & Makinen, J. A. (2013). Forgiveness and reconciliation in emotionally focused therapy for couples: The client change process and therapist interventions. *Journal of Marital and Family Therapy, 39*(2), 148–162. doi: 10.1111/j.1752-0606.2012.00287.x

Experiential Case Study: Child Sexual Abuse

Brad and Sophie have sought counseling because they have just discovered that a female babysitter recently sexually abused their 12-year-old daughter, Briana. A report was made to child protective services, and the babysitter, who is 16, is currently being charged with abuse. Briana has become socially withdrawn and reports intrusive thoughts about the abuse. The couple, who are both practicing lawyers, report increased arguing over the past year since Sophie has had to travel more for work and Brad has had to pick up more of the child-care duties. Sophie feels guilty about the abuse because her travel schedule necessitated the increased use of babysitters.

After an initial consultation, an Satir-based family therapist developed the following case conceptualization.

SATIR HUMAN GROWTH MODEL CASE CONCEPTUALIZATION

For use with individual, couple, or family clients.

Date: 4/15/18   **Clinician:** Sharee Lee   **Client/Case #:** 1020

Introduction to Client & Significant Others

List all significant others for client:

Adults/Parents: Select identifier/abbreviation for use in rest of case conceptualization

AM1: Adult Male   Age: 36   Other   Married heterosexual   Occupation: Lawyer Other identifier: Armenian American, second generation

AF1: Adult Female   Age: 36   European American   Married heterosexual   Occupation: Lawyer Other identifier: Greek American, second generation; reports being diagnosed with bipolar disorder but that it is currently managed with medicaiton.

Children/Adult Children: Select identifier/abbreviation for use in rest of case conceptualization

CF1: Child Female   Age: 12   Multiethnic/Biracial   Grade: 7th School: Greenwood School Other identifier: Socially and academically engaged in school.

None Age: ___ Select Ethnicity Grade: Select Grade School: ___ Other identifier: _____

Others: _____

Presenting Concerns

Describe each significant person's description of the problem:

Adult Male: Although he does not blame AF36 for the abuse, he is concerned about the weakening of AF36's relationship with CF12 over the past year or two due to her increased focus at work. Reports feeling guilty that they made the decision to have AF work because "this might not have happened." Feels helpless in terms of knowing how to help CF12.

Adult Female : Blames self for abuse and feels guilty about pursuing her career; feels as though she has no other choice. At the same time, she is angry that AM is not more supportive of her career, since she has had been the priority for the most of CF12's infancy and elementary school years.

Child Female: Feels supported by parents and is relieved that her parents believed her; reports feeling increasingly uncomfortable around her peers and less social; having nightmares and intrusive thoughts. Feels somewhat neglected by mother since she started traveling more.

Select Person: _____

Broader System: Description of problem from extended family, referring party, school, legal system, etc.:

Extended Family: AF35 and AM36's parents are supportive yet also hint that this could have been prevented if AF36 stayed home with CF12 more rather than try to pursue a career.

Child Protective Services Social Worker: <u>Believes CF12's report and has referred her for therapy to</u> <u>address trauma issues.</u>

Name: _____

Background Information

Trauma/Abuse History (recent and past): <u>Six months ago a female babysitter began molesting CF12,</u> <u>which continue for almost two months before it escalated to a point where CF12 told her parents. Her</u> <u>parents promptly made a report and swift action was taken by CPS.</u>

Substance Use/Abuse (current and past; self, family of origin, significant others): <u>No significant sub-</u> <u>stance issues reported.</u>

Precipitating Events (recent life changes, first symptoms, stressors, etc.): <u>AF36 began traveling more</u> <u>for work a year ago, which necessitated hiring more babysitters for CF12 after school and on weekends.</u> <u>AF36 and AM36 have been arguing more since she has been traveling, and her relationship with CF12</u> <u>has reportedly weakened during this period also.</u>

Related Historical Background (family history, related issues, previous counseling, medical/mental health history, etc.): <u>AF36 was diagnosed with bipolar, as was her mother and sister, and has had prior</u> <u>therapy related to the mood disorder. She is currently taking medications and reports being stable.</u> <u>There have been several divorces by AM36 and AF36's siblings, which alarms them both.</u>

Communication and Validation Patterns

Describe the communication and validation patterns for all significant persons related to client:

Adult Male: *Stance(s) when feels invalidated:* ☐ Placating ☐ Blaming ☒ Superreasonable ☐ Irrelevant

Relational dynamics that triggers survival stance: <u>Survival stance triggered when AM has to engage</u> <u>difficult emotions in himself or other or when he feels attacked by AF or family of origin.</u>

Relational/family belief or rule that informs this triggering dynamic: <u>People should be logical and</u> <u>make sense; men should not have to take care of the children; that is a woman's job. Taking care of chil-</u> <u>dren has less value than achieving at work.</u>

Relational dynamics that enable person to communicate congruently: <u>AM is generally able to be</u> <u>congruent when discussing practical issues, such as work and child-care responsibilities, even when</u> <u>having to solve practical problems.</u>

Adult Female: *Stance(s) when feels invalidated:* ☐ Placating ☒ Blaming ☐ Superreasonable ☐ Irrelevant

Relational dynamics that triggers survival stance: <u>Survival stance triggered when her needs are not</u> <u>recognized in the family or when AM tries to make her feel guilty; also triggered by family of origin,</u> <u>particularly her mother, when she feels they disapprove of her in some way.</u>

Relational/family belief or rule that informs this triggering dynamic: <u>One must be perfect and high</u> <u>achieveing to have worth. It is not fair; everyone else has it easier than me.</u>

(continued)

Communication and Validation Patterns (*continued*)

Relational dynamics that enable person to communicate congruently: When AF36 believes others are not blaming her or when she is not silently blaming or doubting herself.

Child Female: *Stance(s) when feels invalidated:*   ☒ Placating   ☐ Blaming   ☐ Superreasonable   ☐ Irrelevant

Relational dynamics that triggers survival stance: Whenever she feels disapproval from parents or others.

Relational/family belief or rule that informs this triggering dynamic: One must be perfect and high achieving to have worth.

Relational dynamics that enable person to communicate congruently: With AM36 and AF36's support in conjunction with therapeutic services, CF12 can develop a voice to advocate for herself.

Select Person: *Stance(s) when feels invalidated:*   ☐ Placating   ☐ Blaming   ☐ Superreasonable   ☐ Irrelevant

Relational dynamics that triggers survival stance: _____.

Relational/family belief or rule that informs this triggering dynamic: _____.

Relational dynamics that enable person to communicate congruently: _____.

Self-Worth and Self-Esteem

Describe the dynamics of each person's sense of self-worth and self-esteem, including contexts in which each has greater or lesser sense of worth:

Adult Male: AM36 prides himself on his professional identity, which is the primarily source of his self-worth. However, his recent need to participate more in CF12's life while AF36 has been away has compromised his view of self, as his views of gender roles have been challenged.

Adult Female: AF36's self-worth comes from both her professional success and—prior to the abuse—from her role as a mother. However, her sense of self-worth was significantly impacted upon hearing about abuse toward CF12. AF36's identity as a mother has been called into question, and she feels guilty for neglecting CF12 while on business trips, yet also is unable to justify stopping the pursuit of her career.

Child Female: CF12's self-worth has been based on external sources—the approval of her parents and on school achievement—and thus is not consistent or stable. The experience of abuse has done further damage to her sense of worth and may be why she is avoiding her peers.

Select Person: _____

Describe dynamics of social location, such as cultural, gender, social class, or other diversity factors, that inform evaluation of self: Since both AM36 and AF36 financially provide for family, the system's gender roles are nontraditional. AF36's belief that she has duties to maintain both a strong professional identity as well as a significant maternal role create a demanding lifestyle. Fortunately both parents' incomes allow for financial stability and access to useful resources. As is common in second-generation European immigrants from collectivist cultures (Greek and Armenian), both parents have a strong work ethic and focus on the success of the next generation, much like their parents did for them. They have a strong sense of connection to their broader ethnic community that also provides a sense of worth and meaning.

Relational Life Chronology

Describe significant events, specifically those that may relate to sense of validation and worth, in family and/or relational life; please list in chronological order:

Year: 2004   Event: CF12 born   Significance: Created family system and AM36 and AF36's roles as father and mother

Year: 2010   Event: AM36 promoted   Significance: AM36's professional identity strengthened and validated

Year: 2014   Event: AF36 promoted   Significance: AF36's professional success threatened AM36's role as breadwinner and shifted more child-care responsibilities to AM36

Year: 2015   Event: Sexual abuse toward CF12   Significance: CF12 began to question her self-worth, which led to difficulty engaging in positive socialization at school

Year: _____   Event: _____   Significance: _____

Year: _____   Event: _____   Significance: _____

Relational/Family Dynamics

Describe salient dynamics:

☒ **Power struggle/coalitions in family:** Describe: With both AM36 and AF36 as working parents, traditional gender roles are challenged and duties as breadwinner and child-caregiver must be negotiated.

☒ **Parental conflicts:** Describe: AM36 feels resentful for having to take on more child-care responsibilities while AF36 is away on business, since he also works full-time.

☒ **Expression of intimacy/warmth between parents/children and/or within couple:** Describe: Both parents are able to show warmth to their daughter, although AF has been more distant through the

Relational/Family Dynamics (*continued*)

recent turmoil due to her own guilt; the couple struggles with showing the same level of warmth toward each other because resentment and guilt have made it difficult for them to connect.

☒ Describe salient family/relational roles:

☒ Martyr: AF often describes herself as a martyr; in the past it was being a professional working mother without help from husband. Now it is that she must travel for work.

☒ Victim/helpless: CF12's placating stance contributes to her victimization and feeling incapable of managing her life

☐ Rescuer: _____

☐ Good/bad child: _____

☒ Good/bad parent: AM36 is the "good" parent for stepping in to take care of CF12, while AF36 is the "bad" parent for engaging in increased work demands and neglecting family

☐ Other: _____

Describe cultural, gender, social class, or other diversity factors that inform these dynamics: AM36 and AF36 are struggling to define gender roles as a duel career couple with demanding jobs. AM is wanting more traditional Armenian gender roles, with his career the priority, and AF is wanting a more American egalitarian relationship. She believes she had to sacrifice her career for the past 12 years when CF was young; now that she is older, AF feels entitled to pursue her career.

Role of Symptom in System

Hypothesized homeostatic function of presenting problem: How might the symptom serve to maintain connection, create independence/distance, establish influence, reestablish connection, or otherwise help create a sense of balance in the family? The abuse allegations have served as a stabilizing mechanism that creates connection by distracting AM and AF from the power struggle within the marriage regarding gender roles and the division of work/home labor and instead they are able to rally together around the issue of protecting their daughter.

GENOGRAM

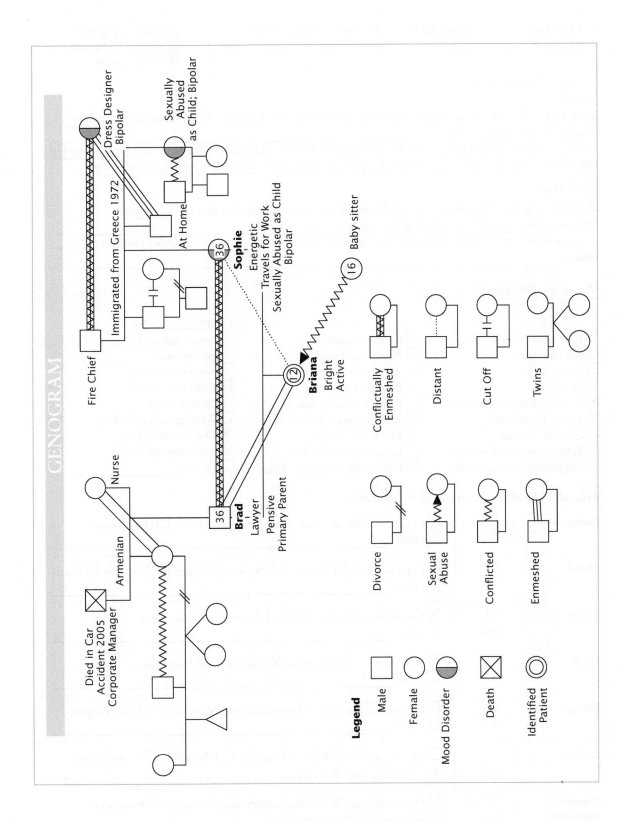

Legend

Male

Female

Mood Disorder

Death

Identified Patient

CLINICAL ASSESSMENT

Clinician: Sharee Lee	Client ID #: 1020	Primary configuration: ☐ Individual ☐ Couple ☒ Family	Primary Language: ☒ English ☐ Spanish ☒ Other: Greek

List client and significant others
Adult(s)

Adult Male   Age: 36   Other Married heterosexual   Occupation: Lawyer   Other identifier: Armenian American, second generation

Identified Patient: Adult Female   Age: 36   Multiethnic/Biracial   Married heterosexual   Occupation: Lawyer
Other identifier: Greek American, second generation; reports being diagnosed with bipolar disorder

Child(ren)

Identified Patient: Child Female Age: 12 European American   Grade: 7th School: Greenwood
Other identifier: Socially and academically engaged at school

Select Gender   Age: ___   Select Ethnicity   Grade: Select Grade School: _____   Other identifier: _____
Others: _____

Presenting Problem(s)

Complete for children:

☒ Depression/hopelessness ☒ Couple concerns ☒ School failure/decline performance
☐ Anxiety/worry ☐ Parent/child conflict ☐ Truancy/runaway
☐ Anger issues ☐ Partner violence/abuse ☐ Fighting w/peers
☒ Loss/grief ☐ Divorce adjustment ☐ Hyperactivity
☐ Suicidal thoughts/attempts ☐ Remarriage adjustment ☐ Wetting/soiling clothing
☒ Sexual abuse/rape ☐ Sexuality/intimacy concerns ☒ Child abuse/neglect
☐ Alcohol/drug use ☒ Major life changes ☒ Isolation/withdrawal
☐ Eating problems/disorders ☐ Legal issues/probation ☐ Other: _____
☐ Job problems/unemployed ☒ Other: Nightmares; trauma

Mental Status Assessment for Identified Patient

Interpersonal	☐ NA	☐ Conflict ☐ Enmeshment ☒ Isolation/avoidance ☐ Harassment ☐ Other: _____
Mood	☐ NA	☒ Depressed/Sad ☒ Anxious ☐ Dysphoric ☐ Angry ☒ Irritable ☐ Manic ☐ Other: _____
Affect	☐ NA	☒ Constricted ☐ Blunt ☐ Flat ☐ Labile ☐ Incongruent ☐ Other: _____
Sleep	☐ NA	☐ Hypersomnia ☐ Insomnia ☒ Disrupted ☒ Nightmares ☐ Other: _____
Eating	☒ NA	☐ Increase ☐ Decrease ☐ Anorectic restriction ☐ Binging ☐ Purging ☒ Other: _____
Anxiety	☐ NA	☐ Chronic worry ☐ Panic ☐ Phobias ☐ Obsessions ☐ Compulsions ☒ Other: Intrusive thoughts
Trauma symptoms	☐ NA	☒ Hypervigilance ☒ Flashbacks/Intrusive memories ☐ Dissociation ☒ Numbing ☐ Avoidance efforts ☐ Other: _____

Psychotic Symptoms	☒ NA	☐ Hallucinations ☐ Delusions ☐ Paranoia ☐ Loose associations ☐ Other: _____
Motor activity/ Speech	☐ NA	☒ Low energy ☐ Hyperactive ☐ Agitated ☐ Inattentive ☐ Impulsive ☐ Pressured speech ☐ Slow speech ☐ Other: _____
Thought	☐ NA	☐ Poor concentration ☐ Denial ☐ Self-blame ☐ Other-blame ☒ Ruminative ☐ Tangential ☐ Concrete ☐ Poor insight ☐ Impaired decision making ☐ Disoriented ☐ Other: _____
Sociolegal	☒ NA	☐ Disregards rules ☐ Defiant ☐ Stealing ☐ Lying ☐ Tantrums ☐ Arrest/incarceration ☐ Initiates fights ☐ Other: _____
Other Symptoms	☒ NA	

Diagnosis for Identified Patient

Contextual Factors considered in making diagnosis: ☒ Age ☒ Gender ☒ Family dynamics ☒ Culture ☒ Language ☒ Religion ☒ Economic ☒ Immigration ☐ Sexual/gender orientation ☒ Trauma ☐ Dual diagnosis/comorbid ☐ Addiction ☐ Cognitive ability ☐ Other: _____

Describe impact of identified factors on diagnosis and assessment process: _____

DSM-5 Level 1 Cross-Cutting Symptom Measure (optional): Elevated scores on: (free at psychiatry.org)

☒ I Depression ☐ II Anger ☐ III Mania ☒ IV Anxiety ☐ V Somatic ☐ VI Suicide ☐ VII Psychosis ☒ VIII Sleep ☐ IX Memory ☐ X Repetitive ☒ XI Dissociation ☐ XII Personality ☐ XIII Substance ☐ Not administered

DSM-5 Code	Diagnosis with Specifier *Include Z/T-Codes for Psychosocial Stressors/Issues*
1. F43.10	1. Posttraumatic stress disorder
2. Z69.020	2. Encounter for mental health services for victim of nonparental child sexual abuse
3. _____	3. _____
4. _____	4. _____
5. _____	5. _____

List Specific DSM-5 Criterion Met for Diagnosis

1. Life-threatening trauma: Sexually molested for 3 months
2. Intrusive thoughts and nightmares most days
3. Detachment from others; social withdrawal
4. Restricted affect
5. Exaggerated startle response; difficulty falling and staying asleep
6. Symptoms for more than 1 month

Medical Considerations

Has patient been referred for psychiatric evaluation? ☒ Yes ☐ No

Has patient agreed with referral? ☒ Yes ☐ No ☐ NA

Psychometric instruments used for assessment: ☐ None ☒ Cross-cutting symptom inventories ☐ Other: _____

Client response to diagnosis: ☒ Agree ☐ Somewhat agree ☐ Disagree ☐ Not informed for following reason:_____

(continued)

Diagnosis for Identified Patient (*continued*)

Current Medications (psychiatric & medical) ☒ NA
1. _____ ; dose _____ mg; start date: _____
2. _____ ; dose _____ mg; start date: _____
3. _____ ; dose _____ mg; start date: _____
4. _____ ; dose _____ mg; start date: _____

Medical Necessity: *Check all that apply*
☒ Significant impairment ☒ Probability of significant impairment ☒ Probable developmental arrest
Areas of impairment:
☒ Daily activities ☒ Social relationships ☐ Health ☒ Work/school ☐ Living arrangement ☐ Other: _____

Risk and Safety Assessment for Identified Patient

Suicidality
☒ No indication/Denies
☐ Active ideation
☐ Passive ideation
☐ Intent without plan
☐ Intent with means
☐ Ideation in past year
☐ Attempt in past year
☐ Family or peer history
  of completed suicide

Homicidality
☒ No indication/Denies
☐ Active ideation
☐ Passive ideation
☐ Intent without means
☐ Intent with means
☐ Ideation in past year
☐ Violence past year
☐ History of assaulting others
☐ Cruelty to animals

Alcohol Abuse
☒ No indication/denies
☐ Past abuse
☐ Current; Freq/Amt: _____

Drug Use/Abuse
☒ No indication/denies
☐ Past use
☐ Current drugs: _____
Freq/Amt: _____
☐ Family/sig.other use

Sexual & Physical Abuse and Other Risk Factors
☒ Childhood abuse history: ☒ Sexual ☐ Physical ☐ Emotional ☐ Neglect
☐ Adult with abuse/assault in adulthood: ☐ Sexual ☐ Physical ☐ Current
☐ History of perpetrating abuse: ☐ Sexual ☐ Physical ☐ Emotional
☐ Elder/dependent adult abuse/neglect
☐ History of or current issues with restrictive eating, binging, and/or purging
☐ Cutting or other self-harm: ☐ Current ☐ Past: Method: _____
☐ Criminal/legal history: _____
☐ Other trauma history: _____
☐ None reported

Indicators of Safety
☐ NA
☒ At least one outside support person
☐ Able to cite specific reasons to live or not harm
☐ Hopeful
☐ Willing to dispose of dangerous items
☒ Has future goals
☐ Willingness to reduce contact with people who make situation worse
☒ Willing to implement safety plan, safety interventions
☐ Developing set of alternatives to self/other harm
☐ Sustained period of safety: _____
☐ Other: _____

Elements of Safety Plan
☐ NA
☐ Verbal no harm contract
☐ Written no harm contract
☒ Emergency contact card
☒ Emergency therapist/agency number
☐ Medication management
☐ Plan for contacting friends/support persons during crisis
☐ Specific plan of where to go during crisis
☒ Specific self-calming tasks to reduce risk before reach crisis level (e.g., journaling, exercising, etc.)
☐ Specific daily/weekly activities to reduce stressors
☐ Other: _____

Legal/Ethical Action Taken: ☐ NA ☒ Action: Report to Child Protective Services; report taken by Susan Roth 7:30 pm 9/4/09

Case Management

Collateral Contacts
- Has contact been made with treating *physicians or other professionals:* ☐ NA ☒ Yes ☐ In process. Name/Notes: Pediatrician, Dr. Maria Garcia.
- If client is involved in mental health *treatment elsewhere,* has contact been made? ☒ NA ☐ Yes ☐ In process. Name/Notes: _____
- Has contact been made with *social worker:* ☐ NA ☒ Yes ☐ In process. Name/Notes: Child protective services assigned case worker, Danielle Garcia.

Referrals
- Has client been referred for *medical assessment:* ☒ Yes ☐ No evidence for need
- Has client been referred for *social services:* ☒ NA ☐ Job/training ☐ Welfare/Food/Housing ☐ Victim services ☐ Legal aid ☐ Medical ☐ Other: _____
- Has client been referred for *group* or other support services: ☐ Yes: _____ ☐ In process ☒ None recommended
- Are there anticipated *forensic/legal processes* related to treatment: ☐ No ☒ Yes; describe: CPS case

Support Network
- Client social support network includes: ☒ Supportive family ☐ Supportive partner ☒ Friends ☒ Religious/spiritual organization ☐ Supportive work/social group ☐ Other: _____
- Describe anticipated effects treatment will have on others in support system (Children, partner, etc.): Parents will participate in treatment.
- Is there anything else client will need to be successful? Family dynamics must be addressed.

Expected Outcome and Prognosis
☒ Return to normal functioning ☐ Anticipate less than normal functioning ☐ Prevent deterioration

Client Sense of Hope: 6

Evaluation of Assessment/Client Perspective
How were assessment methods adapted to client needs, including age, culture, and other diversity issues? Created safe space for CF to talk; used age-appropriate language; asked about language preference; cultural norms for emotional expression and family boundaries considered when making diagnosis and evaluating family; involved family, honoring cultural norms for involvement.

Describe actual or potential areas of client–clinician agreement/disagreement related to the above assessment: Family agrees with PTSD diagnosis and agrees that "something" needs to change in family dynamics to get "back on track."

_____, _____ _____
Clinician Signature License/Intern Status Date

_____, _____ _____
Supervisor Signature License Date

SATIR TREATMENT PLAN

Date: 04/10/2018   **Case/Client #:** 1020

Clinician Name: Sharee Lee   **Theory:** Satir Growth Model

Modalities planned: ☐ Individual Adult ☒ Individual Child ☒ Couple ☒ Family ☐ Group: _____

Recommended session frequency: ☒ Weekly ☐ Every two weeks ☐ Other: _____

Expected length of treatment: 6 months

Treatment Plan with Goals and Interventions

Early-Phase Client Goal

1. Increase <u>sense of physical and emotional safety and sense of normalcy</u> to reduce <u>nightmares and intrusive thoughts.</u>

   Measure: Able to sustain sense of safety for period of 2 ☒ wks ☐ mos with no more than one mild episodes of nightmares or intrusive thoughts.

   a. <u>Explore mind–body connections and the six levels of experiencing related to CF's abuse experience to help her identify how the abuse has affected her coping, feelings, feelings about those feelings, perceptions, expectations and yearnings; also explore levels of experiencing for both parents to help family members communicate and support one another.</u>

   b. <u>Role-playing and sculpting to reinforce sense of being able to protect self and begin to envision healing, including the use of touch to create a physical sense of safety within the family.</u>

Working-Phase Client Goals

1. Increase <u>CF12 sense of safety and esteem in peer relationships</u> to reduce <u>social withdrawal and depressed/anxious mood.</u>

   Measure: Able to sustain engagement in pre-abuse social activities for period of 1 ☒ wks ☐ mos with no more than two mild episodes of withdrawal.

   a. <u>Analyze the ingredients of peer interactions to help identify beliefs from the abuse that may be interfering with her peer relationships and then develop new ways to relate to peers.</u>

   b. <u>Coaching and role play on how to interact with others and maintain safety and boundaries.</u>

2. Increase <u>congruent communication and direct contact between CF12 and parents to reduce CF's depressed mood and anxiety.</u>

   Interventions:

   a. <u>Sculpting to enable family members to better understand how others experience them and to help identify new and more satisfying ways of relating.</u>

   b. <u>Coaching on congruent communication to help family more directly connect.</u>

3. Increase <u>emotional engagement and congruent communication within marriage</u> to reduce <u>triangulation and parental conflict and couple's overfocus on CF.</u>

   Measure: Able to sustain direct, congruent communication for period of ☒ wks ☐ mos with no more than two mild episodes of conflict and triangulation.

   a. <u>Coaching couple to communicate congruently in session and "make contact" with each other.</u>

b. Sculpting gender roles to help couple understand the emotional reality of the other and explore more satisfying ways to divide labor and emotionally connect with partner; compare and contrast with gender roles in their parents' and daughter's generation to create three-generation and cross-cultural perspective.

Closing-Phase Client Goals

1. Increase CF12's sense of self-worth and agency as she enters adolescence to reduce low self-esteem.

   Measure: Able to sustain sense of **agency and worth** for period of 2 ☐ wks ☒ mos with no more than two mild episodes of **placating** and feeling like "damaged goods."

   a. Use levels of experience (iceberg) to facilitate intrapsychic congruence and increase sense of self-approval and decrease reliance on external definition of worth.

   b. Sculpting various ways of being to enable CF to make more conscious life choices and to take actions that enable her to be more congruent with who she wants to be.

2. Increase cohesion of survival triad to create developmentally appropriate supportive relationship with parents as CF transitions to adolescence to reduce conflict.

   Measure: Able to sustain sense of **cohesion in survival triad** for period of 2 ☐ wks ☒ mos with no more than two mild episodes of distance.

   a. Sculpt relationships highlight survival stance vs. congruent stance to experience the difference; sculpt family as they imagine it to be in 5 years to facilitate developmentally appropriate family structure as CF enters adolescence.

   b. Soften and redefine family roles about success, emotions, and how to define a person's worth.

Treatment Tasks

1. Develop working therapeutic relationship using theory of choice.
   Relationship building approach/intervention:

   a. Make contact using warmth and empathy. Clearly establish hope that CF12 will have a normal life and that therapy will help with that process.

2. Assess individual, relational, community, and broader cultural dynamics using theory of choice.

   Assessment strategies:

   a. "Before and after" sculpting of each person's perspective of how the family changed both relative to AF36 increasing travel and the abuse incidents.

   b. Assess each member's survival communication stance and how they are affecting individuals and family since abuse; role of the symptom; family dynamics; chronology; quality of survival triad; levels of experiencing; and self-worth of members.

3. Identify needed referrals, crisis issues, collateral contacts, and other client needs.
   a. *Crisis assessment intervention(s):* Reduce nightmares and other PTSD symptoms; monitor for other crisis behavior throughout treatment.
   b. *Referral(s):* Connect CF12 with available resources for abuse victims, including Victims of Crime, and work with CPS and other authorities on reporting and investigation.

(continued)

Diversity Considerations

Describe specifically how treatment plan, goals, and interventions were adapted to address each area of diversity (Note: Identify specific ethnicity, e.g., Italian American rather than white):

Age: Language appropriate to age and education level will be utilized.

Gender/Sexual Orientation: Particularly since this case involves sexual abuse, extra sensitivity will be utilized when discussing CF12's experiences and symptoms pertaining to presenting issue. The conflict parents are experiencing related to gender roles will be addressed to help them emotionally reconnect with one another.

Race/Ethnicity Religion/Class/Region: Therapeutic factors pertaining to multicultural family environment, which includes Armenian American and Greek American descent, will be considered, including accessibility to emotional exploration, sensitivity to spiritual beliefs, traditionaly vs. contemporary gender roles, and respect for elder generations. Additionally, the legacy of immigration and the related family myths will be explored, including those related to socioeconomic success as primary life focus.

Other factors: The socioeconomic and ethnic/immigrant dynamics of CF's school as well as the school culture itself will be explored as part of helping CF adjust at school.

Evidence-Based Practice (Optional)

Summarize evidence for using this approach for this presenting concern and/or population: The Satir approach has a strong evidence base for the quality of the therapeutic relationship, which is strongly correlated with positive therapeutic outcomes. A warm, supportive relationship is particularly important due to CF's recent sexual abuse experience and should be a good cultural fit for the parents, who are Greek and Armenian, cultures that typically have high emotional expression.

Client Perspective (Optional)

Has treatment plan been reviewed with client: ☒ Yes ☐ No; If no, explain: _____

Describe areas of Client Agreement and Concern: Clients are particularly enthusiastic about wanting family sessions, especially early in therapy.

_____, _____   _____ _____, _____ _____
Therapist's Signature Intern Status Date   Supervisor's Signature License Date

PROGRESS NOTE

Date: 5/12/2018 **Time:** 1:00 ☐ am/pm   **Session Length:** ☐ 45 min. ☒ 60 min. ☐ Other:__minutes

Present: ☒ Adult Male ☒ Adult Female ☐ Child Male ☒ Child Female ☐ Other:_____

Billing Code: ☐ 90791 (eval) ☐ 90834 (45 min. therapy) ☐ 90837 (60 min. therapy) ☒ 90847 (Family) ☐ Other _____

Symptoms(s)	Duration and Frequency Since Last Visit	Progress:
1: Nightmares/intrusive thoughts	1 nightmare this week; intrusive thoughts last for less than 1 minute — 2–3 times/day	**Progressing**
2: Social withdrawal	CF spent lunch with friends all days this week	**Progressing**
3: Depression/anxiety	CF reports mild depression or anxiety; most days but for shorter periods than last week (2–4 hours).	**Progressing**

Explanatory Notes on Symptoms: Report CF feeling "safer" and engaging more socially; intrusive memories and nightmares less of an issue and CF is using techniques from prior weeks to manage. AF still traveling for work but more open to finding ways to minimize the effect it has on CF and AM.

In-Session Interventions and Assigned Homework

Facilitated sharing of each person's emotional response to reported progress and changes. Coached family members on congruent communication, helping each to reduce use of survival stance and defenses. Used ingredients of an interaction related to AF's work schedule to facilitate each person's sharing of personal experience to increase connection and identify better ways to stay connected when AF travels.

Client Response/Feedback

Family engaged eagerly in and responsive to communication coaching and report trying to use what learned in session at home. CF able to meaningfully discuss layers of experience.

Plan

☐ Continue with treatment plan: plan for next session: _____

☒ Modify plan: Couple session next week to discuss gender roles and balancing work and home; following week CF alone. _____

Next session: Date: 5/19 Time: 1:00 ☐ am/ ☒ pm

Crisis Issues: ☒ No indication of crisis/client denies ☐ Crisis assessed/addressed: describe below

_____, _____ _____
Clinician's Signature   License/Intern status   Date

(continued)

SATIR PROGRESS NOTE *(continued)*

Case Consultation/Supervision ☐ Not Applicable

Notes: Now that CF is more stabilized, supervisor encouraged separate couple and child sessions to reinforce generational boundaries and allow CF to discuss more personal issues related to the abuse in private.

Collateral Contact ☐ Not Applicable

Name: Sara Klausner, CPS Social Worker   Date of Contact: 5/12 Time: ____ : ____ ☐ am/ ☐ pm
☒ Written release on file: ☒ Sent/ ☐ Received ☒ In court docs ☐ Other: _____

Notes: Returned social worker's call; requested update on progress.

_____ , _____ _____
Clinician's Signature   License/Intern Status   Date

_____ , _____ _____
Supervisor's Signature   License   Date

C H A P T E R

7

Intergenerational and Psychoanalytic Family Therapies

Learning Objectives

After reading this chapter and a few hours of focused studying, you should be able to:

- **Theory:** Describe the following elements of intergenerational and psychoanalytic family therapies:

  - Process of therapy
  - Therapeutic relationship
  - Case conceptualization
  - Goal setting
  - Interventions

- **Case conceptualization and treatment plan:** Complete theory-specific case conceptualizations and treatment plans for intergenerational and psychoanalytic family therapies using templates that are provided.

- **Research:** Provide an overview of significant research findings for intergenerational and psychoanalytic family therapies.

- Diversity: Analyze strengths, limitations, and appropriate applications for using intergenerational and psychoanalytic family therapies with clients in relation to their social location/diverse identities, including but not limited to ethnic, racial, and/or sexual/gender identity diversity.

- Cross-theoretical comparison: Compare how intergenerational and psychoanalytic family therapies utilize interpersonal patterns (IPs) with other approaches described in this book.

Bowen theory is really not about families per se, but about life.
—Friedman (1991, p. 134)

Lay of the Land

Although distinct from each other, Bowenian intergenerational therapy and psychoanalytic family therapy share the common roots of: (a) psychoanalytic theory and (b) systemic theory. A psychoanalytically trained psychiatrist, Bowen (1985) developed a highly influential and unique approach to therapy that is called Bowen intergenerational therapy. Drawing heavily from object relations theory, psychoanalytic or psychodynamic family therapies have developed several unique approaches, including *object relations family therapy* (Scharff & Scharff, 1987), *family-of-origin therapy* (Framo, 1992), and *contextual therapy* (Boszormenyi-Nagy & Krasner, 1986). These therapies share several key concepts and practices:

- Examining a client's early relationships to understand present functioning
- Tracing transgenerational and extended family dynamics to understand a client's complaints
- Promoting insight into extended family dynamics to facilitate change
- Identifying and altering destructive beliefs and patterns of behavior that were learned early in life in one's family of origin

Bowen Intergenerational Therapy

In a Nutshell: The Least You Need to Know

Bowen intergenerational theory is more about the nature of being human than it is about families or family therapy (Friedman, 1991). The Bowen approach requires therapists to work from a broad perspective that considers the evolution of the human species and the characteristics of all living systems. Therapists use this broad perspective to conceptualize client problems and then rely primarily on the therapist's use of self to effect change. As part of this broad perspective, therapists routinely consider the *three-generational emotional process* to better understand the current presenting symptoms. The process of therapy involves increasing clients' awareness of how their current behavior is connected to multigenerational processes and the resulting family dynamics. The therapist's primary tool for promoting client change is the therapist's personal level of *differentiation,* the ability to distinguish self from other and manage interpersonal anxiety.

The Juice: Significant Contributions to the Field

If you remember a couple of things from this chapter, they should be the following:

Differentiation

Differentiation is one of the most useful concepts for understanding interpersonal relationships, although it can be difficult to grasp at first (Friedman, 1991). An *emotional* or *affective* concept, differentiation refers to a person's ability to separate intrapersonal and interpersonal distress:

- Intrapersonal: Separate thoughts from feelings in order to *respond* rather than *react*; often referred to as self-regulation in contemporary contexts.
- Interpersonal: Know where oneself ends and another begins without loss of self; this typically takes the form of being able to manage conflict without reactivity.

Bowen (1985) also described differentiation as the ability to balance two life forces: the need for *togetherness* and the need for *autonomy*. Differentiation is conceptualized on a *continuum* (Bowen, 1985): a person is more or less differentiated rather than differentiated or not differentiated. Becoming more differentiated is a lifelong journey that is colloquially referred to as "maturity" in the broadest sense.

A person who is more differentiated is better able to handle the ups and downs of life and, more importantly, the vicissitudes of intimate relationships. The ability to clearly separate thoughts from feelings and self from others gives one a greater ability to self-regulate in the face of the challenges that come with increasing levels of intimacy. For example, when one's partner expresses disapproval or disinterest, this does not cause a differentiated person's world to collapse or inspire hostility. Of course, feelings may be hurt, and the person experiences that pain. However, he or she doesn't immediately *act on* or *act out* that pain. Differentiated people are able to reflect on the pain: clearly separate out what is their part and what is their partner's part and identify a respectful way to move forward. In contrast, less-differentiated people feel compelled to react immediately and to express their feelings before thinking or reflecting on what belongs to whom in the situation. Partners with greater levels of differentiation are able to tolerate differences between themselves and others, allowing for greater freedom and acceptance in all relationships. A recent extensive review of 75 years of research on self-regulation, which is a key element of differentiation, concluded that the ability to self-regulate is transmitted intergenerationally, both behaviorally and genetically in a complex reciprocal pattern in which parent and child behavior continually interact to reinforce either higher or lower levels of self-regulation (Bridgett et al., 2015).

Because differentiated people do not immediately react in emotional situations, a common misunderstanding is that differentiation implies lack of emotion or emotional expression (Friedman, 1991). In reality, highly differentiated people are actually able to engage *more* difficult and intense emotions because they do not overreact and instead can thoughtfully reflect on and tolerate the ambiguity of their emotional lives.

It can be difficult to assess a client's level of differentiation because it is expressed differently depending on the person's culture, gender, age, and personality (Bowen, 1985). For example, to the untrained eye, emotionally expressive cultures and genders may look more undifferentiated and emotionally restricted people and cultures may appear more differentiated. However, emotional coolness often is a result of *emotional cutoff* (see "Emotional Cutoff," below), which is how a less-differentiated person manages intense emotions. Therapists need to assess the actual functioning intrapersonally (ability to separate thought from feeling) and interpersonally (ability to separate self from other) to sift through the diverse expressions of differentiation.

Genograms

The **genogram** has become one of the most commonly used family assessment instruments (McGoldrick, Gerson, & Petry, 2008). At its most basic level, a genogram is a type of family tree or genealogy that specifically maps key multigenerational processes that illuminate for both therapist and client the emotional dynamics that contribute to the reported symptoms.

New therapists are often reluctant to do genograms. When I ask students to do their own, most are enthusiastic. However, when I ask them to do one with a client, most are reluctant. They may say, "I don't have time" or "I don't think these clients are the type who would want to do a genogram." Yet after completing their first genogram with a client, they almost always come out saying, "That was more helpful than I thought it was going to be." Especially for newer therapists—and even for seasoned clinicians—genograms are always helpful in some way. Although originally developed for the intergenerational work in Bowen's approach, the genogram is so universally helpful that many therapists from other schools adapt it for their approach, creating solution-focused genograms (Kuehl, 1995) or culturally focused genograms (Hardy & Laszloffy, 1995; Rubalcava & Waldman, 2004).

The genogram is simultaneously: (a) an assessment instrument and (b) an intervention, especially in the hands of an intergenerational therapist. As an assessment instrument, the genogram helps the therapist identify intergenerational patterns that surround the problem, such as patterns of parenting, managing conflict, and balancing autonomy with togetherness. As an intervention, genograms can help clients see their patterns more clearly and how they may be living out family patterns, rules, and legacies without conscious awareness. As a trainee, I worked with one client who had never spoken to her parents about how her grandfather had sexually abused her and had no intention of doing so because she believed it would tear the family apart. This changed the day we constructed her genogram. I had her color in each person she knew he had also abused. When she was done, the three-generation genogram had over 12 victims colored in red; she went home and spoke to her mother that night and began a multigenerational process of healing for her family.

Rumor Has It: The People and Their Stories

Murray Bowen

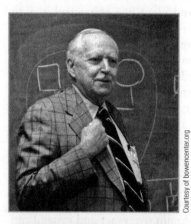

A psychoanalytically trained psychiatrist, Bowen (1966, 1972, 1976, 1985) began working with people diagnosed with schizophrenia at the Menninger Clinic in the 1940s and continued his research in the 1950s at the National Institute for Mental Health (NIMH), where he hospitalized entire families with schizophrenic members to study their emotional processes. He then spent the next 30 years at Georgetown University developing one of the most influential theories of family and natural systems, which has influenced generations of family therapists.

Georgetown Family Center: Michael Kerr

A longtime student of Bowen, Michael Kerr has also been one of his most influential students and has served as director of the Georgetown Family Center, where Bowen refined his clinical approach.

The Center for Family Learning: Philip Guerin and Thomas Fogarty

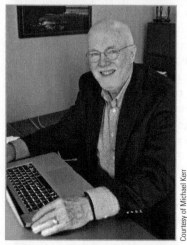

Guerin and Fogarty cofounded the Center for Family Learning in New York, one of the premier training centers for family therapy. Both Guerin and Fogarty have written extensively on the clinical applications of Bowen's model.

Monica McGoldrick and Betty Carter

Betty Carter and Monica McGoldrick (1999) used Bowen's theory to develop their highly influential model of the *family life cycle,* which

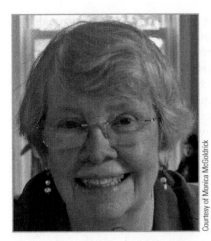

Courtesy of Monica McGoldrick

uses the Bowenian concept of balancing the need for togetherness and independence to understand how families develop. McGoldrick's work with genograms is the definitive work on this tool subject (McGoldrick et al., 2008).

David Schnarch

Grounded in Bowen's intergenerational approach, Schnarch developed a unique approach to working with couples, the sexual crucible model, which is designed to increase a couple's capacity for intimacy by increasing their level of differentiation. One of the hallmarks of this approach is harnessing the intensity in the couple's sexual relationship to promote the differentiation process.

The Big Picture: Overview of Treatment

Much like other approaches that have psychodynamic roots, intergenerational therapy is a *process*-oriented therapy that relies heavily on the *self-of-the-therapist,* most specifically the therapist's level of differentiation, to promote client change (Kerr & Bowen, 1988). This therapy does not emphasize techniques and interventions. Instead, therapists use genograms and assessment to promote insight and then intervene as differentiated persons. For example, when one partner tries to get the therapist to take his or her side in an argument, the therapist responds by simultaneously modeling differentiation and gently promoting it in the couple. By refusing to take sides and also helping the couple tolerate their resulting anxiety (their problem is still not fixed, and neither partner has been "validated" by the therapist), the therapist creates a situation in which the couple can increase their level of differentiation: they can use self-validation to soothe their feelings and learn how to tolerate the tension of difference between them. Change is achieved through alternately using insight and the therapeutic relationship to increase clients' levels of differentiation and tolerance for anxiety and ambiguity.

Making Connections: The Therapeutic Relationship

Differentiation and the Emotional Being of the Therapist

More than in any other family therapy approach, in intergenerational therapy the therapist's level of differentiation (Bowen, 1985; Kerr & Bowen, 1988) and emotional being (Friedman, 1991) are central to the change process. Intergenerational therapists focus on developing a therapeutic relationship that encourages all parties to further their differentiation process: "*the differentiation of the therapist is technique*" (Friedman, 1991, p. 138; emphasis in original). Intergenerational therapists believe that clients can differentiate only as much as their therapists have differentiated (Bowen, 1985). For this reason, the therapist's level of differentiation is often the focus of supervision early in training, and therapists are expected to continually monitor and develop themselves so that they can be of maximum assistance to their clients. Bowen therapists assert that the theory cannot be learned through books (such as this one) but can be learned only through a relationship with a supervisor or teacher who uses these ideas to interact with the student (Friedman, 1991).

A Nonanxious Presence

The greater a therapist's level of differentiation, the more the therapist can maintain a **nonanxious presence** with clients (Kerr & Bowen, 1988). This is not a cold, detached stance but rather an emotionally engaged stance that is *nonreactive,* meaning that the therapist does not react to attacks, "bad" news, and so forth without careful reflection. The therapist does not rush in to rescue clients from anxiety every time they feel overwhelmed by anger, sadness, or another strong emotion; instead, the therapist calmly wades right into the muck the client is trying to avoid and guides the client through the process of separating self from other and thought from feelings (Friedman, 1991). The therapist's calm center is used to help clients move through the differentiation process in a safe, contained environment in which differentiation is modeled. When clients are upset, the "easiest" thing to do is to soothe and calm their anxieties, fears, and strong emotions; this makes everyone calmer sooner, but nothing is learned. The intergenerational therapist instead shepherds clients through a more difficult process, slowly coaching them through that which they fear or detest in order to facilitate growth.

The Viewing: Case Conceptualization and Assessment

Viewing is the primary "intervention" in intergenerational therapy because the approach's effectiveness relies on the therapist's ability to accurately assess the family dynamics and thereby guide the healing process (Bowen, 1985). Although this is true with all therapies, it is truer with intergenerational therapies because the therapist's level of differentiation is critical to the ability to accurately "see" what is going on.

Emotional Systems

Bowen viewed families, organizations, and clubs as **emotional systems** that have the same processes as those found in all natural systems: "Bowen has constantly emphasized over the years that we have more in common with other forms of protoplasm (i.e., life) than we differ from them" (Friedman, 1991, p. 135). He viewed humans as part of an *evolutionary emotional process* that goes back to the first cell that had a nucleus and was able to differentiate its functions from other cells (i.e., human life begins with one cell that divides to create new cells, which then differentiate to create the different systems and structures of the body: blood, muscle, neurons, etc.). This process of differentiating yet remaining part of a single living organism (system) is a primary organizing concept in Bowen's work, and the family's emotional processes are viewed as an extension (not just a metaphor) of the differentiation process of cells. Thus, Bowen's theory of natural systems focuses on the relationship between the human species and all life past and present.

Of particular interest in family therapy are natural systems that have developed emotional interdependence (e.g., flocks of birds, herds of cattle, and human families; Friedman, 1991). The resulting system or emotional field profoundly influences all of its members, defining what is valued and what is not. When a family lacks sufficient differentiation, it may become emotionally fused, an undifferentiated family "ego mass." Intergenerational therapists focus squarely on a family's unique emotional system rather than on environmental or general cultural factors, and they seek to identify the rules that structure the particular system.

This approach is similar to other systemic conceptualizations of the family as a single organism or system; however, Bowen emphasizes that it is fundamentally an *emotional* system. Because this system has a significant impact on a person's behavior, emotions, and symptoms, one must always assess this context to understand a person's problems. For example, in the case study at the end of this chapter, the therapist explores how Wei-Wei's panic attacks fit within the broader fabric of the family system, her immigration history, and her professional life, rather than focusing solely on the medical and psychological aspects of the attacks.

Chronic Anxiety

Bowen viewed **chronic anxiety** as a biological phenomenon that is present in all natural systems. Chronic anxiety involves automatic physical and emotional reactions that are not mediated through conscious, logical processes (Friedman, 1991). Families exhibit chronic anxiety in their responses to crises, loss, conflict, and difficulties. The process of differentiation creates a clear-headedness that allows individuals and families to reduce the reactivity and anxiety associated with survival in natural systems and to instead make conscious choices about how to respond. For example, chronic anxiety in a family may result from a mother feeling guilty about a child's lack of success, in which case it is the therapist's job to help the mother increase her level of differentiation so that she can respond to the child's situation from a clear, reasoned position rather than with a blind emotional reactivity that rarely helps the situation. In the case study at the end of this chapter, the therapist works with the mother to reduce her anxiety and panic as her son finishes medical school and begins his independent life as an adult.

Multigenerational Transmission Process

The **multigenerational transmission process** is based on the premise that emotional processes from prior generations are present and "alive" in the current family emotional system (Friedman, 1991). In this process, children may emerge with higher, equal, or lower levels of differentiation than their parents (Bowen, 1985). Families with severe emotional problems result from a multigenerational process in which the level of differentiation has become lower and lower with each generation. The negative effects of significant family events such as immigration, trauma, major loss, violence, substance abuse, and other legacies commonly are transmitted across three or more generations, such as the intergenerational effects of slavery (Graff, 2014). Some research indicates that interpersonal violence is transmitted intergenerationally (Rivera & Fincham, 2015). Similarly, another study found that individuals whose family was abusive or violent are more likely to have generalized anxiety disorder and their own romantic relationship distress (Priest, 2015). In another study, researchers found that lower levels of differentiation were correlated with high levels of jealousy, providing an excellent example of what Bowen meant by fusion (Lans, Mosek, & Yagil, 2014).

Bowen's approach is designed to help an individual create enough distance from these processes to comprehend the more universal processes that shape human relationships and individual identities (Friedman, 1991). Thus, in the case study at the end of this chapter, the therapist will assess the emotional content of the parents' prior life in China, which is viewed as an ongoing aspect of the family's current reality.

Try It Yourself

By yourself or with a partner, try to identify significant multigenerational transmissions that might be alive in your family today.

Multigenerational Patterns

Intergenerational therapists assess **multigenerational patterns**, specifically those related to the presenting problem. Using a genogram or oral interview, the therapist identifies patterns of depression, substance use, anger, conflict, the parent–child relationship, the couple's relationship, or whatever issues are most salient for the client. The therapist then identifies how the current situation fits with these patterns. Is the client replicating or rebelling against the pattern? How has the pattern evolved with this generation? The therapist thereby gains greater clarity into the dynamics that are feeding the problem. In cases of immigration, such as that at the end of this chapter, the historic family patterns may change because of different cultural contexts (e.g., the family attempts or is forced to blend and adapt), may be rigidly the same (e.g., the family wants to adhere to traditions), or may be radically different (e.g., the family wants to "break" from the past).

Level of Differentiation (Also see "The Juice," above)

When differentiation is used as part of case conceptualization, the therapist assesses the client's level of differentiation along a continuum, which Bowen developed into a differentiation scale that ranges from 1 to 100, with lower levels of differentiation represented by lower numbers (Bowen, 1985). Bowen maintained that people rarely reach higher than 70 on this scale.

Although there are pen-and-paper measures such as the Chabot Emotional Differentiation Scale (Licht & Chabot, 2006), most therapists simply note patterns of where and how a person is able or unable to separate self from other and thought from emotion. What is most useful for treatment is not some overall score or general assessment of differentiation, but rather the specific areas in which clients need to increase their level of differentiation to resolve the presenting problem. For example, a couple may need to increase their ability to differentiate self from other in the area of sex so that they can create a better sexual relationship that allows each person to have preferences, discuss them, and find ways to honor these preferences without becoming emotionally overwhelmed.

Emotional Triangles

Bowen identified **emotional triangles** as one of the most important dynamics to assess because they are the basic building block of families (Bowen, 1985; Friedman, 1991; Kerr & Bowen, 1988). A triangle is a process in which a dyad draws in a third person (or some thing, topic, or activity) to stabilize the primary dyad, especially when there is tension in the dyad. Because triangles use a third person or topic to alleviate tension, the more you try to change the relationship with the third entity, ironically, the more you reinforce the aspects you want to change. Thus, therapists assess triangles to identify the primary relationship that needs to be targeted for change.

Bowen maintained that triangulation is a fundamental process in natural systems (Bowen, 1985). Everyone triangulates to some degree: going down the hall to complain about your boss or coworker is triangulation. However, when this becomes the primary means for dealing with dyadic tension and the members of the dyad never actually resolve the tension themselves, then pathological patterns emerge. The more rigid the triangle, the greater the problems.

The classic family example of a triangle is a mother who becomes overinvolved with her children to reduce unresolved tension in the marriage. This overinvolvement can take the form of positive interactions (overinvolvement in school and social activities, emotional intimacy, constant errands or time devoted to the child) or negative interactions (nagging and worrying about the child; the therapist suspects that this is what is going on in the case study at the end of this chapter). Another common form of triangulation is seen in divorced families, in which both parents often triangulate the child, trying to convince the child to take their side against the other parent. Triangulation can also involve using alcohol or drugs to create dyadic stability, complaining or siding with friends or family of origin against one's spouse, or two siblings siding against a third.

Family Projection Process

The **family projection process** describes how parents "project" their immaturity onto one or more children (Bowen, 1985), causing decreased differentiation in subsequent generations. The most common pattern is for a mother to project her anxiety onto one child, focusing all her attention on this child to soothe her anxiety, perhaps becoming overly invested in the child's academic or sporting activities. The child or children who are the focus of the parent's anxiety will be less differentiated than the siblings who are not involved in this projection process.

Emotional Cutoff

A particularly important process to assess is **emotional cutoff**—situations in which a person no longer emotionally engages with another in order to manage anxiety; this usually occurs between children and parents. Emotional cutoff can take the form of no longer seeing or speaking to the other or, alternatively, being willing to be at the same family event with virtually no interaction. Often people who display cutoff from their family believe that doing so is a sign of mental health (e.g., "I have set good boundaries") or even a sign of superiority (e.g., "It makes no sense for me to spend time with *that type* of person"). They may even report that this solution helps them manage their emotional reactivity. However, cutoff is almost always a sign of lower levels of differentiation (Bowen, 1985). Essentially, the person is so emotionally fused with the other that he or she must physically separate to be comfortable. The higher a person's level of differentiation, the less need there is for emotional cutoff. This does not mean that a highly differentiated person does not establish boundaries. However, when differentiated people set boundaries and limit contact with family, they do so in a way that is respectful and preserves emotional connection, rather than out of emotional reactivity (e.g., after an argument).

Emotional cutoff requires a little more attention in assessment because it can "throw off" an overall assessment of differentiation and family dynamics. People who emotionally cut themselves off as a means of coping often appear more differentiated than they are; it may also be harder to detect certain family patterns because in some cases the client "forgets" or honestly does not know the family history. However, at some times and in certain families, more cutoff is necessary because of extreme patterns of verbal, emotional, or childhood abuse. In such cases, in which contact is not appropriate or possible, the therapist still needs to assess the *emotional* part of the cutoff. The more people can stay emotionally engaged (e.g., have empathy and cognitive understanding of the relational dynamics) without harboring anger, resentment, or fear, the healthier they will be, and this should be a therapeutic goal.

Sibling Position

Intergenerational therapists also look at **sibling position** as an indicator of the family's level of differentiation; all things being equal, the more the family members exhibit the expected characteristics of their sibling position, the higher the level of differentiation (Bowen, 1985; Kerr & Bowen, 1988). The more intense the family projection process is on a child, the more that child will exhibit characteristics of an infantile younger child. The roles associated with sibling positions are informed by a person's cultural background, with immigrants generally adhering to more traditional standards than later generations. Most often, older children identify with responsibility and authority, and later-born children respond to this domination by identifying with underdogs and questioning the status quo. The youngest child is generally the most likely to avoid responsibility in favor of freedom.

Societal Regression

When a society experiences sustained chronic anxiety because of war, natural disaster, economic pressures, and other traumas, it responds with emotionally based reactive decisions rather than rational decisions (Bowen, 1985) and regresses to lower levels of functioning, just like families. These Band-Aid solutions to social problems generate a vicious cycle of increased problems and symptoms. Societies can go through cycles in which their level of differentiation rises and falls.

Targeting Change: Goal Setting

Two Basic Goals

Like any theory with a definition of health, intergenerational therapy has clearly defined long-term therapeutic goals that can be used with all clients:

1. To increase each person's level of differentiation (in specific contexts)
2. To decrease emotional reactivity to chronic anxiety in the system

Increasing Differentiation

Increasing differentiation is a general goal that should be defined operationally for each client. For example, "increase AF's and AM's level of differentiation in the marital relationship by increasing the tolerance of difference while increasing intimacy" is a better-stated goal than "increase differentiation."

Decreasing Emotional Reactivity to Chronic Anxiety

Decreasing anxiety and emotional reactivity is closely correlated with the increasing differentiation. *As differentiation increases, anxiety decreases.* Nonetheless, it can be helpful to include these as separate goals to break the process down into smaller steps. Decreasing anxiety generally precedes increasing differentiation and therefore may be included in the working rather than the termination phase of therapy. As with the general goal of increasing differentiation, it is clinically helpful to tailor this to an individual client. Rather than stating the general goal of "decrease anxiety," which can easily be confused with treating an anxiety disorder (as may or may not be the case), a more useful clinical goal would address a client's specific dynamic: "decrease emotional reactivity to child's defiance" or "decrease emotional reactivity to partner in conversations about division of chores and parenting."

The Doing: Interventions

Theory versus Technique

The primary "technique" in Bowen intergenerational theory is the therapist's ability to embody the theory. The premise is that if therapists understand Bowen's theory of natural systems and work on their personal level of differentiation, they will naturally interact with clients in a way that promotes the clients' level of differentiation (Friedman, 1991). Thus, understanding—"living" the theory—is the primary technique for facilitating client change.

Process Questions

Intergenerational therapists' embodiment of the theory most frequently expresses itself through **process questions**, questions that help clients see the systemic process or the dynamics that they are enacting. For example, a therapist can use process questions to help clients see how the conflict they are experiencing with their spouse is related to patterns they observed in their own parents' relationship: "How do the struggles you are experiencing with your spouse now compare with those of each of your parents? Are they similar or different? Is the role you are playing now similar to that of one of your parents in their marriage? Is it similar to the type of conflict you had with your parents when you were younger? Who are you most like? Least like?" These questions are generated naturally from the therapist's use of the theory to conceptualize the client's situation.

Encouraging Differentiation of Self

According to Bowenian theory, families naturally tend toward togetherness and relationship as part of survival. Thus, therapeutic interventions generally target the counterbalancing force of differentiation (Friedman, 1991) by encouraging clients to use *"I" positions* to maintain individual opinions and mood states while in relationships with others. For example, if spouses are overreactive to each other's moods, every time one person is angry or unhappy, the other feels there is no other choice but to also be in that mood. Therapists promote differentiation by coaching the second spouse to maintain his or her emotional state without undue influence from the other. In this chapter's case study, the therapist will work with Wei-Wei, who is having panic attacks, to increase her sense of differentiation, particularly in relationship to her son but also in relationship to her husband, from whom she has become distant.

Genograms

The genogram is used both as an assessment tool and an intervention (McGoldrick et al., 2008). As an intervention, the genogram identifies not only problematic intergenerational patterns but also alternative ways for relating and handling problems. For example, if a person comes from a family in which one or more children in each generation has strongly rebelled against their parents, the genogram can be used to identify this pattern, note exceptions in the larger family, and identify ways to prevent or intervene in this dynamic. The genogram's visual depiction of the pattern across generations often inspires a greater sense of urgency and commitment to change than when the dynamics are only discussed in session. Constructing the genogram often generates a much greater sense of urgency and willingness to take action as compared with relying strictly on process questions and a discussion of the dynamics. Chapter 11 includes a brief description of how to construct a genogram and use it in session.

Try It Yourself

Create a three- or four-generation genogram of your family. What patterns do you notice? Does anything surprise you?

Detriangulation

Detriangulation involves the therapist maintaining therapeutic neutrality (differentiation) in order to interrupt a client's attempt to involve the therapist or someone else in a triangle (Friedman, 1991). Whether working with an individual, a couple, or a family, most therapists at some point will be "invited" by clients to triangulate with them against a third party who may or may not be present. When this occurs, the therapist "detriangulates" by refusing to take a side, whether literally or more subtly. For example, if a client says, "Don't you think it is inappropriate for a child to talk back?" or "Isn't it inappropriate for a husband to go to lunch with a single woman who is attracted to him?," the quickest way to relieve the client's anxiety is to agree: this makes the relationship between the client and therapist comfortable, allowing the client to immediately feel "better," "understood," and "empathized with." However, by validating the client's position and taking the client's side against another, the therapist undermines the long-term goal of promoting differentiation. Thus, if therapy becomes "stuck," therapists must first examine their role in a potential triangle (Friedman, 1991).

Rather than take a side, the therapist invites clients to validate *themselves,* examine their own part in the problem dynamic, and take responsibility for their needs and wants. There is often significant confusion in the therapeutic community about "validating" a client's feelings. *Validation* implies approval; however, approval from the therapist undermines a client's sense of autonomy. Intergenerational therapists emphasize that when therapists "validate" by saying "It is normal to feel this way," "It sounds like he really hurt you," or in some way imply "You are entitled to feel this way," they close down the opportunity for differentiation. Instead, clients are coached to approve or disapprove of their own thoughts and feelings and then take responsibility and action as needed.

Relational Experiments

Relational experiments are behavioral homework assignments designed to reveal and change unproductive relational processes in families (Guerin et al., 1996). These experiments interrupt triangulation processes by increasing direct communication between a dyad or by reversing pursuer/distancer dynamics that are fueled by lack of differentiation.

Going Home Again

Most adults are familiar with this irony: you seem to be a balanced person who can manage a demanding career, an educational program, and a complex household; yet when you go home to visit family for the holidays, you find yourself suddenly acting like a teenager—or worse. Intergenerational therapists see this difference in functioning as the result of unresolved issues with the family of origin that can be improved by increasing differentiation. Even if you cannot change a parent's critical comments or a sibling's arrogance, you can be in the presence of these "old irritants" and not regress to past behaviors but instead keep a clear sense of self. As clients' level of differentiation grows, they are able to maintain a stronger and clearer sense of self in the nuclear family. The technique of "going home" refers to when therapists encourage clients to interact with family members while maintaining a clearer boundary between self and other and to practice and/or experience the reduced emotional reactivity that characterizes increases in differentiation (Friedman, 1991).

Interventions for Special Populations

The Sexual Crucible Model

One of the most influential applications of Bowen intergenerational theory is the Sexual Crucible Model developed by David Schnarch (1991). The model proposes that marriage functions as a "crucible," a vessel that physically contains a volatile transformational process. In the case of marriage, the therapist achieves transformation by helping both partners differentiate (or more simply, forcing them to "grow up"). As with all crucibles, the contents of marriage must be contained because they are unstable and explosive.

Schnarch views sexual and emotional intimacy as inherently intertwined in the process of differentiation. He directs partners to take responsibility for their individual needs rather than demand that the other change to accommodate their needs, wants, and desires. To remain calm, each person learns to self-soothe rather than demand that the other change. Schnarch also includes exercises like "hugging to relax" in which he helps couples develop a greater sense of physical intimacy and increased comfort with being "seen" by the other. He has developed this model for therapists to use with clients and has also made it accessible to general audiences (Schnarch, 1998).

Schnarch has developed a comprehensive and detailed model for helping couples create the type of relationship most couples today expect: a harmonious balance of emotional, sexual, intellectual, professional, financial, parenting, household, health, and social partnerships. However, Schnarch points out that this multifaceted intimacy has never been the norm in human relationships. His model is most appropriate for psychologically minded clients who are motivated to increase intimacy.

Scope It Out: Cross-Theoretical Comparison

Using Tomm's IPscope described in Chapter 3 (Tomm et al., 2014), this theory approaches the conceptualization of systemic, interpersonal patterns as discussed below.

Theoretical Conceptualization

Bowen's approach is one of the few that examine pathologizing interpersonal patterns (PIPs) across generations. When conceptualizing PIPs, the focus is on how anxiety is managed and the level of differentiation in these cycle. For example, when conceptualizing couples conflict, Bowenian therapists would conceptualize not just the PIPs the couple presents as a problem, but also the PIPs in each family of origin. When conceptualizing the specific PIP, the therapist asks: What anxiety is generating the PIP (e.g., fear of rejection, perfectionism), and how is the lack of differentiation expressing itself (e.g., my partner must approve of me at all times)?

Goal Setting

Intergenerational theory has two basic goals—increasing differentiation and decreasing emotional reactivity—which means wellness interaction patterns (WIPs) include these basic elements in some way, such as "taking responsibility for own emotions/supporting partner in taking responsibility."

Facilitating Change

When facilitating change, intergenerational therapists primarily use transformative interaction patterns (TIPs) that promote insight related to differentiation and anxiety patterns. Going home again may provide an opportunity for a healing interaction pattern (HIP) for some clients. Sociocultural patterns may be introduced through the genogram if the practitioner chooses to do so.

Putting It All Together: Case Conceptualization and Treatment Plan Templates

Areas for Theory-Specific Case Conceptualization: Bowen

When conceptualizing client **cases,** contemporary Bowenian therapists typically use the following dynamics **to inform their treatment plan.** Go to MindTap® to access a digital version of the theory-specific case conceptualization, along with a variety of digital study tools and resources that complement this text and help you be more successful in your course and career. If your instructor didn't assign MindTap, you can find out more about it at Cengagebrain.com. You can also download the form at masteringcompetencies.com.

The Family Projection Process

- *Describe evidence of parental projection onto their child(ren), such as emotionally reactive behavior between family members; describe how it relates to symptoms, etc.*

Patterns of Differentiation and Fusion

- *Describe how the couple/family promotes togetherness and separateness; provide examples.*
- *Describe each person's relative level of differentiation and ability to effectively manage conflict without reactivity; provide examples.*
- *Describe patterns of fusion, in current and past generations; provide examples.*

Emotional Triangles and Cutoff

- Triangles within current partnership
- Triangles with family of origin
- Other triangles
- Emotional cutoffs in extended family

Sibling Position

- *Describe sibling position patterns that seem to be relevant for the family, current, and earlier generations.*

Multigenerational Transmission Process

- *Describe multigenerational transmission of functioning, attending to acculturation issues, residual effects of trauma and loss, significant legacies, use of alcohol and drugs, etc.*

Multigenerational Patterns Informed by Diversity Factors
- *Describe how multigenerational patterns are informed by relevant diversity factors, including those related to cultural, ethnicity, racial, immigration, acculturation, gender, religious, socioeconomic, ability, and sex/gender identity.*

Intergenerational Patterns from Genogram
Construct a family genogram and include all relevant information including:
- Names, ages, and birth/death dates
- Relational patterns
- Occupations
- Psychiatric disorders and alcohol/substance abuse
- Abuse history
- Personality adjectives

Attach genogram to this case conceptualization. Summarize key findings below:

- Substance/Alcohol Abuse: ☐ NA ☐ History: _____
- Sexual/Physical/Emotional Abuse: ☐ NA ☐ History: _____
- Physical/Mental Disorders: ☐ NA ☐ History: _____
- History Related to Presenting Problem: ☐ NA ☐ History: _____

Describe family strengths, such as the capacity to self-regulate and to effectively manage stress.

TREATMENT PLAN TEMPLATE FOR INDIVIDUAL WITH DEPRESSION/ANXIETY: BOWEN

📄 You can download a blank treatment plan (with or without measures) at www.cengagebrain.com or www.masteringcompetencies.com. The following treatment plan template can be used to help you develop individualized treatments for use with individuals with depressive or anxiety symptoms.

Bowen Treatment Plan: Client Goals with Interventions

Initial-Phase Client Goals
1. Reduce *triangulation* between client and [specify] to reduce depression and anxiety.
   a. *Detriangulate* by maintaining therapeutic neutrality and refocusing client on his or her half of problem interactions.
   b. *Relational experiments*—go home and practice relating directly rather than triangulating.

Working-Phase Client Goals
1. Decrease *chronic anxiety* and *reactivity* to stressors to reduce anxiety.
   a. *Encourage differentiated* responses to common anxieties and triggers.
   b. *Relational experiments* to practice responding rather than simply reacting to perceived anxieties and stressors.

2. Decrease mindless repetition of unproductive *multigenerational patterns* and increase consciously chosen responses to stressors to reduce depression and hopelessness.
   a. Use *genogram* to identify multigenerational patterns and intergenerational transmissions related to presenting problems.
   b. Use *process questions* to help clients see the multigenerational processes and make *differentiated* choices instead of mindlessly repeating pattern.

3. Decrease *emotional cutoffs* and reengage in difficult relationships from a differentiated position to reduce anxiety.
   a. Use *process questions* to identify the fusion underlying cutoffs.
   b. Use *going home again* exercise to help client reengage in cutoff relationships from a differentiated position.

Closing-Phase of Client Goals
1. Increase client's ability to *balance need for togetherness and autonomy* in intimate relationships to reduce depression and anxiety.
   a. Use *process questions* to explore how togetherness and autonomy can both be honored.
   b. Use *relational experiments* to practice relating to others from a differentiated position.

2. Increase ability to respond to family-of-origin interactions from a position of engaged *differentiation* to reduce to depression and sense of helplessness.
   a. *Encourage differentiated responses* when engaging family of origin.
   b. Use *going home again* exercises to redefine relationship with family of origin

Treatment Tasks
1. Develop working therapeutic relationship.
   a. Engage with client from a *differentiated* position, conveying a *nonanxious presence*.

2. Assess individual, systemic, and broader cultural dynamics.
   a. Use a *three-generation genogram* to identify *multigenerational patterns, chronic anxiety, triangles, emotional cutoff, family projection process,* and *sibling position.*
   b. Assess client's and significant other's levels of *differentiation* in current crisis/problem situation and in the past.

3. Identify needed referrals, crisis issues, collateral contacts, and other client needs.
   a. *Crisis assessment intervention(s):* Address crisis issues such as self harm, suicidal ideation, substance use, risky sexual behavior, etc.
   b. *Referral(s):* Connect client with *resources* in client's *community* that could be supportive; make collateral contacts as needed.

TREATMENT PLAN TEMPLATE FOR DISTRESSED COUPLE/FAMILY: BOWEN

You can download a blank treatment plan (with or without measures) at www.cengagebrain.com or www.masteringcompetencies.com. The following treatment plan template can be used to help you develop individualized treatments for use with couples and families who report relational distress.

Bowen Treatment Plan: Client Goals with Interventions

Early-Phase Client Goals
1. Reduce *triangulation* between [specify] and [specify] to reduce conflict.
   a. *Detriangulate* in session by maintaining therapeutic neutrality and refocusing each person on his or her half of problem interactions.
   b. Use *process questions* to increase awareness of how triangulation is used to unsuccessfully manage conflict.

Working-Phase Client Goals
1. Decrease *chronic anxiety* in system and *reactivity* to stressors to reduce conflict.
   a. *Encourage differentiated* responses to common anxieties and triggers.
   b. Use *relational experiments* to practice responding rather than simply reacting to perceived anxieties and stressors.

2. Decrease mindless repetition of unproductive *multigenerational patterns* and increase consciously chosen responses to stressors to reduce conflict.
   a. Use *genogram* to identify multigenerational patterns and intergenerational transmissions related to presenting problems.
   b. Use *process questions* to help clients see the multigenerational processes and make *differentiated* choices instead of mindlessly repeating pattern.

3. Decrease *emotional cutoffs* and reengage in difficult relationships from a differentiated position to reduce conflict.
   a. Use *process questions* to identify the fusion underlying cutoffs.
   b. Use *going home again* exercises to help clients reengage in cutoff relationships from a differentiated position.

Closing-Phase Client Goals

1. Increase each person's ability to *balance need for togetherness and autonomy* in intimate relationships to reduce conflict and increase intimacy.
   a. Use *process questions* to explore how togetherness and autonomy can both be honored within the relationship; discuss needs of each person and how they may differ and be accommodated.
   b. Use *relational experiments* to practice relating to others from a differentiated position.

2. Increase ability to respond to family-of-origin interactions from a position of engaged *differentiation* to reduce conflict and increase intimacy.
   a. *Encourage differentiated responses* when engaging family-of-origins.
   b. Use *going home again* exercises to redefine relationships with family of origin.

Treatment Tasks

1. Develop working therapeutic relationship.
   a. Engage with each client from a *differentiated* position, conveying a *nonanxious presence*.

2. Assess individual, systemic, and broader cultural dynamics.
   a. Use a *three- to four-generation genogram* to identify *multigenerational patterns, chronic anxiety, triangles, emotional cutoff, family projection process,* and *sibling position*.
   b. Assess client's and significant other's levels of *differentiation* in current crisis/problem situation and in the past.

3. Identify needed referrals, crisis issues, collateral contacts, and other client needs.
   a. *Crisis assessment intervention(s):* Address crisis issues such as psychological abuse, intimate partner violence, hidden affair, self harm, suicidal ideation, substance use, etc.
   b. *Referral(s):* Connect client with *resources* in client's *family and community* that could be supportive; make collateral contacts as needed.

Psychoanalytic Family Therapies
In a Nutshell: The Least You Need to Know

Many of the founders of family therapy were trained in psychoanalysis, including Don Jackson, Carl Whitaker, Salvador Minuchin, Nathan Ackerman, and Ivan Boszormenyi-Nagy. Although some disowned their academic roots as they developed methods for working with families, others, such as Ackerman and Boszormenyi-Nagy, did not. In the 1980s, renewed interest in object relations therapies led to the development of *object relations family therapy* (Scharff & Scharff, 1987).

These therapies use traditional psychoanalytic and psychodynamic principles that describe inner conflicts and extend these principles to external relationships. In contrast to individual psychoanalysts, psychoanalytic family therapists focus on the family as a nexus of relationships that either support or impede the development and functioning of its members. As in traditional psychoanalytic approaches, the process of therapy involves analyzing intrapsychic and interpersonal dynamics, promoting client insight, and working through these insights to develop new ways of relating to self and others. Some of the more influential approaches are *contextual therapy* (Boszormenyi-Nagy & Krasner, 1986), *family-of-origin therapy* (Framo, 1992), and *object relations family therapy* (Scharff & Scharff, 1987).

The Juice: Significant Contributions to the Field

If you remember one thing from this chapter, it should be this:

Ethical Systems and Relational Ethics

Ivan Boszormenyi-Nagy (Boszormenyi-Nagy & Krasner, 1986) introduced the idea of an **ethical system** at the heart of families that, like a *ledger,* keeps track of *entitlement* and *indebtedness.* Families use this system to maintain trustworthiness, fairness, and loyalty between family members; its breakdown results in individual and/or relational symptoms. Thus, the goal of therapy is to reestablish an ethical system in which family members are able to trust one another and to treat one another with fairness.

Clients often present in therapy with a semiconscious awareness of this ethical accounting system. Their presenting complaint may be that things are no longer fair in the relationship; parents are not sharing their duties equitably or one child is being treated differently than another. In these cases, an explicit dialogue about the family's ethical accounting system—what they are counting as their entitlement and what they believe is owed them—can be helpful in increasing empathy and understanding among family members.

Rumor Has It: The People and Their Stories

Nathan Ackerman and the Ackerman Institute

A child psychiatrist, Nathan Ackerman (1958, 1966) was one of the earliest pioneers in working with entire families, which he posited were split into factions, much the way an individual's psyche is divided into conflicting aspects of self. After developing his family approach at the Menninger Clinic in the 1930s and at Jewish Family Services in New York in the 1950s, he opened his own clinic in 1960, now known as the Ackerman Institute, which has remained one of the most influential family therapy institutes in the country. With Don Jackson, he cofounded the field's first journal, *Family Process.*

Ivan Boszormenyi-Nagy

With one of the most difficult names to pronounce in the field (Bo-zor-ma-nee Naj), Boszormenyi-Nagy was an early pioneer in psychoanalytic family therapy. His unique contribution was his idea that families had an ethical system, which he conceptualized as a *ledger of entitlement and indebtedness* (Boszormenyi-Nagy & Krasner, 1986).

James Framo

A student of Boszormenyi-Nagy, James Framo is best known for developing *family-of-origin therapy;* as part of treatment with individuals, couples, and families, he invited a client's entire family of origin in for extended sessions (Boszormenyi-Nagy & Framo, 1965/1985; Framo, 1992). Framo located the primary problem not only in the family unit but also in the larger extended family system.

David and Jill Scharff

Husband-and-wife team David and Jill Scharff (1987) developed a comprehensive model for object relations family therapy. Rather than focusing on individuals, they apply principles from traditional object relations therapy to the family as a unit.

The Women's Project

Bowenian-trained social workers Marianne Walters et al. (1988) reformulated many foundational family therapy concepts through a feminist lens. Their work challenged the field to examine gender stereotypes that were being reinforced in family therapy theory and practice, within and beyond the practice of Bowen family therapy.

The Big Picture: Overview of Treatment

The psychodynamic tradition includes a number of different schools that share the same therapeutic process. The first task is to create a caring therapeutic relationship, or *holding environment* (Scharff & Scharff, 1987), between the therapist and client. Then the therapist analyzes the intrapsychic and interpersonal dynamics—both conscious and unconscious, current and transgenerational—that are the source of symptoms (Boszormenyi-Nagy & Krasner, 1986; Scharff & Scharff, 1987). The therapist's next task is to promote client insight into these dynamics, which requires getting through client defenses. Once clients have achieved insights into the intrapsychic and interpersonal dynamics that fuel the problem, the therapist facilitates *working through* these insights to translate them into action in clients' daily lives.

Making a Connection: The Therapeutic Relationship

Transference and Countertransference

A classic psychoanalytic concept, **transference** refers to when a client projects onto the therapist attributes that stem from unresolved issues with primary caregivers; therapists use the immediacy of these interactions to promote client insight (Scharff & Scharff, 1987). **Countertransference** refers to when therapists project back onto clients, losing their therapeutic neutrality and having strong emotional reactions to the client; these moments are used to help the therapist and client better understand the reactions the client brings out in others. In therapy with couples and families, the processes of transference and countertransference vacillate more than in individual therapy because of the complex web of multiple relationships.

Contextual and Centered Holding

In contrast to traditional psychoanalysts, who are viewed as neutral "blank screens," object relations family therapists are more relationally focused, creating a nurturing relationship they call a **holding environment**. They distinguish between two aspects of holding in family therapy: contextual and centered (Scharff & Scharff, 1987). **Contextual holding** refers to the therapist's handling of therapy arrangements: conducting sessions competently, expressing concern for the family, and being willing to see the entire family. **Centered holding** refers to connecting with the family at a deeper level by expressing empathetic understanding to create a safe emotional space.

Multidirected Partiality

The guiding principle for relating to clients in contextual family therapy is **multidirectional partiality**, that is, being "partial" with all members of the family (Boszormenyi-Nagy & Krasner, 1986). Therapists must be accountable to everyone who is potentially affected by the interventions, including those not present, such as extended family members. This principle of inclusiveness means that the therapist must bring out the humanity of each member of the family, even the "monster member" (Boszormenyi-Nagy & Krasner, 1986). In practice, multidirectional partiality generally involves *sequential siding* with each member by empathizing with each person's position in turn.

The Viewing: Case Conceptualization and Assessment

Interlocking Pathologies

Expanding the classic psychodynamic view of symptomatology, Ackerman (1956) held that the constant exchange of unconscious processes within families creates **interlocking or interdependent pathologies** and that any individual's pathology reflects those family distortions and dynamics; this position is similar to that of systemic therapies. Thus, when working with a family, the therapist seeks to identify *how* the identified patient's symptoms relate to the less overt pathologies within the family.

Defense Mechanisms

Defense mechanisms are automatic responses to perceived psychological threats and are often activated on an unconscious level (Luborsky, O'Reilly-Landry, & Arlow, 2008). When the ego is unable to reconcile tensions between the id and the superego and/or manage unacceptable drives, it may use one or more defense mechanisms to manage the seemingly irreconcilable conflict. When used periodically, defense mechanisms can be adaptive ways of coping with stress; when used regularly, they become quite problematic. Freud began identifying these early in his work, and later theorists have continued adding to the list. Some of the more salient defense mechanisms when working with couple and family relationships are discussed below.

Splitting

The more intense the anxiety resulting from frustration related to the primary caregiver, the greater the person's need to split these objects, separating good from bad by repressing the rejecting and/or exciting objects, thus leaving less of the *ego,* or conscious self, to relate freely. To the degree that splitting is not resolved, there is an "all good" or "all bad" quality to evaluating relationships. In couples, splitting often results in seeing the partner as "perfect" (all good) in the early phases of the relationship, but when the partner no longer conforms to expectations, the partner becomes the enemy (all bad). In families, splitting can also take the form of the perfect versus the problem child.

Projection

Projection refers to falsely attributing one's own unacceptable feelings, impulses, or wishes onto another, typically without being aware of what one is doing (e.g., seeing others as greedy but not recognizing this characteristic in oneself; Mitchell & Black, 1995). In clinical practice, this is often seen when one partner thinks of cheating and then projects these intentions onto the faithful partner.

Projective Identification

In couples and other intimate relationships, clients defend against anxiety by projecting certain split-off or unwanted parts of themselves onto the other person, who is then manipulated to act according to these projections (Scharff & Scharff, 1987). For example, a husband may project his interest in other women onto his wife in the form of jealousy and accusations of infidelity; the wife then decides to hide innocent information that may feed the husband's fear, but the more she tries to calm his fears by hiding information, the more suspicious and jealous he becomes.

Repression/Suppression

Object relations therapists maintain that children must *repress* anxiety when they experience separation from their primary caregiver (attachment object), which results in less of the ego being available for contact with the outside world. Until this repressed material is made conscious, the adult unconsciously replicates these repressed-object relationships. One of the primary aims of psychoanalytic therapy is to bring repressed material to the surface.

Repression

A central concept in Freud's approach and considered one of the two basic defenses (along with splitting) by Kernberg (1976), **repression** describes the *unconscious process* that occurs when the superego seeks to *repress* the id's innate impulses and drives (St. Clair, 2000). In drive theory, repression is the cause of a wide range of neurotic symptoms, such as obsessions, compulsions, hallucinations, psychosomatic complaints, anxiety, and depression. Because it happens outside of awareness, repression is considered more pathological than suppression, in which the person consciously pushes the impulse out of his or her mind.

Suppression

Unlike repression, **suppression** is the *intentional* avoidance of difficult inner thoughts, feelings, and desires. When thoughtfully chosen, this defense can be very useful when facing difficult emotions over extended periods of time, such as grief, complicated loss, and so on.

Minimizing

Minimizing is used to reduce the intensity of a situation, protecting the person from painful and difficult-to-accept realities. For example, women who are battered often minimize the violence in their heads and to others to avoid facing the drastic implications of fully acknowledging the situation.

Displacement

Displacement refers to unconsciously redirecting intense emotion from a threatening object to a less-threatening object (Ziegler, 2016). This occurs commonly in families, such as when a parent is angry with a boss or situation at work and then redirects this anger onto a partner or children.

Try It Yourself

By yourself or with a partner, identify times you or someone you know has used each of the above defenses in some way. Which defenses do you use most often?

Attachment and Self-Object Relations Patterns

Object relations therapists emphasize the basic human need for relationship and **attachment** to others. Thus, they assess **self-object relations:** how people relate to others based on expectations created by early experiences with primary attachment objects, particularly mothers (Scharff & Scharff, 1987). As a result of these experiences, external objects are experienced as ideal, rejecting, or exciting:

- Ideal object: An internal mental representation of the primary caretaker that is desexualized and deaggressivized and maintained as distinct from its rejecting and exciting elements

- Rejecting object: An internal mental representation of the caregiver when the child's needs for attachment were rejected, leading to anger
- Exciting object: An internal mental representation of the caretaker formed when the child's needs for attachment were overstimulated, leading to longing for an unattainable but tempting object

Parental Introjects

Framo (1976) believes that the most significant dynamic affecting individual and family functioning is parental introjects, the internalized negative aspects of parents. People internalize these attributes and unconsciously strive to make all future intimate relationships conform to them, such as when they hear a parent's critical comments in the neutral comments of a partner. Therapists help clients become conscious of these introjects to increase their autonomy in intimate relationships.

Transference between Family Members

Similar to the way they assess transference from client to therapist, object relations therapists assess for transference from one family member onto another (Scharff & Scharff, 1987). Transference between family members involves one person projecting onto other members introjects and repressed material. The therapist's job is to help the family disentangle their transference, using interpretation to promote insight into intrapsychic and interpersonal dynamics. It is often easier to promote insight into transference patterns in family therapy than in individual therapy because these patterns happen "live" in the room with the therapist, thus reducing the potential for a client to rationalize or minimize them.

Ledger of Entitlement and Indebtedness

Boszormenyi-Nagy (Boszormenyi-Nagy & Krasner, 1986) conceptualized the moral and ethical system within the family as a **ledger of entitlements and indebtedness,** or more simply, a *ledger of merits*—an internal accounting of what you believe is due to you and what you owe others. Of course, because in families each person has his or her own internal accounting system that has a different bottom line, tensions arise over who is entitled to what, especially if there is no consensus on what is fair and how give-and-take should be balanced in the family.

- Justice and fairness: The pursuit of justice and fairness is viewed as one of the foundational premises of intimate relationships. Monitoring fairness is an ongoing process that keeps the relationship *trustworthy.* A "just" relationship is an ideal, and all relationships strive to achieve this never fully attainable goal.
- Entitlements: **Entitlements** are "ethical guarantees" to merits that are earned in the context of relationships, such as the freedom that parents are entitled to because of the care they extend to children. The person's sense of entitlement may be evident only in a crisis or an extreme situation, such as a parent suddenly becoming ill. **Destructive entitlements** result when children do not receive the nurturing to which they are entitled and later project this loss onto the world, which they see as their "debtors."
- Invisible loyalties: Family ledgers extend across generations, fostering **invisible loyalties.** For example, new couples may have unconscious commitments to their family of origin when starting their partnership. Invisible loyalties may manifest as indifference, avoidance, or indecisiveness in relation to the object of loyalty, blocking commitment in a current relationship.
- Revolving slate: A **revolving slate** is a destructive relational process in which one person takes revenge (or insists on entitlements) in one relationship based on the relational transactions in another relationship. Instead of reconciling the "slate" or

account in the relationship in which the debt was accrued, the person treats an inno-cent person as if he or she were the original debtor.

- Split loyalties: This term refers to when a child feels forced to choose one parent (or significant caregiver) over another because of mistrust between the caregivers. Com-mon in divorces, this highly destructive dynamic results in pathology in the child.

- Transgenerational Legacy: Each person inherits a *legacy*, a transgenerational mandate that links the endowments of the current generation to its obligations to future gen-erations. "Legacy is the present generation's ethical imperative to sort out what in life is beneficial for posterity's quality of survival" (Boszormenyi-Nagy & Krasner, 1986, p. 418). Legacy is a positive force in the chain of survival.

Try It Yourself

By yourself or with a partner, review your current relationship with a partner or family, and examine your ledger of entitlements and debts. How does your ledger compare with that of your partner/family members? Can you imagine a way of discussing these to help each appreciate the other more?

Mature Love: Dialogue versus Fusion

Boszormenyi-Nagy and Krasner (1986) describes mature love as a form of dialogue be-tween two people who are conscious of the family dynamics that have shaped their lives. This type of love is quite different from fusion, experienced as an amorphous "we" simi-lar to an infant and its caregiver. Thus, clients are encouraged to make invisible loyalties overt so that they can be critically examined, allowing for conscious choice and action rather than the fear and anxiety that characterize fused relationships.

Targeting Change: Goal Setting

Goals in psychoanalytic therapies include several long-term changes in both individual and relational functioning (Boszormenyi-Nagy & Krasner, 1986; Scharff & Scharff, 1987). General goals include the following:

- Increase autonomy and ego-directed action by making unconscious processes conscious.
- Decrease interactions based on projections or a revolving slate of entitlements.
- Increase capacity for intimacy without loss of self (fusion with object).
- Develop reciprocal commitments that include a fair balance of entitlements and indebtedness.

The Doing: Interventions

Listening, Interpreting, and Working Through

In general, psychoanalytic therapies use three generic interventions:

- Listening and empathy: The primary tool of psychoanalytic therapists is listening objectively to the client's story without offering advice, reassurance, validation, or confrontation. Empathy may be used to help the family to nondefensively hear the therapist's interpretation of their unconscious dynamics.
- Interpretation and promoting insight: Like other psychoanalytic therapists, family psychoanalytic therapists encourage insights into interpersonal dynamics by offering interpretations to the client, such as by analyzing self–object relations or analyzing ledgers of entitlement and indebtedness.

- Working through: Working through is the process of translating insight into new action in family and other relationships. Changing one's behavior on the basis of new insight is often the most difficult part of therapy. Understanding that you are projecting onto your partner feelings and expectations that really belong in your relationship with your mother is not too difficult; changing how you respond to your partner when you feel rejected and uncared for is more challenging.

Eliciting

In contextual therapy, **eliciting** uses clients' spontaneous motives to move the family in a direction that is mutually beneficial and dialogical (Boszormenyi-Nagy & Krasner, 1986). The therapist facilitates this process by integrating the facts of the situation, each person's individual psychology, and interactive transitions to help the family rework the balances of entitlement and indebtedness, helping each member to reinterpret past interactions and identify new ways to move forward.

Detriangulating

Like other systemic therapists, psychoanalytic therapists identify situations in which the parents have triangulated a symptomatic child into the relationship to deflect attention away from their couple distress (Framo, 1992). Once the child's role is made clear, the therapist dismisses the symptomatic child from therapy and proceeds to work with the couple to address the issues that created the need for the child's symptoms.

Family-of-Origin Therapy

Framo (1992) developed a three-stage model for working with couples that involved couples therapy, couples group therapy, and family-of-origin therapy. Therapists begin working with the couple alone to increase insight into their personal and relational dynamics. Next, the couple join a couples group, where they receive feedback from other couples and also view their dynamics; for many couples, insight comes more quickly when they see their problem dynamically acted out in another couple. Finally, each individual member of the couple is invited to have a four-hour-long session with his or her family of origin without the other partner present. These extended family-of-origin sessions are used to clarify and work through past and present issues, thereby freeing individuals to respond to their partners and children without the "ghosts" of these past attachments.

Scope It Out: Cross-Theoretical Comparison

Using Tomm's IPscope described in Chapter 3 (Tomm et al., 2014), this theory approaches the conceptualization of systemic, interpersonal patterns as discussed below.

Theoretical Conceptualization

Psychodynamic family therapists identify PIPs in the current relationship as well as the family of origin and look for patterns of interlocking pathologies, such as a couple made up of a narcissist and a people-pleaser. In addition, psychodynamic therapists may also identify PIPs by examining how attachment patterns interconnect (such as anxious and avoidant) or how each party's defenses match up (denying/projecting).

Goal Setting

In psychodynamic theory, WIPs are characterized as interactions in which each person uses ego-directed action instead of defense mechanisms as well as interactions in which the dyad experiences intimacy without loss of self, a goal that is similar to intergenerational differentiation.

Facilitating Change

Similar to Bowen intergenerational therapists, psychodynamic family therapists primarily use TIPs that promote insight into PIPs across generations. They also use TIPs that help clients examine how their defense mechanisms maintain PIPs and encourage them to learn to more authentically and directly connect with others.

Putting It All Together: Case Conceptualization and Treatment Plan Templates

Areas for Theory-Specific Case Conceptualization: Psychodynamic

When conceptualizing client **cases**, contemporary psychodynamic family therapists typically use the following dynamics **to inform their treatment plan**. Go to MindTap® to access a digital version of the theory-specific case conceptualization, along with a variety of digital study tools and resources that complement this text and help you be more successful in your course and career. If your instructor didn't assign MindTap, you can find out more about it at Cengagebrain.com. You can also download the form at masteringcompetencies.com.

Self–Object Relations Patterns

Identify self–object relation patterns for each person in the family:

- Ideal object
- Rejecting object
- Exciting object

Defenses

Describe internal conflicts and defenses commonly used by client, significant other, and/or key family members:

- Splitting
- Projection/Projective Identification
- Repression/Suppression
- Minimizing
- Displacement

Attachment Patterns

- Describe when (if at all), client(s) feel securely connected in their current attached relationship(s); regularity of secure attachment; relational conditions for secure attachment.
- Describe typical attachment behavior when person does not feel secure in relationships: anxious, avoidant, anxious avoidant; frequency.

Self–Object Relations Patterns, Parental Introjects and Transference

- Describe self–object relation patterns and parental introjects for client, significant other, and/or key family members, especially patterns those related to managing anxiety, criticism, conflict, vulnerability, intimacy, etc.

Interlocking Pathologies

- Based on above analysis, describe unconscious interlocking pathologies between the client(s) and significant others:

Describe the basic pattern of how these interlocking pathologies affect the interaction patterns related to the presenting problem: ☐ Pursuing/Distancing ☐ Criticizing/Defending ☐ Controlling/Resisting ☐ Other: _____

- Start of Tension: _____
- Conflict/Symptom Escalation: _____
- Return to "Normal"/Homeostasis: _____
- Expression of Interlocking Pathologies: _____
- Describe how the clients' social location—age, gender race, ethnicity, sexual orientation, gender identity, social class, religion, geographic region, language, family configuration, abilities, etc.—affects the relational dynamics: _____
- Describe transference of parental introjects and repressed material onto others in the couple/family.

TREATMENT PLAN TEMPLATE FOR INDIVIDUAL WITH DEPRESSION/ANXIETY: PSYCHODYNAMIC

The following treatment plan template can be used to help you develop individualized treatments for use with individuals with depressive or anxiety symptoms. You can download a blank treatment plan (with or without measures) from MindTap at www.cengagebrain.com or www.masteringcompetencies.com.

Psychodynamic Treatment Plan: Client Goals with Interventions

Early-Phase Client Goals

1. Increase awareness of *self–object patterns* and reduce *splitting, idealizing,* or *other defense strategies* to reduce depressed mood and anxiety.
   a. *Listen to and interpret for* client *self–object patterns* and *defense patterns* related to depressed mood and anxiety.
   b. Identify one relationship/area of life in which the client can begin to *work through* the assessed patterns.

Working-Phase Client Goals

1. Decrease interactions based on *projections* and/or a *revolving slate of entitlements* to reduce depressed mood/anxiety.
   a. Offer *interpretations* of *projection patterns* and *revolving slate issues* to increase client awareness.
   b. Use in-session examples of *transference* to help client *work through* projection patterns.

2. Reduce influence of *negative parental introjects* to enable authentic relating to reduce hopelessness and depressed mood.
   a. *Detriangulate* to help client separate negative parental interjects from interpretations and assumptions in current relationships.
   b. Identify one to two relationships in which client can *work through negative parental interjects.*

3. Increase *autonomy* and *ego-directed action* by making unconscious processes conscious to reduce depression and anxiety.
   a. *Eliciting* to develop client motivation to work in productive directions in relationships.
   b. Identify one to two relationships/areas of life in which client can *work through* dynamics increase autonomy and goal-directed action.

Closing-Phase Client Goals

1. Increase capacity for *intimacy* and *mature love* without loss of self to reduce depression and anxiety.
   a. *Interpret defenses and projections* that hinder capacity for mature love.
   b. Identify one to two opportunities to *work through* issues that block capacity for intimacy.

2. Develop *reciprocal commitments* that include a *fair balance of entitlements and indebtedness* to increase capacity for intimacy.
   a. Identify *legacies, loyalties, and revolving slate patterns* that have imbalanced current relationships.
   b. Examine the *ledger of entitlements/indebtedness* to identify more appropriate and balanced calculations of what is due and what is owed.

Treatment Tasks

1. Develop working therapeutic relationship.
   a. Create a *holding environment* that includes *contextual* issues as well as client's dynamics.
   b. Work through client *transference* and monitor therapist *countertransference*.

2. Assess individual, systemic, and broader cultural dynamics.
   a. Identify *self-object relation patterns, splitting, projective identification, repression, parental interjects,* and *defense patterns*.
   b. Identify *interlocking pathologies, transference with partner/family, ledger of entitlements and indebtedness,* and *capacity for mature love*.

3. Identify needed referrals, crisis issues, collateral contacts, and other client needs.
   a. Crisis assessment intervention(s): Address crisis issues such as self harm, suicidal ideation, substance use, risky sexual behavior, etc.
   b. Referral(s): Connect client with *resources* in client's *community* that could be supportive; make collateral contacts as needed.

TREATMENT PLAN TEMPLATE FOR DISTRESSED COUPLE/FAMILY: PSYCHODYNAMIC

The following treatment plan template can be used to help you develop individualized treatments for use with couples and families who report relational distress. You can download a blank treatment plan (with or without measures) from MindTap at www.cengagebrain.com or www.masteringcompetencies.com.

Psychodynamic Treatment Plan: Client Goals with Interventions

Initial-Phase Client Goals

1. Increase awareness of *self–object patterns* and *transference between couple/family members* and reduce *splitting, idealizing, or other defense strategies* to reduce conflict.
   a. *Listen to and interpret for* client *self–object patterns, transference within system,* and *defense patterns* related to conflict in couple/family.
   b. Identify one aspect of relationship in which each person can take action to *work through* the assessed patterns.

Working-Phase Client Goals

1. Decrease couple/family interactions based on *projections* and/or a *revolving slate of entitlements* to reduce conflict.
   a. Offer *interpretations* of *projection patterns* and *revolving slate issues* to increase each person's awareness of dynamics.
   b. Use in-session examples of *transference* both between members and with therapist to help clients *work through* projection patterns.

2. Reduce influence of *negative parental introjects* to enable authentic relating to reduce hopelessness and depressed mood.
   a. *Detriangulation* to help client separate negative parental interjects from interpretations and assumptions in current relationships.
   b. Identify one to three relationships in which client can *work through negative parental interjects*.

3. Increase *autonomy* and *ego-directed action* by making unconscious processes conscious to reduce conflict.
   a. *Elicit* to develop client motivation to work in productive directions in relationship.
   b. Identify areas of relationship in which each member can *work through* dynamics increase autonomy and goal-directed action.

Closing-Phase Client Goals

1. Increase each member's capacity for *intimacy* and *mature love* without loss of self to reduce conflict and increase intimacy.
   a. *Interpret defenses and projections* that hinder capacity of mature love.
   b. Identify opportunities for each member to *work through* issues that block capacity for intimacy.

2. Develop *reciprocal commitments* that include a *fair balance of entitlements and indebtedness* to increase capacity for intimacy.
   a. Identify *legacies, loyalties, and revolving slate patterns* that have imbalanced current relationships.
   b. Examine the *ledger of entitlements/indebtedness* to identify more appropriate and balanced calculations of what is due and what is owed.

Treatment Tasks

1. Develop working therapeutic relationship.
   a. Create a *holding environment* for all members that includes *contextual* issues as well as client's dynamics.
   b. Work through client *transference* and monitor therapist *countertransference* with each member of the system.

2. Assess individual, systemic, and broader cultural dynamics.
   a. Identify each client's *self-object relation patterns, splitting, projective identification, repression, parental interjects,* and *defense patterns.*
   b. Identify *interlocking pathologies, transference within couple/family system, ledger of entitlements and indebtedness,* and *each person's capacity for mature love.*

3. Identify needed referrals, crisis issues, collateral contacts, and other client needs.
   a. Crisis assessment intervention(s): Address crisis issues such as psychological abuse, intimate partner violence, hidden affair, self-harm, suicidal ideation, substance use, etc.
   b. Referral(s): Connect client with *resources* in client's *family and community* that could be supportive; make collateral contacts as needed.

Tapestry Weaving: Working with Diverse Populations

Gender Diversity: The Women's Project

Trained as social workers, Betty Carter, Olga Silverstein, Peggy Papp, and Marianne Walters (Walters et al., 1988) joined together to promote a greater awareness of women's issues in the field of family therapy. They raised the issue of gender power dynamics within traditional families and identified how family therapists were reinforcing stereotypes that were detrimental to women. In particular, they explicated how the misuse of power and control in abusive and violent relationships made it impossible for women to end or escape their victimization, a perspective that is now accepted by most therapists and the public at large. They also asserted that therapists should be *agents of social change,* challenging sexist attitudes and beliefs in families.

Walters et al. (1988) made several suggestions for how family therapists can reduce sexism in their work with couples and families:

* Openly discuss the *gender role expectations* of each partner and parent and point out areas where the couple or family hold beliefs that are unfair or unrealistic.

- Encourage women to take *private time* for themselves to avoid losing their individual identity to the roles of wife and mother.
- Use the self-of-the-therapist to model an *attitude of gender equality.*
- Push men to take on equal responsibility both in family relationships and in the household, as well as for scheduling therapy, attending therapy with children, and/or arranging for babysitting for couples sessions.

Ethnicity and Cultural Diversity

Apart from the work of the Women's Project (Walters et al., 1988; see "Women's Project" above), the application of Bowen intergenerational and psychoanalytic therapies to diverse populations has not been widely explored or studied. In general, these therapies are aimed at "thinking" or psychologically minded clients (Friedman, 1991). Thus, minority groups who prefer action and concrete suggestions from therapists may have difficulty with these approaches. However, the therapist's stance as an expert fits with the expectations of many immigrant and marginalized populations. The work of Bowen, Framo, and Boszormenyi-Nagy that emphasizes the role of extended family members and intergenerational patterns may be particularly useful with diverse clients whose cultural norms value the primacy of the extended family over the nuclear family system. In these families, the nuclear family is expected to subordinate their will to that of the larger family system. In addition, research on the concept of differentiation of self provides initial support for its cross-cultural validity (Skowron, 2004).

In general, the greatest danger in using Bowenian or psychoanalytic therapies with diverse clients is that the therapist may use inappropriate cultural norms to analyze family dynamics, thereby imposing a set of values and beliefs that are at odds with the clients' culture. For example, if a therapist, without reflection, proceeds on the Bowenian premise that the nuclear family should be autonomous and develops therapeutic goals to move an immigrant family in that direction, the therapist could put the client in the difficult situation of being caught between the therapist's goals and the extended family's expectations. Similarly, if the therapist assumes that attachment looks the same in all cultures, the client may be inaccurately and unfairly evaluated, resulting in therapy that is ineffective at best and destructive at worst. Because these theories have highly developed systems of assessing "normal" behavior, therapists must be mindful when working with clients who do not conform to what the therapist considers to be common cultural norms.

Immigration and Intergenerational Conflict

A particularly useful application of Bowen's theory is working with immigrant families who often experience significant struggles between generations. Lui (2015) conducted a meta-analysis of over 60 research studies on Asian and Latino immigrants and found that intergenerational cultural conflict is correlated with acculturation mismatch between parents and children and that this is not always resolved after adolescence. Unlike intergenerational conflict in nonimmigrant families, in Asian and Latino families, intergenerational conflict related to acculturation is significantly correlated with internalizing symptoms, adaptive functioning, and educational outcomes but not externalizing symptoms; women and second-generation immigrant offspring are affected the most. Lui (2015) also found that Southeast Asians were more negatively affected in terms of mental health than their East Asian or Mexican peers. In another study with Asian immigrant families, higher levels of perceived discrimination were associated with more intergenerational conflict, presumably because of intergenerational disagreement about how to respond to discrimination; when the conflict was with the mother, the child was more likely to become depressed (Cheng, Lin, & Cha, 2015). Bowen therapists can use genograms and analysis of intergenerational processes to help parents and children increase their understanding of and empathy for the other and find common understandings that allow them to move forward, feeling supported by their family, which is one of the best predictors of positive acculturation.

Sexual and Gender Identity Diversity

Because the issue of a child's sexual orientation and gender identity has implications for the entire family system, Bowenian therapists working with lesbian, gay, bisexual, transgendered, and questioning (LGBTQ) clients should pay particular attention to intergenerational relationships. One study found that gay and lesbian parents lived closer to and received more support from their own parents (Koller, 2009). In contrast, gays and lesbians who were not parents reported stronger connections with their friend networks, some times referred to as families-of-choice (Koller, 2009). Thus, therapists should pay particular attention to the role of these friendship relationships with LGBTQ clients. Another study considered the effects of parental disapproval on lesbian relationships, which was found to have both positive and negative effects on the relationship (Levy, 2011). The negative effects included amount and quality of time spent as a couple, stress on the couple relationship, emotional impact on the couple, fear/uncertainty, communication problems, and sexual effects. The positive effects of parental disapproval of the relationship included increased closeness, communication, patience, maturity, and valuing of the relationship on the part of the couple. In a study that compared three-generation genograms of heterosexual and homosexual males found that overall there were more similarities than differences but that twice as many parents of gay/lesbian children had significant marital issues and twice as many heterosexual men had more distant relationships with their fathers than did gay men (Feinberg & Bakeman, 1994).

Psychodynamic therapy has long been criticized for its pathologizing of same-sex attraction, and thus psychodynamic family therapists working with gay and lesbian couples should consider using gay-affirmative psychodynamic approaches (Rubinstein, 2003). Rubinstein recommends that psychodynamic therapists working with LGBTQ clients consider a multifaceted identity formation that includes, biological sex, gender identity, social sex-role, and sexual orientation. He suggests that social sex-role confusion is usually the most salient issue for gay and lesbian clients, who often feel conflicted over conforming to culturally approved behaviors for maleness and femaleness. In addition, psychoanalytic therapy can be used to help LGTBQ clients address their internalized homophobia by exploring their personal meaning of being attracted to same-sex partners.

Research and the Evidence Base

The focus of research on Bowenian and psychoanalytic therapies has not been on outcome, as is required to be labeled as empirically validated studies (Chapter 2); instead the focus of research has been on the validity of the concepts. Miller, Anderson, and Keala (2004) provide an overview of the research on the validity of the intergenerational theoretical constructs. They found that research supports the relation between differentiation and: (a) chronic anxiety, (b) marital satisfaction, and (c) psychological distress. However, there was little support for Bowen's assumption that people marry a person with a similar level of differentiation or his theories on sibling position; his concept of triangulation received partial empirical support.

Of particular interest to researchers is Bowen's concept of differentiation of self, which has been the focus of scores of research studies on topics such as client perceptions of the therapeutic alliance (Lambert, 2008), adolescent risk-taking behaviors (Knauth, Skowron, & Escobar, 2006), parenting outcomes in low-income urban families (Skowron, 2005), and adult well-being (Skowron, Holmes, & Sabatelli, 2003). Lawson and Brossart (2003) conducted a study that predicted therapeutic alliance and therapeutic outcome from the therapist's relationship with his or her parents, providing support for the Bowenian emphasis on the self-of-the-therapist. Another study considering a psychometric measure of differentiation identifies two aspects of differentiation: (a) affect regulation (the ability to regulate one's expressed mood), and (b) the ability to negotiate interpersonal togetherness with separateness (Jankowski & Hooper, 2012). Most recently, researchers validated a Chinese version of the Differentiation of Self Inventory (Lam & Chan-So, 2015).

With regard to psychoanalytic family therapies, significant research has been conducted on the nature of attachment in problem formation (Wood, 2002). The concept of attachment is also central to two empirically supported family therapies: emotionally focused therapy (see Chapter 6; Johnson, 2004) and multidimensional therapy (Chapter 4; Liddle et al., 2001). Research is needed on the outcomes and effectiveness of Bowenian and psychoanalytic family therapies so that these models can be refined and further developed. More generally, brief psychodynamic therapy for specific conditions, such as depression, rather than general personality restructuring (the original focus of psychoanalytic therapies) has a solid evidence base. In addition, recent process research on psychodynamic therapy supported the "Goldilocks" hypothesis: moderate-intensity interventions are more effective than gentle or intense (McCarthy, Keefe, & Barber, 2016).

QUESTIONS FOR PERSONAL REFLECTION AND CLASS DISCUSSION

1. Differentiation requires the ability to regulate your emotions and behaviors even when you feel threatened in a relationship and to clearly identify your contributions to the situation rather than blame others. Compare this concept to secure attachment.

2. One of the fundamental goals of Bowen intergenerational therapy is to reduce emotional reactivity in the relational system to enable members to take responsibility for their half of negative interactions by consciously choosing to engage in more effective interactions. If a Bowen therapist worked with you and your relationships, what would need to change?

3. How might differentiation look different based on race, ethnicity, gender, socioeconomic status, level of education, and age? Do you believe differentiation is a concept that can or should be used with all populations? Who might it marginalize?

4. Describe an experience with triangulation in your life. What was your role in it, and how did it affect the primary dyad's relationship?

5. Describe an experience you have had with transference or countertransference, either in therapy or your personal life. Describe its effects on both parties and the relationship.

6. Looking at your family of origin, describe interlocking pathologies (Hint: Look for the most opposite personalities or defenses). Describe how they reinforced each other's behavior in negative interaction cycles.

7. Nagy describes mature love as occurring between two people who are conscious of the dynamics in the families of origin and are differentiated enough to not be driven by invisible loyalties rather than being fused with and reactive to their partners. What are your thoughts on his definition of mature love?

ONLINE RESOURCES

Ackerman Institute: Psychoanalytic Therapy and Family Therapy Training
www.ackerman.org

The Bowen Center
thebowencenter.org

Georgetown Family Center: Bowen Center for the Study of the Family
www.thebowencenter.org

Family Process: Journal
www.familyprocess.org

Sexual Crucible Model
www.passionatemarriage.com

Go to MindTap® for an eBook, videos of client sessions, activities, practice quizzes, apps, and more—all in one place. If your instructor didn't assign MindTap, you can find out more information at CengageBrain.com.

REFERENCES

*Asterisk indicates recommended introductory readings.

Ackerman, N. W. (1956). Interlocking pathology in family relationships. In S. Rado & B. G. Daniels (Eds.), *Changing conceptions of psychoanalytic medicine* (pp. 135–150). New York: Grune & Stratton.

Ackerman, N. W. (1958). *The psychodynamics of family life.* New York: Basic Books.

Ackerman, N. W. (1966). *Treating the troubled family.* New York: Basic Books.

Boszormenyi-Nagy, I., & Framo, J. L. (1965/1985). *Intensive family therapy: Theoretical and practical aspects.* New York: Brunner/Mazel.

*Boszormenyi-Nagy, I., & Krasner, B. R. (1986). *Between give and take: A clinical guide to contextual therapy.* New York: Brunner/Mazel.

Bowen, M. (1966). The use of family theory in clinical practice. *Comprehensive Psychiatry 7,* 345–374.

Bowen, M. (1972). Being and becoming a family therapist. In A. Ferber, M. Mendelsohn, & A. Napier (Eds.), *The book of family therapy.* New York: Science House.

Bowen, M. (1976). Theory in practice of psychotherapy. In P. J. Guerin (Ed.), *Family therapy: Theory and practice.* New York: Gardner.

*Bowen, M. (1985). *Family therapy in clinical practice.* New York: Jason Aronson.

Bridgett, D. J., Burt, N. M., Edwards, E. S., & Deater-Deckard, K. (2015). Intergenerational transmission of self-regulation: A multidisciplinary review and integrative conceptual framework. *Psychological Bulletin, 141*(3), 602–654. doi:10.1037/a0038662

*Carter, B., & McGoldrick, M. (1999). *The expanded family life cycle: Individual, family, and social perspectives* (3rd ed.). Boston, MA: Allyn & Bacon.

Cheng, H., Lin, S., & Cha, C. H. (2015). Perceived discrimination, intergenerational family conflicts, and depressive symptoms in foreign-born and U.S.-born Asian American emerging adults. *Asian American Journal Of Psychology, 6*(2), 107–116. doi:10.1037/a0038710

Feinberg, J., & Bakeman, R. (1994). Sexual orientation and three generational family patterns in a clinical sample of heterosexual and homosexual men. *Journal of Gay & Lesbian Psychotherapy, 2*(2), 65–76. doi:10.1300/J236v02n02_04

Framo, J. L. (1976). Family of origin as a therapeutic resource for adults in marital and family therapy: You can and should go home again. *Family Process 15*(2), 193–210.

*Framo, J. L. (1992). *Family-of-origin therapy: An intergenerational approach.* New York: Brunner/Mazel.

Friedman, E. H. (1991). Bowen theory and therapy. In A. S. Gurman & D. P. Kniskern (Eds.), *Handbook of family therapy* (vol. 2, pp. 134–170). Philadelphia, PA: Brunner/Mazel.

Graff, G. (2014). The intergenerational trauma of slavery and its aftermath. *Journal of Psychohistory, 41*(3), 181–197.

Guerin, P. J., Fogarty, T. F., Fay, L. F., & Kautto, J. G. (1996). *Working with relationship triangles: The one-two-three of psychotherapy.* New York: Guilford.

Hardy, K. V., & Laszloffy, T. A. (1995). The cultural genogram: Key to training culturally competent family therapists. *Journal of Marital and Family Therapy, 21,* 227–237.

Jankowski, P. J., & Hooper, L. M. (2012). Differentiation of self: A validation study of the Bowen theory construct. *Couple and Family Psychology: Research and Practice,* doi:10.1037/a0027469

Johnson, S. M. (2004). *The practice of emotionally focused marital therapy: Creating connection* (2nd ed.). New York: Brunner/Routledge.

*Kernberg, O. (1976). *Object relations theory and clinical psychoanalysis.* New York: Aronson.

*Kerr, M., & Bowen, M. (1988). *Family evaluation.* New York: Norton.

Knauth, D. G., Skowron, E. A., & Escobar, M. (2006). Effect of differentiation of self on adolescent risk behavior. *Nursing Research, 55,* 336–345.

Koller, J. (2009). A study on gay and lesbian intergenerational relationships: A test of the solidarity model. *Dissertation Abstracts International Section A, 70,* 1032.

Kuehl, B. P. (1995). The solution-oriented genogram: A collaborative approach. *Journal of Marital and Family Therapy, 21,* 239–250.

Lam, C. M., & Chan-So., P. C. Y. (2015). Validation of the Chinese version of Differentiation of Self Inventory (C-SDI). *Journal of Marital and Family Therapy, 41,* 86–101.

Lambert, J. (2008). Relationship of differentiation of self to adult clients' perceptions of the alliance in brief family therapy. *Psychotherapy Research, 18,* 160–166.

Lans, O., Mosek, A., & Yagil, Y. (2014). Romantic jealousy from the perspectives of Bowen's concept of differentiation and gender differences. *Family Journal, 22*(3), 321–331. doi: 10.1177/1066480714530835

Lawson, D. M., & Brossart, D. F. (2003). Link among therapist and parent relationship, working alliance, and therapy outcome. *Psychotherapy Research, 13,* 383–394.

Levy, A. (2011). The effect of parental homo-negativity on the lesbian couple. *Dissertation Abstracts International, 71,* 5132.

Licht, C., & Chabot, D. (2006). The Chabot Emotional Differentiation Scale: A theoretically and psychometrically sound instrument for measuring Bowen's intrapsychic aspect of differentiation. *Journal of Marital and Family Therapy, 32*(2), 167–180.

Liddle, H. A., Dakof, G. A., Parker, K., Diamond, G. S., Barrett, K., & Tejeda, M. (2001). Multidimensional family therapy for adolescent drug abuse: Results of a randomized clinical trial. *American Journal of Drug and Alcohol Abuse, 27,* 651–688.

Luborsky, E. B., O'Reilly-Landry, M., & Arlow, J. A. (2008). Psychoanalysis. In R. J. Corsini & D. Wedding (Eds.), *Current psychotherapies* (8th ed.; pp. 15–62). Pacific Grove, CA: Thompson.

Lui, P. P. (2015). Intergenerational cultural conflict, mental health, and educational outcomes among Asian and Latino/a Americans: Qualitative and meta-analytic review. *Psychological Bulletin, 141*(2), 404–446. doi:10.1037/a0038449

McCarthy, K. S., Keefe, J. R., & Barber, J. P. (2016). Goldilocks on the couch: Moderate levels of psychodynamic and process-experiential technique predict outcome in psychodynamic therapy. *Psychotherapy Research, 26*(3), 307–317. doi: 10.1080/10503307.2014.973921

*McGoldrick, M., Gerson, R., & Petry, S. (2008). *Genograms: Assessment and intervention* (3rd ed.). New York: Norton.

Miller, R. B., Anderson, S., & Keala, D. K. (2004). Is Bowen theory valid? A review of basic research. *Journal of Marital and Family Therapy, 30,* 453–466.

Mitchell, S. A., & Black, M J. (1995). *Freud and beyond: A history of modern psychoanalytic thought.* New York: Basic Books.

Priest, J. (2015). A Bowen family systems model of generalized anxiety disorder and romantic relationship distress. *Journal of Marital and Family Therapy, 41*(3), 340–353.

Rivera, P., & Fincham, F. (2015). Forgiveness as a mediator of the intergenerational transmission of violence. *Journal of Interpersonal Violence, 30*(6), 895–910.

Rubalcava, L. A., & Waldman, K. M. (2004). Working with intercultural couples: An intersubjective-constructivist perspective. *Progress in Self Psychology, 20,* 127–149.

Rubinstein, G. (2003). Does psychoanalysis really mean oppression? Harnessing psychodynamic approaches to affirmative therapy with gay men. *American Journal of Psychotherapy, 57*(2), 206–218.

*Scharff, D., & Scharff, J. (1987). *Object relations family therapy.* New York: Aronson.

Schnarch, D. M. (1991). *Constructing the sexual crucible: An integration of sexual and marital therapy.* New York: Norton.

Schnarch, D. M. (1998). *Passionate marriage: Keeping love and intimacy alive in committed relationships.* New York: Holt.

Skowron, E. A. (2004). Differentiation of self, personal adjustment, problem solving, and ethnic group belonging among persons of color. *Journal of Counseling and Development, 82,* 447–456.

Skowron, E. A. (2005). Parental differentiation of self and child competence in low-income urban families. *Journal of Counseling Psychology, 52,* 337–346.

Skowron, E. A., Holmes, S. E., & Sabatelli, R. M. (2003). Deconstructing differentiation: Self regulation, interdependent relating, and well-being in adulthood. *Contemporary Family Therapy, 25,* 111–129.

*St. Clair, M. (2000). *Object relations and self psychology: An introduction.* Belmont, CA: Brooks/Cole.

Tomm, K., St. George, S., Wulff, D., & Strong, T. (2014). *Patterns in interpersonal interactions: Inviting relational understandings for therapeutic change.* New York: Routledge.

*Walters, M., Carter, B., Papp, P., & Silverstein, O. (1988). *The invisible web: Gender patterns in family relationships.* New York: Guilford.

*Wood, B. L. (2002). Attachment and family systems (Special issue). *Family Process, 41.*

Ziegler, D. J. (2016). Defense mechanisms in rational emotive cognitive behavior therapy personality theory. *Journal of Rational-Emotive & Cognitive-Behavior Therapy, 34*(2), 135–148. doi:10.1007/s10942-016-0234-2

Intergenerational Case Study: Panic, Launching Children, and an Adult Survivor of Sexual Abuse

Wei-Wei is seeking therapy because she recently started having panic attacks. She lives with her husband, who is a surgeon, and reports that life has been going well: she was recently promoted to rank of full professor at a prestigious university, and her only son recently finished medical school. She reports no particular stress at the moment and is unsure why she is having these attacks. Her only prior history of mental disorders was anorexia as a teen as a way of coping with being sexually abused by an uncle while growing up in China.

After an initial consultation, an intergenerational family therapist developed the following case conceptualization.

BOWEN INTERGENERATIONAL FAMILY THERAPY CONCEPTUALIZATION

For use with individual, couple, or family clients.

Therapist: Mei Zhou   **Client/Case #:** 1121   **Date:** 2/3/18

Introduction to Client & Significant Others

Identify significant persons in client's relational/family life who will be mentioned in case conceptualization:

Adults/Parents: Select identifier/abbreviation for use in rest of case conceptualization

AF1: 53 (IP), Professor of Dance; Immigrated from China to seek graduate education

AM1: 55, Surgeon; Immigrated from China to seek education; met Wei-wei in school

Children/Adult Children: Select identifier/abbreviation for use in rest of case conceptualization

CM1: 26, Recently graduated from medical school; starting residency in Oregon; girlfriend moved with him.

Presenting Concerns

Describe each significant person's description of the problem:

AF53: Reports not knowing why she is having panic attacks; reports that life is otherwise "fine."

AM55: Believes that panic is related to AF53's perfectionism and loss of CM26 at home.

CM26: Describes AF53 as "high-strung" and always wanting things to be perfect.

Broader System: Description of problem from extended family, referring party, school, legal system, etc.:

Extended Family: The couple has not involved their families in their current issues.

AF's friend: Believes AF53 is having a mid-life crisis with CM26 leaving home and having finally reached her last major professional goal: tenure.

Background Information

Trauma/Abuse History (recent and past): AF53 reports being sexually abused by her uncle as a child growing up in Beijing, China. Her parents were active in the communist party and were very concerned about how they were viewed in the community; when she told them about the abuse, they did not believe her. The abuse continued until she was old enough to fight him off at around 16.

Substance Use/Abuse (current and past; self, family of origin, significant others): None reported.

Precipitating Events (recent life changes, first symptoms, stressors, etc.): After a period of positive life transitions—she was promoted at a prestigious university last year and her son finished his residency six months prior—AF53 had her first panic attack 4 months ago while at the opera with her husband. She reports feeling suddenly overwhelmed and had to leave in the middle of the performance. Since then she has had an attack every 2-4 weeks with no identifiable trigger.

Related Historical Background (earlier incidents, family history, related issues, prior treatment, etc.): When she was an adolescent, she reports eating very little to gain a sense of control over her life. She made it a goal to get a visa to study in the United States, which she did at 22. Lee is also an immigrant from China, coming to the nited States to study. The couple met in college through the Chinese student association. The couple sees their extended families every 4–5 years, AF53 rarely communicating with hers any longer.

Family Projection Process

Describe evidence of parental projection onto their child(ren), such as emotionally reactive behavior between family members; describe how it relates to symptoms, etc.: AF has projected her perfectionist anxiety onto her son; she has typically reacted harshly to his poor performance in any area of life. She also takes extreme pride in his accomplishments.

Patterns of Differentiation and Fusion

Describe how the couple/family promotes togetherness and separateness; provide examples: AF and AM have always shared similar life goals and a similar work ethic. The family has typically been close and supportive of one another, to the point that most members are involved with even minor decisions others make. They have their most separateness in their professional lives, with CM having autonomy in this area as long as he performs well.

Describe each person's relative level of differentiation and ability to effectively manage conflict without reactivity; provide examples: AF is probably the least differentiated in the family, being the most reactive to both AM and CM. CM is likewise very reactive to AF, and still prefers to have her take on tasks such as his laundry, clothes shopping, and doctors appoints than do it himself. AM is the most differentiated, but still can be reactive to AF if they disagree on a subject.

Describe patterns of fusion, in current and past generations; provide examples: AF's family of origin was very fused, with her parents expecting to take on their values and to bear sexual abuse for the sake of the family's reputation. AF continues with this pattern with her son. AM's parents fought constantly, and he has vowed not to do this, but he has also not learned how to resolve conflict well with AF. He generally tries to avoid or deny conflict, but at times he explodes, similar to his father. CM seems to be adopting a similar pattern to AM's role in system.

Emotional Triangles and Cutoff

☒ Triangles within current partnership: Describe: AF and AM have triangulated CM, who has been the glue of their relationship

☐ Triangles with family of origin: Describe: _____

☐ Other triangles: _____

☒ Emotional cut-offs in extended family: Describe all: AF has cut off from her mother in China because of her handling of the child abuse and her mother's otherwise cold distant personality.

(continued)

Sibling Position

Describe sibling position patterns that seem to be relevant for the family, current, and earlier generations: All members of the family are only children, and fit the pattern of being responsible and seeking roles of authority.

Multigenerational Transmission Process

Describe multigenerational transmission of functioning, attending to acculturation issues, residual effects of trauma and loss, significant legacies, use of alcohol and drugs, etc.: This family has experienced significant trauma and loss. AF's family were part of the cultural revolution in China, a period of intense fear in which families turned against each other and it was difficult to know who to trust. Within this context, AF also experienced sexual abuse and no one felt safe enough to risk creating more trauma. The pattern was to just shut down emotions and deny that anything is wrong. AF has continued this pattern, and this may be related to her panic attacks that appear to have no trigger. Both AM and AF immigrated without significant financial support from their families and had to make it on their own, learning the language and the culture. Their coping strategy was to work hard and just keep moving. AM's father died while he was in the States, and he never got to say goodbye to him. He has guilt about this, but has never shared it with anyone.

Multigenerational Patterns Informed by Diversity Factors

Describe how multigenerational patterns are informed by relevant diversity factors, including those related to cultural, ethnicity, racial, immigration, acculturation, gender, religious, socio-economic, ability, and sex/gender identity: Both AM and AF are from middle-class families in China, with AF's father having a higher social status due to his political involvement. AF embraces her feminine side in her area of study, dance; but otherwise, she has adopted a more formal and distant relational style, similar to her mother. AM has tried to not be like his father, who was often hot-headed, and instead tries to remain cool and calm. Both AM and AF have embraced traditional Chinese values, such as putting the children's needs first, avoiding public shame for the family, and pushing children to excel. As immigrants, they had to work hard to survive and did so by achieving financial and professional success.

Intergenerational Patterns from Genogram

Construct a family genogram and include all relevant information including:
- Names, ages, and birth/death dates
- Relational patterns
- Occupations
- Psychiatric disorders and alcohol/substance abuse
- Abuse history
- Personality adjectives

Genogram should be attached to report. Summarize key findings below:

Substance/Alcohol Abuse: ☒ NA ☐ History: _____

Sexual/Physical/Emotional Abuse: ☐ NA ☒ History: AF sexually abused by mother's brother;

                                                                                                                    abuse was ignored by family

Physical/Mental Disorders: ☒ NA ☐ History: _____

History Related to Presenting Problem: ☒ NA ☐ History: AF had eating disorder in childhood

Describe family strengths, such as the capacity to self-regulate and to effectively manage stress: The
entire family self-regulates—or at least is stoic—in public and professional settings. The family has
overcome many challenges and issues of self-regulation primarily limited to their private lives.

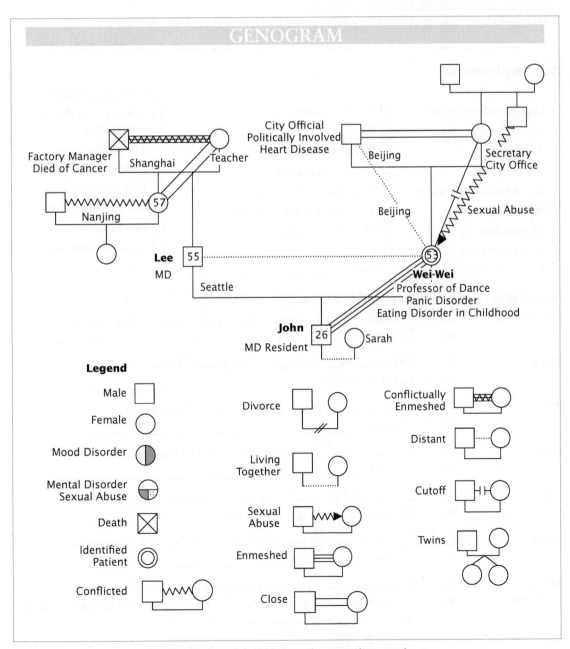

GENOGRAM

CLINICAL ASSESSMENT

Clinician: Me Zhou	Client ID #: 1121	Primary configuration: ☐ Individual ☒ Couple ☐ Family	Primary Language: ☐ English ☐ Spanish ☒ Other: Mandarin

List client and significant others

Adult(s)

Adult Female   Age: 53   Asian American   Married heterosexual   Occupation: Professor of dance   Other identifier: Immigrated from Beijing to pursue education.

Adult Male   Age: 55   Asian Amereican   Married heterosexual   Occupation: Surgeon   Other identifier:

Immigrated from Shanghai to pursue education.

Child(ren)

Child Male   Age: 26   Asian Amereican Grade: Select Grade School: Medical School   Other identifier: Currently in MD residency; lives with girlfriend.

Select Gender   Age:___   Select Ethnicity Grade: Select Grade School:___   Other identifier:_____

Others: _____

Presenting Problem(s)

☐ Depression/hopelessness
☒ Anxiety/worry
☐ Anger issues
☒ Loss/grief
☐ Suicidal thoughts/attempts
☒ Sexual abuse/rape
☐ Alcohol/drug use
☐ Eating problems/disorders
☐ Job problems/unemployed

☐ Couple concerns
☐ Parent/child conflict
☐ Partner violence/abuse
☐ Divorce adjustment
☐ Remarriage adjustment
☐ Sexuality/intimacy concerns
☒ Major life changes
☐ Legal issues/probation
☐ Other: _____

Complete for children:
☐ School failure/decline performance
☐ Truancy/runaway
☐ Fighting w/peers
☐ Hyperactivity
☐ Wetting/soiling clothing
☐ Child abuse/neglect
☐ Isolation/withdrawal
☐ Other: _____

Mental Status Assessment for Identified Patient

Interpersonal	☐ NA	☐ Conflict ☒ Enmeshment ☐ Isolation/avoidance ☐ Harassment ☐ Other: Disengagement
Mood	☐ NA	☐ Depressed/Sad ☒ Anxious ☐ Dysphoric ☐ Angry ☐ Irritable ☐ Manic ☐ Other:
Affect	☐ NA	☒ Constricted ☐ Blunt ☐ Flat ☐ Labile ☐ Incongruent ☐ Other:
Sleep	☐ NA	☐ Hypersomnia ☐ Insomnia ☒ Disrupted ☐ Nightmares ☐ Other:
Eating	☐ NA	☐ Increase ☐ Decrease ☐ Anorectic restriction ☐ Binging ☐ Purging ☒ Other: Hx of anorexia in adolescence
Anxiety	☐ NA	☐ Chronic worry ☒ Panic ☐ Phobias ☐ Obsessions ☐ Compulsions ☐ Other:
Trauma Symptoms	☐ NA	☐ Hypervigilance ☐ Flashbacks/Intrusive memories ☐ Dissociation ☒ Numbing ☐ Avoidance efforts ☒ Other: Untreated childhood sexual ab use

Psychotic Symptoms	☒ NA	☐ Hallucinations ☐ Delusions ☐ Paranoia ☐ Loose associations ☐ Other: _____
Motor Activity/ Speech	☐ NA	☒ Low energy ☐ Hyperactive ☐ Agitated ☐ Inattentive ☐ Impulsive ☐ Pressured speech ☐ Slow speech ☐ Other: _____
Thought	☐ NA	☐ Poor concentration ☐ Denial ☐ Self-blame ☐ Other-blame ☐ Ruminative ☐ Tangential ☐ Concrete ☒ Poor insight ☐ Impaired decision making ☐ Disoriented ☐ Other: _____
Sociolegal	☒ NA	☐ Disregards rules ☐ Defiant ☐ Stealing ☐ Lying ☐ Tantrums ☐ Arrest/incarceration ☐ Initiates fights ☐ Other: _____
Other Symptoms	☒ NA	_____

Diagnosis for Identified Patient

Contextual Factors considered in making diagnosis: ☒ Age ☒ Gender ☒ Race/Ethnicity ☒ Language ☒ Religion ☒ Social class ☒ Immigration ☐ Sexual/gender orientation ☐ Cognitive ability ☐ Other: _____

Describe impact of identified factors on diagnosis and assessment process: <u>Services provided in Mandarin Chinese; Chinese norms for emotional expression and interpersonal connection considered when assessing family; untreated childhood trauma considered in assessing current symptoms</u>

DSM-5 Level 1 Cross-Cutting Symptom Measure (optional): Elevated scores on: (free at psychiatry.org)
☐ I Depression ☐ II Anger ☐ III Mania ☒ IV Anxiety ☒ V Somatic ☐ VI Suicide ☐ VII Psychosis
☒ VIII Sleep ☐ IX Memory ☐ X Repetitive ☒ XI Dissociation ☐ XII Personality ☐ XIII Substance
☐ Not administered

DSM-5 Code	Diagnosis with Specifier *Include Z/T-Codes for Psychosocial Stressors/Issues*
1. <u>F41.0</u> 2. <u>Z69.810</u> 3. <u>Z60.0</u> 4. _____ 5. _____	1. <u>Panic Disorder</u> 2. <u>Personal past history of sexual abuse in childhood; R/O PTSD</u> 3. <u>Phase of life issue</u> 4. _____ 5. _____

List Specific DSM-5 Criterion Met for Diagnosis

1. <u>Panic attacks: palpitations, sweating, trembling, shortness of breath, feeling of choking, chest pain, dizziness, fear of losing control</u>

2. <u>Worry about implications of attacks; fear of another attack</u>

3. _____

4. _____

5. _____

Medical Considerations

Has patient been referred for psychiatric evaluation? ☒ Yes ☐ No

Has patient agreed with referral? ☒ Yes ☐ No ☐ NA

Psychometric instruments used for assessment: ☐ None ☒ Cross-cutting symptom inventories
☐ Other: _____

Client response to diagnosis: ☒ Agree ☐ Somewhat agree ☐ Disagree ☐ Not informed for following reason: _____

(continued)

Diagnosis for Identified Patient (*continued*)

Current Medications (psychiatric & medical) ☐ **NA**
1. <u>Xanax</u>; dose <u>0.5</u> mg;   start date: <u>2/15</u>
2. _____; dose _____ mg; start date: _____
3. _____; dose _____ mg; start date: _____
4. _____; dose _____ mg; start date: _____

Medical Necessity: *Check all that apply*
☒ Significant impairment ☐ Probability of significant impairment ☐ Probable developmental arrest
Areas of impairment:
☒ Daily activities ☒ Social relationships ☒ Health ☒ Work/School ☐ Living arrangement ☐ Other: _____

Risk and Safety Assessment for Identified Patient

Suicidality	**Homicidality**	**Alcohol Abuse**
☒ No indication/denies	☒ No indication/denies	☒ No indication/denies
☐ Active ideation	☐ Active ideation	☐ Past abuse
☐ Passive ideation	☐ Passive ideation	☐ Current; Freq/Amt: _____
☐ Intent without plan	☐ Intent without means	**Drug Use/Abuse**
☐ Intent with means	☐ Intent with means	☒ No indication/denies
☐ Ideation in past year	☐ Ideation in past year	☐ Past use
☐ Attempt in past year	☐ Violence past year	☐ Current drugs: _____
☐ Family or peer history of completed suicide	☐ History of assaulting others	Freq/Amt: _____
	☐ Cruelty to animals	☐ Family/sig.other use

Sexual & Physical Abuse and Other Risk Factors

☒ Childhood abuse history: ☒ Sexual ☐ Physical ☐ Emotional ☐ Neglect
☐ Adult with abuse/assault in adulthood: ☐ Sexual ☐ Physical ☐ Current
☐ History of perpetrating abuse: ☐ Sexual ☐ Physical ☐ Emotional
☐ Elder/dependent adult abuse/neglect
☒ History of or current issues with restrictive eating, binging, and/or purging
☐ Cutting or other self-harm: ☐ Current ☐ Past: Method: _____
☐ Criminal/legal history: _____
☐ Other trauma history: _____
☐ None reported

Indicators of Safety

☐ NA
☒ At least one outside support person
☒ Able to cite specific reasons to live or not harm
☐ Hopeful
☐ Willing to dispose of dangerous items
☐ Has future goals
☐ Willingness to reduce contact with people who make situation worse
☒ Willing to implement safety plan, safety interventions
☐ Developing set of alternatives to self/other harm
☐ Sustained period of safety: _____
☐ Other: _____

Elements of Safety Plan

☐ NA
☐ Verbal no harm contract
☐ Written no harm contract
☒ Emergency contact card
☒ Emergency therapist/agency number
☒ Medication management
☐ Plan for contacting friends/support persons during crisis
☒ Specific plan of where to go during crisis
☒ Specific self-calming tasks to reduce risk before reach crisis level (e.g., journaling, exercising, etc.)
☐ Specific daily/weekly activities to reduce stressors
☐ Other: _____

Legal/Ethical Action Taken: ☐ NA ☐ Action: <u>Consulted with lawyer about abuse reporting in foreign country; adivsed that since in past and no potential identified victions, no action needs to be taken.</u>

Case Management

Collateral Contacts

- Has contact been made with treating *physicians or other professionals*: ☐ NA ☒ Yes ☐ In process. Name/ Notes: <u>MD prescribed medication; ruled out other medical causes, including hormonal changes due to</u> <u>menopause.</u>
- If client is involved in mental health *treatment elsewhere*, has contact been made? ☒ NA ☐ Yes ☐ In process. Name/Notes: _____
- Has contact been made with *social worker*: ☒ NA ☐ Yes ☐ In process. Name/Notes: _____

Referrals

- Has client been referred for *medical assessment*: ☒ Yes ☐ No evidence for need
- Has client been referred for *social services*: ☒ NA ☐ Job/training ☐ Welfare/Food/Housing ☐ Victim services ☐ Legal aid ☐ Medical ☐ Other: _____
- Has client been referred for *group* or other support services: ☐ Yes: _____ ☒ In process ☐ None recommended
- Are there anticipated *forensic/legal processes* related to treatment: ☒ No ☐ Yes; describe: _____

Support Network

- Client social support network includes: ☐ Supportive family ☒ Supportive partner ☐ Friends ☐ Religious/spiritual organization ☒ Supportive work/social group ☐ Other: _____
- Describe anticipated effects treatment will have on others in support system (Children, partner, etc.): <u>Husband will attend sessions to help couple transition effectively to empty nest.</u>
- Is there anything else client will need to be successful? <u>Expand social network.</u>

Expected Outcome and Prognosis
☒ Return to normal functioning ☐ Anticipate less-than-normal functioning ☐ Prevent deterioration

Client Sense of Hope: <u>5 Moderate hope</u>

Evaluation of Assessment/Client Perspective
How were assessment methods adapted to client needs, including age, culture, and other diversity issues?

<u>Services provided in Mandarin; use of family life cycle to contextualize panic; honor Chinese value of</u>
<u>saving face by avoiding blame and using medical explanations where possible; also refer for possible</u>
<u>hormone issues related to menopause.</u>

Describe actual or potential areas of client–clinician agreement/disagreement related to the above assessment: <u>Client is largely in agreement, but not sure if childhood issues could be relevant.</u>

_____, _____   _____
Clinician Signature   License/Intern Status   Date

_____, _____   _____
Supervisor Signature   License   Date

TREATMENT PLAN

Clinician Name: Mei Zhou   **Date:** 2/3/18

Case/Client: #1121   **Theory:** Bowen Intergenerational Therapy

Modalities planned: Individual Adult Individual Child ☒ Couple ☒ Family Group:

Recommended session frequency: ☒ Weekly Every two weeks Other:

Expected length of treatment: 6 months

Treatment Plan with Goals, Measures, and Interventions

Early-Phase Client Goal

1. Decrease daily stress and *chronic anxiety* to reduce potential for panic attacks.

   Measure: Able to sustain low stress levels for period of 2 ☐ wk ☒ mo with no more than 2 mild episodes of panic.
   a. Identify most obvious sources of stress and identify ways to increase AF53's responsibility for her own thoughts and feelings, thereby increasing her level of *differentiation.*
   b. Develop plan with AF53 and AM55 for how to identify panic warning signs and how best to manage, encouraging them to increase their *emotional connection* while maintaining *clear boundaries.*

Working-Phase Client Goals

1. Increase AF53's awareness of impact of launching CM26 to reduce *enmeshment* with CM26 and the related *anxiety.*

   Measure: Able to sustain greater acceptance of change for period of 2 ☐ wk ☒ mo with no more than __ mild episodes of diffuse boundaries and relational anxiety.
   a. *Process questions* to help AF53 identify impact of CM26 leaving home; compare with her leaving her parents and never returning.
   b. Encourage *relational experiments* to reduce enmeshment and take action on insight.

2. Increase couple's *emotional intimacy* and connection to reduce disengagement and anxiety.

   Measure: Able to sustain emotional connection for period of 2 ☐ wk ☒ mo with no more than two mild episodes of disengagement.
   a. Detriangulate CM26 and work from marital relationship by increasing conversations about each other's emotional and personal lives.
   b. Process questions to help couple identify how their lack of conflict is symptomatic of disconnection and how immigration and abuse history have contributed to fear of intimacy.

Closing-Phase Client Goals

1. Increase AF53's ability to maintain *emotional center in anxious moments* to reduce anxiety and panic.

   Measure: Able to sustain increased *differentiation* for period of 3 ☐ wk ☒ mo with no more than mild episodes of anxiety (no panic attacks).
   a. *Process questions* to help AF53 identify her emotional responses and how to effectively manage so that panic attacks are not triggered.
   b. Promote *differentiation* by helping AF53 and AM55 envision a hopeful future after launching CM26 and rediscovering each other as marital partners.

2. Increase each person's ability to *balance need for togetherness and autonomy* in family relationships to increase intimacy.
   a. *Process questions* to explore how togetherness and autonomy can both be honored within the relationship; discuss needs of each person and how they may differ and be accommodated.
   b. *Relational experiments* to practice relating to others from a differentiated position.

Treatment Tasks

1. Develop working therapeutic relationship.
   a. Use *nonanxious presence*, respecting culture and education level.

2. Assess individual, systemic, and broader cultural dynamics.
   a. Use *3-to-4 generation genogram* to identify *multigenerational patterns, chronic anxiety, triangles, emotional cut-off, family projection process, and sibling position.*
   b. Assess each family member's level of *differentiation* in current crisis/problem situation and in the past.

3. Identify needed referrals, crisis issues, collateral contacts, and other client needs. Note:
   c. *Referrals/Resources/Contacts:* Encourage AF53 to work with psychiatrist in managing medications and keeping open communication with psychiatrist about progress and side effects.

Diversity Considerations

Describe how treatment plan, goals, and interventions were adapted to address each area of diversity:

Age: *Include developmental tasks, cognitive ability, family life cycle, generational differences, etc.:*

A significant element of the treatment plan is to help the family, particularly AF, transition to empty-nest phase of family life cycle by helping AF develop identity that is less centered on CM and to help AF and AM strengthen their marital relationship. Also will address generational differences regarding acculturation.

Gender/Sexual Orientation: *Include specific gender role identity (e.g., working mother, traditional male, male–female transsexual, etc.), sexual orientation, ethnically based gender roles, etc.:*

As is common in Chinese families, AF's identity has been closely tied to CM's success and activities; as he transitions to greater independence and possibly marriage, AF will need to examine how to maintain her sense of identity as a mother without emotional fusion to CM. AM maintains traditional male identity, with minimal emphasis on emotional connection; this may need to softened as he and AF transition to empty nest.

Race/Ethnicity/Religion/Class/Region: *Include race, ethnicity (i.e., Italian American rather than White), immigration-status, religious beliefs, socio economic status, and geographic region:*

Interventions will be designed to be consistent with Chinese values of saving face and will include scientific and theoretical explanations where possible to attend to couples' level of education and backgrounds in research fields.

Other factors: *Identify any other significant diversity considerations, such as school, work, community, etc.:*

Will explore possible resources for expanding AF's social network in the Chinese American community or at the university.

(continued)

Evidence-Based Practice (Optional)

Summarize evidence for using this approach for this presenting concern and/or population: <u>Bowen approaches have been used frequently with immigrant Asian and Latino families to address differences in generational acculturation. In addition, the Bowenian construct of differentiation has been correlated with chronic anxiety, marital satisfaction, and psychological distress, all of which are significant issues for AF as she transitions to empty nest. Furthermore, differentiation is also correlated with affect regulation and the ability to negotiate interpersonal togetherness and separateness, which are directly related to AF's presenting issues of panic and life transition. Finally, a Chinese version of the Differentiation of Self Inventory has been validated for populations in China and can provide culturally appropriate assessment of differentiation.</u>

Client Perspective (Optional)

Has treatment plan been reviewed with client: ☒ Yes ☐ No; If no, explain: _____

Describe areas of Client Agreement and Concern: <u>AF is willing to explore potential of CM's launching as having an effect on her panic as it one of the only recent changes, although she is not 100% convinced it is the cause; couple willing to discuss how they will redefine relationship without CM at home.</u>

PROGRESS NOTE

Date: 3/10/16 **Time:** 2:00 ☐ am/ ☒ pm   **Session Length:** ☒ 45 min. ☐ 60 min. ☐ other: __ minutes

Present: ☒ Adult Male ☒ Adult Female ☐ Child Male ☐ Child Female ☐ Other: _____

Billing Code: ☐ 90791 (eval) ☒ 90834 (45 min. therapy) ☐ 90837 (60 min therapy) ☐ 90847 (family)

☐ Other: _____

Symptom(s)	Duration and Frequency Since Last Visit	Progress
1. Panic attack	None this week; second week in a row	**Progressing**
2. Worry/general stress	Mild-moderate 5 days	**Progressing**
3. Emotional connection	Couple had date night	**Progressing**

Explanatory Notes on Symptoms: AF reports no panic attack this week even during active weekend. Report she has been successful in eliminating several small daily stressors. Couple report had good date night without discussing CM

In-Session Interventions and Assigned Homework

Process questions to explore dynamics between AF and CM and AF and AM; triangulation process. Therapist used self and nonanxious presence to detriangulate from couple and to avoid overreacting to AF wanting therapist to side with her on issues related to CM. Design relational experiment for next call with CM this weekend.

Client Response/Feedback

Clients respond well to insight-oriented discussion about dynamics, although are more resistant to taking action on insights. Still some hesitancy from AF on reducing focus on CM both personally and within marriage.

Plan

☒ Continue with treatment plan: plan for next session: Follow-up on relational experiment. _____
☐ Modify plan: _____

Next session: Date: 3/17 Time: 2:00 ☐ am/ ☒ pm

Crisis Issues: ☒ No indication of crisis/client denies ☐ Crisis assessed/addressed: describe below

_____, _____   _____

Clinician's Signature   License/Intern Status   Date

(continued)

PROGRESS NOTE (*continued*)

Case Consultation/Supervision ☐ Not Applicable

Notes: Supervisor reviewed genogram; continued focus on helping AF clarify boundaries with

AM and CM

Collateral Contact ☐ Not Applicable

Name: Dr. Debi Brown Date of Contact: 3/9 Time: _____ : _____ ☐ am/ ☐ pm

☐ Written release on file: ☒ Sent/ ☐ Received ☐ In court docs ☐ Other: ____

Notes: Faxed clinical update to psychiatrist

_____ , _____ _____
Clinician's Signature   License/Intern Status   Date

_____ , _____ _____
Supervisor's Signature   License   Date

CHAPTER
8

Cognitive–Behavioral and Mindfulness-Based Couple and Family Therapies

Learning Objectives

After reading this chapter and a few hours of focused studying, you should be able to:

- **Theory:** Describe the following elements of cognitive–behavioral family therapy:
  - Process of therapy
  - Therapeutic relationship
  - Case conceptualization
  - Goal setting
  - Interventions

- **Case conceptualization and treatment plan:** Complete theory-specific case conceptualizations and treatment plans for cognitive–behavioral family therapy using templates that are provided.

- **Research:** Provide an overview of significant research findings for cognitive–behavioral family therapy and describe key elements of the following evidence-based treatments: integrative behavioral couples therapy and multifamily groups.

- **Diversity:** Analyze strengths, limitations, and appropriate applications for using cognitive–behavioral family therapy with clients in relation to their social location/diverse identities, including but not limited to ethnic, racial, and/or sexual/gender identity diversity.

- **Cross-theoretical comparison:** Compare the use of cognitive–behavioral family therapy interpersonal patterns (IPs) against the other approaches described in this book.

The key thread that binds these diverse perspectives [behavioral therapies] is a demand for continual empirical challenge. Every strategy, and every case, is subjected to empirical scrutiny that aims to define the specific therapeutic ingredients that facilitate the achievement of the specific benefits desired by the family. In other words, every family presents a new experiment with the potential to advance therapeutic frontiers.
—*Falloon (1991, p. 65)*

Lay of the Land

Behavioral and cognitive–behavioral couple and family therapies (in this book called cognitive–behavioral family therapy, or CBFT—to save trees) are a group of related therapies based on the behavioral and cognitive–behavioral approaches originally developed for working with individuals. The most influential of these therapies are the following:

- Behavioral couple and family therapies: Separate behavioral models for couple therapy (Jacobson & Christensen, 1996) and family therapy (Patterson & Forgatch, 1987) have been developed and continue to be researched and refined.
- Cognitive–behavioral couple and family therapy: This therapy was developed by several therapists to integrate cognitive elements into therapy with couples and families (Dattilio, 2005; Epstein & Baucom, 2002).
- Integrative behavioral couples therapy (IBCT): An enhanced version of *behavioral couples therapy,* IBCT integrates the humanistic principle of *accepting* one's partner to improve long-term outcomes (Jacobson & Christensen, 1996).
- Gottman method couple therapy: This scientific approach to couple therapy is based on Gottman's 30 years of research on the key differences between happy and unhappy marriages (Gottman, 1999). Although Gottman's approach is not an empirically supported treatment, its treatment goals are supported by research data.
- Mindfulness-based therapies: The newest kids on the block, mindfulness-based therapies use either mindfulness mediation practice or principles based on this practice to help clients alter their relationship with—rather than fix—problem thoughts, emotions, and behaviors.
- Multicouple and multifamily groups therapies: Several evidence-based multicouple and multifamily groups therapies have been developed to address issues such as severe mental illness, intimate partner violence, relationship enhancement, and parenting.

Cognitive–Behavioral Family Therapies

In a Nutshell: The Least You Need to Know

In the field of general mental health, cognitive–behavioral therapies (CBTs) are some of the most commonly used therapeutic approaches. They have their roots in behaviorism—Pavlov's research on stimulus–response pairings with dogs and Skinner's research on rewards and punishments with cats—the premises of which are still widely used with phobias, anxiety, and parenting. Broadly speaking, CBT has been described as having three waves, each building upon and expanding the previous: (a) behavioral, (b) cognitive and social learning, and (c) contextual and experiential (Hayes, 2004). CBFTs have followed this same trajectory. Until the 1980s, most of the CBFTs were primarily behavioral: behavioral family therapy (Falloon, 1991) and behavioral couple therapy (Holtzworth-Munroe & Jacobson, 1991). Next, CBFT entered the second wave with approaches that more directly incorporate cognitive components: cognitive–behavioral family therapy (Epstein & Baucom, 2002; Dattilio, 2005) and Gottman method couple therapy approach (1999). Most recently, CBFTs are entering the "third wave," which includes integrative behavioral couples therapy and mindfulness-based couple and family therapy.

CBFTs integrate systemic concepts into standard cognitive–behavioral techniques by examining how family members—or any two people in a relationship—*reinforce* one another's behaviors to maintain symptoms and relational patterns. Therapists generally assume a directive, "teaching," or "coaching" relationship with clients, which is quite different from other approaches, which include "joining" or "empathizing" with clients to form a relationship. Because this approach is rooted in experimental psychology, research is central to its practice and evolution, resulting in a substantial evidence base.

The Juice: Significant Contributions to the Field

If you remember one thing from this chapter, it should be the following:

Parent Training

Arguably, CBFT's greatest influence has been in the area of parenting (Patterson & Forgatch, 1987). Most therapists who work with families with young children, regardless of their primary orientation, use classic behavioral concepts of reinforcement and consistency to help improve parental efficiency (Dattilio, 2005; Patterson & Forgatch, 1987). The basic behavioral principle of *reinforcement*—that the positive or negative responses from the environment shape future behavior—is hardwired into reptilian and mammalian nervous systems and, to a large extent, all living creatures. Therefore, if a dog is given a treat each time it sits on command, it learns the command by pairing compliance with the positive reinforcer, the treat. *Consistency*—reinforcing every time—is the key, especially in the beginning. Kids, employees, graduate students, and, to a lesser extent, spouses work essentially on the same principle.

Patterson and Forgatch (1987) developed one of the most prominent approaches to parent training. Their approach is based on the following key concepts and techniques:

- Teaching compliance and socialization: Therapists aim to teach children to comply with parental requests, with the broader goal of teaching children to function in society.
- Improving parental requests: Parental requests should be: (a) few in number, (b) polite, (c) statements rather than questions, (d) made only once before enforcing a consequence, (e) specific, and (f) well timed.
- Monitoring and tracking: Parents must monitor their children's behavior away from home by always asking four basic questions: Who? Where? What? When?
- Creating a contingent environment: Parents are encouraged to use *point charts* to develop positive contingencies (rewards) that encourage desired behavior in children.
- Five-minute work chore: Parents are taught to assign a lesser punishment, such as the five-minute work chore, with initial infractions before removing privileges or using harsher punishments.

Being consistent and reinforcing behaviors are not the only skills parents need to master, but they are essential and therefore used widely when child behavior is a presenting concern. In the case study at the end of this chapter, the therapist includes parent training to help treat attention-deficit/hyperactivity disorder (ADHD) in a seven-year-old boy.

Rumor Has It: The People and Their Stories

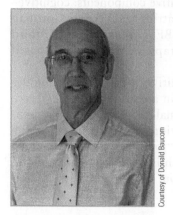

Donald Baucom

A professor at the University of North Carolina at Chapel Hill, Donald Baucom has researched the efficacy of cognitive–behavioral couples for over four decades, collaborating closely with Norman Epstein (Baucom et al., 2015; Epstein & Baucom, 2002; Epstein, Dattilio, & Baucom, 2016).

Frank Dattilio

Frank Dattilio (2005) developed *cognitive–behavioral family therapy,* adopting traditional cognitive therapy. Specifically, his work adapts Aaron Beck's (1976, 1988) concept of schemas—underlying core beliefs—for working with families.

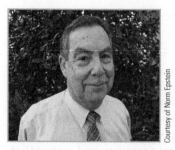

Norman Epstein

A professor at the University of Maryland, Norman Epstein has been a leader in developing cognitive–behavioral approaches for working with couples (Epstein, 1982; Epstein & Baucom, 2002) and families (Epstein, Schlesinger, & Dryden, 1988; Freeman, Epstein, & Simon, 1987). His most recent work, enhanced couple cognitive–behavioral therapy, expands the scope of CBFT to include stress-and-coping theory to expand the focus to include a broader ecological perspective (Epstein & Baucom, 2002).

John Gottman

For over 30 years, John Gottman (1999) has studied key factors in couples' communication, divorce, and marital satisfaction. On the basis of this research, he has developed a scientifically based couples therapy, originally called the marriage clinic approach, that reduces behaviors that predict divorce and increases those that predict long-term marital satisfaction. He has written several books for the general public, including *The Seven Principles for Making Marriages Work* (Gottman, 2002) and *And Baby Makes Three* (Gottman & Gottman, 2008).

Neil Jacobson and Andrew Christensen

In the early 1970s, Neil Jacobson developed behavioral couple therapy, which was later recognized as an empirically validated treatment (Jacobson & Addis, 1993; Jacobson & Christensen, 1996). Although effective in improving couple functioning in the short term, therapeutic gains were generally lost by the two-year follow-up. Therefore, Jacobson decided to add a more affective, humanistic focus that emphasizes *acceptance* of one's partner, calling this new model "integrative behavioral couples therapy." Christensen has carried on the development of this approach since Jacobson's death in 1999.

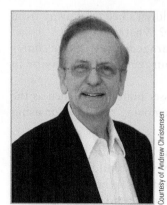

Gerald Patterson and Marion Forgatch

Researchers at the Oregon Social Learning Center, Patterson and Forgatch (1987) have developed one of the most influential behavioral parent training programs.

The Big Picture: Overview of Treatment

The therapy process for most CBFTs includes the following steps:

Step 1. Assessment: Obtain a detailed behavioral and/or cognitive assessment of *baseline functioning*, including the frequency, duration, and context of problem behaviors and thoughts. Many CBFT practitioners use formal self-report questionnaires, such as the Dyadic Adjustment Scale, as part of their assessment (Epstein & Baucom, 2002; see also Chapter 14).

Step 2. Target behaviors and thoughts for change: Cognitive–behavioral therapists identify *specific* behaviors and thoughts for intervention (e.g., rather than using the general goal of "improve communication," the therapist targets tantrum frequency, name calling, curfew noncompliance, and other problem behaviors).

Step 3. Educate: Therapists educate clients on their irrational thoughts and dysfunctional patterns.

Step 4. Replace and retrain: Interventions are designed to replace dysfunctional behaviors and thoughts with more productive ones.

Making a Connection: The Therapeutic Relationship

Directive Educator and Expert

Although the affective quality of connection exhibited by CBFT therapists varies greatly (i.e., from cool and detached to warm and friendly), the primary role of the therapist is the same: to serve as an expert who *directs* and *educates* the client and family on how to better manage their problems (Falloon, 1991). Following the classic medical model, traditional CBFT therapists maintained a distance from clients, much like medical doctors today, simply diagnosing and prescribing interventions without achieving much emotional connection. Influenced by recent research such as the common factors model, which indicates that the affective quality of the therapeutic relationship is a strong predictor of positive outcomes (see Chapter 2), many CBFT therapists are increasing their use of empathy and warmth to create a connection with their clients.

Empathy in Cognitive–Behavioral Therapy

True to their research foundations, cognitive–behavioral therapists increasingly use empathy, warmth, and a nonjudgmental stance to build a therapeutic alliance; this approach is based on research results that indicate these therapist qualities predict positive outcomes (Meichenbaum, 1997; see also, "Common Factors" in Chapter 2). However, *the reason a cognitive–behavioral therapist uses empathy is quite different from the reason a humanistic therapist uses empathy.* This is frequently misunderstood, so I am going to say it again in case your mind was wandering: *cognitive–behavioral therapists use empathy for entirely different reasons than humanistic therapists.* Cognitive–behavioral therapists use empathy to create *rapport,* which then allows them to get to the "real" interventions that will change a client's behaviors, thoughts, and emotions. In dramatic contrast, for experiential therapists, empathy *is* the intervention: they maintain that empathy is a curative process in and of itself (Rogers, 1961). Cognitive–behavioral therapists who use empathy should not be seen as "manipulative," because in most cases the idea is to make clients feel more comfortable with the process, not to trick them. They should also not be seen as "integrating" experiential concepts, because they are not using an experiential concept in the way experiential therapists would use it. Instead, they are *adapting* it to work within their philosophical assumptions about therapy and the change process.

Contemporary Cognitive–Behavioral Alliance

Judith Beck (2005) describes five practices for fostering the therapeutic alliance that reflect more contemporary sensibilities:

- *Actively collaborate with the patient:* Decisions about counseling should be jointly made with the client.
- *Demonstrate empathy, caring, and understanding:* Expressing empathy helps clients trust the therapist.
- *Adapt one's therapeutic style:* Interventions, self-disclosure, and directiveness should be adjusted for each client based on personality, presenting problem, etc.
- *Alleviate distress:* Demonstrating clinical effectiveness by helping clients solve problems and improving their moods enhances the therapeutic relationship.
- *Elicit feedback at the end of the session:* By asking clients, "How did it go?" at the end of each session, therapists can intervene early in cases of alliance rupture.

By building a collaborative and engaged alliance, therapists are more likely to be effective and work through possible dysfunctional beliefs the client may have about counseling or the therapist that interfere with the process, such as "My therapist doesn't understand me" or "This will never work."

Written Contracts

CBFT therapists are perhaps the most businesslike of all therapists in their relationship with clients (Holtzworth-Munroe & Jacobson, 1991), at least in their written descriptions—and more than other therapists, they put this relationship on paper. CBFT therapists frequently use *written contracts* that spell out goals and expectations to help structure the relationship and to increase clients' motivation and dedication. Putting goals and agreements in writing and having clients sign it to show that they agree can be a very motivating experience that creates commitment to the process.

The Viewing: Case Conceptualization and Assessment

Problem Definition

From a CBFT therapist's perspective, most families do not come in with usefully defined problems. When a CBFT therapist hears, "We don't communicate anymore" or "My son is defiant," the therapist still has not heard a problem description. Problem analysis is the process of taking these vague descriptions and developing them into a clear description of behavioral interactions and their emotional consequences.

Problem analysis focuses on *present-day* behaviors, emotions, and cognitions. When clients tell their story about relationship distress or personal disappointments, CBFT therapists listen for the: (a) behaviors, (b) emotions, and (c) thoughts that make the situation a problem. For example, if a client says that she is feeling depressed that her husband has left her, the therapist focuses on specific problematic *behaviors* (e.g., she no longer wants to see her friends), *feelings* (e.g., feeling worthless and hopeless), and *thoughts* (e.g., I will never find anyone again). These concrete, definable symptoms, not that she is divorced, are the "problem." The focus of treatment is on reducing these undesirable thoughts, feelings, and behaviors and increasing more desirable ones. For example, in the case study at the end of the chapter, the child is diagnosed with ADHD; however, the therapist does not rely on this generic description of the problem but instead works with the family to define clear, specific behaviors that can be targeted for change, such as "not able to do more than 15 minutes of homework," or "gets up out of seat during in-class reading periods."

Analysis of Interaction Patterns

Once therapists have a clearly defined problem, they conduct a functional analysis of the interaction patterns related to the presenting problem (Epstein & Baucom, 2002; Falloon,

1991). CBFT therapists often use a combination of client self-report and observation. Similar to other couple and family therapists, CBFT practitioners track the negative interaction patterns, but they focus closely, more so than other therapists, on how the couple or family *mutually reinforces* these behaviors. CBFT therapists always obtain a behavioral description of the problem interaction patterns, and they often also identify the problematic cognitions associated with the interaction. For example, the therapist might first ask a couple to describe their behaviors related to their nag/withdraw pattern: first she asks for him to help; he says no because of another commitment; she gets angry and calls him lazy and unreliable; he responds by saying she is unreasonable and then leaves the room. After getting a behavioral description, the therapist can go back and ask about attributions and beliefs that informed each party's behavior, such as "you don't care whether you don't help when asked" or "you treat me like a child." As part of this process, they gather information about the frequency, duration, severity, triggers, and consequences.

More recently, some CBFT therapists are also obtaining descriptions of how each person's stress response is activated during the problem interaction patterns (Dattilio, 2010). The stress, or fight–flight–freeze response is designed to enable humans to quickly react to life-and-death situations, such as a bear attack, by triggering very strong emotions of fear or anger and priming the body for physical defense. As part of this defense system, activity in the prefrontal cortex is reduced because its reliance on language and logical analysis makes it too slow for surviving physical threats. However, the same response is triggered with psychological threats. Thus, when couples and families argue, once their stress responses are triggered they are more likely to perceive the others as threats and their emotional reactivity reduces their capacity for language, reason, and problem-solving, which explains why heated arguments so rarely solve problems. By identifying where and how the stress response is triggered for each party during the interaction cycle, therapists can more precisely identify where and how to intervene, most often with a time-out.

Functional Analysis: Role of the Symptom

Originating in systemic theory, **functional analysis** identifies the precise contexts, antecedents, and consequences of the problem behavior (Falloon, 1991). However, family interactions are rarely as simple as the basic formula that works with laboratory rats: antecedent → behavior → consequence. Thus, Falloon (1991, p. 76) recommends the following questions to facilitate functional analysis in families:

FUNCTIONAL ANALYSIS QUESTIONS FOR FAMILIES

- How does this specific problem handicap this person (and/or the family) in everyday life?
- What would happen if the problem were reduced in frequency?
- What would this person (and his or her family) gain if the problem were resolved?
- Who (or what) reinforces the problem with attention, sympathy, and support?
- Under what circumstances is the specific problem reduced in intensity?
- Under what circumstances is the specific problem increased in intensity?
- What do family members currently do to cope with the problem?
- What are the assets and deficits of the family as a problem-solving unit?

When assessing couples, Holtzworth-Munroe and Jacobson (1991) recommend the following:

FUNCTIONAL ANALYSIS QUESTIONS FOR COUPLES

1. *Strengths and skills of the relationship*
   - What are the major strengths of the relationship?
   - What is each spouse's capacity to reinforce the other?
   - What behaviors are highly valued by the other?
   - What activities and interests do the couple currently share?
   - What relational competencies does each possess?

2. *Presenting problems*
   - What are the primary complaints (defined behaviorally)?
   - What behaviors occur too frequently? Under what circumstances and with what reinforcements do they occur?
   - What behaviors occur too infrequently? Under what circumstances and with what reinforcements do they occur?
   - How did these problems develop over time?
   - Is there consensus about what needs to change?

3. *Sex and affection*
   - Is either unsatisfied with the frequency or quality of their sex life? What behaviors are associated with the dissatisfaction?
   - Is either unsatisfied with the frequency or quality of nonsexual physical affection? What behaviors are associated with the dissatisfaction?
   - Is either in an extramarital affair? Is there a history of affairs?

4. *Future prospects*
   - Are both seeking to improve the relationship, or is one or are both contemplating separation?
   - Have steps been taken toward separation or divorce?

5. *Social environment*
   - What are the alternatives to this relationship, and how attractive are they?
   - Is their social network supportive of separation?
   - If there are children, what are the current effects, and what might be the effects of divorce?

6. *Individual functioning*
   - Does either have a significant mental or physical health disorder?
   - What is the relationship history of each, and how does it affect the present relationship?

Adapted from Holtzworth-Munroe & Jacobson, 1991, pp. 106–107.

When conducting a functional analysis, the therapist also looks for mutually reinforcing behaviors between parties and examines how these patterns are maintaining the symptom. This concept is similar to the systemic therapy concept of seeing the family's interactional patterns as interlocking steps in a dance. For example, if a parent inconsistently reinforces a child's problematic behavior (e.g., sometimes sets a consequence for talking back and sometimes does not), the behavior is likely to continue (e.g., because of an intermittent schedule of reinforcement); in the case study at the end of this chapter, the therapist is equally interested in assessing *how* the parents respond to their son's hyperactivity as she is in assessing the child's behaviors because the parents' responses reinforce—for better or worse—the son's behavior. Similarly, if a wife's depression results in less conflict in the marriage, this creates a positive reinforcement for the depression.

Try It Yourself

With a partner or on your own, conduct a functional analysis of a recent couple or family issue in your life or the life of a client. Does a direction for intervention become clearer?

Expectations and Standards

Epstein and colleagues (Baucom et al., 1989; Dattilo, 2010; Epstein, Chen, & Beyder-Kamjou, 2005) have identified five major types of cognition that influence how couples emotionally and behaviorally respond to one another.

- Selective perceptions: Focusing on certain events or information to the exclusion of others
- Attributions: Inferences about the causes of positive and negative aspects of the relationship
- Expectancies: Predictions about the likelihood of certain events in the relationship; these are often informed by one's family of origin as well as racial/ethnic background.
- Assumptions: Basic beliefs or assumptions about the characteristics of the partner and/or the relationship
- Standards: Beliefs about the characteristics that the relationship and each partner "should" have; these are often shaped by one's family of origin as well as gendered ethnic and racial standards of behavior.

Cognitive Distortions

The cognitive therapy of Aaron Beck (1976) focused on identifying and changing the **cognitive distortions** that were fueling the problems in an individual's life, such as the belief that one must be perfect or that life should be fair. Drawing on Beck's work, Dattilo (2005, 2010) has developed a system for assessing cognitive distortions related to relationships, of which we all have two sets: (a) beliefs about our family of origin, and (b) beliefs about couples and families in general:

1. Arbitrary inference: A belief based on little evidence (e.g., assuming your child is trying to hide something because he did not answer the cell phone immediately)
2. Selective abstraction: Focusing on one detail while ignoring the context and other obvious details (e.g., believing you've failed as a parent because your child is doing poorly in school)
3. Overgeneralization: Just like it sounds, generalizing one or two incidents to make a broad sweeping judgment about another's essential character (e.g., believing that because your son listens to acid rock he is not going to college and will end up on drugs)

4. Magnification and minimization: Going to either extreme of overemphasizing or underemphasizing based on the facts (e.g., ignoring two semesters of your child's poor grades is minimizing; hiring a tutor for one low test score is magnification)

5. Personalization: A particular form of arbitrary influence in which external events are attributed to oneself; especially common in intimate relationships (e.g., my spouse has lost interest in me because she did not want to have sex tonight)

6. Dichotomous thinking: All-or-nothing thinking: always/never, success/failure, or good/bad (e.g., if my husband isn't "madly in love" with me, he really doesn't love me at all)

7. Mislabeling: Assigning a personality trait to someone based on a handful of incidents, often ignoring exceptions (e.g., saying one's husband is lazy because he does not help immediately upon being asked)

8. Mind reading: A favorite in family and couple relationships: believing you know what the other is thinking or will do based on assumptions and generalizations; becomes a significant barrier to communication, especially when related to disagreements and hot topics such as sex, religion, money, and housework (e.g., before your spouse says a word, you are defending yourself).

Schemas

Beck (1976) identified **schemas** as the fundamental source of cognitive distortions and automatic thoughts. Schemas refer to long-held basic assumptions about how the world and relationships work and a person's place in it (Dattilio, 2010). When working with couples and families, CBFT therapists can identify three basic types of schemas:

- Schemas about self: These tend to address themes of worth, needs, should, roles, etc., such as "I am only a worthwhile person when I am in an intimate relationship."
- Schemas about others/relationships: These can be shared by family members or held solely by one person, and they typically define expectations, shoulds, valuing of others, roles, etc., such as "if someone loves you, they always put you first."
- Schemas about life: Life schemas address basic assumptions about life, good/bad, safety, etc., such as "Life should be easy."

Try It Yourself

With a partner or on your own, identify key schemas that have shaped your life.

Baseline Assessment with Child Behaviors

At the beginning of treatment with children, CBFT therapists conduct a **baseline assessment** of functioning, which provides a starting point for measuring change. They ask clients to log the: (a) frequency, (b) duration, and (c) severity of specific behavioral symptoms, such as tantrums, anger, social withdrawal, or conflict. Therapists may also identify antecedent events that may have triggered the symptoms. Patterson and Forgatch (1987) use monitoring and tracking charts to help parents obtain a baseline description of their child's behavior. Although clients' verbal recall of their symptoms may seem sufficient, usually a baseline assessment provides more detailed and accurate information than recall alone, especially when remembering a child's behavior. A baseline log may look like this:

SAMPLE BASELINE LOG

PROBLEM BEHAVIOR	WHEN?	HOW LONG?	HOW SEVERE?	EVENTS BEFORE?	EVENTS AFTER?
Tantrum when did not get candy at grocery store; cried, said, "I hate you" to mother; refused to follow instructions	Before lunch and after doing several other errands	5 minutes of crying; 1 hour pouting afterward	Moderate; stopped crying when left store	Very hot day; slept poorly night before; fight with brother earlier; mother did not give in to his first two requests	Another fight with brother in afternoon; mother yelled at him once got in car; refused to go to bed on time

Targeting Change: Goal Setting

Specific treatment goals are identified through the previously discussed assessment procedures. Goals are stated in behavioral and measurable terms, such as "reduce arguments to no more than one per month." When working with couples and families, therapists use their authoritative role to identify goals that are agreeable to all (Holtzworth-Munroe & Jacobson, 1991). Immediately after clear goals are agreed upon, therapists also obtain a commitment from the couple or family to follow instructions and complete out-of-therapy assignments, often with a written contract. Getting clients to promise to complete assignments greatly increases the likelihood that they will follow through.

Examples of Middle-Phase CBFT Goals

- Reduce CM tantrums by replacing positive and inconsistent reinforcements of tantrums with effective schedule of consistent consequences designed to extinguish the behaviors.
- Replace perfectionist beliefs about child school performance with more realistic expectations.
- Reduce generalizations and mind reading between mother and father in their parenting discussions.

Examples of Late-Phase CBFT Goals

- Develop positive mutual reinforcement cycle to reduce negativity and labeling.
- Redefine family schemas to increase tolerance of difference between members.
- Redefine couple schemas to reduce pressure for perfection and increase tolerance of weaknesses in other.

The Doing: Behavioral Interventions

Classical Conditioning: Pavlov's Dogs

Used primarily to treat anxiety disorders, **classical conditioning** was developed by Ivan Pavlov (1932) in his famous experiments with salivating dogs. Pavlov was able to train dogs to salivate at the sound of a bell by pairing the dog's natural response to salivate at the sight of food with a bell. When the bell was rung each time food was presented, the dog learned that the bell signaled that food was coming and began salivating. After enough repetition, the dog began to salivate with just the sound of the bell (as anyone who has owned more than one dog knows, the speed at which the dog learns this is highly breed-specific). This procedure is technically described as *conditioned and unconditioned stimuli and responses.*

How Classical Conditioning Works

1. **The Natural State of Affairs**

   Food (unconditioned stimulus; UCS) →
   Salivation (unconditioned response; UCR)

2. **Process of Pairing Conditional Stimulus with Response**

   Food (UCS) + *Bell* (conditioned stimulus; CS) →
   Salivation (conditioned response: CR)

3. **Resulting Pairing**

   Bell (conditioned stimulus; CS) →
   Salivation (conditioned response: CR)

Operant Conditioning and Reinforcement Techniques: Skinner's Cats

The bread and butter of parent training is *operant conditioning.* Interventions based on operant conditioning use the principles identified by B. F. Skinner (1953) to modify human behavior, whether one's own or another's. The essential principle is to reward behavior in the direction of the desired behavior using small, incremental steps, a process called *shaping behavior.* Once a certain set of skills has been mastered, the bar is raised for which behavior will be reinforced (positively and/or negatively), with ever-closer approximations to the desired behavior. Thus, if parents are trying to teach a child to complete homework independently, they may begin by overseeing when, where, and how the child completes homework and reinforcing success and failure under these conditions. Once the child regularly succeeds with full oversight, the child is given an area of responsibility to master—perhaps when the homework is done—and reinforced for success in this area. Next, the child may be rewarded for managing the list of homework assignments without oversight. This process continues until the child completes homework independently, much to the parents' delight. This type of reinforcement plan was used in the case study at the end of this chapter.

Forms of Reinforcement and Punishment

In operant conditioning, desired behaviors can be positively or negatively reinforced or punished, depending on the behavior. The following four options are used alone or in combination to shape desired behavior.

Four Options for Shaping Behavior

- **Positive reinforcement or reward:** Rewards desired behaviors by *adding* something desirable (e.g., a treat)
- **Negative reinforcement:** Rewards desired behaviors by *removing* something *un*desirable (e.g., relaxing curfew)

- **Positive punishment:** Reduces undesirable behavior by *adding* something *un*desirable (e.g., assigning extra chores)
- **Negative punishment:** Reduces undesirable behavior by *removing* something desirable (e.g., grounding)

SUMMARY OF OPERANT CONDITIONING

	INCREASE DESIRED BEHAVIOR	DECREASE UNDESIRABLE BEHAVIOR
Add Something	**Positive reinforcement;** reward	**Positive punishment**
Remove Something	**Negative reinforcement**	**Negative punishment**

Frequency of Reinforcement and Punishment

The frequency of reinforcement and punishment is key to increasing or decreasing behavior.

- Immediacy: The more immediate the reinforcement or punishment, the quicker the learning, especially with young children.
- Consistency: The more consistent the reinforcement or punishment, the quicker the learning. Consistency involves rewarding or punishing a behavior every time it occurs or on a consistent schedule (e.g., every other time) to create predictability.
- Intermittent reinforcement: Random and unpredictable reinforcement increases the likelihood of a behavior, but not always the behavior you want. Inconsistent reinforcement of desired behaviors often *increases undesired behaviors;* thus, if a parent inconsistently reinforces curfew, the child is more likely to break it. However, random positive reinforcement of well-established desired behaviors helps sustain them (e.g., randomly reinforcing positive grades with periodic privileges).

The principles of positive and negative reinforcement and reward are incorporated into the following interventions.

Encouragement and Compliments

Patterson and Forgatch (1987) strongly encourage *positive reinforcement* to increase desired behavior with children. When working with distressed relationships, they coach families to increase compliments and expressions of appreciation to increase positive reinforcement.

Contingency Contracting

Contingency contracting can be used to promote new behaviors by creating a contingency that must be met to receive a desired reward. Parents can use contingency contracting with children that detail how privileges will be earned and lost (Falloon, 1988, 1991; Patterson & Forgatch, 1987). For example, if a child's grade point average (GPA) is above 3.0, the parents agree to an 11:00 p.m. curfew on Friday and Saturday.

Point Charts and Token Economies

Generally used with younger children, point charts (Patterson & Forgatch, 1987) or **token economies** (Falloon, 1991) are used to shape and reward positive behaviors by allowing children to build up points that they can apply to privileges, treats, or purchases. Because the rewards must be motivating for each particular child, siblings may have different rewards. In addition, the rewards should be appropriate and readily approved by the parent. For example, if parents offer a reward that is too expensive or takes too much time from their schedule, they will have difficulty keeping up their half of the bargain. In most cases, punishment is added to a token economy by having the child lose points for poor behavior. In the case study at the end of this chapter, the therapist implements such a system to help a family whose son has been diagnosed with ADHD.

Behavior Exchange and Quid Pro Quo

When working with couples, mutual behavior exchanges—called **quid pro quo** ("this for that") arrangements—can be useful to help the partners negotiate relational rules (e.g., "If you make dinner, I will do the dishes"; Holtzworth-Munroe & Patterson, 1991). However, research indicates that couples who rely primarily on quid pro quo arrangements tend to have lower levels of marital satisfaction (Gottman, 1999). Does that mean that using this technique is harmful when working with couples? Although a well-designed research study would best answer this question, it is wise to use behavior exchange judiciously with couples, balancing it with more affective techniques to increase understanding and acceptance and to avoid framing marriage as a business deal. To this end, Holtzworth-Munroe and Jacobson (1991) recommend having each partner select a behavior to "give" rather than have each "ask" for what he/she wants.

Communication and Problem-Solving Training

To help couples and families solve their problems, CBFT therapists also provide training in communication using the following guidelines (Epstein & Baucom, 2002; Falloon, 1991; Holtzworth-Munroe & Jacobson, 1991):

- Begin with the positive: When introducing a problem, each is instructed to begin with a statement of appreciation or a compliment.
- Single subject: The communication training begins by identifying only one problem for the problem-solving session.
- Specific, behavioral problems: Problems are defined in specific behavioral terms rather than in global statements of feelings, characteristics, or attitudes (e.g., "he doesn't care" or "she's a nag").
- Describe impact: When describing a complaint, the partner is encouraged to share the emotional impact of the behavior.
- Take responsibility: Partners are encouraged to take responsibility for their half of the problem interaction.
- Paraphrase: After one person has spoken, the other summarizes what was heard so that misunderstandings can be immediately clarified.
- Avoid mind reading: Clients are to avoid making inferences about the other's motivations, attitudes, or feelings.
- Disallow verbal abuse: Insults, threats, and other forms of verbal abuse are not allowed; the therapist redirects the couple in appropriate directions.

Psychoeducation

A hallmark of CBFT therapy, **psychoeducation** involves teaching clients psychological and relational principles about their problems and how best to handle them (Falloon,

1988, 1991; Patterson & Forgatch, 1987). Psychoeducation can be done in individual or group sessions. The content typically falls into one of four categories:

- Problem-oriented: Information about the patient's diagnosis or situation, such as ADHD, divorced, alcohol dependence, or depression. Therapists use this type of education to motivate clients to take new action.
- Change-oriented: Information about how to reduce problem symptoms, such as by improving communication, reducing anger, or decreasing depression. Therapists use this type of education to help clients actively solve their problems. For such education to be successful, clients need to be highly motivated, and therapists need to introduce the new behavior in small, practical steps using everyday language.
- Bibliotherapy: *Bibliotherapy* is a fancy term for assigning clients readings that will be: (a) motivating and (b) instructional for dealing with their presenting problem. Typically, therapists assign a self-help or popular psychology book, but they may also assign fiction or professional literature.
- Cinema therapy: Similar to bibliotherapy, cinema therapy involves assigning clients to watch a movie that will speak to the problem issues (Berg-Cross, Jennings, & Baruch, 1990).

TIPS FOR EFFECTIVELY PROVIDING PSYCHOEDUCATION

- *Practice!* Yes, I'm serious. There aren't too many skills I recommend new therapists "practice" on family and friends, but psychoeducation is the major exception. Try explaining concepts and research outcome to people who haven't read books like this one. Notice the types of questions they ask after you explain a concept. That will help you learn what you might be leaving out, what type of jargon needs defining, and what people actually find useful.

- *Ask first.* Perhaps the single greatest secret to making psychoeducation work is *timing:* providing information when the client is in a receptive state. How do you know when they are ready? Ask them. "Would you be open to learning more about X?" If you fail to ask, you may not find a receptive audience.

- *Keep it very, very brief.* During a 50-minute session, I recommend keeping total psychoeducation time to 1 to 2 minutes—that's the max—and I am not exaggerating. Any other brilliant information you have to share should be saved for the following week, because most clients cannot meaningfully integrate and act upon more than a single principle at once.

- *Make one point—and one point only.* Teach only one concept, point, or skill in a session. Anything else is too much to be *practically* useful.

- *Ensure understanding and acceptance:* After briefly providing information, *directly ask* if clients understand and if they believe it is useful and realistic for their life.

- *Apply it immediately.* After you provide information, immediately identify how it can be practically applied in the clients' life to address a problem that occurred in the past week or upcoming week.

(continued)

> ## TIPS FOR EFFECTIVELY PROVIDING PSYCHOEDUCATION (*CONTINUED*)
>
> - *Give step-by-step tasks:* After offering 2 minutes of psychoeducation, the following 48 minutes involve step-by-step instructions on how to apply the information to solve a current problem. Get specific: who does, what, when and where? Also work with the client to identify potential roadblocks and resistance? potential roadblocks.
> - *Follow up on tasks:* The next time you meet, ask the client if they used the information to any extent; if not, why; and if so, what happened.

Homework Tasks

CBFT therapists often assign homework tasks that are designed to solve the clients' problem (Dattilio, 2005; Falloon, 1991; Holtzworth-Munroe & Jacobson, 1991). For example, to reduce a couple's conflict, therapists may assign communication tasks, such as using a timer to take turns listening to and summarizing what the other is saying. They may also develop tasks for reducing depression, such as journaling positive thoughts or increasing recreational and social activities. In CBFT, the tasks are logical solutions to reported problems.

Homework Compared with Strategic Directives

CBFT tasks are linear and literal. In contrast, strategic and other systemic therapists assign tasks designed to: (a) metaphorically make the covert overt (metaphorical task), (b) interrupt the problem interaction or behavioral pattern enough to allow the system to develop a new pattern (directive), or (c) make the uncontrollable controllable (paradox).

Homework Compared with Solution-Focused Tasks

In contrast to CBFT tasks, solution-focused tasks are designed to enact the *solution* rather than reduce the problem (see Chapter 9). In addition, solution-focused tasks are: (a) broken into small steps, (b) developed from clients' ideas and past successes, and (c) designed to increase motivation and hope as much as to solve the problem.

The Doing: Cognitive and Affective Interventions

Challenging Irrational Beliefs

Challenging irrational beliefs involves confronting unhelpful beliefs that are creating or sustaining the problem (Ellis, 1994). This can be done in session by the therapist or out of session with a thought record (see "Thought Records," below). A therapist challenges a client's irrational belief in two ways:

- Direct confrontation: The client is explicitly told that the belief is irrational.
- Indirect confrontation: The therapist uses a series of questions to help the client see how the belief or idea is irrational and/or contributing to the creation of the problem.

The decision to use a direct or indirect approach depends on the therapeutic relationship, the therapist's style, and the client's receptiveness to a particular approach; cultural and gender issues of the client and therapist also significantly affect this dynamic. The direct approach generally requires that the therapist use and the client accept a more hierarchical, expert stance, whereas the indirect approach typically is more appropriate when the therapeutic relationship is less hierarchical and the client has a greater need for autonomy.

Socratic Method and Guided Discovery

Using the **Socratic method**, sometimes referred to as **guided discovery** or inductive reasoning, to gently encourage clients to question their own beliefs, cognitive therapists use open-ended questions that help clients "discover" for themselves that their beliefs are either illogical (i.e., contrary to obvious evidence) or dysfunctional (i.e., not working for them; Beck, 2005). A less confrontational approach than other techniques, when questioning the validity of belief, therapists generally take a relatively neutral stance, allowing the client's own logic, evidence, and reason to do the majority of the convincing. Although the term *change* is used to describe what happens, in actuality, tightly held beliefs are slowly eroded over time by the client questioning and requestioning his or her validity in different situations.

QUESTIONS FOR EVALUATING THE VALIDITY OF BELIEFS

- What evidence do you have to support your belief? What evidence is there to the contrary? So, what might be a realistic middle ground?
- What does respected person X or Y or Z say about your situation? How could they all be wrong?
- If your child [or another significant person] were to say the same thing, how would you respond?
- What is the realistic likelihood that things will really go *that* badly? What is a more realistic outcome?
- You bring up one possible reason for X. Have you considered another explanation? Perhaps . . .?
- How likely is it that Person X's behavior was 100% directed at you? What else might have played a role in his/her behavior?

Thought Records

Originally developed by Albert Ellis (1962) to analyze irrational thinking with individuals, the A-B-C theory has also been applied to working with families (Ellis, 1978, 1994). In this model, A is the "activating event," B is the "belief" about the meaning of that event, and C is the emotional or behavioral "consequence" based on the belief.

ELLIS'S A-B-C THEORY

A = Activating event → **B** = Belief about A → **C** = Emotional and behavioral consequence

---

Most clients come in able to see only the connection between A and C, and thus report that A *causes* C: "I am depressed *because* my husband does not help out with the kids" or "I am *angry* because my son doesn't listen to me." The therapist's job is to help the client identify the B belief that the client does not put into the equation, such as "If he does not help with the children in the ways I want him to, he really does not care about me" or "Good kids follow through on parental requests without questioning the parent."

These irrational beliefs are identified in assessment and targeted for change in the intervention phase.

Using Ellis's A-B-C Theory, therapists often ask clients to confront their own irrational thinking and problem behaviors by assigning "thought records" (Dattilio, 2005). A type of structured journaling, thought records provide a means for clients to analyze their own cognitions and behaviors and develop more adaptive responses. Before assigning these as homework, therapists usually practice in session on a whiteboard to demonstrate the process. Thought records generally include the following information:

- Trigger situation (e.g., argument with spouse)
- "Automatic" or negative thoughts (e.g., "she will never change"; "he is so selfish")
- Emotional response: How automatic thoughts made person feel (e.g., hurt, rejected, betrayed)
- Evidence for: Evidence that supports the automatic or negative thoughts and interpretations (e.g., "he has done this before"; "she has not changed and does not seem to be trying")
- Evidence against: Evidence that counters the automatic thoughts (e.g., "she did seem genuinely sorry"; "he has been really trying in other areas")
- Cognitive distortions: Depending on the evidence, different types of cognitive distortions (e.g., arbitrary inference, selective abstraction, overgeneralization, magnification, minimization, personalization, dichotomous thinking, mislabeling, mind reading)
- Alternative thought: A more balanced perspective that incorporates both forms of "evidence" and corrects the cognitive distortion (e.g., "This is an area where we really seem to have differences; but we really do get along in so many other ways that are important to me; we are both trying to make this better")

SAMPLE THOUGHT RECORD

TRIGGER SITUATION	AUTOMATIC THOUGHT	EMOTIONAL RESPONSE	EVIDENCE FOR	EVIDENCE AGAINST	COGNITIVE DISTORTIONS	REALISTIC ALTERNATIVE
Argument over household chores	He'll never change; he's selfish and lazy	Hurt, anger, betrayal	Has done this before; not changing	Genuinely sorry; made progress in other areas; problem less frequent	Magnification; overgeneralization; selective abstraction	We have differences in this area; we are both trying to adjust to the other's need; he will probably never be exactly what I want in this area

With *relational issues* it is helpful to add the following:

- What did I do to contribute to this problem interaction? (e.g., I came on strong and blaming in the beginning; would not accept apology)
- What can I do differently next time? (e.g., be gentler when presenting my concern; listen with an open mind)

With *behavioral issues* the following can be added:

- Problem behaviors (e.g., yelling)
- Alternative behaviors (e.g., take time out, count to 10, take a deep breath)

Try It Yourself

Identify a recent stressful event and do a thought record to analyze the event and identify the cognitions that informed your response. What alternatives can you identify?

Scope It Out: Cross-Theoretical Comparison

Using Tomm's IPscope described in Chapter 3 (Tomm et al., 2014), this theory approaches the conceptualization of systemic, interpersonal patterns as follows:

Theoretical Conceptualization

CBFT therapists identify pathologizing interpersonal patterns (PIPs) by tracking both the behaviors and the cognitions in the PIP. They use functional analysis to carefully analyze the mutual reinforcement and purpose of the symptom in the system.

Goal Setting

Wellness interaction patterns (WIPs) are conceptualized as behaviors and cognitions that do not cause symptoms or relational distress. Although skill training related to communication, problem solving, and parenting are offered, the focus is symptom reduction and long-term maintenance of gains rather than mastering a specific set of skills (so, clients don't have become "perfect" at skills, they just need to learn enough to navigate life without distress).

Facilitating Change

CBFT therapists use two primary transformative interpersonal patterns (TIPs) to facilitate change: education and guided discovery. Psychoeducation is offered on a range of topics to help clients either view their situation differently or learn more effective actions. Therapists also use cognitive techniques such as guided discovery, Socratic dialogue, and thought records to help clients discover for themselves more effective ways of viewing their situation.

Putting It All Together: Case Conceptualization and Treatment Plan Templates

Areas for Theory-Specific Case Conceptualization: CBFT

When conceptualizing client *cases,* contemporary CBFT therapists typically use the following dynamics *to inform their treatment plan.* Go to MindTap® to access a digital version of the theory-specific case conceptualization, along with a variety of digital study tools and resources that complement this text and help you be more successful in your course and career. If your instructor didn't assign MindTap, you can find out more about it at Cengagebrain.com. You can also download the form at masteringcompetencies.com.

Analysis of the Problem Interaction Pattern

Identify the Problem Interaction Pattern

* Describe each person's observable behavior at the start of tension.
* Describe each person's observable behavior during conflict/symptom escalation.
* Describe each person's observable behavior at the return to "normal"/homeostasis.

Frequency and Duration

* Frequency of problem interaction pattern
* Duration of problem interaction pattern
* Severity of problem interaction pattern
* Triggers of problem interaction pattern
* Consequences/Reinforcements of problem interaction pattern:

Neurobiological Dynamics of Problem Interaction Pattern (Describe when and how the stress response is triggered for each person during the interaction.)

* Typical triggers of stress response for each person involved in PIP:
* Typical behaviors when stress response is triggered:
* What helps each to calm down once stress response is triggered:

Functional Analysis: Role of the Symptom

Identify mutually reinforcing behaviors that sustain symptom.

* How does this specific problem handicap this person (and/or the family) in everyday life?
* What would happen if the problem were reduced in frequency?
* What would this person (and his or her family) gain if the problem were resolved?
* Who (or what) reinforces the problem with attention, sympathy, and support?
* Under what circumstances is the specific problem reduced in intensity?
* Under what circumstances is the specific problem increased in intensity?
* What do family members currently do to cope with the problem?
* What are the assets and deficits of the family as a problem-solving unit?
* What behaviors need to increase? Decrease?

Patterns of Cognitive Distortions

Identify cognitive distortions in automatic thoughts and beliefs for client(s); provide examples:

* Arbitrary inference
* Selective abstraction
* Overgeneralization
* Magnification and minimization
* Personalization
* Dichotomous thinking
* Mislabeling
* Mind reading

Relational Cognition Patterns

Describe cognitive patterns that specifically relate to how client(s) see significant others:

* Selective perceptions
* Attributions

- Expectancies
- Assumptions
- Standards

Schemas

Describe schemas for client(s) underlying problem interaction pattern or other high affect situation; for more than one client, list schemas for each.

- Schemas about self (e.g., worth, needs, shoulds, roles, etc.):
  I am   .
- Schemas about others (e.g., expectations, shoulds, valuing of, role of, etc.):
  People are.
- Schemas about life (e.g., good/bad, optimistic vs. pessimistic, safe/unsafe, etc.):
  The world/life is.

TREATMENT PLAN FOR INDIVIDUAL WITH DEPRESSION/ ANXIETY: CBFT

The following treatment plan template can be used to help you develop individualized treatments for use with individuals with depressive or anxiety symptoms. You can download a blank treatment plan (with or without measures) from MindTap at www .cengagebrain.com or www.masteringcompetencies.com.

CBFT Treatment Plan: Client Goals with Interventions

Early-Phase Client Goals
1. Reduce *cognitive distortions* related to anxiety to reduce anxiety.
   a. *Psychoeducation* about the nature of anxiety and how to change it.
   b. *Thought records (homework)* for developing more realistic beliefs.

Working-Phase Client Goals
1. Reduce *cognitive distortions* related to depression to reduce depressed mood.
   a. *Psychoeducation* about the nature of depression and how to change it.
   b. Identify and *challenge cognitive distortions* underlying depression.
   c. *Thought records (homework)* to continue process of developing realistic schemas and beliefs.

2. Reduce use of *negative schemas* to interpret daily events to reduce depressed mood and anxiety.
   a. *Socratic dialogue* to allow client to discover the irrational beliefs that fuel depression and anxiety.
   b. Assign *homework tasks* that require action that is based on more realistic schemas about life and relationships.

3. Reduce *mutually reinforcing negative patterns* that trigger negative moods to reduce depression and anxiety.
   a. *Communication training* to improve client's half of negative interactions with others.
   b. *Change consistency and frequency of reinforcement* patterns for both desired and undesired relational interactions.

Closing-Phase Client Goals
1. Increase ability to make *realistic interpretations* of daily life and identify when thoughts are irrational to reduce depression and anxiety and increase sense of wellness.
   a. *Problem-solving training* to help client manage ongoing daily challenges.
   b. *Thought records* and *Socratic dialogue* with self to continue identifying and debunking unrealistic beliefs.

2. Increase ability to *relate to others using realistic relational schemas* to reduce depression and increase capacity for intimacy.
   a. *Thought records* to identify and counter unrealistic expectations of significant relationships.
   b. *Bibliotherapy* to develop more realistic expectations and beliefs

Treatment Tasks

1. Develop working therapeutic relationship.
   a. Develop an *empathic, supportive* working relationship with family in which therapist is able to effectively provide *education* from a position of *expertise*.

2. Assess individual, systemic, and broader cultural dynamics.
   a. Conduct *baseline assessment* of depressive and anxiety symptoms and *functional analysis* of the role of depression/anxiety in client's life/relationships.
   b. Identify *cognitive distortions, family schemas,* and *core beliefs* that are the source of depressive and anxious thinking.

3. Identify needed referrals, crisis issues, collateral contacts, and other client needs.
   a. *Crisis assessment intervention(s):* Address crisis issues such as self-harm, suicidal ideation, substance use, risky sexual behavior, etc.
   b. *Referral(s):* Connect client with *resources* in client's *community* that could be supportive; make collateral contacts as needed. Introduce possibility of *mindfulness-based cognitive therapy group* or similar group.

TREATMENT PLAN FOR COUPLES/FAMILIES IN CONFLICT: CBFT

You can download a blank treatment plan (with or without measures) from MindTap at www.cengagebrain.com or www.masteringcompetencies.com. The following treatment plan template can be used to help you develop individualized treatments for use with couples and families who report relational distress.

CBFT Treatment Plan: Client Goals with Interventions

Early-Phase Client Goals

1. Reduce *mutually reinforcing negative patterns* that trigger negative moods to reduce conflict.
   a. *Psychoeducation* about the nature of couple/family conflict and how to change it.
   b. Identify *quid pro quo* agreements for issues on which couple/family is willing to negotiate.
   c. Identify *unrealistic expectations* members have of each other.

Working-Phase Client Goals

1. Reduce *unrealistic expectations of partner/child/parents* and increase acceptance to reduce conflict.
   a. *Psychoeducation* about relationships and realistic expectations.
   b. Identify and *challenge cognitive distortions* underlying expectations of others and relationships in general.

2. Increase ability to *communicate* respectfully and effectively to reduce conflict.
   a. *Psychoeducation and communication training* to increase skills and knowledge.
   b. *Homework tasks* that help family to practice new communication skills.

3. Increase ability to effectively *problem-solve* to reduce conflict.
   a. *Problem-solving training* to help couple/family learn skills and strategies for effectively solving problems.
   b. *Homework tasks* to practice problem solving with initially minor and then increasingly difficult issues.

Closing-Phase Client Goals

1. Increase ability to *relate to partner/family members using realistic relational schemas* to reduce conflict and increase capacity for intimacy.
   a. *Thought records* to identify and counter unrealistic expectations of significant relationships.
   b. *Bibliotherapy* to develop more realistic expectations of relationships, such as John Gottman's *The Seven Principles for Making Marriage Work* (2002) or Dan Siegel's *The Whole-Brain Child* (2012).

2. Increase each member's ability to make *realistic interpretations* of daily life and identify when thoughts are irrational to reduce conflict and increase sense of wellness.
   a. *Problem-solving training* to help client manage ongoing daily challenges.
   b. *Thought records* and *Socratic dialogue* with self to continue identifying and debunking unrealistic beliefs.

Treatment Tasks

1. Develop working therapeutic relationship.
   a. Develop an *empathic, supportive* working relationship with all members of system in which therapist is able to effectively provide *education* from a position of *expertise*.

2. Assess individual, systemic, and broader cultural dynamics.
   a. *Analysis of interaction patterns* and *functional analysis* of the presenting complaints in significant relationships.
   b. Identify each person's and jointly held *cognitive distortions, family schemas,* and *core beliefs* that are the source of relational conflict.

3. Identify needed referrals, crisis issues, collateral contacts, and other client needs.
   a. Crisis interventions: potential for domestic violence, child abuse/neglect, etc.
   b. Referrals/resources/contacts: Introduce possibility of *mindfulness-based couple or parenting group* or similar CBT group.

Clinical Spotlight: Integrative Behavioral Couples Therapy

In a Nutshell: The Least You Need to Know

Part of the third wave of CBFTs, integrative behavioral couple therapy (IBCT) has evolved over the years, originally beginning as a primarily behavioral approach (Jacobson & Christensen 1996; Christensen, Dimidjian, & Martell, 2015). To improve long-term outcomes, Jacobson and Christensen (1996) integrated more affective aspects, particularly acceptance of one's partner, to the original behavioral model. In one study, couples in IBCT maintained their improved communication skills two years after termination of therapy better than did couples in traditional CBFT (Baucom et al., 2011). Today, along with emotionally focused couple therapy (see Chapter 6), IBCT is widely recognized as one of the major evidence-based treatments for couple therapy (Lebow et al., 2012). IBCT is based on an assumption that is fundamentally different from that of most couple therapies; namely, all couples experience areas of difference and disagreement (so, it's not just you). What distinguishes couples who become distressed is *how* they engage these differences. The primary focus of IBCT is to help couples *accept the differences* between them and learn not to take these differences personally; instead, couples learn to develop more effective relational patterns to accommodate these differences. Specifically, the focus is on changing one's self rather than one's partner (probably the one thing every person initially coming to couples therapy secretly hopes for: "please, fix my partner but don't ask me to change." I call it the first session prayer.).

The Big Picture: Overview of Treatment

Phases of Treatment

As an evidence-based treatment, IBCT has a recommended structure that can be tailored as needed to individual couples (Christensen et al. 2015). Similar to emotionally focused therapy (EFT), the course of treatment is brief, with a typical range of 15 to 26 sessions. Weekly sessions are recommended in order to provide continuity and focus. The sessions are typically organized as follows:

- Initial assessment: three sessions with both individual and couple sessions
- Feedback session: fourth session
- Intervention: Remaining sessions before termination
- Termination: One to two final sessions to summarize and review process

Overarching Goals

There are two fundamental goals in IBCT:

1. Increase each partner's ability to understand and accept his/her partner as an individual.
2. Enable the couple to work together to change their patterns and improve the quality of the relationship.

The Viewing: Case Conceptualization

Initial Assessment

The initial assessment is a comprehensive and structured process that involves both conjoint couple sessions and individual sessions. Typically, several self-report questionnaires are used, including the couples satisfaction index, marital status inventory, and revised conflict tactics scale (Christensen et al., 2015). Similar to EFT, the course of treatment is typically brief, with 26 sessions for moderately distressed couples (Christensen et al., 2015).

True to their behavioral roots, IBCT therapists conduct a functional assessment (see "Case Conceptualization" in the general CBFT section above) around areas of dissatisfaction, focusing on not only the problem behavior but the other partner's response to that behavior. In addition, the therapist takes a relationship history, which includes early attraction, dating, development of the problem, and the current situation. During the initial assessment, the therapist strives to answer these six guiding questions:

1. How distressed is this couple?
2. How committed is this couple to the relationship?
3. What issues divide the partners (the theme or themes of the couple)?
4. Why are these issues such a problem for them (the DEEP [see "Case Formulation: DEEP Analysis," below] analysis of those themes)?
5. What are the strengths holding them together?
6. What can treatment do to help them? (Christensen et al., 2015, p. 71)

Case Formulation: DEEP Analysis

Based on the initial assessment, therapists generate a case formulation, which is shared with the couple typically in the fourth session (Christensen et al., 2015). An effective case formulation helps each partner reduce blame and criticism of the other and increase willingness for change and acceptance. The case formulation has four basic parts, which are referred as DEEP analysis:

1. Differences and incompatibilities: the theme: Generally focused on a difference between the couple, the theme describes a basic-underlying focus of conflict and provides a link between seemingly disparate areas of struggle in the relationship. Common themes include:
   - Distance/closeness: Conflict over needs for closeness vs. separation
   - Control/responsibility: Conflict over power in one or more areas
   - Artist/scientist: Conflict over predictability vs. spontaneity
2. Emotional reaction, sensitivities, and vulnerabilities: In addition to identifying themes, therapists also identify potential sources for each partner's sensitivity or vulnerability in this area, such as an overbearing or detached parent. Identifying vulnerabilities invites an empathetic response from each partner and can also serve to reduce viewing differences as a personal attack.
3. External circumstances and stressors: The next area of focus is external circumstances and stressors that exacerbate the conflict around differences, such as work, social, child, scheduling, or extended family issues.
4. Patterns of communication and interactions: The final element of the case conceptualization is to identify the systemic interaction patterns that occur when conflict about the theme begins. Because most people want to eliminate problematic differences in their partner, many couples become polarized around the theme, which results in the unintended effect of strengthening and exaggerating the differences even more. The *polarization process* refers to how attempts to change one's partner tends make the differences more entrenched and irreconcilable. The effects of the polarization process is that both partners feel mutually trapped and stuck in the relationship.

The Doing: Interventions

IBCT involves three basic types of interventions: acceptance strategies, tolerance strategies, and change strategies (Christensen et al., 2015).

Acceptance Strategies

Two basic strategies are used to help couples foster acceptance: empathic joining and unified detachment. Therapists facilitate empathic joining between the couple by helping each to reformulate their expression of pain *without* blaming or accusing the other, which is often achieved by using the theme. Similarly, the therapist can help couples to express their feelings by framing them without "hard emotions," such as anger and resentment, and instead use "soft emotions," such as sadness or fear, or the "emotion behind the emotion" (similar to but not the same as primary and secondary emotions in emotionally focused therapy; see Chapter 6).

The other acceptance strategy, unified detachment, refers helping the partners develop enough emotional distance to allow for intellectual analysis of their conflicts, similar to mindfulness principles of "accepting what is" (see "Mindfulness-Based Therapies," above). Therapists help promote unified detachment by referring back to the theme in the case formulation. Similarly, therapists can ask the couple to analyze a recent argument and identify the specific elements of the interaction pattern, including how each responded to the other and escalated the conflict.

Tolerance Building

Similar to acceptance strategies, tolerance building requires that the partners let go of fruitless conflicts and attempts to change one another with regard to basic personality differences. Obviously, certain behaviors need to change, such as violence, substance abuse, affairs, or other destructive behaviors. Some ways therapists increase partners' tolerance of differences in their partner include:

- Pointing out positive aspects of the "negative" behavior (virtually any behavior is a strength in one context and a weakness in another; see Chapter 11)
- Practicing "negative" behavior in session to desensitize and reframe
- Faking negative behaviors at home when you do not naturally feel like doing it (similar to symptom prescription; see Chapter 4)
- Promoting tolerance through self-care

Change Techniques

Finally, IBCT therapists incorporate some traditional behavioral techniques to facilitate change when appropriate. Typically, IBCT therapists start with acceptance and tolerance interventions to build a greater sense of collaboration and willingness to change. Commonly used change techniques in IBCT include communication and problem-solving skills and behavior exchange or quid pro quo.

Web-Based Module: Our Relationship

An 8-hour web-based course based on IBCT, OurRelationship, has been developed to make couples therapy accessible to more couples (Doss et al., 2013). Designed to help couples work through a specific issue, the course is based on IBCT principles that help couples develop emotional acceptance of their partner differences; this is then translated to behavioral change. The curriculum is divided into three parts: observe, understand, and respond. The partners work separately through each part to develop material for a joint conversation at the end of each of the three segments. In one randomized control study with 300 couples using the OurRelationship program, couples reported significant improvement in relationship satisfaction, relationship confidence, and negative relationship quality as well as improvements in individual functioning, including depressive symptoms, anxiety, perceived health, work functioning, and quality of life (Doss et al., 2016).

Clinical Spotlight: Gottman Method Couples Therapy Approach
In a Nutshell: The Least You Need to Know

Gottman (1999) developed his scientifically based marital therapy from observational and longitudinal research on communication differences between couples who stayed together and ones who divorced. In the therapy based on these findings, the therapist coaches couples to develop the interaction patterns that distinguish successful marriages from marriages that end in breakup. Gottman's model is one of the few therapy approaches that are grounded entirely in research results rather than theory. However, a "scientifically based" therapy differs from an empirically supported treatment (see Chapter 2) in that the former uses research to set therapeutic goals, whereas the latter requires research on treatment outcomes. He revised his original theory, the sound marital house (Gottman, 1999) to include the element of trust (Gottman, 2011).

Debunking Marital Myths
Myth 1: Communication Training Helps

Gottman's (1999) research debunks several myths, including the myth that improving communication helps couples stay together. His research indicates that better communication produces short-term gains but that training couples to talk using "I" statements and "nonblaming" statements does not significantly affect whether or not they stay together. Instead, he found that both happily and unhappily married couples engage in defensiveness, criticism, and stonewalling (three of the Four Horsemen; contempt, the fourth, is seen mostly in marriages heading for divorce; see "The Four Horsemen of the Apocalypse," below). However, those who stay together maintain a ratio of 5:1 positive-to-negative interactions during conflict (20:1 during nonconflict conversations). Thus, simply improving communication is not as important as increasing the ratio of positive-to-negative interactions during conflict.

Myth 2: Anger Is a Dangerous Emotion

Contrary to what many therapists and the public may assume, Gottman (1999) found that expressing anger did not predict divorce; however, contempt (feeling superior to one's partner) and defensiveness do. Furthermore, although anger was associated with lower marital satisfaction in the short term, it was associated with increased marital satisfaction over the long term.

Myth 3: Quid Pro Quo Error

Gottman (1999) also found that quid pro quo ("this for that"; see "Behavior Exchange and Quid Pro Quo," above) actually characterizes *unhappy* marriages. Thus, he argued that contingency contracting is *not* appropriate when treating couples.

The Big Picture: Overview of Treatment

Gottman (1999) uses a highly detailed assessment system with numerous written and oral assessment tools to assess couples and to target areas for change. The intervention process involves extensive psychoeducation about what works and what does not, as well as structured exercises that sometimes include videotaping the couple's conversations, replaying them for analysis, and identifying where and how improvements can be made. Gottman also believes that couples therapy should be characterized as the following:

- A positive affect experience: Therapy should primarily be a positive affect experience; it should be enjoyable for clients, and therapists should avoid criticizing or implying blame.
- Primarily dyadic: Therapy should primarily be a dyadic experience between the couple rather than triadic with the therapist moderating all interactions.
- Emotional learning: Learning is state-dependent, meaning that in order to change an emotional state, couples must be in that emotional state and then work through it; thus, couples have difficult conversations in session to learn how to handle them differently.
- Easy: Interventions should seem easy and nonthreatening.
- Nonidealistic: Therapists should not be idealistic about the potential for marital bliss and instead aim for realistic goals, such as reducing conflict.

Making a Connection: The Therapeutic Relationship

Therapist as Coach

The therapist serves as a relationship coach, empowering couples to take ownership of their relationship (Gottman, 1999). The therapist does not soothe the couple during difficult conversations but rather coaches them on how to soothe themselves and each other.

The Viewing: Case Conceptualization and Assessment

Assessing Divorce Potential

After studying couples for over 30 years, Gottman (1999) can predict a couple's potential for divorce in the next 5 years with 97.5% accuracy with only five variables, an impressive achievement. Furthermore, his careful research has identified several key predictors of divorce, the most notorious of which are the Four Horsemen of the Apocalypse.

The Four Horsemen of the Apocalypse

In Gottman's studies, the presence of the following four behaviors during a couple's argument predicted divorce with 85% accuracy.

1. Criticism: A statement that implies something is globally wrong with the partner (e.g., "always," "never," or a statement about personality). Women tend to criticize more than men.
2. Defensiveness: Used to ward off attack, defensiveness claims, "I'm innocent."
3. Contempt: The *single best predictor of divorce,* contempt is seeing oneself as superior to one's partner (e.g., "you are incapable of an intelligent thought"). Happy marriages had zero incidents of contempt.
4. Stonewalling: Stonewalling is when the listener withdraws from interaction, either physically or mentally. Men are more likely to stonewall than women.

5:1 Ratio

Most couples criticize, defend, and stonewall to a certain extent. The difference between those who stay together and those who do not lies in the ratio of positive-to-negative interactions during conflict conversations. Stable couples have five times as many positive interactions as negative interactions during conflict; distressed couples may have a 1:1 ratio. Many couples find this research result very helpful in learning how to improve their marriage.

Negative Affect Reciprocity

Negative affect reciprocity is the increased probability that one partner's emotions will be negative *immediately following* negativity in the other. Otherwise stated, "My negativity is *more predictable* after my partner has been negative than it ordinarily would be" (Gottman, 1999, p. 37). Negative affect reciprocity is the most consistent correlate of marital satisfaction and dissatisfaction, regardless of the culture studied, and it is a far superior measure than the total amount of negative affect in the relationship.

Repair Attempts

Repair attempts refer to when one partner tries to "make nice" and end the conflict, soothe the other, or soften the complaint. Because happy couples are more responsive to repair attempts, they need fewer of them. Distressed couples frequently reject repair attempts, resulting in a higher number of total attempts. When failed repair attempts are combined with the Four Horsemen, Gottman (1999) can predict with 97.5% accuracy whether a couple will divorce in the next five years.

Accepting Influence

Marriages in which men are unwilling to accept influence from their wives (e.g., suggestions, requests) are 80% more likely to end in divorce, making this the single best predictor of divorce.

Harsh Startup

Harsh startup is raising an issue using negative affect in the first minute of a conversation. For 96% of couples, only the first minute of data is necessary to predict divorce or stability, and harsh startup is one of several key variables in predicting divorce in that first minute (Gottman, 1999). Relationships in which the woman uses harsh startup are more likely to end in divorce.

Distance and Isolation Cascade

What if there are no horsemen in sight? Does that mean a couple is doing well? Not necessarily. If problems go unresolved, often couples become emotionally disengaged, starting the **distance-and-isolation cascade** (Gottman, 1999). These couples often say, "Everything is okay," but there is underlying tension and sadness. These couples are characterized by an absence of emotional expression, lack of friendship, unacknowledged tension, high levels of physiological arousal in conflict, and few efforts to soothe the other.

Typologies of Happy Marriages

Gottman (1999) has identified three different types of stable, happy marriages, which means that there is more than one way to get marriage right. All maintain the 5:1 ratio of positive-to-negative interactions but do so at different rates.

- Volatile couples: Volatile couples are more emotionally expressive, expressing more positive and negative emotions. Passionate fighting and passionate loving characterize their relationships.
- Validating couples: Validating couples have moderate emotional expression and strong marital friendships.
- Conflict-avoiding couples: Conflict-avoiding couples have the least emotional expression, minimize problems, prefer to talk about the strengths of their marriage, and end conversations on a note of solidarity.

THE SOUND RELATIONSHIP HOUSE

Gottman (1999) maintains that marriages that work have two elements:
- An overall sense of positive affect
- An ability to reduce negative affect during conflict

He has designed a marriage therapy to increase these two qualities in ailing marriages in a model he terms *the sound marital house*, which has seven key aspects:

1. **Love maps:** A cognitive understanding of who your partner is and what makes him or her happy is a basic component of marital friendship.
2. **Fondness and admiration system:** This refers to the amount of respect and affection partners feel for each other and are willing to express.
3. **Turning toward versus turning away:** The Emotional Bank Account: This is a habitual turning toward and opening to each other emotionally in nonconflict interactions (e.g., wanting to share stories, spend time together).
4. **Positive sentiment override:** This refers to giving your partner "the benefit of the doubt," as compared with negative sentiment override, in which even neutral comments are interpreted negatively.

(continued)

> ## THE SOUND RELATIONSHIP HOUSE (CONTINUED)
>
> 5. **Problem solving:** Another myth that Gottman's research has caused therapists to reconsider is that couples need to improve their problem-solving skills. That is only half the story, or more precisely, 31%. Gottman's research indicates that both successful and unsuccessful couples argue about the same topics 69% of the time; he calls these the perpetual problems, which are due to inherent personality differences.
>
>   - **Solving the solvable:** Stable couples are able to successfully resolve solvable problems.
>
>   - **Dialogue with perpetual problems:** Happy couples avoid gridlock and instead find a way to continue talking about their perpetual problems and core personality differences. Because it is impossible not to have perpetual problems, selecting a partner is really about choosing a particular set of perpetual problems.
>
>   - **Physiological soothing:** In successful marriages, partners are able to soothe themselves and their partner, enabling everyone to "calm down."
>
> 6. **Making dreams come true:** Couples avoid gridlock, especially around perpetual problems, by working together to make each partner's dreams come true.
>
> 7. **Creating shared meaning:** Happy couples develop a marital "culture," with rituals of connection and shared meanings, roles, and goals.

Trust

In 2011, Gottman revised his theory to include the concept of trust, which he defines as specific action, not a feeling or personality trait. He defines trust as being able to count on one's partner to act on one's behalf without regard to his or her personal payoff, especially when couples are engaged in conflict in which both are being nasty (nasty–nasty conflict). More simply stated, how much can one count on one's partner to act to benefit one, especially during conflict? Unhappy couples get stuck in nasty–nasty conflict because they do not have sufficient trust for either to move toward repair. Gottman helps couples learn how to emotionally attune to each other to build trust, similar to the process of emotionally focused therapy (see Chapter 6).

The Doing: Interventions

Session Format

Therapy begins with a highly structured assessment process. In the intervention phase, the typical session follows this format:

- Catch-up: The couple check in on marital events, homework, and major issues; they are directed to talk to one another, not report to the therapist.
- Preintervention marital interaction: the boxing round: The couple interact for 6 to 10 minutes, usually by discussing a difficult topic.
- Give an intervention: After the interaction, the therapist asks the couple for an intervention before suggesting one, based on the premise that people tend to be more accepting of their own ideas.

- The spouses make the intervention on their own: The couple discuss their thoughts on how to improve their interactions, with the therapist facilitating and educating as necessary to help them master the process.
- Got resistance? If there is resistance, the therapist needs to address the source of these concerns.
- No resistance? Once the couple has a viable plan for altering their interaction, the therapist instructs them to engage in another 6-minute interaction to practice the suggested changes.
- Homework: Tasks are assigned based on the interactions in session.

Specific Interventions

Gottman uses highly detailed interventions that are outlined in *The Marriage Clinic* (Gottman, 1999). Some of the more notable interventions are as follows.

Love Maps

Couples are encouraged to develop their knowledge of each other by answering the following questions (Gottman, 1999, p. 205):

- Who are your partner's friends?
- Who are your partner's potential friends?
- Who are the rivals, competitors, "enemies" in your partner's world?
- What are the recent important events (in your partner's life)?
- What are some important upcoming events?
- What are some current stresses in your partner's life?
- What are your partner's current worries?
- What are some of your partner's hopes and aspirations for self and others?

Soften Startup

Gottman teaches couples to use the following rules to help soften startup.

- Be concise: Keep the initial statement brief and to the point.
- Complain but don't blame: Complain about a specific incident rather than blame or label.
- Start with something positive: Pose problems by starting with something positive.
- Use "I" instead of "you" statements: Start statements with "I" rather than "you" to avoid blaming and to increase personal responsibility.
- Describe what is happening rather than judge: Keep statements behavioral rather than global.
- Ask for what you need: Clearly describe the behavioral changes you desire.
- Be polite and appreciative: Express appreciation for what your partner does do, and be respectful.
- Express vulnerable emotions: When possible, describe more vulnerable than blaming emotions.

Dreams within Conflict

When working with the gridlock created by perpetual problems, the therapist asks each partner about the deeper meanings and dreams that are beneath his/her rigid stance in the gridlock. In session, partners are directed to ask each other the following questions in relation to a perpetual problem or gridlock issue (Gottman, 1999, p. 248):

- What do you believe about this issue?
- What do you feel about it? Tell me all of your feelings about it.

- What do you want to happen?
- What does this *mean* to you?
- How do you think your goals can be accomplished?
- What dreams or symbolic meanings (e.g., freedom, hope, caring) are behind your position on this issue?

Negotiating Marital Power

Gottman facilitates couple discussion of gender roles using an extensive checklist (Gottman, 1999, pp. 298–300). He does not advocate a particular division of labor but instead helps the couple arrive at their own definition of "fair and equitable." The purpose of this exercise is to increase respect for the roles and duties of each partner.

Evidence-Based Couple and Family Group Therapies

Lay of the Land

Several evidence-based group therapy models have been developed for couples and families, mostly based on CBFT principles. These models include multicouple/multifamily groups for the following presenting concerns:

- Severe mental illness
- Partner abuse and domestic violence
- Marital enrichment
- Parent training

Psychoeducational Multifamily Groups for Severe Mental Illness

Family psychoeducation has been used as part of treatment in schizophrenia, bipolar, and childhood mood disorders (Luckstead et al., 2012). Numerous controlled, clinical studies have demonstrated that patients diagnosed with schizophrenia whose families receive psychoeducation have reduced incidents of psychotic relapse and rehospitalization (McFarlane et al., 2002). The relapse rate for these patients is about 15%, less than half the rate of those who receive individual therapy and medication or medication alone (for which the relapse rate is 30 to 40%). Several comparison studies indicate that multifamily groups are more effective than single-family sessions in which the family learns the same psychoeducational material, making groups not only the more cost-effective treatment but also the more effective treatment overall. Multifamily groups lead to lower relapse rates and higher rates of employment than single-family sessions, probably because of the enhanced support that group settings offer. There is sufficient evidence at this time to consider family psychoeducation for families with a schizophrenic member as an *evidence-based practice* (Luckstead et al., 2012; McFarlane et al., 2002).

The U.S. Substance Abuse and Mental Health Services Administration (SAMHSA) describes multifamily psychoeducational groups as being characterized by the following (Luckstead et al., 2012):

- Assumes involved family members of persons diagnosed with schizophrenia need information, assistance, and support
- Assumes the way relatives behave toward a consumer with a mental illness affects the individual's well-being and clinical outcomes
- Combines information, cognitive, behavioral, problem-solving, emotional, coping, and consultation elements
- Is created and led by mental health professionals

- Is offered as part of a clinical treatment plan for the diagnosed individual
- Focuses on improving the diagnosed individual's outcomes but also addressed family member outcomes
- Includes at least the following content:
  - Illness, medication, and treatment management
  - Problems accessing health care
  - Services coordination
  - Attention to all parties' expectations, emotional experiences, and distress
  - Improving family communication
  - Structured problem-solving instructions
  - Expanding social support networks
  - Explicit crisis planning
- Are generally diagnosis-specific, although some cross-diagnosis programs are being developed.

Research indicates that psychodynamic and insight-oriented therapies are counterindicated (not recommended) with families that have a member diagnosed with schizophrenia.

The *psychoeducational curriculum* for multifamily groups for families with a member diagnosed with schizophrenia typically includes the following:

- Education about the illness, prognosis, psychological treatment, and medication
- The biological, psychological, and social factors related to the illness
- Education on the role of high emotional expression in the home in increasing the likelihood of relapse (Hooley, Rosen, & Richters, 1995)
- Possible social isolation and stigmatization
- The financial and psychological burden on the family
- The importance of developing a strong social network to support the family
- Problem-solving skills

The *process* aspect of multifamily groups includes the following:

- Creating a forum for mutual aid and support
- Normalizing the family's experience
- Reducing the sense of stigma
- Creating a sense of hope by seeing how other families have coped
- Socializing with each other outside the group context

When families participate in these groups, the patient and the family have fewer social problems, fewer clinical management problems, reduced secondary stress (stress caused by the hospitalization of the patient), increased employment, and decreased relapse and rehospitalization. In the past decade, several studies have been conducted in countries outside the United States, primarily in Asia and Europe, with some showing positive outcomes similar to those in the United States and some not showing significant differences; thus, more exploration into cultural adaptation and applicability is needed (Luckstead et al., 2012).

Although most of the research on groups has been done with schizophrenic and schizoaffective disorders, several studies have used multifamily psychoeducation groups as a component of treatment for other severe mental health disorders (McFarlane et al., 2002), including the following:

- Bipolar disorder
- Dual diagnosis (e.g., substance abuse and an Axis I diagnosis)
- Obsessive–compulsive disorder
- Depression
- Posttraumatic stress disorder in veterans
- Alzheimer's disease
- Suicidal ideation in adolescents

- Congenital abnormalities
- Intellectual impairment
- Child molesters and pedophilia
- Borderline personality disorder

Groups for Intimate Partner Abuse

A widespread and difficult-to-treat phenomenon with numerous physical and emotional effects on children, women, and families, physical abuse of one's partner is increasingly targeted for intervention by state and local authorities. Today, most states mandate therapy in cases of partner abuse, a specific form of domestic violence. Treatment is most frequently delivered in the form of gender-based group therapy (i.e., groups for male or female batterers and groups for male or female victims of abuse; Stith et al., 2012; Stith, Rosen, & McCollum, 2002). However, increasingly, couple-based approaches are being researched as alternative approaches, with initial studies indicating that carefully designed couple-based approaches to partner violence have comparable outcomes to the traditional gender-based groups, with no evidence of an increased potential for violence (Stith et al., 2002; Stith, Rosen, & McCollum, 2002).

Traditional Gender-Based Groups for Partner Abuse

The traditional gender-based groups for partner abuse are based on the work of Lenore Walker (1979) and the closely related Duluth Model (Pence & Paymar, 1993). These models are psychoeducational cognitive–behavioral groups grounded in feminism that are widely used in the criminal justice system. Lenore Walker used the *cycle of violence* to describe the dynamics of the abuse relationship. The cycle has three phases: honeymoon, tension-building, and acting out:

- Honeymoon phase: This is the phase in which the batterer pursues the victim, asking forgiveness, promising to stop the violence, and attempting to woo the victim back.
- Tension-building phase: Victims often describe the tension-building phase as a state of "living on eggshells." During this period, conflict and tension are rising and the victim tries to avoid behaviors that will "set off" the perpetrator.
- Acting out or explosion: The final phase is characterized by a physically violent episode; after this episode, the cycle repeats as the batterer tries to repair the relationship in the honeymoon phase.

In the early years of violent relationships, the cycle typically moves slowly, perhaps with only one or two mildly violent episodes per year (e.g., pushing, shoving, throwing objects, one slap). Over time, the frequency and severity of the violent episodes increase.

In addition to the cycle of violence, the Duluth Model uses the idea of the *wheel of power and control,* which describes the means by which batterers are believed to maintain control over their partners. The eight spokes of the wheel are as follows:

- Coercion and threats
- Intimidation
- Emotional abuse
- Isolation
- Minimizing, denying, and blaming
- Using children
- Economic abuse
- Male privilege

Although the Duluth Model is one of the most frequently used models for treating batterers, Dutton and Corvo (2006, 2007) note studies on the effectiveness of batterer intervention groups indicate a high recidivism rate, with 40% of participants remaining nonviolent. In comparison, untreated batterers have a 35% chance of remaining nonviolent, indicating that typical batterer intervention programs made very little impact on recidivism, which is why therapists are looking for other alternatives (Stith et al., 2012).

Conjoint Treatment of Partner Abuse

Because of the limitations of the Duluth Model, therapists and researchers have explored other models of treatment, including conjoint couples therapy (Stith et al., 2002), narrative therapy (Jenkins, 1990) and solution-focused therapy (Lipchik & Kubicki, 1996; Milner & Singleton, 2008; Stith et al., 2002). Of these, conjoint couples therapy has been the best researched (Stith et al., 2012).

Until recently, couples therapy was considered "inappropriate" for the treatment of domestic violence, largely because of the assumption that there is a significant struggle for power, control, and dominance in all battering relationships. However, as already noted, there is little research to support this assumption (Dutton & Corvo, 2006, 2007) and there is increased interest in and funding for this new approach (Stith et al., 2012).

Emerging research indicates that there is more than one type of batterer (Holtzworth-Munroe & Stuart, 1994): (a) those who are violent only within their families; (b) those who have more severe pathology, such as depression or borderline personality disorder, and (c) those who are generally violent and have antisocial characteristics. Conjoint couples therapy is designed for only one type of batterer: *family-only batterers without apparent psychopathology*. Arguments for using conjoint couples treatment for mild cases of family-only battering include the following (Stith, Rosen, & McCollum, 2002):

- It is estimated that as many as 67% of all couples presenting for couples therapy have a history of violence. Therapists may begin treating a couple for other issues before discovering violence; stopping therapy because of this revelation can result in the couple choosing not to pursue further treatment.
- Statistics show that 50 to 70% of wives who are battered return to the abusive partner after separating or going to a shelter; conjoint couples therapy provides one of the few safe forums for these couples to safely discuss their relationship.
- The majority of violent relationships are *bidirectional,* with both parties committing acts of violence. Because cessation of violence by one partner is highly dependent on the cessation of violence by the other, conjoint treatment, in which both parties are deescalating violence, has a greater likelihood of reducing bidirectional violence.

Conjoint Couples Treatment

Several approaches for working conjointly with couples have been developed; most combine couple-only sessions with multicouple groups (Stith, Rosen, & McCollum, 2002). The common characteristics of conjoint couples treatment of partner violence include the following:

- Each partner is carefully screened to determine whether the couple should participate in couple sessions or multicouple group sessions. Couples in which there has been serious injury to one or both partners are excluded. In addition, in private screening interviews, both partners must state that they prefer couples therapy and that they are not afraid of speaking freely in session with their partner.
- The primary goal is decreasing violence and emotional abuse, not saving the marriage or relationship.
- Partners are encouraged to take responsibility for their own violence.
- The skill-building component emphasizes identifying when one is angry, knowing how to deescalate self and other, and taking time-outs.
- The effectiveness of the program is measured by the reduction or elimination of violence.

Effectiveness of Conjoint Couples Treatment

Although the research is relatively new, several forms of conjoint couples treatment and multicouple group treatment of partner violence appears to be *more effective* than traditional gender-based models in reducing physical violence (Stith et al., 2012). For men in particular, the multicouple groups had more positive outcomes than single-couple sessions. In the carefully designed conjoint programs studied, there was no evidence that women in conjoint couples treatment for domestic violence were more likely to be abused than when the batterers were treated separately; thus, if thoughtfully approached, it does not appear that conjoint couples treatment increases the incidence of violence (Stith et al., 2002). Furthermore, using conjoint couples treatment when the batterer also had a substance abuse issue was superior to individual treatment in reducing violence (Stith et al., 2012).

Relationship Enhancement Programs

One of the most common forms of multicouple group sessions, relationship enhancement programs are preventive interventions for nondistressed couples who want to improve the quality of their relationship (Halford et al., 2002; Markman & Rhoades, 2012). These programs are typically offered as multicouple psychoeducational groups, which are generally grounded in cognitive–behavioral therapies. These groups may include lectures, demonstrations, audiovisual programs, practice, and discussion. Some of the more prominent programs include the following:

- Relationship Enhancement (RE) (Guerney, 1987)
- Prevention and Relationship Enhancement Program (PREP) (Markman, Stanley, & Blumberg, 2001)
- Minnesota Couples Communication Program (MCCP) (Miller, Nunnally, & Wackman, 1976)
- Practical Application of Intimate Relationship Skills (PAIRS) (DeMaria & Hannah, 2002)

All these programs promote positive communication, conflict management, and positive expression of affection. Variations in the curriculum include the following:

- Preventing destructive conflict (emphasized in PREP)
- Developing empathy for one's partner (emphasized in RE)
- Strong emphasis on conflict management (emphasized in MCCP and RE)
- Commitment, respect, love, and friendship (emphasized in PREP)

Effectiveness of Multicouple Relationship Enhancement Programs

In the research literature on these programs, most couples report high satisfaction, rating skill training in communication as the most helpful intervention (Halford et al., 2002; Markman & Rhoades, 2012). Meta-analyses report an effect size of 0.44 (a difference of almost half a standard deviation from control groups) for communication at follow-up, which is impressive when you consider that they were not distressed initially, with stronger findings for more rigorously designed studies (Markman & Rhoades, 2012). In addition, skill-based relationship enhancement results in a significant increase in relationship skills upon completion of the program. Studies vary from no improvement to modest improvement in relationship satisfaction immediately following completion of a course. However, there is limited research on the long-term effectiveness of these programs. Such research has been conducted only on skill-based groups that met for four to eight sessions and that targeted dating, engaged, or recently married couples. These long-term studies indicate the following:

- Relational skills learned in the group are maintained for a period of several years but begin to trail off in 5 to 10 years.

- PREP participants reported enhanced relationship satisfaction and functioning 2 to 5 years after the course.
- PREP participants reported fewer incidents of violence at the 5-year follow-up than those who did not participate.
- Certain effects, such as increased satisfaction and decreased divorce rate, seemed to become evident at the 4- to 5-year mark, meaning that the difference between couples who participated in PREP and those who began marriage without an enrichment program became detectable only several years later.
- In one study involving older, more distressed couples, PREP was not effective, indicating that enrichment programs that work early in a relationship might not be equally effective for more established or more distressed couples.

Guidelines

Based on their review of the research literature, Halford et al. (2002) propose the following as best practices in relationship enhancement:

- Assess risk and protective factors: Before admitting couples to a relationship-enhancement group, therapists should screen them for risk factors associated with higher stress and divorce, such as parental divorce, age, previous marriages, length of time the partners have known each other, cohabitation history, and the presence of stepchildren. In addition, therapists should consider protective factors and strengths, such as clear communication and realistic relationship expectations.
- Encourage high-risk couples to attend: Relationship enhancement is more likely to benefit high-risk couples early in their relationships because they are more likely to need better skills to manage their stressors.
- Assess and educate about relationship aggression: Because physical and verbal aggression occur at high rates early in couple relationships, education about aggression and how to handle it can better prepare couples to reduce hostile and dangerous behavior.
- Offer relationship education at change points: In addition to the beginning of a relationship, couples can benefit from relationship enhancement at numerous other life and developmental transition points, such as the birth of a child, relocation, major illness, and unemployment.
- Promote early presentation of relationship problems: Because long-standing distress predicts poor response to couples therapy, couples should be encouraged to address mild distress as it emerges rather than allow the relationship to deteriorate further.
- Match content to couples with special needs: Program enhancement needs to be adapted to fit a couple's special needs, such as a major mental health diagnosis, alcohol or substance abuse, and stepfamily issues.
- Enhance accessibility of evidence-based relationship education programs: Programs can be made more accessible by increasing the formats in which they are offered: weekly, on weekends, or online.

Parent Training

Parent training is a cognitive–behavioral intervention that has shown effectiveness in treating a wide range of childhood problems. It is the treatment of choice for oppositional defiant disorder (ODD) and the only treatment that produces normalization of functioning in a child with ADHD (Kaslow, Broth, Smith & Collins, 2012). Parent training has been shown to be effective with both individual families and multifamily groups (DeRosier & Gilliom, 2007; van den Hoofdakker, van der Veen-Mulders, & Sytema, 2007).

Parent training group curricula include elements similar to those of parent training with individual families:

- Encouraging positive reinforcement to shape desired behaviors
- Using natural and logical consequences whenever possible
- Improving parents' ability to listen and communicate understanding to their child
- Increasing parents' use of "I" statements
- Providing multiple-choice options for children in negotiations when appropriate
- Training parents in emotional coaching to help their children identify, express, and appropriately manage their emotions
- Using contingency contracting and point systems to motivate children
- Training in how to use time-outs and other punishments to reduce negative behaviors

Mindfulness-Based Therapies

In a Nutshell: The Least You Need to Know

Described as a leading force in the third wave of behavioral therapy (with "pure" behavioral therapy the first wave and cognitive–behavioral therapy the second), mindfulness-based approaches add a paradoxical twist to cognitive-behavioral approaches: accepting difficult thoughts and emotions in order to transform them (Hayes, 2004). Therapists using mindfulness-based approaches encourage clients to curiously and compassionately observe difficult thoughts and feelings without the intention to change them. By changing *how* they relate to their problems—with curiosity and acceptance rather than avoidance—clients experience new thoughts, emotions, and behaviors in relation to the problem and thus have many new options for coping and resolving issues.

In couple and family therapy, **mindfulness** has been used to help couples and families become more accepting of one another, improve their communication, and increase intimacy (Carson et al., 2004; Duncan, Coatsworth, & Greenberg, 2009; Gehart, 2012). Mindfulness-based practices are rooted in Buddhist psychology, which is essentially a constructivist philosophy, making it theoretically most similar to postmodern (see Chapter 10) and systemic (see Chapter 4) therapies (Gehart, 2012). Therapists working with these therapies may find that the concepts naturally fit with their approach. These practices require therapists to have their own mindfulness practice and training before trying to teach clients to do the same.

A Brief History of Mindfulness in Mental Health

Mindfulness has an unusual history as a cognitive–behavioral approach: it was not developed in a researcher's lab or from a Western philosophical tradition. Instead, mindfulness comes from religious and spiritual traditions, making it a surprising favorite for cognitive–behavioral therapists, who ground themselves almost exclusively in Western scientific traditions. Most commonly associated with Buddhist forms of meditation, mindfulness is found in virtually all cultures and religious traditions, including Christian contemplative prayer (Keating, 2006), Jewish mysticism, and the Islamic-based Sufi tradition. Although it has religious roots, mindfulness entered mental health as a nonreligious stress-reduction technique and was intentionally separated from religion and spiritual elements and adapted for use in behavioral health settings (Kabat-Zinn, 1990).

Over 30 years ago, Jon Kabat-Zinn (1990) began researching the Mindfulness-Based Stress Reduction (MBSR) program at the University of Massachusetts, which has been highly influential in making mindfulness a mainstream practice in behavioral medicine. The MBSR program is an eight-week group curriculum that teaches participants how to practice mindful breathing, mindful yoga postures, and mindful daily activities. Participants are encouraged to practice daily at home for 20 to 45 minutes per day.

MBSR shows great promise as an effective treatment for a wide range of physical and mental health disorders, including chronic pain, fibromyalgia, psoriasis, depression, anxiety, ADHD, eating disorders, substance abuse, compulsive behaviors, and personality disorders (Baer, 2003; Gehart, 2012).

Teasdale, Segal, and Williams (1995) have adapted the MBSR curriculum for depression relapse in their program, Mindfulness-Based Cognitive Therapy (MBCT). With 50% of "successfully" treated cases of depression ending in relapse within a year, MBCT therapists are using mindfulness to reduce the high relapse rate, with promising results.

In addition to including mindfulness-based stress reduction (Kabat-Zinn, 1990) and mindfulness-based cognitive therapy (Teasdale et al., 1995), mindfulness has been integrated into two therapeutic approaches that have also shown great promise in treating a wide range of clinical conditions: dialectic behavioral therapy (Linehan, 1993) and acceptance and commitment therapy (Hayes, Strosahl, & Wilson, 1999).

Mindfulness Basics

The most common form of mindfulness involves observing the breath (or focusing on a repeated word, a *mantra*) while quieting the mind of inner chatter and thoughts (Kabat-Zinn, 1990). Focus is maintained on the breath, grounding the practitioner in the present moment *without judging* the experience as good or bad, preferred or not preferred. Usually within seconds, the mind loses focus and wanders off—thinking about the exercise, a fight that morning, to-do lists, past memories, future plans; feeling an emotion or itch; or hearing a noise in the room. At some point, the practitioner realizes that the mind has wandered off and then returns to the object of focus without berating the self for "failing" to focus but rather with compassionate understanding that the loss of focus is part of the process—refraining from beating oneself up is usually the most difficult part. This process of focusing–losing focus–regaining focus–losing focus–regaining focus continues for an established period of time, usually 10 to 20 minutes.

Gehart and McCollum (2007, 2008; McCollum, 2015; McCollum & Gehart, 2010; Gehart, 2012) have used mindfulness to help first-year therapists and seasoned therapists learn how to develop therapeutic presence, with encouraging reports from trainees who say that they notice significant changes both in and out of the therapy session. Trainees report being better able to be emotionally present with clients, less anxious in session, and better able to respond in difficult moments. Most report that their overall level of stress noticeably decreases within two weeks of practicing five days per week for 2 to 10 minutes; they also report better relationships and a greater sense of inner peace. Not bad for an investment of 10 to 15 minutes per week You might want to give it a try.

STARTING YOUR PERSONAL MINDFULNESS PRACTICE

1. **Find a regular time:** The most difficult part of doing mindfulness is finding time—2 to 10 minutes—several days a week. My colleague Eric and I have our students do five days per week. It is best to "attach" mindfulness practice to some part of your regular routine, such as before or after breakfast or while working out, brushing your teeth, seeing clients, coming home, or going to bed (if you are not too tired).

2. **Find a partner or group (optional):** If possible, find a partner or meditation group with whom you can practice on a regular basis. The camaraderie will help keep you motivated.

(continued)

STARTING YOUR PERSONAL MINDFULNESS PRACTICE (*CONTINUED*)

3. **Use a timer (highly advisable):** Using a timer helps structure the mindfulness session, and many find it helps them focus better because they don't wonder whether time is up. Most mobile phones have alarms and timers that work well; you can also purchase meditation apps with Tibetan chimes for iPhones and other smartphones. Digital egg timers work well too—avoid the ones that tick.

4. **Sit comfortably:** When you are ready, find a comfortable chair to sit in. Ideally, you should not rest your back against the chair, but rather sit toward the front so that your spine is erect. If this is too uncomfortable, sit normally with your spine straight—but not rigid.

5. **Breathe:** Set your timer for 2 minutes initially. Watch yourself breathe while quieting the thoughts and any other discourse in your mind.

   - Don't try to change your breathing; just notice its qualities, not judging it as good or bad.

   - Know that your mind will wander off numerous times—both to inner and outer distractions. Each time it does, gently notice it without judging—perhaps imagine it disappearing like a cloud drifting off, soap bubbles popping, or say "ah, that too"—and then gently return your focus to watching your breath.

   - Accept your mind as it is each time you practice; some days it is easier to focus than others. The key is to practice acceptance of "what is," rather than fall into the common pattern of being frustrated with what is not happening.

   - The goal is *not* to have extended periods without thinking but rather to practice nonjudgmental acceptance and cultivate a better sense of how the mind works.

6. **Notice:** When the bell rings, notice how you feel. The same, more relaxed, more stressed? Try only to notice without judging. You may or may not feel much difference; the most helpful effects are cumulative rather than immediate. If you happen to notice you wish to go on, go ahead and add a minute or two the next time you practice. Slowly, you will add minutes until you find a length of time that works well for you. Don't extend the time until you feel a desire to do so.

7. **Repeat:** Our students report the best outcomes with shorter regular practices rather than longer but infrequent practices. Thus, doing five 2-minute practices is likely to produce better outcomes than one 10-minute session each week.

Resources to Support Your Practice

- *Free meditation podcasts:* You can download free guided mindfulness meditations and other free resources to support your practice from my website, www.dianegehart.com, and from UCLA's Mindfulness Awareness Research Center, www.marc.ucla.edu.

- *Workbooks: Mindfulness for Therapists* (McCollum, 2015), *The Mindfulness-Based Stress Reduction Workbook* (Stahl & Goldstein, 2010) and *Get Out of Your Mind and Into Your Life: The New Acceptance and Commitment Therapy* (Hayes & Smith, 2005) are excellent workbooks to teach you practical techniques.

Try It Yourself

Using the instructions above, practice two to five minutes of mindfulness.

Specific Mindfulness Approaches

Mindfulness-Based Stress Reduction and Mindfulness-Based Cognitive Therapy

Not primarily about teaching how to become a good meditation practitioner, these mindfulness-based group treatments are designed to help clients change how they relate to their thoughts and internal dialogue. Using a highly structure group process, clients are introduced to mindfulness breathing (similar to the instructions above), as well as mindful yoga (stretching) positions, and mindful daily activities (e.g., washing dishes mindfully, walking, etc.; Kabat-Zinn, 1990). Depending on the group's focus, clients may be taught to apply mindfulness to physical conditions, difficult emotions, depressive thinking, etc. The group format is ideal for motivating clients to practice regularly at home and report back to the group on progress.

The eight groups in MBSR cover the following:

- Session 1: Introduction to mindfulness: Foundations of mindfulness and body scan meditation
- Session 2: Patience: Working with perceptions and dealing with the "wandering mind"
- Session 3: Nonstriving: Introduction to breathing meditation; mindful lying yoga; qualities of attention
- Session 4: Nonjudging: Responding versus reacting; awareness in breathing meditation; standing yoga; research on stress
- Session 5: Acknowledgment: Group check-in on progress; sitting meditation
- Session 6: Let it be: Skillful communication; loving kindness meditation; walking meditation; day-long retreat
- Session 7: Everyday mindfulness: Mindful movement and everyday applications; practicing on one's own life
- Session 8: Practice never ends: Integrating with everyday life

The eight groups of MBCT cover the following (Segal, Williams, & Teasdale, 2002):

- Session 1: Automatic pilot: Introduce mindfulness; eating mindfulness exercise; mindfulness body scan
- Session 2: Dealing with barriers: Explore mental chatter using the body-scan exercise
- Session 3: Mindfulness of the breath: Introduce mindfulness breathing focus and three-minute breathing space exercise
- Session 4: Staying present: Link mindfulness to automatic thoughts and depression
- Session 5: Allowing and letting be: Introduce acceptance and "allowing" things to just be
- Session 6: Thoughts are not facts: Reframe thoughts as "just thoughts" and not facts
- Session 7: How can I best take care of myself?: Introduce specific techniques for depressive thoughts
- Session 8: Using what has been learned to deal with future moods?: Motivate to continue practice

Through these mindfulness exercises, clients learn to:

- Deliberately direct their attention and thereby better control their thoughts
- Become curious, open, and accepting of their thoughts and feelings, even those that are unpleasant
- Develop greater acceptance of self, other, and things as they are
- Live in and experience themselves in the present moment

Dialectical Behavior Therapy

Originally developed for treating borderline suicidal clients, dialectical behavior therapy (DBT; Linehan, 1993) is named for the fundamental dialectical tension between change and acceptance: "The paradoxical notion here is that therapeutic change can only occur in the context of acceptance of what is; however, 'acceptance of what is' is itself change" (p. 99). In contrast to other cognitive–behavioral approaches, this approach is based on the premise that emotion *precedes* the development of thought and that strong emotions, traumatic experiences, and attachment wounds are the source of psychopathology. In a nutshell, the process of DBT helps clients be present with, tolerate, and accept strong emotions in order to transform them. In a sense, it is a client's desperate attempts to avoid painful emotions that are the root of the problem.

DBT therapists help clients "be with" difficult emotions by encouraging clients to manage dialectical tension, the tension between two polar opposites, such as both loving and hating someone. Rather than retreat to either pole, the therapist encourages clients to experience how they can both simultaneously feel love and dislike by acknowledging the multiple levels of truth and reality in a given situation. These contradictory feelings and thoughts are first tolerated, then explored, and eventually synthesized so that the reality of the two extremes can be recognized. For example, an adult might come to acknowledge both ultimately loving a critical parent but at the same time hating how that parent speaks to her. As the client becomes able to accept having both loving and hateful feelings toward the parent, she will find herself less reactive and emotional about the situation. The process of DBT involves helping clients learn to increase balance in their lives by better managing the inherent dialectical tensions in life:

- Being able to both seek to improve oneself as well as accept oneself
- Being able to accept life as it is and also seek to solve problems
- Taking care of one's own needs as well as those of others
- Balancing independence and interdependence

Acceptance and Commitment Therapy

A behavioral approach that shares philosophical assumptions with postmodern and narrative approaches (see Chapter 10), acceptance and commitment therapy (ACT, pronounced "act," not A-C-T) is based on the postmodern premise that we construct our realities through language, which shapes our thoughts, feelings, and behaviors. ACT practitioners believe that human suffering is in large measure created and sustained through language; "It is not that people are thinking the wrong thing—the problem is thought itself and how the verbal community (contemporary culture) supports its excessive use as a mode of behavioral regulation" (Hayes et al., 1999, p. 49). Unlike traditional cognitive–behavioralists, ACT practitioners assert that attempts to control thoughts and feelings and avoid direct experience are the *problem,* not the solution. Instead, they advocate mindfulness-based *experiencing* to promote acceptance of the full range of human emotions: "In the ACT approach, a goal of healthy living is not so much to feel *good,* but rather to *feel* good. It is psychologically healthy to feel bad feelings as well as good feelings" (p. 77; emphasis in source).

THE SAME ACRONYM, ACT, IS USED TO OUTLINE THE PROCESS OF THERAPY

A = Accept and embrace difficult thoughts and feelings

C = Chose and commit to a life direction that reflects who the client truly is

T = Take action steps toward this life direction.

The first phase in ACT is for clients to accept and embrace the very thoughts and feelings they have been trying to avoid via their symptoms: accepting loss, feeling fear, and acknowledging anger. Therapists caution clients to not "buy into" their thoughts and to challenge them to see the flimsy link between reasons (aka, excuses) and causes of their behavior. At the same time, they help clients to develop a *willingness* to experience difficult thoughts and feelings with their *observing self*. Through this process of observation, clients are better able to identify their true values and selves, which helps them not only readily identify a life direction but also to commit to pursuing it. As you might imagine, this is not as simple as it sounds. In the action phase, most clients reexperience the resistance to experience and negative thoughts that brought them to therapy in the first place. However, with increased ability to accept these and a renewed commitment to pursue a meaningful life direction, the therapist can work with the client when obstacles arise in pursuing new action.

Mindfulness in Couple and Family Therapy

Family therapists are just beginning to explore the potential of mindfulness in couple and family therapy both in group format and traditional couple/family therapy sessions (Carson et al., 2004; Gehart, 2012; Gehart & McCollum, 2007). Several studies provide support for the idea that cultivating mindfulness may be particularly helpful for couples. In a study by Wachs and Cordova (2008), mindfulness is positively correlated with marital adjustment. Similarly, Barnes et al. (2008) found that the personality trait of mindfulness predicted greater marital satisfaction, lower emotional stress after conflict, and better communication. Block-Lerner et al. (2008) found that mindfulness training increased empathetic responding in couples, and Carson et al. (2008) found that couples in a mindfulness-based relationship enhancement group demonstrated greater relationship satisfaction and less relational distress.

Similarly, mindfulness has been used to enhance parent–child relationships as well as to help children with ADHD and other conduct issues. Several mindfulness-based parenting programs have been developed and researched, including mindful parenting (Duncan et al., 2009), mindfulness-based parenting training (Dumas, 2005), and mindfulness-based childbirth and parenting (Duncan & Bardacke, 2010). Furthermore, mindfulness has been enthusiastically studied as a potential non-medication–based treatment for ADHD that may actually "correct" brain functioning by increasing activity in the prefrontal cortex and decreasing activity of the limbic system (Zylowska, Smalley, & Schwartz, 2009). Finally, mindfulness has been used with adolescents to decrease aggressiveness and improve their ability to regulate emotion (Singh et al., 2007).

Loving Kindness Meditation

When working with couples and families to improve their relationships, therapists often emphasize *loving-kindness meditation* rather than mindfulness breath meditation (Carson et al., 2004; Gehart, 2012). Loving kindness meditation involves sending well wishes to various people, typically an acquaintance, a significant other, a person with whom one has a difficult relationship, and one's self. The therapist can guide couples in this practice in session and invite them to practice at home with a recording or using the basic formula below:

LOVING KINDNESS MEDITATION

Acquaintance: Bring to mind an acquaintance.
May this person be happy and joyful.
May this person be free from suffering.
May this person experience radiant health.
May this person have ease of well-being.
May this person be deeply at peace.
May this person be at peace with people in his/her life.

Continue this with each of the following:
- A significant other (just one; you can do others later)
- A person with whom you have a difficult relationship
- Yourself
- All beings

Based on Gehart (2012, p. 169).

Tapestry Weaving: Working with Diverse Populations
Ethnic, Racial, and Cultural Diversity

Because CBFT defines behavioral norms (e.g., each culture defines "rational" differently), therapists must apply this approach carefully with diverse populations to avoid conflicts in values and relational styles. CBFT's emphasis on the expert stance in relation to clients has strengths and weaknesses when working with diverse populations. Men and certain cultural groups, such as Latinos, Asians, and Native Americans, often prefer active, directive therapy (Gehart & Lyle, 2001; Pedersen et al., 2002). However, hierarchical differences may cause a rebellious reaction in some clients (e.g., highly educated adults or teens) or an overly compliant and withholding response in others (e.g., women who have a habit of people-pleasing; Gehart & Lyle, 2001).

By design, cognitive–behavioral therapies aim to help clients conform to dominant cultural values, because that is equated with "functional" within a given society. Therefore, therapists need to carefully evaluate treatment goals prior to intervention to ensure that they do not clash with religious, cultural, racial, socioeconomic, or other values and realities and to consider how the various cultures of which a client is a part may have conflicting values. Researchers are just now exploring the specific effects of ethnicity in CBT practice, identifying in which contexts ethnicity plays the greatest role. For example, initial studies have found no significant difference when using CBT for depression with European Americans, Latino, and Asian Americans (Marchand et al., 2010); however, another study found that ethnicity played a significant role in the strength of the therapeutic relationship over the course of therapy with perpetrators of domestic violence (Walling et al., 2012). Thus, ongoing research will further refine our understanding of how best to use CBT with diverse populations. Based on this emerging research and clinical expertise, CBT therapists have begun developing recommendations for specific ethnic groups.

Hispanic and Latino Clients

CBFT is generally considered to be culturally consistent and appropriate for working with Hispanic and Latino clients (Organista & Muñoz, 1996). Therapists have developed several suggestions for successfully working with Hispanic and Latino clients using CBFT.

- *Addressing language needs:* Language issues are central when working with many immigrant Latino families, who often prefer to discuss private and emotional issues in their native language (most people prefer to discuss emotional issues in their native language, and Spanish speakers are particularly passionate about this). In addition, Spanish-speaking therapists need to consider how to translate not just words but concepts across cultures; for example, in one CBT program for Latinos the A-B-C method for disputing irrational beliefs was streamlined and translated as the *Si, Pero* (Yes, But . . .) technique (Piedra & Byoun, 2012).
- *Increasing experiential components:* When modifying standard CBT or CBFT curricula, therapists often increase the applied and experiential components: rather than talk about it, do it (Piedra & Byoun, 2012).
- *Respecting cultural value of* familismo: Family is highly valued, with individual interests often placed second to family needs; thus, CBFT therapists need to be careful to avoid labeling a Latino or Latina's choice to put family above personal needs as "irrational" (Duarté-Vélez, Bernal, & Bonilla, 2010; González-Prendes, Hindo, & Pardo, 2011).
- *Respecting cultural value of* personalismo: Latino culture values warm and trusting personal relationships, which therapists need to integrate into the therapeutic relationship (González-Prendes et al., 2011). To create a context of *personalism,* therapists can begin their initial session in "small talk," sharing their background in addition to learning about the client's (Organista & Muñoz, 1996).
- *Respecting the cultural value of* respeto: Latino families are typically hierarchical, with formal expectations of respect to parents and elders; in addition, clients may prefer to be addressed with formal titles, Señor or Señora (González-Prendes et al., 2011; Organista & Muñoz, 1996).
- *Respecting the cultural value of* machismo: Often misunderstood in its negative extreme, within its native culture, machismo refers to a man's sense of leadership, loyalty, and responsibility to provide and care for the family (Duarté-Vélez et al., 2010; González-Prendes et al., 2011).
- *Working with spirituality:* Many Hispanic/Latino clients have a strong sense of spirituality, most often Roman Catholic (Duarté-Vélez et al., 2010). Prayer, church, and the church community are resources that therapists can tap into; however, therapists should also discuss the use of prayer to ensure that it facilitates active problem solving rather than reduce the client's sense of efficacy or responsibility (Organista & Muñoz, 1996).
- *Working with attitudes to gay/lesbian relationships:* Their strong religious beliefs may lead Hispanic families to have a highly negative response to a child's coming out, often viewing same-sex attraction as a "sin"; this can create significant cultural dissonance and rejection for gay Latino youth (Duarté-Vélez et al., 2010).
- *Addressing immigration, migration, and acculturation:* Many Hispanics have complex immigration and migration patterns, often moving back and forth between cultures multiples times and having family members who live in different countries at the same time. In addition, acculturation is often an issue between parents and children, and CBFT therapists need to help clients to address this (Piedra & Byoun, 2012).

African American Clients

Many experts also consider CBFT an appropriate choice for working with African Americans because it helps them directly dispute problematic social beliefs and focus on present behaviors (Kelly, 2006; McNair, 1996). Recommendations for adaptation include:

- *Forming a collaborative relationship:* Clients should be invited to work with the therapist in setting goals and agreeing on time frames; this relationship should be used to foster a greater sense of self-efficacy in the client (Kelly, 2006; McNair, 1996).
- *Focusing on behaviors and skills:* Rather than analyzing the past, therapists should focus on problems that are being experienced in the present and are of immediate importance and relevance to the client (McNair, 1996).
- *Enabling empowerment:* CBFT therapists can help empower clients by working with them to develop coping and communication skills and to expand the support networks (Kelly, 2006). Furthermore, clients can be taught how to use thought records and other strategies to solve their own problems without the therapist.
- *Disputing stereotypes and expectations:* CBFT therapists can use the techniques of the approach to help African Americans identify and logically dispute many of the stereotypes and expectations they have internalized from the broader culture—such as having to be twice as good to be good enough—and to increase their personal sense of purpose and opportunities (McNair, 1996).
- *Addressing discrimination:* Therapists can help African Americans mitigate the effects of discrimination by specifically identifying how they cope with discrimination and how it relates to how they perceive and relate to the world (McNair, 1996).
- *Using functional analysis:* Functional analysis that examines the symptom in behavioral terms can help circumvent potential therapist bias and prejudice and can help clients do the same (Kelly, 2006).

Chinese American Clients

Therapists have also considered how best to use cognitive–behavioral approaches with Chinese Americans. Hwang and colleagues (2006) recommend they do the following:

1. Explicitly educate the client about the process and goals of therapy to increase his or her understanding and acceptance.
2. Learn more about the client's cultural background and its significance to the client.
3. Clearly establish goals and measures of improvement early in treatment to reduce confusion about the process.
4. Focus on psychoeducational aspects and reinforce efforts to learn to reduce stigma and empower clients.
5. Use *cultural bridging* to link Western psychological concepts to the client's cultural beliefs and practices (e.g., discussing Qi [life energy] when discussing depression)
6. Present him or herself as an expert; this is often helpful to Chinese American clients.
7. Explicitly discuss the therapist–client relationship to clarify roles and set realistic expectations.
8. Attend to cultural differences in communication and deference to authority.
9. Spend extra time joining with client and learning about immigration history and family background.
10. Respect the family orientation of the Chinese culture, and involve family whenever possible.

11. Be sensitive to the social stigma associated with mental illness in Chinese community and the desire to keep the diagnosis private.
12. Be patient, because the Chinese people may not be comfortable discussing emotions.
13. Be aware of the push–pull between the client's culture of origin and the culture of therapy.
14. Integrate Chinese cultural healing traditions, such as Qigong or acupuncture, into the treatment plan.
15. Be aware of the ethnic differences in expressing distress, with the Chinese notion of self involving a closer relationship between mind and body than in the Western culture.

Sexual and Gender Identity Diversity

Several authors have considered how to adapt CBT and CBFT for working with lesbian, gay, bisexual, transgendered, and questioning (LGBTQ) clients. Safren and Rogers (2001) note that typically therapists either overestimate or underestimate the impact that sexual orientation and difference have on a client's presenting problems; therefore, they recommend that therapists begin by examining their own beliefs and schemas related to sexual orientation and identity. Furthermore, Safren and Rogers (2001) encourage CBT therapists to examine the role that societal norms and stigma play in the development of client's beliefs and schemas.

When working with LGBTQ youth and adults, therapists need to assess additional areas of stress and functioning:

* Overt acts of harassment, abuse, and violence (Safren et al., 2001)
* **Internalized homophobia** (Safren et al., 2001)
* Existence of social support networks (Safren & Rogers, 2001)
* Development of identity as a sexual minority (Safren et al., 2001)
* Disclosure of sexual orientation to family, friends, and others (Safren et al., 2001)
* Development of platonic and romantic relationships with other gay, lesbian, bisexual, or transgendered persons (Safren et al., 2001)
* Stress due to social stigma (Glassgold, 2009)
* Stress due to concealing stigma and distress (Glassgold, 2009)

Mylott (1994) has identified common irrational beliefs with which gay, lesbian, and bisexual adults frequently struggle; these beliefs are largely informed by societal norms and include:

* I need to be loved.
* I can't stand rejection.
* Because people will often accept or reject me on the basis of my physical attractiveness, age, socioeconomic status, masculinity, or femininity, I have to use these same criteria to accept or reject myself.
* It will be awful if I grow old without a lover.
* I can't stand being alone, and since I can't stand being alone, it is better to be in an emotionally and even physically damaging relationship than to be alone.
* When gay people are the victims of homophobia, I have to get very angry and upset about it; I also have to become enraged at homophobic individuals, groups, and institutions.
* I can accept my homosexuality only if I know for certain that it is genetically determined, or that "God made me gay." Otherwise, I cannot accept myself.
* It's awful if people (family, friends, the church, etc.) don't accept my homosexuality.

CBT therapists help clients to learn how to adapt more realistic beliefs about their life, sexuality, and others using techniques such as thought records or Socratic dialogue.

When working with families whose children are coming out, Willougby and Doty (2010) adapted Datillo's (2005) work to help the family adjust. In their case study, they began working with the parents for four sessions without the child present in order to identify schemas and automatic thoughts that were triggered by the child's coming out. In addition, the CBFT therapist invited the parents to explore expectations and attributions about being gay or lesbian from their parents and families of origin. In the second and later sessions, the therapist challenged the parents' negative beliefs about sexual orientation. In the third and fourth session, the therapist made direct suggestions for alternative behaviors. Finally, in fifth and sixth sessions, the therapist invited the child in to facilitate more effective communication with the parents.

Research and the Evidence Base

Because CBFT's conceptual home is in experimental psychology, research is part of its culture; therefore, CBFT therapies are some of the best-researched approaches in family therapy. More individually focused CBT along with CBFTs are the most frequently listed evidence-based approach in the Substance Abuse and Mental Health Services Administration Registry of Evidenced-Based Practices (www.nrepp.samhsa.gov)—high on the list for individual issues such as depression and anxiety.

Over the years, CBFT theorists have modified their approach—sometimes dramatically—on the basis of research outcomes to incorporate more affective and relational components. Behavioral couples therapy is the premier example of this trend. Because of good short-term but poor long-term outcomes, Jacobson and Christensen (1996) reformulated their couples therapy to include more affective aspects; the new approach is called *integrative behavioral couples therapy.* Similarly, because research indicates that a nonjudgmental therapeutic alliance is crucial, CBFT therapists have become increasingly attentive to this aspect of therapy (Beck, 2005).

Although CBFT has an extensive research history, therapists should not assume that it is therefore superior to other approaches in every case or even in general. As discussed in Chapter 2, when confounding factors such as researcher allegiance are controlled for, no therapy is consistently found to be superior to any other (Sprenkle & Blow, 2004). Furthermore, for certain issues, such as adolescent conduct, systemic approaches have been found to be superior to CBT (see Chapter 4). Finally, many therapists have critiqued CBT because its claims to superiority have more to do with the volume of research by CBT proponents than any substantive advantage (Loewenthal & House, 2010). Along those lines, Miller (2012) reports that a massive effort to transform all mental health in Sweden to CBT resulted in no effect on overall outcome of those diagnosed with depression and anxiety, with over 25% dropping out of treatment; in addition, a significant number of these clients who were not considered disabled prior to treatment *became* disabled, costing the government more money. The Swedish government soon ended its attempt to systematically institute CBT, instead encouraging new approaches. Thus, although CBT does have the most extensive evidence base in the field, it is by no means a panacea and has by no means provided a simple answer the question of what works best in therapy.

QUESTIONS FOR PERSONAL REFLECTION AND CLASS DISCUSSION

1. CBFT therapists take a more directive and expert position. What are the strengths and limitations of such a stance? How might client gender, race, ethnicity, or sexual/gender orientation affect this dynamic?

2. CBFT therapists do a detailed analysis of how couple and family behaviors, cognitions, and emotions mutually reinforce each other. How is this similar to or different from other systemic approaches?

3. Identify some expectations and standards from your family of origin. With which of these do agree? With which do you not agree? Have you enacted any expectations in your own life or relationships that surprised you?

4. Do you think "training" couples to communicate or problem-solve better is useful? Why or why not? Can there be one right way?

5. Do you think mindfulness is a realistic practice for most couples or families? Why or why not?

6. One of the couples approaches with the best-documented outcomes, IBCT focuses on increasing acceptance and tolerance of one's partner and the differences between partners. Why do you think this approach works?

7. Marriages in which men who do not accept influence from their wives have an 80% chance of divorce. Why do you think this is? Why do you think some men do not accept influence from their wives?

8. CBFT has one of the most robust evidence bases of any couple or family therapy. Why do you think this is? Do you think these approaches are significantly different from others in this text? Why or why not?

ONLINE RESOURCES

Frank Dattilio
www.dattilio.com

Gottman Relationship Institute
www.gottman.com

Integrative Behavioral Couples Therapy
http://ibct.psych.ucla.edu

Oregon Social Learning Center: Patterson and Forgatch Parenting Program
www.oslc.org

OurRelationship: Online Couples Therapy Module
www.ourrelationship.com

Substance Abuse and Mental Health Services Administration National

Registry of Evidenced-Based Programs and Practices
www.nrepp.samhsa.gov

UCLA Mindfulness Awareness Research Center
www.marc.ucla.edu

UMass Center for Mindfulness: Jon Kabat-Zinn
www.umassmed.edu/cfm/mbsr

Go to MindTap® for an eBook, videos of client sessions, activities, practice quizzes, apps, and more—all in one place. If your instructor didn't assign MindTap, you can find out more information at CengageBrain.com.

REFERENCES

*Asterisk indicates recommended introductory readings.

Baer, R. A. (2003). Mindfulness training as a clinical intervention: A conceptual and empirical review. *Clinical Psychology: Science and Practice, 10*(2), 125–143.

Barnes, S., Brown, K. W., Krusemark, E., Campbell, W. K., & Rogge, R. D. (2008). The role of mindfulness in romantic relationship satisfaction and responses to relationship stress. *Journal of Marital and Family Therapy, 33,* 482–500.

Baucom, D. H., Epstein, N. B., Kirby, J. S., & LaTaillade, J. J. (2015). Cognitive-behavioral couple therapy. In A. S. Gurman, J. L. Lebow, D. K. Snyder, (Eds.), *Clinical handbook of couple therapy* (5th ed.) (pp. 23–60). New York: Guilford.

Baucom, D., Epstein, N., Sayers, S., & Sher, T. (1989). The role of cognitions in marital relationships: Definitional methodological, and conceptual issues. *Journal of Family Psychology, 10,* 72–88.

Baucom, K. J. W., Sevier, M., Eldridge, K. A., Doss, B. D., & Christensen, A. (2011). Observed communication in couples 2 years after integrative and traditional behavioral couple therapy: Outcome and link with 5-year follow-up. *Journal of Consulting and Clinical Psychology, 79,* 565–576.

Beck, A. T. (1976). *Cognitive therapy and the emotional disorders.* New York: International Universities Press.

*Beck, A. T. (1988). *Love is never enough.* New York: Harper & Row.

*Beck, J. (2005). *Cognitive therapy for challenging problems: What to do when the basic don't work.* New York: Guilford.

Berg-Cross, L., Jennings, P., & Baruch, R. (1990). Cinematherapy: Theory and application. *Psychotherapy in Private Practice, 8,* 135–157.

Block-Lerner, J., Adair, C., Plumb, J. C., Rhatigan, D. L., & Orsillo, S. M. (2008). The case for mindfulness-based approaches in the cultivation of empathy: Does nonjudgmental, present-moment awareness increase capacity for perspective-taking and empathic concern? *Journal of Marital and Family Therapy, 33,* 501–516.

Carson, J. W., Carson, K. M., Gil, K. M., & Baucom, D. H. (2004). Mindfulness-based relationship enhancement. *Behavior Therapy, 35*(3), 471–494. doi: 10.1016/S0005-7894(04)80028-5

Carson, J. W., Carson, K. M., Gil, K. M., & Baucom, D. H. (2008). Self expansion as a mediator of relationship improvements in a mindfulness intervention. *Journal of Marital and Family Therapy, 33,* 517–526.

Christensen, A., Dimidjian, S., & Martell, C. R. (2015). Integrative behavioral couple therapy. In A. S. Gurman, J. L. Lebow, D. K. Snyder, A. S. Gurman (Eds.), *Clinical handbook of couple therapy* (5th ed.) (pp. 61–94). New York: Guilford.

*Dattilio, F. M. (2010). *Cognitive-behavioral therapy with couples and families: A comprehensive guide for clinicians.* New York: Guilford.

*Dattilio, F. M. (2005). Restructuring family schemas: A cognitive-behavioral perspective. *Journal of Marital and Family Therapy, 31,* 15–30.

DeMaria, R., & Hannah, M. (2002). *Building intimate relationships: Bridging treatment, education and enrichment through the PAIRS Program.* New York: Brunner/Routledge.

DeRosier, M. E., & Gilliom, M. (2007). Effectiveness of a parent training program for improving children's social behavior. *Journal of Child and Family Studies, 16,* 660–670.

Doss, B. D., Benson, L. A., Georgia, E. J., & Christensen, A. (2013). Translation of integrative behavioral couple therapy to a web-based intervention. *Family Process, 52,* 139–152.

Doss, B. D., Cicila, L. N., Georgia, E. J., Roddy, M. K., Nowlan, K. M., Benson, L. A., & Christensen, A. (2016). A randomized controlled trial of the web-based OurRelationship program: Effects on relationship and individual functioning. *Journal or Consulting and Clinical Psychology, 84,* 285–296.

Duarté-Vélez, Y., Bernal, G., & Bonilla, K. (2010). Culturally adapted cognitive-behavioral therapy: Integrating sexual, spiritual, and family identities in an evidence-based treatment of a depressed Latino adolescent. *Journal of Clinical Psychology, 66*(8), 895–906. doi:10.1002/jclp.20710

Dumas, J. E. (2005). Mindfulness-based parent training: Strategies to lessen the grip of automaticity in families with disruptive children. *Journal of Clinical Child and Adolescent Psychology, 34*(4), 779–791. doi:10.1207/s15374424jccp3404_20

Duncan, L. G., & Bardacke, N. (2010). Mindfulness-based childbirth and parenting education: Promoting family mindfulness during the perinatal period. *Journal of Child and Family Studies, 19*(2), 190–202. doi:10.1007/s10826-009-9313-7

Duncan, L. G., Coatsworth, J., & Greenberg, M. T. (2009). A model of mindful parenting: Implications for parent–child relationships and prevention research. *Clinical Child and Family Psychology Review, 12*(3), 255–270. doi:10.1007/s10567-009-0046-3

Dutton, D. G., & Corvo, C. (2006). Transforming a flawed policy: A call to revive psychology and science in domestic violence research and practice. *Aggression and Violent Behavior, 11,* 457–483.

Dutton, D. G., & Corvo, C. (2007). The Duluth Model: A data-impervious paradigm and a failed strategy. *Aggression and Violent Behavior, 12,* 658–667.

Ellis, A. (1962). *Reason and emotion in psychotherapy.* New York: Stuart.

Ellis, A. (1978). Family therapy: A phenomenological and active-directive approach. *Journal of Marriage and Family Counseling, 4,* 43–50.

Ellis, A. (1994). Rational-emotive behavior marriage and family therapy. In A. M. Horne (Ed.), *Family counseling and therapy* (pp. 489–514). San Francisco, CA: Peacock.

Epstein, N. (1982). Cognitive therapy with couples. *American Journal of Family Therapy, 10,* 5–16.

Epstein, N., & Baucom, D. (2002). *Enhanced cognitive-behavioral therapy for couples: A contextual approach.* Washington, DC: American Psychological Association.

Epstein, N., Chen, F., & Beyder-Kamjou, I. (2005). Relationship standards and marital satisfaction in Chinese and American couples. *Journal of Marital and Family Therapy, 31,* 59–74.

Epstein, N. B., Dattilio, F. M., & Baucom, D. H. (2016). Cognitive-behavior couple therapy. In T. L. Sexton, J. Lebow, (Eds.) , *Handbook of family therapy* (pp. 361–386). New York: Routledge/Taylor & Francis.

Epstein, N., Schlesinger, S., & Dryden, W. (1988). *Cognitive-behavioral therapy with families.* New York: Brunner/Mazel.

*Falloon, I. R. H. (Ed.). (1988). *Handbook of behavioral family therapy.* New York: Guilford.

Falloon, I. R. H. (1991). Behavioral family therapy. In A. S. Gurman & D. P. Kniskern (Eds.), *Handbook of family therapy* (vol. 2, pp. 65–95). Philadelphia, PA: Brunner/Mazel.

Freeman, A., Epstein, N., & Simon, K. (1987). *Depression in the family.* New York: Routledge.

Gehart, D. (2012). *Mindfulness and acceptance in couple and family therapy.* New York: Springer.

Gehart, D. R., & Lyle, R. R. (2001). Client experience of gender in therapeutic relationships: An interpretive ethnography. *Family Process, 40,* 443–458.

*Gehart, D., & McCollum, E. (2007). Engaging suffering: Towards a mindful re-visioning of marriage and family therapy practice. *Journal of Marital and Family Therapy, 33,* 214–226.

Gehart, D., & McCollum, E. (2008). Teaching therapeutic presence: A mindfulness-based approach. In S. Hicks (Ed.), *Mindfulness and the healing relationship.* New York: Guilford.

Glassgold, J. M. (2009). The case of Felix: An example of gay-affirmative, cognitive-behavioral therapy. *Pragmatic Case Studies in Psychotherapy, 5*(4), 1–21.

González-Prendes, A., Hindo, C., & Pardo, Y. (2011). Cultural values integration in cognitive-behavioral therapy for a Latino with depression. *Clinical Case Studies, 10*(5), 376–394. doi: 10.1177/1534650111427075

*Gottman, J. M. (1999). *The marriage clinic: A scientifically based marital therapy.* New York: Norton.

Gottman, J. M. (2002). *The seven principles for making marriage work.* New York: Three Rivers.

Gottman, J. M. (2011). *The science of trust.* New York: Norton.

Gottman, J. M., & Gottman, J. S. (2008). *And baby makes three.* New York: Three Rivers.

Guerney, B. G. (1987). *Relationship enhancement manual.* Bethesda, MD: Ideal.

Halford, W. K., Markman, H. J., Stanley, S., & Kline, G. H. (2002). Relationship enhancement. In D. Sprenkle (Ed.), *Effectiveness research in marriage and family therapy* (pp. 191–222). Alexandria, VA: American Association for Marriage and Family Therapy.

Hayes, S. C. (2004). Acceptance and commitment therapy, relational frame theory, and the third wave of behavioral and cognitive therapies. *Behavior Therapy, 35*(4), 639–665. doi:10.1016/S0005-7894(04)80013-3

Hayes, S. C., & Smith, S. (2005). *Get out of your mind and into your life.* Oakland, CA: New Harbinger.

*Hayes, S. C., Strosahl, K. D., & Wilson, K. G. (1999). *Acceptance and commitment therapy: An experiential approach to behavior change.* New York: Guilford.

Holtzworth-Munroe, A., & Jacobson, N. S. (1991). Behavioral marital therapy. In A. S. Gurman & D. P. Kniskern (Eds.), *Handbook of family therapy* (vol. 2, pp. 96–133). Philadelphia, PA: Brunner/Mazel.

Holtzworth-Munroe, A., & Stuart, G. L. (1994). Typologies of male batterers: Three subtypes and the differences among them. *Psychological Bulletin, 116,* 476–497.

Hooley, J. M., Rosen, L. R., & Richters, J. E. (1995). Expressed emotion: Toward clarification of a critical construct. In G. A. Miller (Ed.), *The behavioral high-risk paradigm in psychopathology* (pp. 88–120). New York: Springer.

Hwang, W., Wood, J. J., Lin, K., & Cheung, F. (2006). Cognitive-behavioral therapy with Chinese Americans: Research, theory, and clinical practice. *Cognitive and Behavioral Practice, 13,* 293–303.

Jacobson, N. S., & Addis, M. E. (1993). Research on couples and couples therapy: What do we know? Where are we going? *Journal of Consulting and Clinical Psychology, 57,* 5–10.

*Jacobson, N. S., & Christensen, A. (1996). *Integrative couple therapy.* New York: Norton.

Jenkins, A. (1990). *Invitations to responsibility: The therapeutic engagement of men who are violent and abusive.* Adelaide, Australia: Dulwich Centre.

Kabat-Zinn, J. (1990). *Full catastrophe living: Using the wisdom of your body and mind to face stress, pain, and illness.* New York: Delta.

Keating, T. (2006). *Open mind open heart: The contemplative dimension of the gospel.* New York: Continuum International.

Kelly, S. (2006). Cognitive-behavioral therapy with African Americans. In P. A. Hays & G. Y. Iwamasa (Eds.), *Culturally responsive cognitive-behavioral therapy: Assessment, practice, and supervision* (pp. 97–116). Washington, DC: American Psychological Association. doi:10.1037/11433-004

Kaslow, N., Broth, M., Smith, C., & Collins, M. (2012). Family-based interventions for child and adolescent disorders. *Journal of Marital and Family Therapy, 38,* 82–100.

*Linehan, M. M. (1993). *Cognitive-behavioral treatment of borderline personality disorder.* New York: Guilford.

Lebow, J., Chambers, A., Christensen, A., & Johnson, S. (2012). Research on the treatment of couple distress. *Journal of Marital and Family Therapy, 38,* 145–168.

Lipchik, E., & Kubicki, A. (1996). Solution-focused domestic violence views: Bridges toward a new reality in couples therapy. In S. D. Miller, M. A. Hubble, & B. L. Duncan (Eds.), *Handbook of solution-focused brief therapy* (pp. 65–97). San Francisco, CA: Jossey-Bass.

Loewenthal, D. & House, R. (2010). *Critically engaging CBT.* Berkshire, UK: Open University Press.

Luckstead, A., McFarlane, W., Downing, D., & Dixon L. (2012). Recent developments in family psychoeducation as an evidence-based practice. *Journal of Marital and Family Therapy, 38,* 101–121.

Marchand, E., Ng, J., Rohde, P., & Stice, E. (2010). Effects of an indicated cognitive-behavioral depression prevention program are similar for Asian American, Latino, and European American adolescents. *Behaviour Research and Therapy, 48*(8), 821–825. doi:10.1016/j.brat.2010.05.005

Markman, H., & Rhoades, G. (2012). Relationship education research: Current status and future directions. *Journal of Marital and Family Therapy, 38,* 169–200.

Markman, H., Stanley, S., & Blumberg, S. (2001). *Fighting for your marriage.* San Francisco, CA: Wiley.

McCollum, E. E. (2015). *Mindfulness for therapists: Practice for the heart.* New York: Routledge/Taylor & Francis.

McCollum, E., & Gehart, D. (2010). Using mindfulness to teach therapeutic presence: A qualitative outcome study of a mindfulness-based curriculum for teaching therapeutic presence to master's level marriage and family therapy trainees. *Journal of Marital and Family Therapy, 36,* 347–360. doi: 10.1111/j.1752-0606.2010.00214.x

McFarlane, W. R., Dixon, L., Lukens, E., & Luckstead, A. (2002). Severe mental illness. In D. Sprenkle (Ed.), *Effectiveness research in marriage and family therapy* (pp. 255–288). Alexandria, VA: American Association for Marriage and Family Therapy.

McNair, L. D. (1996). African American women and behavior therapy: Integrating theory, culture, and clinical practice. *Cognitive and Behavioral Practice, 3*(2), 337–349. doi:10.1016/ S1077-7229(96)80022-8

Meichenbaum, D. (1997). The evolution of a cognitive-behavior therapist. In J. K. Zeig (Ed.) *The evolution of psychotherapy: Third conference* (pp. 95–106). New York: Brunner/Mazel.

Miller, S. (2012, May 12). Revolution in Swedish mental health practice: The cognitive behavioral therapy monopoly gives way. Retrieved from www.scott-miller.com/?q=node%F160.

Miller, S. L., Nunnally, E. W., & Wackman, D. B. (1976). A communication training program for couples. *Social Casework, 57,* 9–18.

Milner, J., & Singleton, T. (2008). Domestic violence: Solution-focused practice with men and women who are violent. *Journal of Family Therapy, 30*(1), 29–53.

Mylott, K. (1994). Twelve irrational ideas that drive gay men and women crazy. *Journal of Rational-Emotive & Cognitive Behavior Therapy, 12*(1), 61–71. doi:10.1007/BF02354490

Organista, K. C., & Muñoz, R. F. (1996). Cognitive behavioral therapy with Latinos. *Cognitive and Behavioral Practice, 3*(2), 255–270. doi:10.1016/ S1077-7229(96)80017-4

Patterson, G., & Forgatch, M. (1987). *Parents and adolescents: Living together: Part 1: The Basics.* Eugene, OR: Castalia.

Pavlov, I. P. (1932). Neuroses in man and animals. *Journal of the American Medical Association, 99,* 1012–1013.

Pedersen, P. B., Draguns, J. G., Lonner, W. J., & Trimble, J. E. (Eds.). (2002). *Counseling across cultures* (5th ed.) Thousand Oaks, CA: Sage.

Pence, E., & Paymar, M. (1993). *Education groups for men who batter: The Duluth Model.* New York: Springer.

Piedra, L. M., & Byoun, S. (2012). Vida Alegre: Preliminary findings of a depression intervention for immigrant Latino mothers. *Research on Social Work Practice, 22*(2), 138–150. doi: 10.1177/1049731511424168

Rogers, Carl. (1961). *On becoming a person: A therapist's view of psychotherapy.* London: Constable.

Safren, S. A., Hollander, G., Hart, T. A., & Heimberg, R. G. (2001). Cognitive-behavioral therapy with lesbian, gay, and bisexual youth. *Cognitive and Behavioral Practice, 8*(3), 215–223. doi:10.1016/S1077-7229(01)80056-0

Safren, S. A., & Rogers, T. (2001). Cognitive-behavioral therapy with gay, lesbian, and bisexual clients. *Journal of Clinical Psychology, 57*(5), 629–643. doi:10.1002 /jclp.1033

Segal, Z. V., Williams, J. G., & Teasdale, J. D. (2002). *Mindfulness-based cognitive therapy for depression: A new approach to preventing relapse.* New York: Guilford.

Siegel, D. & Bayne, T. (2012). *The whole-brain child.* New York: Bantam.

Skinner, B. F. (1953). *Science and human behavior.* New York: MacMillan.

Singh, N. N., Lancioni, G. E., Joy, S., Winton, A. W., Sabaawi, M., Wahler, R. G., & Singh, J. (2007). Adolescents with conduct disorder can be mindful of their aggressive behavior. *Journal of Emotional and Behavioral Disorders, 15*(1), 56–63. doi: 10.1177/10634266070150010601

Sprenkle, D. H., & Blow, A. J. (2004). Common factors and our sacred models. *Journal of Marital and Family Therapy, 30,* 113–129.

Stahl, B., & Goldstein, B. (2010). *A mindfulness-based stress reduction workbook.* New York: New Harbinger.

Stith, S., McCollum, E., Amanor-Boadu, Y., & Smith, D. (2012). Systemic perspectives on intimate partner violence treatment. *Journal of Marital and Family Therapy, 38,* 220–240.

Stith, S. M., McCollum, E. E., Rosen, K. H., & Locke, L. D. (2002). Multicouple group treatment for domestic violence. In F. Kaslow (Ed.), *Comprehensive textbook of psychotherapy* (vol. 4). New York: Wiley.

Stith, S. M., Rosen, K. H., & McCollum, E. E. (2002). Domestic violence. In D. Sprenkle (Ed.), *Effectiveness research in marriage and family therapy* (pp. 223–254). Alexandria, VA: American Association for Marriage and Family Therapy.

Teasdale, J. D., Segal, Z. V., & Williams, J. M. C. (1995). How does cognitive therapy prevent depressive relapse and why should attentional control (mindfulness) help? *Behaviour Research and Therapy, 33,* 25–39.

Tomm, K., St. George, S., Wulff, D., & Strong, T. (2014). *Patterns in interpersonal interactions: Inviting relational understandings for therapeutic change.* New York: Routledge.

van den Hoofdakker, B. J., van der Veen-Mulders, L., & Sytema, S. (2007). Effectiveness of behavioral parent training for children with ADHD in routine clinical practice: A randomized controlled study. *Journal of the American Academy of Child and Adolescent Psychiatry, 46,* 1263–1271.

Wachs, K., & Cordova, J. V. (2008). Mindful relating: Exploring mindfulness and emotional repertoires in intimate relationships. *Journal of Marital and Family Therapy, 33,* 464–481.

Walker, Lenore E. (1979). *The battered woman.* New York: Harper & Row.

Willougby, B.L.B, & Doty, N.D. (2010). Brief cognitive behavioral family therapy following a child's coming out: A case report. *Cognitive and Behavioral Practice, 17*(1), 37–44. doi:10.1016/j.cbpra.2009.04.006

Walling, S., Suvak, M. K., Howard, J. M., Taft, C. T., & Murphy, C. M. (2012). Race/ethnicity as a predictor of change in working alliance during cognitive behavioral therapy for intimate partner violence perpetrators. *Psychotherapy, 49*(2), 180–189. doi:10.1037/a0025751

Zylowska, L. L., Smalley, S. L., & Schwartz, J. M. (2009). Mindful awareness and ADHD. In F. Didonna (Ed.), *Clinical handbook of mindfulness* (pp. 319–338). New York: Springer. doi:10.1007/978-0-387-09593-6_18

Cognitive–Behavioral Case Study: ADHD and Blended Family

Diamond and Tom are seeking counseling for their seven-year-old son Albert, who was just diagnosed with ADHD. They have been married for six years, and each has children from a prior marriage. Diamond has two daughters from her prior marriage, Sharie (14) and Debbie (10), and Tom has a son from a former relationship, Desmond (10). The couple report reluctantly agreeing to put Albert on medications at the doctor's recommendation, but that they would like to find a better solution. They report that he is hyperactive at home and does not follow directions; he also has similar problems at school that have led to lower grades than they expect. They report the household as "hectic," with Diamond and Tom both working long, odd hours and Albert's siblings in and out of the house to visit with their other parents.

After meeting with the family, a cognitive–behavioral family therapist developed the following case conceptualization.

COGNITIVE–BEHAVIORAL FAMILY THERAPY CASE CONCEPTUALIZATION

For use with individual, couple, or family clients.

Date: 6/22/16   **Clinician:** Sally Wright   **Client #:** 8007

Introduction to Client & Significant Others

Identify significant persons in client's relational/family life who will be mentioned in case conceptualization:

Adults/Parents: Select identifier/abbreviation for use in rest of case conceptualization

AF1: Female   Age: 34   African American   Occupation: Hairstylist   Other:

AM1: Male   Age: 40   African American/Native American   Occupation: Owns remodeling business
Other identifier:

Children/Adult Children: Select identifier/abbreviation for use in rest of case conceptualization

CF14: Age: 14   African American   Grade: 9 Other: Daughter of AF; Visits bio dad on weekends; honor student; track

CF10: Age: 10   African American   Grade: 5   Other: Daughter of AF; Visits biological Dad on weekends; dance/cheer

CM10: Age: 10   African American   Grade: 5 Other: Son of AM Lives with Mom 60% of time

CM 7: Age: 7   African American   Grade: 2 Other: Identified patient; only biological son of AF1 and AM1

Background Information

Trauma/Abuse History (recent and past): AF was sexually abused as a child by her brother. AF had a highly conflictual divorce with her former husband.

Substance Use/Abuse (current and past; self, family of origin, significant others): No history reported.

Precipitating Events (recent life changes, first symptoms, stressors, etc.): AF34 and AM40 report that CM7 was always an active, energetic child who was difficult to parent. Since starting first grade, things have been difficult: frequent notes and calls from the teacher about his disruptive behavior and his grades have been inconsistent. His teacher requested they take him to the doctor to be evaluated for ADHD because he was in danger of not passing the second grade. CF14 is in charge of helping him with his homework and typically watches him in the afternoons; CF10 keeps busy with her activities.

Related Historical Background (family history, related issues, previous counseling, medical/mental health history, etc.): AF34 and AM40 married six years ago, after she got pregnant with CM7. AF34 had two children from a prior marriage, ages 14 and 10, and she has a conflictual relationship with their father whom she rarely tries to speak with; the children visit him every other weekend. AM40 has a 10-year-old son from a prior relationship and has physical custody 40% of the time.

(continued)

Functional Analysis of Problem Interactional Patterns

Primary Problem Interaction Pattern (PIPs; A ⇆ B): *Describe dynamic of primary PIP:*

Pursuing/Distancing Criticizing/Defending Controlling/Resisting X Other: <u>Good/bad parent</u>

Describe each person's observable behavior at the start of tension: <u>CM7 and CM10 start fighting over</u> <u>video game, CF10 and CF14 leave the room.</u>

Describe each person's observable behavior during conflict/symptom escalation: <u>AF34 tells them to</u> <u>stop arguing; they ignore her; she then puts them on a time-out; they sneak away before it should be</u> <u>over and go to the garage to help dad on project. When AF34 finds them there, she gives AM40 "the</u> <u>look" and tells him that they were supposed to be on time-out; AM40 takes children's side by saying that</u> <u>they are doing fine now and getting along.</u>

Describe each person's observable behavior at the return to "normal"/homeostasis: <u>AF34 backs</u> <u>down because the boys do seem to be behaving and AM40 has them doing something productive.</u>

- Frequency of PIP: 1–3 times per week
- Duration of PIP: 15 minutes
- Severity of PIP: 5/10
- Triggers of PIP: Conflict between boys; not getting what they want
- Consequences/Reinforcements of PIP: AM provides leniency; AF acquiesces to AM

Neurobiological Dynamics: Describe when and how the stress response is triggered for each during PIP:
Typical triggers of stress response for each person involved in PIP:
AM: Particular look or tone from AF; AF asking for him to do things.
AF: Kids bickering; AM not supporting her; AM not following through on tasks.
CF14 and CF10: Not often involved in the dynamic; but CF14 can have similar dynamic with mother
CM10: Not getting what he wants; having to deal with CM7
CM7: Not getting what he wants; being told no; being told to focus on task
Typical behaviors when stress response is triggered:
AM: Defensiveness toward AF
AF: Backing down to AM; walling self off; yelling at AM or kids
CM10: Disobeying; yelling; ignoring
CM7: Disobeying; tantrum; running away
What helps each to calm down once stress response is triggered:
AM: When AF does not push issue; when he can return focus to a project, TV, or something of interest
AF: Focusing on something else, usually household tasks
CM10: Playing video game; new activity; going to room alone
CM7: Parents helping to calm him down; quiet space; video game.

Functional Analysis: Role of the Symptom

Identify mutually reinforcing behaviors that sustain symptom:

- How does this specific problem handicap this person, couple, and/or family in everyday life? <u>CM7</u> <u>experiences difficulty at home and school; conflict in the house; parents are divided; CM10 and CF10</u> <u>often feel ignored.</u>

- What would happen if the problem were reduced in frequency? <u>CM7 would have greater success at school; less conflict at home; AF and AM would feel they are on same team; other siblings will likely feel they get equal attention and that there is less favoritism.</u>

- What would this person (and his or her family) gain if the problem were resolved? <u>CM7 would be able to perform better at school in terms of his grades and he would be more cooperative at home; more relaxed at home; kids would play more together; couple would support each other.</u>

- Who (or what) reinforces the problem with attention, sympathy, and support? <u>AM not backing AF with setting limits with the kids. Parents feeling guilty due to blended family issues.</u>

- Under what circumstances is the specific problem reduced in intensity? <u>CM7 does homework well in quiet area with someone helping him through each step. Kids do better if parents are there when conflict starts or when CF14 is around.</u>

- Under what circumstances is the specific problem increased in intensity? <u>AF setting harsh consequences; anyone yelling.</u>

- What do family members currently do to cope with the problem? <u>Attend church; AM tries to minimize conflict by redirecting kids.</u>

- What are the assets of the family as a problem-solving unit? <u>Both families of origins are generally close and supportive. School is supportive; CF14 is usually a positive influence.</u>

- Deficits? <u>Adjusting to blended family; parents do not have effective strategy for managing children's behaviors. More structure would be good for CM7.</u>

- What behaviors need to increase? <u>Consistent parenting; kids being more cooperative, doing homework in a quiet area with someone helping CM7 through each step.</u>

- Decrease? <u>Kids fighting over video games; CM7 attention at school; AF setting harsh consequences; AM being too lenient with kids and undermining AF when limits are set.</u>

Expectations and Standards

Describe the following for the client(s):

Selective perceptions of significant others: <u>Both AF and AM see the other as not doing a good job parenting. AF sees AM as being too lenient and AM sees AF as being too strict.</u>

Character attributions to significant others: <u>AM thinks AF is too serious and pushes everyone too hard. AF sees AM as not caring and lazy. CF14 and CM10 think CF7 is being babied and favored.</u>

Expectancies of significant others: <u>AF expects AM to support her and help out more around the house and with children. AM thinks AF should take his views into consideration more.</u>

Assumptions about significant others: <u>AF assumes AM should have her same set of expectations. AM assumes AF should readily agree with him.</u>

(continued)

Expectations and Standards (continued)

Standards for significant others: <u>AF has high standards for the children's performance at school and home; AM wants to see children enjoy themselves and have fun.</u>

Describe any expectations or standards related to the presenting issue that are derived from the client's social location, including ethnic, gender, socioeconomic, sexual orientation, and other relevant contexts: <u>African-American women are often seen as the strength of the family and often take on most of the burden of running a household and raising the children; AF seems to be assuming this pattern. AM reports that his desire to be lenient with the children at times come from an awareness of the challenges and marginalization they will encounter as black males. AF has similar concerns, but sees having high expectations for them as the answer.</u>

Cognitions about Couples and Families

Identify cognitive distortions in automatic thoughts and beliefs for client(s); provide examples:

☐ Arbitrary inference:

☒ Selective abstraction: <u>AF and AM focus on what each other is doing wrong ; everyone focuses on CM7's ADHD behaviors.</u>

☒ Overgeneralization: <u>AF and AM overgeneralize about the support they receive from the other.</u>

☐ Magnification and minimization:

☒ Personalization: <u>AF personalizes CM7's behavior when they are in public; believes it means she is a bad mother.</u>

☐ Dichotomous thinking:

☐ Mislabeling:

☐ Mind reading:

Self and Family Schemas

Describe schemas for client(s) underlying problem interaction pattern or other high affect situation; for more than one client, list out schemas for each.

- Schemas about self (e.g., worth, needs, shoulds, roles, etc.):
  AF: I must prove myself to be worthy to be loved.
  AM: I need to be appreciated and respected for what I do.
  CF14: I must succeed to be loved.
  CF10: I need people to see me.
  CM10: I need others to like me.
  CM7: Something is wrong with me.

- Schemas about others (e.g., expectations, shoulds, valuing of, role of, etc.):
  In relationships, people should not argue. (AM, AF)
  In relationships, the man should be in charge. (AM; in some aspects AF)
  Parents are at fault when children are poorly behaved. (AF)

- Schemas about life (e.g., good/bad, optimistic/pessimistic, safe/unsafe, etc.):
  The world/life is not fair, especially with regard to race. (AF, AM)
  You have to work hard to make it in life. (AF, AM)
  Safety comes from predictability. (AF)

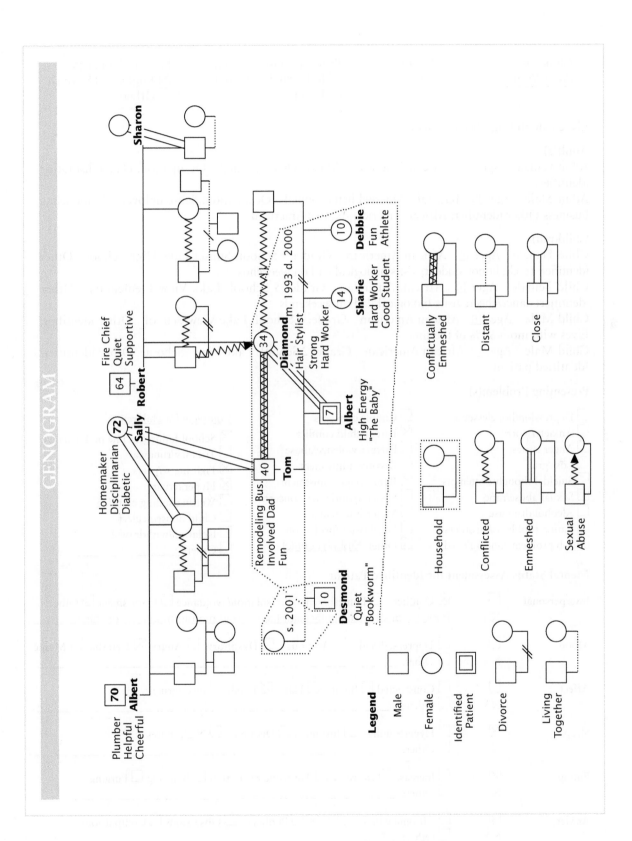

GENOGRAM

Albert
70
Plumber
Helpful
Cheerful

Sally
72
Homemaker
Disciplinarian
Diabetic

Robert
64
Fire Chief
Quiet
Supportive

Sharon

Tom
40
Remodeling Bus.
Involved Dad
Fun

Diamond
34
m. 1993 d. 2000
Hair Stylist
Strong
Hard Worker

Desmond
10
Quiet
"Bookworm"

Albert
7
High Energy
"The Baby"

Sharie
14
Hard Worker
Good Student

Debbie
10
Fun
Athlete

s. 2001

Conflictually
Enmeshed

Distant

Close

Household

Conflicted

Enmeshed

Sexual
Abuse

Legend

Male

Female

Identified
Patient

Divorce

Living
Together

CLINICAL ASSESSMENT

Clinician: Sally Wright	Client ID #: 8007	Primary configuration: ☐ Individual ☐ Couple ☒ Family	Primary Language: ☒ English ☐ Spanish ☐ Other:

List client and significant others

Adult(s)

Adult Female   Age: 34   African American   Married heterosexual   Occupation: Hairstylist Other identifier:

Adult Male   Age: 40   Biracial   Married heterosexual   Occupation: Self-employed—Remodeling business Other identifier: African American/Native American

Child(ren)

Child Female   Age: 14   African American   Grade: 9 School: Sunset Hills High School   Other identifier: track; honor student; visits biological dad on weekends

Child Female   Age: 10   African American   Grade: 5 School: Lake View Elementary   Other identifier: dance/cheer; visits biological dad on weekends

Child Male   Age: 10   African American   Grade: 5 School: Lake View School   Other identifier: Lives with mom 60% of the time

Child Male   Age: 7   African American   Grade: 2 School: Lake View School   Other identifier: Identified patient

Presenting Problem(s)

☐ Depression/hopelessness
☐ Anxiety/worry
☐ Anger issues
☐ Loss/grief
☐ Suicidal thoughts/attempts
☐ Sexual abuse/rape
☐ Alcohol/drug use
☐ Eating problems/disorders
☐ Job problems/unemployed

☐ Couple concerns
☒ Parent/child conflict
☐ Partner violence/abuse
☐ Divorce adjustment
☒ Remarriage adjustment
☐ Sexuality/intimacy concerns
☐ Major life changes
☐ Legal issues/probation
☒ Other: Sibling conflict

Complete for children:
☒ School failure/decline performance
☐ Truancy/runaway
☒ Fighting w/peers
☒ Hyperactivity
☐ Wetting/soiling clothing
☐ Child abuse/neglect
☐ Isolation/withdrawal
☐ Other: _____

Mental Status Assessment for Identified Patient

Interpersonal	☐ NA	☒ Conflict ☐ Enmeshment ☐ Isolation/avoidance ☐ Harassment ☒ Other: Poor social skills; difficulty establishing and maintaining relationships
Mood	☐ NA	☐ Depressed/Sad ☐ Anxious ☐ Dysphoric ☐ Angry ☒ Irritable ☐ Manic ☐ Other: _____
Affect	☐ NA	☐ Constricted ☐ Blunt ☐ Flat ☒ Labile ☐ Incongruent ☐ Other: _____
Sleep	☒ NA	☐ Hypersomnia ☐ Insomnia ☐ Disrupted ☐ Nightmares ☐ Other: _____
Eating	☒ NA	☐ Increase ☐ Decrease ☐ Anorectic restriction ☐ Bingeing ☐ Purging ☐ Other: _____
Anxiety	☒ NA	☐ Chronic worry ☐ Panic ☐ Phobias ☐ Obsessions ☐ Compulsions ☐ Other: _____

Trauma symptoms	☒ NA	☐ Hypervigilance ☐ Flashbacks/Intrusive memories ☐ Dissociation ☐ Numbing ☐ Avoidance efforts ☐ Other: _____
Psychotic symptoms	☒ NA	☐ Hallucinations ☐ Delusions ☐ Paranoia ☐ Loose associations ☐ Other: _____
Motor activity/ Speech	☐ NA	☐ Low energy ☒ Hyperactive ☐ Agitated ☒ Inattentive ☒ Impulsive ☐ Pressured speech ☐ Slow speech ☐ Other: _____
Thought	☐ NA	☒ Poor concentration ☐ Denial ☒ Self-blame ☐ Other-blame ☐ Ruminative ☒ Tangential ☐ Concrete ☐ Poor insight ☒ Impaired decision making ☐ Disoriented ☐ Other: _____
Sociolegal	☐ NA	☐ Disregards rules ☐ Defiant ☐ Stealing ☐ Lying ☐ Tantrums ☐ Arrest/incarceration ☒ Initiates fights ☐ Other: _____
Other Symptoms	☒ NA	_____

Diagnosis for Identified Patient

Contextual Factors considered in making diagnosis: ☒ Age ☒ Gender ☒ Family dynamics ☒ Culture ☐ Language ☒ Religion ☐ Economic ☐ Immigration ☐ Sexual/gender orientation ☐ Trauma ☐ Dual diagnosis/comorbid ☐ Addiction ☒ Cognitive ability ☒ Other: Dx by MD

Describe impact of identified factors on diagnosis and assessment process: Medical doctor's dx used in making dx; considered cultural, SES norms for CM7's behaviors; considered blended family dynamics; religious resources considered as strength that can be used in treatment.

DSM-5 Level 1 Cross-Cutting Symptom Measure (optional): Elevated scores on: (free at psychiatry.org) ☐ I Depression ☐ II Anger ☐ III Mania ☐ IV Anxiety ☐ V Somatic ☐ VI Suicide ☐ VII Psychosis ☐ VIII Sleep ☐ IX Memory ☐ X Repetitive ☐ XI Dissociation ☐ XII Personality ☐ XIII Substance X Not administered

DSM-5 Code	Diagnosis with Specifier *Include Z/T-Codes for Psychosocial Stressors/Issues*
1. F90.2	1. Attention-Deficit/Hyperactivity Disorder, Combined presentation; Moderate
2. Z62.820	2. Parent-Child Relational Problems
3. Z55.9	3. Academic or educational problem
4. _____	4. _____
5. _____	5. _____

List Specific DSM-5 Criterion Met for Diagnosis

1. Inattention: carelessness, difficulty with sustained attention, does not listen, does not follow instructions, loses things, forgetful, distractible
2. Hyperactivity: fidgets, leaves seat, runs in classroom, talks excessively, blurts out answers, interrupts others
3. Grades have dropped from 3.5 to 2.75 GPA
4. Symptoms before age 12

Medical Considerations
Has patient been referred for psychiatric evaluation? ☒ Yes ☐ No
Has patient agreed with referral? ☒ Yes ☐ No ☐ NA
Psychometric instruments used for assessment: ☐ None ☐ Cross-cutting symptom inventories ☒ Other: Initial assessment conducted by MD; Youth Outcome Questionnaire
Client response to diagnosis: ☐ Agree ☒ Somewhat agree ☐ Disagree ☐ Not informed for following reason: _____

(continued)

Diagnosis for Identified Patient *(continued)*

Current Medications (psychiatric & medical) ☐ NA
1. <u>Adderall (school days only)</u>; dose <u>5</u> mg; start date: <u>04/02/2016</u>
2. _____ ; dose _____ mg; start date: _____
3. _____ ; dose _____ mg; start date: _____
4. _____ ; dose _____ mg; start date: _____

Medical Necessity: *Check all that apply* ☒ Significant impairment ☐ Probability of significant impairment
☒ Probable developmental arrest
Areas of impairment:
☒ Daily activities ☒ Social relationships ☐ Health ☒ Work/school ☐ Living arrangement ☐ Other:

Risk and Safety Assessment for Identified Patient

Suicidality
☒ No indication/denies
☐ Active ideation
☐ Passive ideation
☐ Intent without plan
☐ Intent with means
☐ Ideation in past year
☐ Attempt in past year
☐ Family or peer history of completed suicide

Homicidality
☒ No indication/denies
☐ Active ideation
☐ Passive ideation
☐ Intent without means
☐ Intent with means
☐ Ideation in past year
☐ Violence past year
☐ History of assaulting others
☐ Cruelty to animals

Alcohol Abuse
☒ No indication/denies
☐ Past abuse
☐ Current; freq/Amt: _____

Drug Use/Abuse
☒ No indication/denies
☐ Past use
☐ Current drugs:_____
  Freq/Amt: _____
☐ Family/sig. other use

Sexual & Physical Abuse and Other Risk Factors
☐ Childhood abuse history: ☐ Sexual ☐ Physical ☐ Emotional ☐ Neglect
☐ Adult with abuse/assault in adulthood: ☐ Sexual ☐ Physical ☐ Current
☐ History of perpetrating abuse: ☐ Sexual ☐ Physical ☐ Emotional
☐ Elder/dependent adult abuse/neglect
☐ History of or current issues with restrictive eating, binging, and/or purging
☐ Cutting or other self harm: ☐ Current ☐ Past: Method: _____
☐ Criminal/legal history: _____
☐ Other trauma history: _____
☒ None reported

Indicators of Safety
☐ NA
☒ At least one outside support person
☐ Able to cite specific reasons to live or not harm
☒ Hopeful
☐ Willing to dispose of dangerous items
☐ Has future goals
☐ Willingness to reduce contact with people who make situation worse
☐ Willing to implement safety plan, safety interventions
☐ Developing set of alternatives to self/other harm
☐ Sustained period of safety: _____
☐ Other: _____

Elements of Safety Plan
☐ NA
☐ Verbal no harm contract
☐ Written no harm contract
☒ Emergency contact card
☒ Emergency therapist/agency number
☒ Medication management:
☐ Plan for contacting friends/support persons during crisis
☐ Specific plan of where to go during crisis
☒ Specific self-calming tasks to reduce risk before reach crisis behaviors (e.g., journaling, exercising, etc.)
☐ Specific daily/weekly activities to reduce stressors
☐ Other: _____

Legal/Ethical Action Taken: ☒ NA ☐ Action: _____

Case Management

Collateral Contacts
- Has contact been made with treating *physicians or other professionals:* ☐ NA ☒ Yes ☐ In process. Name/Notes: <u>Prescribing physician/pediatrician</u>
- If client is involved in mental health *treatment elsewhere,* has contact been made? ☐ NA ☒ Yes ☐ In process. Name/Notes: <u>Contact with school counselor and psychologist</u>
- Has contact been made with *social worker:* ☒ NA ☐ Yes ☐ In process. Name/Notes: _____

Referrals
- Has client been referred for *medical assessment:* ☒ Yes ☐ No evidence for need
- Has client been referred for *social services:* ☒ NA ☐ Job/training ☐ Welfare/food/housing ☐ Victim services ☐ Legal aid ☐ Medical ☐ Other: _____
- Has client been referred for *group* or other support services: ☒ Yes: <u>Parenting</u> ☐ In process ☐ None recommended
- Are there anticipated *forensic/legal processes* related to treatment: ☒ No ☐ Yes; describe: _____

Support Network
- Client social support network includes: ☒ Supportive family ☐ Supportive partner ☐ Friends ☒ Religious/spiritual organization ☐ Supportive work/social group ☐ Other: _____
- Describe anticipated effects treatment will have on others in support system (Children, partner, etc.): <u>Will work with family to unify parents regarding consequences and limits.</u>
- Is there anything else client will need to be successful? <u>Coordination with teacher</u>

Expected Outcome and Prognosis
☒ Return to normal functioning ☐ Anticipate less than normal functioning ☐ Prevent deterioration

Client Sense of Hope: 6

Evaluation of Assessment/Client Perspective
How were assessment methods adapted to client needs, including age, culture, and other diversity issues?
<u>Contacted MD and schoolteacher; did assessment with entire family present; used child-friendly language; encouraged sharing about religion; discussed racism. Considered blended family issues as significant contibutors to report problems.</u>

Describe actual or potential areas of client–clinician agreement/disagreement related to the above assessment:
<u>AF has made decision to use medicaton; AM is against medications but has agreed to try; parents are willing to work on parenting and family issues to reduce or eliminate need for medication.</u>

_____, | Clinician Signature | License/Intern Status | Date

_____, | Supervisor Signature | License | Date

TREATMENT PLAN

Date: 06/22/2016   **Case/Client #:** 8007

Clinician Name: Sally Wright   **Theory:** Cognitive–Behavioral Family therapy

Modalities planned: ☐ Individual Adult ☐ Individual Child ☐ Couple ☒ Family ☐ Group:
Recommended session frequency: ☒ Weekly ☐ Every two weeks ☐ Other: _____
Expected length of treatment: 3 months

Treatment Plan with Goals and Interventions

Early-Phase Client Goal

1. Increase cooperative and *mutually supportive parent coalition* to reduce children's problem behavior.

   Measure: Able to consistently support each other for a period of 2 months with no more than 2 mild episodes of inconsistent parenting.

   a. *Socratic dialogue* to identify each partner's relational cognition patterns related to coparenting and mutually agree on a set of *shared expectations and standards* for the children's behavior.
   b. *Parent skill training* to develop shared approach to setting consequences and limits with all children.

Working-Phase Client Goals

1. Increase *parental effectiveness* to consistently reinforce CM7's hyperactivity and distracting to reduce disruptive behaviors at home and at school.

   Measure: Able to sustain consistent reinforcement system for a period of 2 months with no more than three mild episodes of failing to support the other or failing to follow through on stated consequence.

   a. *Psychoeducation* on specific parenting techniques for children diagnosed with ADHD.
   b. Couple *problem solving* and *communication training* around parenting issues and family schemas related to parenting.
2. Reduce *cognitive distortions* that blame family members to reduce conflict.

   Measure: Able to sustain nonblaming interactions for a period of 4 weeks with no more than 2 mild episodes of blame.

   a. *Challenging* cognitive distortions and identify more realistic perspectives.
   b. *Problem-solving* skills training to help family identify more effective ways to address differences.
3. Increase CM7 independence with schoolwork to reduce academic failure.

   Measure: Able to sustain doing homework with monitoring only at the beginning and end of homework session for period of 4 weeks with no more than four mild episodes of failure to complete homework.

   a. Use *operant conditioning* to begin increasing CM7's independence with homework.

   b. Increase AM40's involvement in homework and decrease CF14's involvement.

   c. *Token reward system* for turning in homework, studying, and grades.

Closing-Phase Client Goals

1. Increase *realistic relational schemas* for a blended family to reduce conflict.

   Measure: Able to sustain effective family problem solving for period of 2 months with no more than 2 mild episodes of conflict that last for no more than a day.

   a. *Psychoeducation* with blended families to develop realistic expectations.
   b. *Guided discovery* to help family develop more realistic standards and expectations for themselves.

2. Increase each member's ability to make *realistic interpretations* of self, others, and life to reduce conflict and increase sense of wellness.

   a. *Analyze schemas* related to self, other, and life, and identify realistic alternatives.
   b. *Thought records* to continue identifying and debunking unrealistic beliefs.

Treatment Tasks

1. Develop working therapeutic relationship using theory of choice.

   a. Develop an *empathic, supportive* working relationship with family in which therapist is able to effectively and respectfully provide *education* from a position of expertise.

2. Assess individual, relational, community, and broader cultural dynamics using theory of choice.

   a. Conduct *functional analysis* of CM7 symptoms; identify role in system.
   b. Assess *cognitive distortions and family schemas* related to blended family, parenting, sibling relationships, and CM7's behavior.
   c. Administer Youth Outcome Questionnaire
   d. Verbally check in with family every   month to inquire about their perspective on treatment.
   e. Session-rating scales

3. Identify needed referrals, crisis issues, collateral contacts, and other client needs.

   a. *Crisis assessment intervention(s):* Consult with school counselor, teacher
   b. *Referral(s):* Contact prescribing physician and teacher to discuss *baseline functioning* and related treatments. During closing phase of treatment, consult with psychiatrist and teacher about gains and follow-up care; identify school resources to maintain gains there; consider referral for *mindfulness program* for CM and/or entire family to reduce long-term use of ADHD medications.

Diversity Considerations

Describe specifically how treatment plan, goals, and interventions were adapted to address each area of diversity (*Note:* Identify specific ethnicity, e.g., Italian American rather than white):

Age: Use child-friendly, teen-friendly, and parent-appropriate language and activities.

Gender/Sexual Orientation: Attend to gender-role dynamics between AF and AM, especially in relation to child-rearing and household duties. Also, attend to gender and age dynamics between siblings, with older siblings both female and the younger both male. Isomorphic patterns, with females having more responsibility.

Race/Ethnicity/Religion/Class/Region: Consider racial status within broader community; invite discussion of racial differences between family and therapist; identify resources in African American community, school, and extended family; explore gendered racial identity for each.

(continued)

Diversity Considerations *(continued)*

Other Factors: Respectful of their religious beliefs; respectful of their experiences of not feeling respected by school professionals; respectful discussion of goals in language appropriate for family.

Evidence-Based Practice (Optional)

Summarize evidence for using this approach for this presenting concern and/or population: CBFT is often the treatment of choice for ADHD, especially regarding parenting skills and shaping of child behavior. The approach has also been identified as an appropriate fit with African American clients because of the direct approach and focus on present problems

Client Perspective (Optional)

Has treatment plan been reviewed with client ☒ Yes ☐ No; If no, explain: _____

Describe areas of Client Agreement and Concern: Clients asked whether patient will be able to get off all medication; informed client that medication decisions need to be made by a psychiatrist; the current plan is designed to reduce the symptoms being treated by medication. They will need to consult with psychiatrist about need for medication as therapy progresses.

_____, _____ _____ _____, _____ _____
Therapist's Signature   Intern Status   Date   Supervisor's Signature   License   Date

PROGRESS NOTE

Date: 06/29/2016   **Time:** 4:00 ☐ am/☒ pm   **Session Length:** ☐ 45 min. ☒ 60 min. ☐ Other: _____ minutes

Present: ☒ AM ☒ AF ☒ CF14 ☒ CM10 ☒ CF10 ☒ CM7

Billing Code: ☐ 90791 (eval) ☐ 90834 (45 min. therapy) ☐ 90837 (60 min. therapy) ☒ 90847 (family) ☐ Other: _____

Symptom(s)	Duration and Frequency Since Last Visit	Progress
1: Hyperactivity	No "red marks" in class this week	Progressing
2: Inattention/Grades	Turned in all but 1 class assignment; most HW	Progressing
3: Family conflict	CM10 and CM7 one fight on Sat	Progressing

Explanatory Notes on Symptoms: Report role plays have helped with in-class behavior problems; AF and AM report supporting each other with reinforcing behaviors at school and doing homework and that they have had fewer conflicts since parent training session. Continued conflict between CM10 and CM7, but able to resolve more quickly.

In-Session Interventions and Assigned Homework

Reviewed reward system and answered parents' questions related to it. Psychoeducation on blended family issues; used art to have each person depict what he/she likes most about this family and what he/she likes least. Developed plan for family fun night to increase cohesion.

Client Response/Feedback

Parents are eager to discuss problems but children can listen for only so long; all members actively engage in art activity, which brought out playfulness.

Plan

☒ Continue with treatment plan: plan for next session: Parents only, to begin working on increasing CM7 independence with homework

☐ Modify plan: _____

Next session: Date: 7/6   Time: 4:00 ☐ am/☒ pm

Crisis Issues: ☒ No indication of crisis/client denies ☐ Crisis assessed/addressed: describe below

_____

_____,   _____   _____
Clinician's Signature,   License/Intern Status   Date

◇◇

(continued)

PROGRESS NOTE *(continued)*

Case Consultation/Supervision ☐ Not Applicable

Notes: Supervisor provided outline for operant conditioning related to homework.

Collateral Contact ☐ Not Applicable

Name: Ms. Anna Schaerf and Mr. Matt Kloeris   Date of Contact: 6/30/2016   Time: 11:30 ☒ am/☐ pm

☒ Written release on file: ☒ Sent/☐ Received ☐ In court docs ☐ Other: _____

Notes: Teachers report improved behavior in class and with schoolwork. Report continued talking during class but staying seated; less conflict with peers; turning in more classwork.

_____ ,   _____   _____
Clinician's Signature   License/Intern Status   Date

_____ ,   _____   _____
Supervisor's Signature   License   Date

CHAPTER
9

Solution-Based Therapies

Learning Objectives

After reading this chapter and a few hours of focused studying, you should be able to:

- Theory: Describe the following elements of solution-based therapies:
  - Process of therapy
  - Therapeutic relationship
  - Case conceptualization
  - Goal setting
  - Interventions

- Case conceptualization and treatment plan: Complete a theory-specific case conceptualizations and treatment plans for solution-based therapies using templates that are provided.

- Research: Provide an overview of significant research findings for solution-based therapies.

- Diversity: Analyze strengths, limitations, and appropriate applications for using solution-based therapies with clients in relation to their social location/diverse identities, including but not limited to ethnic, racial, and/or sexual/gender identity diversity.

- Cross-theoretical comparison: Compare how solution-based therapies utilize interpersonal patterns (IPs) with other approaches described in this book.

We intend to influence clients' perceptions in the direction of solution through the questions we choose to ask and our careful use of solution language. Reflection upon these questions helps clients to consider their situations from new perspectives.
—*O'Hanlon and Weiner-Davis (1989, p. 80)*

377

Lay of the Land

The most well-known and arguably the first strength-based therapies, solution-based therapies, are positive, active approaches that help clients move toward desired outcomes. The following three main strands of practice share many more similarities than differences:

- Solution-focused brief therapy (SFBT): Developed by Steve de Shazer (1985, 1988, 1994) and Insoo Berg (1994) at the Milwaukee Brief Family Therapy Center, this therapy focuses on the future with minimal discussion of the presenting problem or the past; interventions target small steps in the direction of the solution.
- Solution-oriented therapy: This therapy (O'Hanlon & Weiner-Davis, 1989) and the related approach, *possibility therapy* (O'Hanlon & Beadle, 1999), were developed by Bill O'Hanlon and colleagues to incorporate a similar future orientation while drawing more directly from the language techniques used in the Ericksonian trance. Solution-oriented therapy uses more interventions that draw from the past and present to identify potential solutions than does solution-focused brief therapy.
- Solution-oriented Ericksonian hypnosis: Both solution-focused and solution-oriented therapies were inspired by the work of Milton Erickson (see Chapters 3 and 4), whose strength-oriented trance work is one of the most popular modern approaches to hypnosis.

Because of their numerous commonalities, this chapter presents solution-focused and solution-oriented therapies together under the general term *solution-based therapies;* it then discusses Ericksonian hypnosis.

Solution-Based Therapies

In a Nutshell: The Least You Need to Know

Solution-based therapies are brief therapy approaches that grew out of the work of the Mental Research Institute in Palo Alto (MRI) and Milton Erickson's brief therapy and trance work (de Shazer, 1985, 1988, 1994; O'Hanlon & Weiner-Davis, 1989). The first and leading "strength-based" therapies, solution-based therapies are increasingly popular with clients, insurance companies, and county mental health agencies because they are efficient and respectful of clients. As the name suggests, solution-based therapists spend a minimum of time talking about problems and instead focus on moving clients toward enacting solutions. Rather than being "solution givers," solution-based therapists work with the client to envision potential solutions based on the client's experiences and values. Once the client has selected a desirable outcome, the therapist assists in identifying small, incremental steps toward realizing this goal. The therapist does not solve problems or offer solutions but instead collaborates with clients to develop aspirations and plans that they then translate into real-world action.

Common Solution-Based Therapy Myths

More so than others, solution-based therapists are haunted by myths and misconceptions about what actually happens in session. So let's straighten these out before we go any further.

Myth: Solution-Based Therapists Propose Solutions (a.k.a. Give Advice)

Fact: Solution-based therapists do not suggest logical solutions to clients (O'Hanlon & Beadle, 1999). Instead, the client identifies solutions with the help of the therapist, who identifies exceptions to the problem, descriptions of what is already working, and client resources to help the client envision potential solutions. Once a clear behavioral goal is identified, the therapist works with the client to take small steps in this direction.

Myth: Solution-Based Therapists Never Talk about the Problem

Fact: Solution-based therapists are not psychic; therefore, like all therapists, they must spend some time talking about the problem. However, they spend *less* time talking about the problem than most other therapists, especially solution-focused brief therapy (SFBT) therapists (De Jong & Berg, 2002). Solution-based therapists typically follow their clients' lead in determining how much and how often they need to talk about the problem versus the solution. To add further myth-busting evidence, hallmark techniques, such as *exception questions,* require talking about the problem as part of identifying the solution.

Myth: Solution-Based Therapists Never Talk about the Past

Fact: Again, solution-based therapists are not psychic, and they actually have numerous techniques that are grounded in talking about the past. However, when they talk about the past, they focus on strengths as well as the problem (Bertolino & O'Hanlon, 2002). Talking about the past is one of the most important means of identifying solutions: what has worked and what has not. The past is talked about in ways that facilitate the enactment of solutions.

Myth: Emotions Are Not Discussed

Fact: Solution-based therapists have been criticized for not addressing emotions (Kim & Franklin, 2015; Lipchik, 2002). Unlike humanistic therapists, solution-based therapists do *not* view the expression of negative emotion as curative in and of itself; instead, emotions are used as clues to what works and what does not and where clients want to go (Lipchik, 2002). More to the point, solution-focused practitioners give their attention primarily to positive emotions rather than negative emotions (Kim & Franklin, 2015). In fact, the solution-focused emphasis on positive emotions as a means to reduce negative emotions has a strong evidence base in positive psychology. Specifically, the broaden-and-build theory of positive emotions has a strong evidence base and closely parallels the therapeutic process of solution-focused therapy. This theory involves using positive emotion to help people to broaden their attention to other options when facing a challenge and then build on these alternatives, creating an upward spiral effect.

The Juice: Significant Contributions to the Field

If you remember one thing from this chapter, it should be this:

Assessing Client Strengths

Assessing *client strengths* is one of the key practices in solution-based therapies (Bertolino & O'Hanlon, 2002; De Jong & Berg, 2002; O'Hanlon & Weiner-Davis, 1989). Strengths include resources in a person's life (personally, relationally, financially, socially, or spiritually) and may include family support, positive relationships, and religious faith. Most therapists underestimate the difficulty of identifying strengths. In fact, identifying client strengths is often harder than diagnosing pathology because clients come in with a long list of problems they want fixed and are thus prepared to discuss pathology. Surprisingly, many clients, especially those with depressive or anxious tendencies (the majority of outpatient cases), have great difficulty identifying areas without problems in their lives. Similarly, many couples who have been distressed and arguing for long periods of time, such as Suzie and Jorge in the case study at the end of this chapter, have difficulty identifying positive characteristics in their partners, happy times in the marriage, and in the most desperate of cases, the reasons they got together in the first place. Therefore, therapists often have to ask more subtle questions and attend to vague clues in order to assess strengths well.

Solution-based therapists assess strengths in two ways: (a) by directly asking about strengths, hobbies, and areas of life that are going well; and (b) by listening carefully for exceptions to problems and for areas of unnoticed strength (Bertolino & O'Hanlon, 2002; De Jong & Berg, 2002). Furthermore, I have found that any strength in one context has the potential to be a liability in another context and that the inverse is also true: any weakness in one area is generally a strength in another area (see Client Strengths in Chapter 11). Therefore, if a client has difficulty identifying strengths and more readily discusses weaknesses and problems, a finely tuned solution-focused ear will be able to identify potential areas in which the "weakness" is a strength. For example, a person who is critical, anxious, or negative in a relational context typically excels at detailed or meticulous work and tasks. This insight can be useful in identifying ways for clients to move toward their goals. Solution-based therapists have been at the vanguard of a larger movement within mental health that emphasizes identifying and utilizing client strengths to promote better clinical outcomes (Bertolino & O'Hanlon, 2002). Increasingly, county mental health and insurance companies are requiring assessment of strengths as part of initial intake assessments. The key to successfully assessing strengths is having an unshakable belief that all clients have significant and meaningful strengths no matter how dire and severe their situations appear. It is helpful for therapists to remember that we typically see people at their worst moments; therefore, even if we are not seeing strengths at present, they are undoubtedly there. Solution-based therapists maintain that all people have strengths and resources, and they make it their job to help identify and utilize those strengths in achieving client goals.

Rumor Has It: The People and Their Stories

Behind-the-Scenes Inspiration: Milton Erickson

Milton Erickson served as an inspiration to Bill O'Hanlon's solution-oriented therapy and Steve de Shazer's solution-focused brief therapy. Trained in medicine as a psychiatrist, Erickson was a master therapist who was well known for his brief, rapid, and creative interventions (Erickson & Keeney, 2006; Haley, 1993; O'Hanlon & Martin, 1992). Rather than follow a specific theory, Erickson relied on keen observation while listening with an open mind to each patient's unique story. He frequently employed light trance work to evoke patient strengths and latent abilities (Haley, 1993; O'Hanlon & Martin, 1992). At a time when most therapies focused on the past, Erickson directed his clients to focus on the present and future, often envisioning times without the problem. Although others have meticulously studied his work, there has been no consensus or singular definition of Ericksonian therapy. The influence of his trance work is clearly evident in interventions such as the *miracle question* and the *crystal ball technique,* which rely on a pseudo-orientation to time and the implicit assumption that change *will* occur.

Solution-Focused Brief Therapy: Milwaukee Brief Family Therapy Center

Steve de Shazer

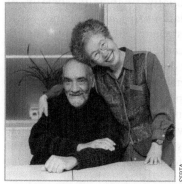

Steve de Shazer was a deeply thoughtful leader in the field. After his early work at the MRI with giants such as Jay Haley, Paul Watzlawick, John Weakland, and Virginia Satir, the late Steve de Shazer developed, with his wife Insoo Kim Berg, solution-focused brief therapy: "An iconoclast and creative genius known for his minimalist philosophy and view of the process of change as an inevitable and dynamic part of everyday life, he was known for reversing the traditional psychotherapy interview process by asking clients to describe a detailed resolution of the problem that brought them into therapy, shifting the focus of treatment from problems to solutions" (Trepper et al., 2006, p. 133). De Shazer was a prolific writer (de Shazer, 1985, 1988, 1994; de Shazer & Dolan, 2007), laying much of the philosophical and theoretical foundations for solution-focused work. His early work was influenced by the trance work of Milton Erickson (de Shazer, 1985, 1988) and his later work by Ludwig Wittgenstein, who viewed language as inextricably woven into the fabric of life (de Shazer & Dolan, 2007). With Berg, de Shazer founded the Solution-Focused Brief Therapy Association and the Milwaukee Brief Family Therapy Center, where they trained therapists until their deaths in 2005 (de Shazer) and 2007 (Berg).

Insoo Kim Berg

Warm and exuberant, Insoo Kim Berg was an energetic developer and leading practitioner of SFBT, cofounding the Milwaukee Brief Family Therapy Center and the Solution-Focused Brief Therapy Association with her husband, Steve de Shazer (Dolan, 2007). She was an outstanding clinician who furthered the development of SFBT, developing solution-focused approaches to working with drinking issues (Berg & Miller, 1992), substance abuse (Berg & Reuss, 1997), family-based services (Berg, 1994), child protective services families (Berg & Kelly, 2000), children (Berg & Steiner, 2003), and personal coaching (Berg & Szabo, 2005).

Scott Miller

Originally trained at the Milwaukee Brief Family Therapy Center with de Shazer and Berg, Scott Miller, along with his colleagues Barry Duncan and Mark Hubble, has been a strong proponent of the *common factors* movement (see Chapter 2; Miller, Duncan, & Hubble, 1997) and client-centered, outcome-informed therapy (see Chapter 14).

Yvonne Dolan

Yvonne Dolan studied and worked with de Shazer and Berg at the Milwaukee Brief Family Therapy Center, specializing in sexual abuse and trauma treatment (Dolan, 1991, 2000).

Linda Metcalf

Linda Metcalf applies solution-focused therapy in school counseling contexts, including solution-focused school counseling (Metcalf, 2008), solution-focused children's groups (Metcalf, 2007), solution-focused parenting (Metcalf, 1998), and solution-focused teaching (Metcalf, 2003).

Solution-Oriented Therapy

Bill O'Hanlon

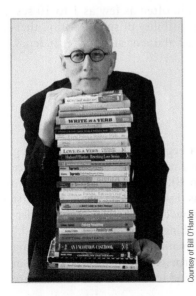

Courtesy of Bill O'Hanlon

A former student of Milton Erickson, Bill O'Hanlon is an energetic and popular leader in solution-oriented, strength-based therapies, including solution-oriented therapy and possibility therapy (O'Hanlon & Beadle, 1999; O'Hanlon & Weiner-Davis, 1989). A prolific and highly accessible writer and speaker, O'Hanlon emphasizes the significance of language, using subtle shifts in language to spark change. His work aims to transform client viewing as well as to solve the problem while attending to broader contextual issues that impact the client's situation (Bertolino & O'Hanlon, 2002). He has written extensively on numerous topics, including solution-oriented couples therapy (Hudson & O'Hanlon, 1991), solution-oriented approaches to treating sexual abuse (O'Hanlon & Bertolino, 2002), solution-oriented hypnosis (O'Hanlon & Martin, 1992), solution-oriented therapy with children and teens (Bertolino & O'Hanlon, 1998), and spirituality in therapy (O'Hanlon, 2006) as well as books for clients and popular audiences (O'Hanlon, 2000, 2005, 2006).

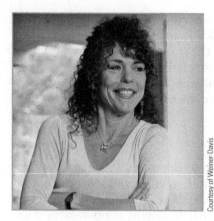

Courtesy of Weiner-Davis

Michele Weiner-Davis

Michele Weiner-Davis developed a highly successful solution-oriented approach to working with divorce that she calls *divorce busting* (Weiner-Davis, 1992). She uses a brief, solution-oriented self-help approach for couples who want to prevent divorce.

Collaborative, Strength-Based Therapy
Matthew Selekman

Grounding his work in solution-oriented therapies and systems theory, Matthew Selekman has developed collaborative, strength-based therapies for working with children, adolescents, families, and self-harming adolescents (Selekman, 1997, 2005, 2006).

Solution-Focused Associations

SFBT has been influential in the United States, Europe, Latin America, and Asia, as discussed below.

- *European Brief Therapy Association:* Founded in 1994, the European Brief Therapy Association serves as a network of brief therapy practitioners in Europe who have worked closely with de Shazer and Berg over the years. They sponsor research projects in brief therapy and meet annually, bringing together therapists from across Europe and the world.
- *Solution-Focused Brief Therapy Association (SFBTA):* In 2001, Steve de Shazer and *Terry Trepper* began organizing the SFBTA to bring together North American SFBT practitioners and researchers. Under the dynamic leadership of Thorana Nelson, Eric McCollum, Terry Trepper, Yvonne Dolan, and others, SFBTA is an active and engaged community of practitioners, educators, and researchers who work to further develop and refine SFBT practices.

The Big Picture: Overview of Treatment

Small Steps to Enacting Solutions

In broad strokes, solution-based therapists help clients identify their preferred solution (by talking about the problem, exceptions, and desired outcomes) and work with clients to take small, active steps in this general direction each week (O'Hanlon & Weiner-Davis, 1989). In some cases, this is a very time-limited approach, often as few as 1 to 10 sessions; solution-focused therapists are advocates of the possibility of single-session therapy. In more complex cases, such as the treatment of sexual abuse or alcohol dependency, therapy may take years (O'Hanlon & Bertolino, 2002).

Making a Connection: The Therapeutic Relationship

The Zen of Viewing: The Beginner's Mind

O'Hanlon and Weiner-Davis (1989) use the concept of a beginner's mind when forming a relationship, referring to the classic Zen saying, "In the beginner's mind there are many possibilities; in the expert's mind there are few" (p. 8). Assuming a position of the beginner's mind involves listening to each client's story as if you are listening for the first time, not filling in blanks with personal or professional knowledge. Most therapists underestimate how hard it is to do this. When a client starts talking about "feeling depressed," most therapists believe they have useful diagnostic information, unthinkingly assuming that clients have read diagnostic manuals and use the term as a professional would. In contrast, solution-oriented therapists bring a beginner's mind to the conversation and are curious about *how this person experiences his or her unique depression*. If you get in the habit of asking, you will find that every depression is surprisingly "one of a kind." Thus, solution-oriented therapists make no assumptions when they are listening; instead, they ask to hear more about clients' unique experiences and understandings.

Echoing the Client's Key Words

Solution-based therapists carefully attend to *client word choice* and echo their key words whenever possible (De Jong & Berg, 2002). For example, rather than teaching clients to use psychiatric terms such as *depression* or *hallucinations* to describe their experience, the therapist prefers to use the clients' own language, such as "feeling blue" or "schizos." Using client language often makes the problem more solvable and engenders greater hope. For many, "ending the blahs" or "getting back to my old self" is a more attainable goal than treating a psychiatrically defined problem of "major depressive disorder, single episode, moderate."

Carl Rogers with a Twist: Channeling Language

O'Hanlon and Beadle (1999) describe how solution-oriented therapists use reflection, including reflection of feelings, with clients to build rapport. This approach is similar to humanistic approaches, such as Carl Rogers's client-centered therapy, but with a twist: solution-oriented reflections *delimit* the difficult feeling, behavior, or thought by reflecting on a time, context, or relational limit. Such reflections generally take one of three forms:

1. Past tense rather than chronic state or characteristic: Therapists reflect statements back to clients in the past tense—for example, "You were feeling down yesterday."
2. Partial rather than global: Therapists reflect global statements back to clients as partial statements—for example, "Your partner sometimes/often (instead of always) does things that annoy you."
3. Perception rather than unchangeable truth: Therapists reflect a client's "truth" or "reality" claim as a perception—for example, in response to "I'll never find anybody," they might say, "There does not seem to be anybody you are interested in right now."

For example, suppose a client is telling a story about how her boyfriend got angry at her for "no reason." A client-centered reflection would be something like, "You aren't feeling understood" (present-focused statement about client's unexpressed emotion), whereas the solution-focused twist to delimit would be, "You were not feeling understood *by your boyfriend last Saturday.*" The solution-oriented twist emphasizes the limited time and relational context in order to: (a) define the problem in more solvable ways and (b) create hope. O'Hanlon and Beadle (1999) refer to this process as "channeling language." This technique helps both the client and the therapist transition to desired outcomes.

Optimism and Hope

Optimism and hope are brilliantly palpable in solution-based therapies (Miller, Duncan, & Hubble, 1996, 1997). With all clients, solution-based therapists assume that change is inevitable and that improvement—in some form—is always possible (O'Hanlon & Weiner-Davis, 1989). Their optimism and hope do not stem from naïveté but rather from their ontology and epistemology: their theory of what it means to be human and how people learn. Because change is always happening—moods, relationships, emotions, and behaviors are in constant flux—change is inevitable (Walter & Peller, 1992). They have hope that the change will be positive because the client is in therapy to make an improvement and because over 90% of clients report positive outcomes in psychotherapy (Miller et al., 1997). Hope is cultivated early in therapy to develop motivation and momentum (Bertolino & O'Hanlon, 2002). For example, in the case study at the end of this chapter, the wife has little hope for the relationship; therefore, the therapist consciously tries to instill this hope early in treatment.

Assumption of Solution and Possibilities

A subtle but essential element of the therapeutic relationship is that the solution-focused therapists view all clients as resilient and capable of enacting solutions to their presenting problems (Franklin et al., 2012). Although philosophical at one level, this assumption is realized in their word choice, descriptions, and verb tense—"when you two are getting along better" or "as you recover from trauma." This belief that clients are fully capable of change tends to inspire clients to believe in themselves and is key to making the interventions associated with this approach work.

The Viewing: Case Conceptualization and Assessment

Strengths and Resources

Assessing strengths and resources is covered in "The Juice: Significant Contributions to the Field," above and in Chapter 11.

Exceptions and "What Works"

Solution-based therapists listen for **exceptions** and examples of what works when clients are talking (de Shazer, 1985, 1988; O'Hanlon & Weiner-Davis, 1989). If you are listening closely, most clients spontaneously offer exceptions and examples of what works: "His ADHD is less of a problem in his math class" or "When his stepbrother helps him with homework, there does not seem to be much of a problem." These exceptions provide clues to what works and therefore what clients need to do more frequently.

Solution-based therapists identify exceptions and descriptions of what works in two ways: (a) indirectly, by listening for spontaneous descriptions, and (b) directly, by asking questions. They listen as carefully for exceptions as medical-model therapists listen for diagnostic symptoms. They then use these exceptions to help clients enact preferred solutions in their lives. They also ask exception questions to gather more information about what works:

EXAMPLES OF EXCEPTION QUESTIONS

- Are there any times when the problem is less likely to occur or be less severe?
- Can you think of a time when you expected the problem to occur but it didn't?
- Are there any people who seem to make things easier?
- Are there places or times when the problem is not as bad?

The vast majority of clients can identify exceptions with questions such as these. The underlying assumption is that the problem varies in intensity; the times when the problem is less severe are considered exceptions and generally provide clues to what works (de Shazer, 1985; O'Hanlon & Weiner-Davis, 1989). Especially with diagnoses such as depression, which is experienced most of the time on most days, therapists need to focus on variations of intensity rather than on the absence of the symptom to identify exceptions. With couples, such as in the case study for this chapter, the therapist listens for times when the two are not fighting, "get along," or get things done, which may be in relation to children, work, extended family, and so forth.

Try It Yourself

Find a partner and take turns asking exception questions and identifying when the problem is less of a problem. Did any ideas for how to improve the situation emerge?

Client Motivation: Visitors, Complainants, and Customers

Steve de Shazer (1988) assessed client motivation for change using three categories: visitors, complainants, and customers.

- **Visitors** do not have a complaint, but others generally have a complaint against them. Visitors are typically brought to therapy by an outside other, such as courts, parents, or spouse.
- **Complainants** identify a problem but expect therapy or some other person to be the primary source of change. They are there to have their problems fixed by an expert.
- **Customers** identify a problem and want to take action toward the solution.

CLIENT MOTIVATIONS

	VISITOR	COMPLAINANT	CUSTOMER
Motivation	Low	Moderate to high	High
Source of Problem or Solution	Outside other (spouse, parent, court) thinks client has a problem.	Problem generally related to outside cause or person; expect therapist or another to be source of solution.	Self as part of problem and active agent in solution.
View of Who Needs to Change	Outside other needs to believe there is no problem.	Outside other needs to change and/or fix it.	Self needs to take action to fix things.
Building Therapeutic Alliance	Therapist identifies areas where client sees a problem and is willing to become a customer for change.	Therapist honors client's view of the situation while identifying specific instances where client can make a difference.	Therapist joins with client by complimenting readiness for change.
Focus of Interventions	Building alliance; understanding client perspective; framing outside request for change as "the problem."	Observation-oriented tasks (e.g., identifying exceptions over the week; Selekman, 1997).	Reframing; identifying what does not work; action-oriented tasks.
Readiness for Action	Not ready for making active changes in life until client believes there is some sort of problem and is motivated to change.	Not ready for action until open to the idea that client's actions can make a difference.	Ready to take action to make changes.

Assessing clients' motivation is helpful for knowing how to join with the client as well as knowing how to proceed. Many new therapists assume that all clients are customers for change: ready to take action to improve their situation simply because they showed up for a therapy session. However, this is often not the case. People come to therapy with mixed emotions and levels of motivation. Generally, most mandated clients are "visitors," and therapists need to find a way to connect with their agenda while still working with the referring party's agenda. This same dynamic is often the case with children, teens, and even one half of a couple. With complainants, therapists need to either find ways for the client to contribute to making a difference or help shift the viewing of the problem to increase the client's willingness to take action. In the case study at the end of this chapter, Suzie is a complainant, seeing her husband as the problem, and Jorge is a visitor, not even aware until now that there was a problem; thus, the therapist will need to adjust the treatment plan to honor how each views the situation and motivate each accordingly.

Targeting Change: Goal Setting

Goal Language: Positive and Concrete

Solution-based therapists state their goals in positive, observable solution-based terms (De Jong & Berg, 2002; Franklin, 2015). Positive goal descriptions emphasize what the client is *going to be doing* rather than focusing on symptom reduction, which is typical in the medical model and cognitive–behavioral therapies. Observable descriptions include clear, specific behavioral indicators of the desired change.

EXAMPLES OF OBSERVABLE AND NONOBSERVABLE GOALS

POSITIVE, OBSERVABLE GOALS	NEGATIVE (SYMPTOM-REDUCING), NONOBSERVABLE GOALS
Increase periods of enjoyable activity, social interaction, and hope for future	Reduce depression
Increase frequency of couple's emotionally intimate conversations	Reduce couple conflict
Increase cooperation and prosocial activities	Reduce defiance

You may have noticed that reading the left column generates more hope and provides greater direction for clinical change than reading the right column. Positive, observable goals provide a constant reminder to the therapist and client of the goal, and reinforce a solution-focused and solution-oriented perspective. Many solution-based techniques, such as scaling questions (discussed below), invite the client to measure goal progress weekly; thus, carefully crafted goal language is particularly critical to success in solution-based therapies.

Solution-based goals should also have the following qualities (Bertolino & O'Hanlon, 2002; De Jong & Berg, 2002):

- Meaningful to client: Goals must be personally important to the client.
- Interactional: Rather than reflect a general feeling (e.g., "feeling better"), the goals should describe how interactions with others will change.
- Situational: Goals are stated in situational terms (e.g., "improved mood at work") rather than in global terms.
- Small steps: Goals should be short term and have identifiable small steps.
- Clear role for client: Goals should identify a clear role for the client rather than for others.

- Realistic: Goals need to be realistic for this client at this time.
- Legal and ethical: Goals should be legal and adhere to client, therapist, and professional ethics.

Miracle and Other Solution-Generating Questions

The original solution-generating question, the **miracle question** serves to both: (a) conceptualize and assess and (b) set goals in solution-based counseling. Legend (and good authority) has it that Insoo Kim Berg developed the miracle question based on a client's desperate and exasperated claim to Insoo that "maybe only a miracle will help." So, Insoo, using the clients' language and worldview, played with the idea and had clients describe how life would be if there were a miracle (de Shazer, 1988; de Shazer et al., 2007). The intervention was so successful that it was crafted into a hallmark intervention that is frequently used early in treatment to identify the focus. Since then, several variations have been developed, including the crystal ball technique (de Shazer, 1985), magic wand questions (Selekman, 1997), and the time machine (Bertolino & O'Hanlon, 2002). When successfully delivered, these questions help clients envision a future without the problem, generating hope, motivation, and goals.

EXAMPLES OF SOLUTION-GENERATING QUESTIONS

- **Miracle questions:** "Imagine that you go home tonight and during the middle of the night a miracle happens: all the problems you came here to resolve are miraculously resolved. However, when you wake up, you have no idea a miracle has occurred. What are some of the first things you would notice that would be different? What are some of the first clues that a miracle has occurred?"

- **Crystal ball questions:** "Imagine I had a crystal ball that allowed us to look into the future to a time when the problems you came here for are already resolved. I hold it up to you, and you look in. What do you see?"

- **Magic wand questions:** "Imagine I had a magic wand (or imagine that this magic wand I have actually works), and after you leave I wave it and all of the problems you came here for are resolved overnight. You of course have no idea that your problems have been solved. When you wake up in the morning, what would be the first clues that something is different? What would you be doing differently? What would others be doing differently?"

- **Time machine questions:** "Imagine I had a time machine that could propel you into the future to the point in time when the problems you came to see me for are totally resolved. Imagine you stepped into the machine: Where do you end up? Who is with you? What is happening? How is your life different? How did your problems go away?"

Successfully delivering one of these solution-generating questions is far more difficult than it appears. As you can imagine, if done poorly, these hit the floor like a lead balloon. To avoid such humiliation, solution-focused experts have several suggestions for successfully delivering the miracle question (Bertolino, 2010; Bertolino & O'Hanlon,

2002: De Jong & Berg, 2002; de Shazer, 1988; de Shazer et al., 2007). In addition, I suggest you think of asking the miracle question as having three specific phases:

- Phase 1: Setup for the miracle
- Phase 2: Delivery of the miracle question
- Phase 3: Facilitation of the answer

Phase 1: Setup for the Miracle—Three Steps with Three Nods

- Phase 1, Step 1: *Obtain Client Agreement and Wait for Nod 1:* The first and most critical step is to prepare clients by changing their state of mind so that they are willing to engage in an atypical conversation. By asking, "May I ask an unusual question?" or "Would you be willing to play along if I ask a somewhat odd question?" The counselor signals clients to change their frame of mind so that they are better able to enter a more fanciful, creative conversation. The counselor waits for the client to say "okay" or nod in agreement.

- Phase 1, Step 2: *Custom Tailor Initial Setup and Wait for Nod 2:* After the client agrees to the odd question, begin delivering the question but customize it to include numerous little details from the client's everyday life to get him or her fully engaged in the story and to enable him or her to better visualize the miracle. For example, you might say, "Let's imagine that after we are done talking here, you get in your car and drive home; you make dinner for the family like you usually do; you clean up dishes like you usually do; and check the kids' homework like you usually do." *Continue describing the typical day and evening until the client starts to nod.*

- Phase 1, Step 3: *Setup for Miracle and Wait for Nod 3:* Once the client nods, continue with, "Then you get the kids to bed, maybe do some minor chores or watch television, and then you finally get to bed and fall asleep." Up to this point, you have only asked the client to imagine a regular day, but this is very important. The goal is to have the client psychologically leave the session and vividly envision being at home, where the miracle is to occur. *Pause and wait for the nod or verbal affirmation before moving on to the miracle; don't move on to the miracle without such confirmation.*

Phase 2: Deliver the Miracle Question—Four Steps with Three Pauses and a Snap

- Phase 2, Step 1: *Introduce the Miracle with Pause 1:* "Then, during the night . . . while you are sleeping . . . a miracle happens" (de Shazer et al., 2007, p. 42). Pause and wait for a reaction that signals surprise or that the client is thinking: a smirk, laugh, tilt of the head, raised eyebrow, or funny look. Insoo reportedly looked intently at the client and smiled; Steve warned that if the pause is too long, the client is likely to respond with, "I don't believe in miracles"; so keep moving.

- Phase 2, Step 2: *Specifically Define the Terms of the Miracle with Optional Snap:* "And it's not just any miracle. This miracle makes the problems that brought you here today disappear . . . just like *that*" (de Shazer et al., 2007, p. 43; emphasis in source). Snapping your fingers at this point is optional but adds flair (you might need extra practice with that part). If you forget to include the "problems that brought you here" part of the question, you most likely will get a wish list appropriate for a genie in a lantern, which is not the answer we want for this question. Without this limit on the miracle, clients will spend a lot of time exploring vague and unrelated goals, and the counselor will spend more time with follow-up questions to get a useful answer.

- Phase 2, Step 3: *Add Mystery with Pause 2:* "However, because you were sleeping, you don't know that *the miracle has happened*" (De Jong & Berg, 2002, p. 85; emphasis in source). If delivered well, most clients start bobbing their heads at this point, stare off into space, or otherwise begin to behave as if they were thinking about the proposition.

- Phase 2, Step 4: *Ask What Is Different, with Pause 3:* "So, you wake up in the morning after the miracle happens during the night. All the problems that brought you here are gone—poof—just like that. What is the very first thing you notice after you wake up? What are the little changes you start to notice that tell you the problem is gone?" (de Shazer et al., 2007, p. 43). At this point, many clients need some time to think about their answer, often becoming quiet, still, and pensive. This is generally a sign that the client is generating new ideas, so it is important that the counselor patiently wait for the response. Rushing clients at this point will likely generate more-of-the-same thinking.

Phase 3: Facilitating the Description of the Miracle: 2 Steps with one List

- Phase 3, Step 1: *Focus Client on Behavior Changes in Positive Language:* Those new to this intervention often imagine their work is done once the question has been asked. For the miracle question to be useful in case conceptualization, the counselor needs to skillfully facilitate the description of the miracle—not just any miracle will do. Once the client begins to describe what is different, the counselor helps focus the answer by asking about *observable behavioral changes* in the client and others. In typical solution-focused style, the counselor is interested not in what the client is *not* doing but instead in what the client *is* doing. For example, if the client says, "I will not be depressed any more," the counselor responds with, "What will you be doing instead?"
- Phase 3, Step 2: *Continue Until You Have Enough to Identify Clear Goals:* Once the client identifies one new behavior, the counselor asks for more: "What else would be different?" The counselor continues until several (three or more) concrete miracle behaviors are identified that can be useful for developing goals and a clear direction for change. In the case study at the end of this chapter, the therapist uses the miracle question with Suzie and Jorge to identify what a satisfying relationship would look like for each.

Try It Yourself

Find a partner and take turns asking the miracle question. What helps the client get into the right frame of mind for this question?

Scaling Questions and the Miracle Scale

If I were challenged to use only one technique to work with clients from start to finish, **scaling questions** would have to top the list of possibilities, as they are arguably one of the most versatile and comprehensive interventions. Therapists can use scaling questions to: (a) assess strengths and solutions, (b) set goals, (c) design homework tasks, (d) measure progress, and (e) manage crises with safety plans (see Scaling for Safety in Chapter 12). They can be used in the first session and reused weekly until the last session. Like many modern-day miracle, all-in-one products—such as shampoo–conditioners, moisturizer–sunscreen–foundations, and car wash-and-waxes—this technique is likely to be one of your go-to techniques for years to come.

As the name indicates, scaling questions involve asking clients to use a scale to define their goals and rate their progress toward them; it is most often a 10-point scale, but sometimes percentages or shorter, nonnumeric versions are used with children (Bertolino, 2010; de Shazer, 1994; O'Hanlon & Weiner-Davis, 1989; Selekman, 1997). de Shazer and Dolan (2007) recommend having 0 represent "when you decided to seek help" rather than when things are "at their worst." When scaling 0 to mean "at their worst," this can refer to decades earlier or have different meanings to different people. Instead, scaling from "when you decided to seek help" allows for a clearer system for measuring progress from the beginning to the end of therapy; de Shazer and Dolan refer to these as "miracle scales" and use them to follow up with the miracle question (see "Solution-Focused Case Conceptualization," below). Others use 0 or 1 to represent things at their worst (Bertolino, 2010).

Two Approaches to Scaling

Miracle Scale: Measures Progress from Beginning of Therapy

When You Decided to Seek Help   *Miracle Situation*

0-------1-------2-------3-------4-------5-------6-------7-------8-------9-------10

Worst-to-Solution Scale: Measures Progress in General

Things at Their Worst   *Solution*

0-------1-------2-------3-------4-------5-------6-------7-------8-------9-------10

Scaling questions can be used early in the therapy process to help identify meaningful long-term goals in much the way the miracle question is used (see below):

Scaling Question for Long-Term Goal Setting (Assessing Solutions and Setting Goals)

If you were to put your situation on a scale from 1 to 10—with 0 being where you were when you decided to seek help (or at their worst) and 10 being where you'd like to be—can you describe to me what you would be doing (*not* what you would *not* be doing) if things were at a 10? Where are you today? What was happening and what were you doing at a 0?

As the client responds, the therapist listens for clear, specific descriptions of what life would be like at a 10, helping the client to paint a clear, behavioral picture: What is the client doing, what are others doing, how does the day go? Once a clear description of the 10 scenario is developed, the therapist can then ask where things are today and obtain a behavioral description of the current situation. A concrete description of when things were at the point at which the client decided to seek help or were at their worst (0 or 1) can also be useful assessment information. Once the big picture is assessed, the same scale can be used to identify what works.

Scaling Question for Assessing What Works

If 0 is where you were when you decided to seek help and 10 is where you would be if the problem you came here for were resolved, where are you today? [If above a 0] What are you doing or what is happening that tells us you are at a 3 and not a 0? How did you get from a 0 to here?

This next set of questions helps identify what works, exceptions, and potential solutions that need to be assessed before more specific interventions can be developed. If the client gets stuck answering any of these questions, it can be helpful to ask how significant others might rate them on the scale. After exploring where a client is this week, where he or she was when deciding to seek counseling, and where he or she would like to be, then it is time to use scaling to identify the next step.

SCALING QUESTION FOR DESIGNING WEEK-TO-WEEK INTERVENTIONS AND TASKS

On a scale from 0 to 10, with 10 being your desired goal, where are you this week? [Client responds and rates: e.g., 3]. If you are at a 3 this week, what things would need to be different in your life for you to come in and say you were at a 4, one step higher (or *half* a step higher if client tends toward pessimism or needs to keep goal smaller)?

This is not an easy question to answer. Often clients rush ahead and describe an 8, 9, or 10 when the next step is really a 4. In such cases, the therapist needs to help clients identify more realistic expectations. In other cases, clients say, "I don't know"; when this happens, therapists need to practice patience, silence, and encouragement to help clients identify mini-steps toward their goal; this is a critical part of the process. The client—not the therapist—is the only person who can answer this question in any meaningful way. Remember, the therapist is not a solution-giver.

Once a clear description of the next step is developed, this information is used to identify specific, small tasks the client can take during the next week to move one step higher on the scale. It generally takes an entire session to fully flesh out concrete steps that are: (a) realistic and meaningful and (b) something that the client is motivated to try. For the intervention to work, the therapist and client need to develop micro-steps that take into account the client's motivation, willingness, schedule, variations in the schedule, reactions of others, etc. The therapist asks questions to identify and listens for potential barriers and pitfalls as well as helpful resources, working with the client to find ways to negotiate these. Together, the client and therapist work together to develop specific homework tasks that client believes will help move him or her toward the goals.

For example, if the client's initial response is that "At a 4, I would feel less anxious," the therapist needs to ask follow-up questions such as, "How would you know you were less anxious?" "What would you be doing differently?" "How would your days be different?" "What changes would other people notice in you?" These questions help the client identify one to two specific, small steps to be taken over the week, such as "invite a friend over," "go to the mall alone," "watch a funny movie," etc. The steps need to be small enough, especially early in the process, that the client thinks the steps are easily attainable.

SCALING QUESTION FOR MEASURING PROGRESS

Last week you said you were at a 3, where would you say you are this week, and why? [If things got better] What did *you do* that helped move you up the scale? [If things stayed the same or got worse] What happened that kept things the same (or made them worse)?

The therapist follows up the next week to see if the homework tasks helped move clients closer to their goals. If so, they explore what helped and how to do more of it. If clients don't report progress or report that things got worse [with or without doing the homework], the therapist does not despair, but simply goes back to more carefully assess whether: (a) the solution has been meaningfully assessed and concretely identified and (b) the task was small enough, concrete enough, and motivating enough. This scale can be used to measure progress from the beginning to the end of the counseling process. In the case study at the end of this chapter, the therapist plans to take very small steps toward change because Suzie's problems have been brewing for years, and she is skeptical and hesitant.

One Thing Different: Client-Generated Change

In the beginning, the key is to do one small thing differently—for example, call one friend, rather than visit with someone every day (de Shazer, 1985, 1988; O'Hanlon, 2000; O'Hanlon & Weiner-Davis, 1989). Similarly, a goal such as "get up and exercise one day this week" is more likely to generate change and motivation for further change than a goal such as "get up and exercise every day this week." In most cases, making this one small change starts a cascade of change events that are inspired by the client's *own* motivation rather than by the prescription of the therapist (or even the co-created solution with the therapist). Ideas generated in therapy are not viewed as the "best," "only," or "correct" solution but rather as activities that will spark clients to identify what works for them.

The Doing: Interventions

Solution-Focused Tenets for Intervention

de Shazer et al. (2007, p. 2) identify basic tenets of solution-focused intervention that therapists can use to guide their work.

- If it isn't broken, don't fix it: Don't use therapeutic theory to determine areas of intervention.
- If it works, do more of it: Amplify and build upon things that are currently working.
- If it's not working, do something different: Even if it's a good idea, if it's not working, find another solution.
- Small steps can lead to big changes: Begin with small doable changes; these typically happen and quickly lead to more change.
- The solution is not necessarily related to the problem: Focus on moving forward, not on understanding why there is a problem.
- The language for solution development is different from that needed to describe a problem: Problem talk is negative and past-focused; solution talk is hopeful, positive, and future-focused.
- No problem happens all the time; there are always exceptions that can be utilized: Even the smallest exception is useful for identifying potential solutions.
- The future is both created and negotiable: Clients have a significant role in designing their future.

Formula First Session Task

As the name implies, the formula first session task (de Shazer, 1985) is typically used in the first session with all clients, regardless of the issue, to increase the client's hope for the therapy process and motivation for change.

EXAMPLE OF A FORMULA FIRST-SESSION TASK

Formula first-session task: "Between now and the next time we meet, we [I] would like you to observe, so that you can describe to us [me] next time,

> what happens in your [pick one: family, life, marriage, relationship] that you want to continue to have happen." (de Shazer, 1985, p. 137)
>
> **Paraphrase with introduction:** "As we are starting therapy, many things are going to change. However, I am sure that there are many things in your life and relationships that you do *not* want to have changed. Over the next week, I want [each of] you to generate a list of the things in your life and relationships that you *do not* want to have changed by therapy. Notice small things as well as big things that are working right now."

This directive stimulates clients to notice what is working, identifies their strengths and resources, and helps generate optimism about their ability to change.

Scaling Questions for Weekly Task Assignments

Scaling questions are used for goal setting (see previous discussion) as well as for developing weekly tasks and homework (O'Hanlon & Weiner-Davis, 1989). Once a client has identified what behaviors would constitute moving up the scale, the therapist works with the client to identify specific activities and behaviors that will make the small changes needed to enact these behaviors. This intervention can be used weekly to develop homework assignments that will move clients step-by-step toward their goals. If clients do not follow through on the assigned tasks, therapists need to reassess by asking the following questions: (a) Am I expecting a complainant to be as motivated for change as a customer? (b) Was the task too big, or can smaller steps be taken? (c) Are the right people involved? and (d) What actually motivates the client to take action and move toward change?

Asking Presuppositional Questions and Assuming a Future Solution

Presuppositional questions and talk that assumes future change help clients to envision a future without the problem, generating hope and motivation (O'Hanlon & Beadle, 1999; O'Hanlon & Weiner-Davis, 1989). Solution-focused therapists assume that things will change based on the observation that all things change: it is impossible for a client's situation to not change. Knowing that change is inevitable and that most clients benefit from therapy, therapists can be confident when they ask presuppositional questions, such as the following:

• What will you be doing differently once we resolve these issues?
• Do you think there are other concerns you will want to address once we resolve these issues?
• When the problem is resolved, what is one of the first things you will do to celebrate?

Questions such as these can be very helpful in cases—such as the one with Suzie and Jorge at the end of this chapter—when one or more parties is feeling hopeless.

Utilization

Drawing on the hypnotic work of Milton Erickson, de Shazer (1988) employed utilization techniques to help clients identify and enact solutions. **Utilization** refers to finding a way to use and leverage whatever the client presents as a strength, interest, proclivity, or habit to develop meaningful actions and plans that will lead in the direction of solutions. For example, if a client has difficulty making friends and close relations but has numerous pets, the therapist will utilize the client's interest in animals to develop more human connections, perhaps by having the client take a dog for a walk in public places, join a dog agility class, or volunteer at a pet shelter.

Coping Questions

Coping questions generate hope, agency, and motivation, especially when clients are feeling overwhelmed (De Jong & Berg, 2002; de Shazer & Dolan, 2007). They are used when the client is not reporting progress, describing an acute crisis, or otherwise feeling hopeless. Coping questions direct clients to identify how they have been coping with a current or past difficult situation.

EXAMPLES OF COPING QUESTIONS

- "This sounds hard—how are you managing to cope with this to the degree that you are?" (de Shazer & Dolan, 2007, p. 10)
- "How have you managed to prevent it from getting worse?" (p. 10)

Compliments and Encouragement

Solution-based therapists use compliments and encouragement to motivate clients and highlight strengths. The key with compliments is to compliment *only* when clients are making progress toward *goals that they have set* or to compliment *specific strengths that relate to the problem*. This is so important that I am going to say it again and put it in a special box so you don't forget.

THERAPEUTIC COMPLIMENTS

Rule for Making Compliments
Compliment only when clients are making progress toward goals they have set, or compliment specific strengths that relate to the problem; compliment their progress, not their personhood.

EXAMPLES

Therapeutic compliment:

- Wow! You made real progress toward your goal this week.

Even better therapeutic compliment:

- I am impressed; you not only followed through on the chart idea we developed last week but you came up with your own additional strategies [setting up a weekend outing with his son] to improve your relationship with your son. (compliments specific behavior toward goal)

Not-so-good therapeutic compliments:

- I really admire what you have done with your life. (too personal and does not clearly relate to the problem; sounds like you are buttering up client)
- You really are a great mom. (nonspecific; evaluating mothering skills globally; discouraging client from evaluating her own behavior and performance as a mother)

When a therapist compliments the client on anything other than the client's goals and strengths, a situation is being set up in which the therapist is rendering judgment, albeit a positive one, on the client or his or her life. Compliments should not be used to be "nice" to clients (De Jong & Berg, 2002). They should be used only to reinforce progress toward goals that clients have set for themselves and stated in such a way that they encourage clients to validate themselves rather than rely on an outside authority figure to do so. When clients can set goals and make progress toward them, they develop a greater sense of *self-efficacy* ("I can do this"), which is a greater predictor of happiness than self-esteem (Seligman, 2004).

Interventions for Specific Problems

Couples Therapy and Divorce Busting

Solution-oriented couples therapy is popular because the emphasis on strength and hope is well suited for working with negative, interpersonal conflict, especially with couples who are in crisis or considering divorce (Hudson & O'Hanlon, 1991; Weiner-Davis, 1992). These solution-oriented couples therapies have several unique interventions.

Videotalk

Videotalk is based on distinguishing among three levels of experience: facts, stories, and experience (Hudson & O'Hanlon, 1991). The *facts* are a behavioral description of what was done and said, what would be recorded on videotape during the couple's interaction. The *story* is the interpretation and meaning that a person associates with the behaviors and words. The *experience* is the internal thoughts and feelings each person had. When couples are having difficulty, therapists can help them sort through their differences by separating the facts from the story and the experience to increase each person's understanding of how he or she is interpreting the situation. Clients are encouraged to use videotalk (e.g., "She asked me three times" or "He went to his study after dinner without saying anything to me") instead of their default interpretations (e.g., "She was nagging" or "He is distant"). By using videotalk to separate the *behaviors* from the *interpretation of the behaviors,* couples become less defensive with one another and are able to engage in conversations in which they better understand each other and can identify meaningful ways to reduce future conflict.

Try It Yourself

Find a partner and take turns using videotalk to describe a problem situation or interaction. How does separating the behavior from the interpretation change how you understand the situation?

From Complaints to Requests

Solution-oriented therapists encourage clients to ask for what they want rather than what they don't want or, in other words, to move from making *complaints* to making *requests* (O'Hanlon & Hudson, 1991; Weiner-Davis, 1992). For example, instead of saying, "You don't do anything romantic anymore" (a global, overgeneralizing complaint), the partner would learn to rephrase the complaint as a request: "I would really enjoy adding romance back into our relationship." These requests need to be behavioral and specific. Thus, the person in this example needs to add a specific behavioral request: "I'd like to go away for a weekend; go to dinner and a movie; go to the beach for a sunset walk" and/or "It would be nice if we went back to giving each other a kiss before we left the house, leaving little love notes, or giving each other massages."

Therapy for Sexual Abuse and Trauma

Yvonne Dolan (1991) and Bill O'Hanlon and Bob Bertolino (2002) use solution-based therapies with child and adult survivors of childhood sexual abuse. Solution-based approaches stand out from traditional approaches to sexual abuse treatment in their optimistic and hopeful stance that emphasizes the resiliencies of survivors. Given that these clients have *survived* such a difficult trauma, solution-oriented therapists harness those strengths in new ways to help them resolve current issues. Some of the distinctive qualities of these approaches include those discussed below.

Honoring the Agency of Survivors

More so than traditional therapists, solution-based therapists honor the agency of survivors, allowing them to decide whether to tell their abuse stories and to determine the pacing of their treatment (Dolan, 1991; O'Hanlon & Bertolino, 2002). Although many therapists insist that survivors cannot heal without sharing the details of their abuse with their therapists, solution-based therapists would not readily agree. Instead, they work with clients to identify whether, when, how, and to whom it is best to tell their stories. By fully honoring their agency, therapists create a relationship in which survivors regain full authority over the private aspects of their lives, reclaiming the autonomy that was lost through the abuse. Therapists who play a more directive role in working with a survivor may unintentionally replicate the abuse pattern by forcing clients to reveal parts of their sexual life in the name of treatment before they are ready to do so, leaving them feeling violated and retraumatized.

The Recovery Scale: Focusing on Strengths and Abilities

Dolan (1991) uses the *Solution-Focused Recovery Scale* to identify the areas of the client's life that were not affected by the abuse, thus reducing the sense that the client's whole life and self have been affected. The success strategies in these areas are used to address areas that are affected by the abuse.

3-D Model: Dissociate, Disown, and Devalue

O'Hanlon and Bertolino (2002) conceptualize the aftereffects of abuse and trauma using the 3-D model, which postulates that abuse leads people to dissociate, disown, and devalue aspects of the self, with the result that they develop symptoms that either inhibit experience (e.g., lack of sexual response, lack of memories, lack of anger) or that create intrusive experiences (e.g., flashbacks, sexual compulsions, or rage). The goal of therapy is to reconnect people with these disowned parts. O'Hanlon and Bertolino (2002) note that many of the symptoms related to sexual abuse are experienced as a sort of *negative trance,* a feeling that the experience is uncontrollable and involves only a part of the self. Solution-oriented therapists use *permissive, validating,* and *inclusive language* to encourage clients to revalue and include the devalued aspects of self that were disowned through the abuse.

Constructive Questions

Dolan (1991, pp. 37–38) uses constructive questions to identify the specifics of clients' unique solutions:

• What will be the first [smallest] sign that things are getting better, that this [the sexual abuse] is having less of an impact on your current life?
• What will you be doing differently when this [sexual abuse trauma] is less of a current problem in your life?

- What will you be doing differently with your time?
- What will you be thinking about [doing] instead of thinking about the past?
- Are there times when these things are already happening to some [even a small] extent? What is different about those times? What is helpful about those differences?
- What differences will these healing changes make when they have been present in your life over an extended period of time [days, weeks, months, years]?
- What do you think your significant other would say would be the first sign that things are getting better? What do you think your significant other will notice first?
- What do you think your [friends, boss, significant other, etc.] will notice about you as you heal even more?
- What differences will these healing changes you've identified make in future generations of your family?

Videotalk (Action Terms)

Because of the intense emotions that characterize abuse and trauma, survivors often have difficulty identifying the effects of abuse in their present life. O'Hanlon and Bertolino (2002) use *videotalk* (discussed above) with survivors to help identify specific actions and patterns of behavior that re-create the traumatic experience, including the sequence of events, antecedents, consequences, invariant actions, repetitive actions, and body responses. Once these recurrent patterns are identified, therapists help clients either change one part of the context to interrupt the cycle and create space for new responses or, if the client feels a certain degree of control over the symptoms, identify new, alternative solution-generating actions.

Scope It Out: Cross-Theoretical Comparison

Using Tomm's IPscope described in Chapter 3 (Tomm et al., 2014), this theory approaches the conceptualization of systemic, interpersonal patterns as described below.

Case Conceptualization

Unique in the field, solution-focused therapists routinely assess only wellness interpersonal patterns (WIPs), although they may track pathologizing or healing interpersonal patterns (PIPs and HIPs) if appropriate or useful for a particular client. However, the focus of their initial assessment is: What will the solution—or wellness—look like? Although not always explicit in the solution-focused literature, solution-focused therapists carefully assess interaction patterns that are associated with the desired solution, typically getting a behavioral description of the WIP first and then going back and getting the meaning or significance that the client attributes to these interactions. For example, a parent I worked with described a solution in which her teen would be more cooperative and use a more respectful tone as part of the "solution"; I then inquired about the parent's half of the interaction in this WIP. Together we identified "making respectful requests"/ "responding with respect" as the wellness pattern; this helped us develop a more complete description of the preferred solution.

Goal Setting

Goal setting in solution-based therapies involves identifying the WIPs and sometimes the HIPs related to the client's preferred solution.

Facilitating Change

When facilitating change, solution-based therapists identify small, behavioral steps clients can take to move them closer to their WIPs. Typically they will have only minimal conversation about PIPs and will carefully assess it only if it seems necessary for a particular client. Similarly, unless a HIP seems warranted in a particular case, such as when one person in the couple has had an affair, the solution-focused therapist will tend to focus on only the WIP. Solution-focused therapists tend to assess sociocultural interpersonal patterns (SCIPs) when assessing for strengths and resources that may be useful in facilitating WIPs.

Putting It All Together: Case Conceptualization and Treatment Plan Templates

Theory-Specific Case Conceptualization: Solution-Based

📝 When conceptualizing client cases, contemporary solution-focused therapists typically use the following dynamics to inform their treatment plan. Go to MindTap® to access a digital version of the theory-specific case conceptualization, along with a variety of digital study tools and resources that complement this text and help you be more successful in your course and career. If your instructor didn't assign MindTap, you can find out more about it at Cengagebrain.com. You can also download the form at masteringcompetencies.com.

Preferred Solution and Miracle Day

- Describe each significant person's description of the solution or miracle day, focusing on *observable,* actual behaviors (what a video camera would see) rather than what would not be happening.
- Significance: What difference do clients say these behaviors and events make? What meanings are ascribed?
- Relational: Who is likely to notice first? What will he or she see? What difference would that make to him or her? What difference does that make for you?

Exceptions

- Identify as many times, places, relationships, context, etc. when the problem is less of a problem or the solution is enacted in part or entirely. Describe these exceptions in detail, including who, where, when, and what and any other factors that might relate to the exception.

Solution Scaling

- On a scale of 0 to 10, where 10 is the miracle day and 0 is the opposite, where were the clients at the initial interview? At the most recent sessions?
- What does one small step on the scale look like in behavioral terms?

Interpersonal Patterns

- Identify one or more solution(s) above, and describe the positive interaction pattern(s) related to the solution, including behavioral descriptions of each person's part of the pattern (e.g., showing affection/appreciating affection) or for individuals, their internal pattern (e.g., thinking positive/trying harder).

Resources for Preferred Solutions

- Personal: Describe potentially useful personal resources and qualities for enacting the preferred solution.
- Relational and social: Describe potentially useful relational and social resources for enacting the preferred solution.

- Community, diversity, and spiritual: Describe potentially useful resources for enacting the preferred solution:
  - Actual or potential supportive social communities, including ethnic, racial, lesbian, gay, bisexual, transgendered, and questioning (LGBTQ), religious, gender, linguistic, local/regional, immigrant, socioeconomic, professional/job-related, etc.
  - Spiritual beliefs and religious practices that are coping resources
- Health and Hobbies: Describe potentially useful resources for enacting the preferred solution:
  - Healthy habits, such as exercising, eating well, regular sleep, stress-reduction strategies, etc.
  - Hobbies, sources of fun, and nonvocational skills

TREATMENT PLAN TEMPLATE FOR INDIVIDUALS WITH SEXUAL ABUSE TRAUMA: SOLUTION-BASED

You can download a blank treatment plan (with or without measures) from MindTap at www.cengagebrain.com or www.masteringcompetencies.com. The following treatment plan template can beμ used to help you develop individualized treatments for use with individuals with sexual abuse trauma symptoms.

Solution-Based Treatment Plan: Client Goals with Interventions

Early-Phase Client Goals

1. Increase *sense* of *control and safety when remembering abuse* to reduce flashbacks, dissociation, and hypervigilance.
   a. *Formula first session task* to identify existing areas of life that are working and can be used when feeling overwhelmed.
   b. *Scaling for safety* (see Chapter 12) to develop a safety plan for when emotions and memories become overwhelming.
   c. *Coping questions* to explore how client has been coping and how to expand these abilities.

Working-Phase Client Goals

1. Increase *client's sense of safety* with friends, family, and at home to reduce hypervigilance and dissociation.
   a. *Scaling questions* to identify small steps to increase sense of trust and openness in safe relationships.
   b. *Constructive questions* to help clients identify the specific behaviors that will characterize more trusting relationships.

2. Increase client's sense of *agency and survivorship* and decrease self-blame related to abuse to reduce sense of victimization, hopelessness, and stigma.
   a. *Permissive, validating, and inclusive language* to help clients reconnect with disowned and undervalued parts of themselves.
   b. *Channeling language* to help clients separate past from the present experience and to delimit the effects of the abuse.
   c. *Exception and coping questions* to enable client to rewrite is perferred term the story of abuse in such a way that includes attempts to avoid the abuser, stop the abuse, ask for help, and/or cope to increase sense of agency and decrease self-blame.

3. Increase client's sense of *positive connection with his or her body and sexuality* to reduce physical symptoms of trauma, sexual issues, body image issues, and/or eating issues.
   a. *Exception questions* to help client identify positive associations with body and sexuality.
   b. *Presuppositional questions* that assume the client will return to a healthy relationship with body and identify strategies for doing so.

Closing-Phase Client Goals

1. Increase client's *sense of agency* and engagement in [specify enjoyable activities] to reduce hopelessness and depressed mood.
   a. *Scaling questions* to identify small, doable steps to reclaiming agency in own life.
   b. *Therapeutic compliments* of client's attempts to take steps toward agency.

2. Increase client's ability to engage in *satisfying intimate relationships* to reduce isolation, hypervigilance, and extreme sense of vulnerability.
   a. *Scaling questions* to identify small steps to forming and/or improving intimate relationships.
   b. *Videotalk* for helping client identify patterns of interpreting partner's behavior based on past trauma rather than on the present situation.

Treatment Tasks

1. Develop working therapeutic relationship.
   a. Intervention: Develop *collaborative* relationship and inspire *hope* and *optimism*, using *beginner's mind* and listening for *strengths*.
   b. Assess individual, systemic, and broader cultural dynamics.
   c. Use *miracle question* to concretely and behaviorally define solutions in positive terms.
   d. Identify *exceptions* to the effects of abuse in all areas of life, times when trauma symptoms are less severe, areas of life not affected by the trauma, *strengths and resources*, supportive relationships, and client level of *motivation*.
   e. Use the *recovery scale* to identify areas of strengths and resources.

2. Identify needed referrals, crisis issues, collateral contacts, and other client needs.

   Crisis assessment intervention(s): Address crisis issues such as self harm, suicidal ideation, substance use, risky sexual behavior, etc.

   Referral(s): Connect client with *resources* in client's *family and community* that could be supportive; make collateral contacts as needed.

TREATMENT PLAN TEMPLATE FOR DISTRESSED COUPLE/FAMILY: SOLUTION-BASED

You can download a blank treatment plan (with or without measures) from MindTap at www.cengagebrain.com or www.masteringcompetencies.com. The following treatment plan template can be used to help you develop individualized treatments for use with couples and families who report relational distress.

Solution-Based Treatment Plan: Client Goals with Interventions

Early-Phase Client Goals

1. Increase engagement in *shared, enjoyable activities* to reduce conflict.
   a. *Formula first session task* to identify existing areas of relationship that are working.
   b. *Exception questions* to identify areas of relationship that are more satisfying and identify between-session tasks for increasing or expanding these activities

Working-Phase Client Goals

1. Increase *satisfying communication* between couple/family to reduce conflict.
   a. *Videotalk* to separate behavior from interpretations and help each person better understand the other.
   b. Suggest clients move from making complaints to *making positive, behavioral requests* of each other.

2. Increase [specify positive couple/family interactions and relational patterns] to reduce conflict.
   a. *Scaling questions* to identify small steps (*one thing different*), with instructions for each member.
   b. *Channeling language* to reduce the sense that other members are "always" a certain way.
   c. *Therapeutic compliments* to encourage small steps toward desired solutions.

3. [For couples] Increase *mutually enjoyable physical and sexual intimacy* to reduce conflict and increase intimacy.
   a. *Exception questions* to help clients' areas of intimate life that are or have been satisfying for both.
   b. *Scaling questions* to identify small, concrete steps each could take to make desired changes.

Closing-Phase Client Goals

1. Increase *sense of shared identity and connection* to reduce conflict and increase sense of intimacy.
   a. *Scaling questions* to identify small, doable steps to reclaiming agency in own life.
   b. *Compliment* client's attempts to take steps toward agency.

Treatment Tasks

1. Develop working therapeutic relationship.
   a. Develop *collaborative* relationship with all members; inspire *hope* and *optimism,* using *beginner's mind* and listening for *strengths.*

2. Assess individual, systemic, and broader cultural dynamics. *Diversity note:*
   a. Use *miracle question* with each person to concretely and behaviorally define solutions in positive terms.
   b. Identify *exceptions* to conflict, times of connection, areas of life not affected by the conflict, *strengths and resources,* supportive relationships, and client level of *motivation.*

3. Identify needed referrals, crisis issues, collateral contacts, and other client needs.
   a. Address crisis issues such as psychological abuse, intimate partner violence, hidden affair, self harm, suicidal ideation, substance use, etc.
   b. *Referral(s):* Connect client with *resources* in client's *family and community* that could be supportive; make collateral contacts as needed.

Solution-Oriented Ericksonian Hypnosis

Solution-oriented hypnosis, also known as Ericksonian hypnosis or naturalistic trance, is a unique form of hypnosis that aims to evoke client strengths and resources to resolve problems (Erickson & Keeney, 2006; Lankton, Lankton, & Matthews, 1991; O'Hanlon & Martin, 1992). As the name suggests, solution-oriented Ericksonian hypnosis grew out of the work of Milton Erickson, *preceding* solution-focused and solution-oriented therapies. Many solution-focused premises and techniques directly evolved from Erickson's approach to hypnosis and therapy, and Lankton et al. (1991) also describe how this approach can be used as a comprehensive approach for working with couples and families.

Difference from Traditional Hypnosis

Solution-oriented hypnosis is different from traditional hypnosis in two significant ways (O'Hanlon & Martin, 1992):

- *Permissive rather than hierarchical:* Traditional hypnosis is hierarchical; the therapist runs the show ("You will become very sleepy"), whereas solution-oriented hypnosis is permissive ("You may find yourself wanting to close your eyes, or you may prefer to keep them open").
- *Evokes client's natural resources:* In traditional hypnosis, the therapist effectively "reprograms" the client once he or she is in a trance; in solution-oriented therapy, the therapist tries to "evoke" or stimulate the client's natural resources for healing, serving more as a midwife who allows the natural process to occur.

The Big Picture: Overview of Treatment

Ericksonian therapy invites the client to go into a trance in order to evoke resources and strengths that the client already has: this may be done with or without a clear induction into a hypnotic trance state. Erickson was known for using stories, analogies, and directives to activate latent abilities to enable clients to resolve their problems (O'Hanlon & Martin, 1992). His work was arguably the first *brief therapy,* developed during a time when psychiatry and psychotherapy were dominated by psychodynamic ideas about problem development and problem resolution (Erickson & Keeney, 2006; O'Hanlon & Martin, 1992). Many of his students have gone on to further develop his work, including Richard Bandler, John Grinder, Jay Haley, Bill O'Hanlon, Ernest Rossi, and Jeffrey Zeig, and the Milton H. Erickson Foundation continues training in his approach.

The Doing: Interventions

Permission

When inviting clients to enter a trance state, Ericksonian therapists give their clients *permission* to think, experience, and feel whatever they are experiencing without any pressure to *do* something (O'Hanlon & Martin, 1992). Clients are given explicit permission to have doubts, allow their mind to chatter, lose focus, entertain distracting thoughts, and accept other thoughts or feelings.

Presuppositions

Ericksonian therapists who are inviting clients into a trance state *presuppose* that clients will enter a trance state by delivering certain questions and comments to the client (O'Hanlon & Martin, 1992); for example, "Have you ever been in a trance before today?" "You can choose to keep your eyes open or closed when you go into a trance." "Don't go into a trance too quickly" (p. 18).

Splitting

The therapist may split into two things that the client may habitually consider to be one, such as the conscious and unconscious mind or the left brain and right brain (O'Hanlon & Martin, 1992). In general, problem-saturated thoughts and feelings are attributed to the conscious mind and positive thoughts to the unconscious to allow the person to trust the trance process. For example, the therapist may attribute doubt or apprehension to the conscious mind and trust to the unconscious mind: "Your conscious mind may doubt that trance is even possible, but your unconscious mind knows exactly what to do."

Class of Problems versus Class of Solutions

To the untrained eye, Erickson often seemed to discuss issues and topics that were totally unrelated to the problem. For example, when working with a child with enuresis, he might spend the entire session chatting about seemingly unrelated topics, such as baseball and digestion, without ever discussing the presenting problem (O'Hanlon and Martin, 1992). Erickson would assess the class of problem (e.g., lack of muscle control) and then identify the class of solution that would most likely solve the problem (e.g., gaining muscle control) (O'Hanlon & Martin, 1992). Similarly, if a person's depressed mood was characterized by pessimism, he would find areas in which the client had hope and optimism; if the client's depression was related to a recent failure, he would find ways to evoke a sense of success, whether actual or potential. Thus, for Erickson, the focus was on evoking the class of solution—*in any other area of the person's life*—rather than trying to solve the literal problem. He would focus on evoking the solution through both dialogue and trance.

Identifying the class of solution is a particularly useful concept when assessing strengths because it highlights that all strengths are not created equal. Erickson draws our attention to the fact that it is most important *to identify client strengths that are in the same class of solutions that relate to the presenting problem.* Thus, if a child is having difficulty following parental requests at home, therapists should carefully listen for other situations in which the client is able to follow rules, whether playing on a soccer team, paying attention in class, or playing board games with a friend.

Tapestry Weaving: Working with Diverse Populations
Ethnic, Racial, and Cultural Diversity

Because it does not use a theory of health to predefine client goals (O'Hanlon & Weiner-Davis, 1989), solution-focused therapy can be adapted to a wide range of populations and value systems. This therapy is widely used with diverse populations in North America, South America, Europe, the Middle East, Asia, and Australia (Gingerich & Peterson, 2013). It has also been studied and found to be effective with a range of clients, including immigrants, African Americans, Hispanics/Latinos, Saudi Arabians, Chinese, and Koreans; and in a wide range of contexts, such as schools, prisons, hospitals, businesses, and colleges (Gingerich & Peterson, 2013; Liu et al., 2015; Suitt, Franklin, & Kim, 2016). When working with diverse clients, solution-focused therapists access the client's unique emotional, cognitive, and social resources, which often relate to issues of diversity.

Corcoran (2000) identifies several reasons why solution-focused therapy is generally a good fit for diverse populations:

- *Behavior considered in context:* The solution-based viewing of behaviors in context allows for a more accurate understanding of the problem behaviors of marginalized populations.
- *Client-generated, behavioral goals:* The goal-setting process of solution-based therapies is a good fit for many ethnic groups because the goals are set in client language, they are concrete and behavioral, and they are generally short term.
- *Behavioral rather than emotional focus:* The focus on behavior rather than emotion is more comfortable and value-consistent for many ethnic minority groups.
- *Future orientation:* The focus on solving problems in the future rather than on understanding the past makes sense to many ethnic minorities.

Asian American Clients

Several therapists have explored using solution-based therapies with Asians and Asian Americans, with the most international research conducted in China (Epstein et al., 2014;

Liu et al., 2015). Hsu and Wang (2011) describe solution-focused therapy as being highly compatible for Asian clients because of its positive reframing (avoids losing face), relation-based perspective, and focus on pragmatic solutions. In a recent meta-analysis of the effectiveness of solution-focused therapy in China, researchers found that this approach had medium to very large effect sizes for adults diagnosed with internalizing disorders, such as depression, anxiety, and self-esteem issues; these effect sizes were larger than is typical in the United States (Kim et al., 2015). Considerations for working with Asian clients include:

- *Filial piety:* Several therapists have used solution-focused therapy to help clients navigate issues of filial piety, a common Asian value in which elders are obeyed and honored (Lee & Mjelde-Mossey, 2004: Hsu & Wang, 2011). Solution-focused approaches help reframe each generation's perspective in positive terms, so the good intentions of each are better understood.
- *Form and content:* Many Asian societies value the *form* (*how* something is done) as much as the *content* (*what* is done) (Berg & Jaya, 1993). This can translate to family members being more concerned about how someone approached a problem as about what was done to solve it.
- *Practical solutions:* Asian cultures generally discourage dramatic displays of emotion, and this often translates to a preference for therapeutic approaches that focus on pragmatic solutions rather than on exploration of feelings and causes (Berg & Jaya, 1993).
- *Saving face:* Solution-focused therapy is unique in that its focus on "what to do from here" rather than on identifying root causes more easily allows for Asian clients to save face. Asian cultures are *shame-based,* not guilt-based, and thus positive reframes and compliments work particularly well with these populations (Berg & Jaya, 1993).
- *Brief treatment:* As therapy is usually a last resort for Asian families, who prefer privacy, the brief approach of solution-focused therapy is an excellent fit (Berg & Jaya, 1993).
- *Complimenting:* When used in China, practitioners avoid too much complimenting, which was a signature strength of Insoo Berg, to make the approach fit cultural values of humility and modesty (Liu et al., 2015).

Muslim American Clients

Solution-focused therapy has been identified as an appropriate approach for Muslim Americans, who face significant discrimination in the United States (Chaudhry & Li, 2011). Similar to others in collectivist cultures, most Muslim Americans prefer to seek advice for personal problems from their family, religious teachers, or ethnic community; when they do seek professional assistance, it is typically for a specific problem. In addition, Muslim Americans have legitimate reasons to be cautious in divulging their personal information, because it may be divulged, accessed, or used against them politically. Based on a religion that is practiced around the world, the Muslim American community is quite diverse, and limited generalizations can be made. Nonetheless, Chaudhry and Li (2011) identify some potential ways that solution-focused therapy may be particularly appropriate for these populations:

- *Minimal self-disclosure:* Unlike psychodynamic or other approaches that emphasize history, solution-focused therapy requires less self-disclosure, which is particularly appropriate when a client fears potential political implications. The focus on practical steps toward client-defined solutions rather than on the client's inner world is likely to be felt safer and more comfortable.
- *Client-defined goals:* Solution-focused therapists typically define the focus of therapy using client language and worldview rather than using their theory to construct a focus of treatment. The goals also tend to be behavioral and practical rather than based on a theoretical construct, and the goals are defined directly by the client, reducing the chance of therapist bias or misunderstanding.

- *Brief:* Muslim Americans, who often have a strong community of support, are likely to be attracted to the brief and focused nature of solution-based therapy rather than to approaches that do not aspire to be short term.
- *Competence-seeking:* As the targets of significant discrimination and attack, Muslim Americans are likely to experience the strength-based approach of solution-based work not only refreshing but essential to creating an effective therapeutic relationship.

Native Americans/American Indians

Solution-based approaches have also been identified as potentially appropriate for working with Native Americans in North and South America (Meyer & Cottone, 2013). Few therapeutic approaches have been applied specifically with this population. Meyer and Cottone (2013) highlight that the social constructionist foundations of solution-based therapies make the approach particularly appropriate for diverse populations that have worldviews that may differ from those of their therapists. They note several ways that solution-based approaches are compatible and can be adapted to work with Native Americans:

- *Change:* The assumption that "change is constant" in solution-focused work is similar to Native American spiritual beliefs that change is continuous and unavoidable.
- *Client solutions:* The solution-focused emphasis on honoring the client's preferred solution easily allows for clients to make use of their unique healing and spiritual traditions.
- *Time orientation:* As a culture that orients to the present moment rather than to the future, techniques such as the miracle question or others that are future-focused need to be adjusted to have a present focus. Meyers and Cottone (2013) recommend altering the miracle question to have the client identify "a time when the client experienced harmony with all people and things" (p. 54).
- *Interruptions:* In most traditional cultures, interrupting another is considered highly rude and culturally inappropriate. Therapists should wait until the client is done speaking before responding and should avoid "helpful" interruptions that might be considered polite in other cultural contexts.
- *Resources versus strengths:* As the Native American culture values humility, solution-focused therapists should focus on client resources rather than strengths; focusing on strengths may make the client uncomfortable. Similarly, rather than a traditional scaling question with "10 being best," therapists working with Native Americans may find using a ranking system based on specific behaviors more effective than standard scaling, which has elements of competition and boastfulness.

Sexual and Gender Identity Diversity

Because solution-based therapies do not have a predefined theory of health and focus on client-defined goals, these models can be appropriate when working with gay, lesbian, bisexual, or transgendered clients. However, to be sensitive to these issues, therapists should inquire with the "beginner's mind" about their possible role in the client's presenting problem rather than assume that because it is not mentioned it is not part of the problem or solution. Little has been written specifically about solution-based therapies and these populations. However, this approach has been used to facilitate adjustment to one's spouse coming out. Treyger and colleagues (2008) found solution-based therapy appropriate for a case in which a woman's spouse announced he was gay. The approach was used to help the client identify her own solutions to the situation in a supportive, nonpathologizing context. They used Buxton's (2004) seven-stage model for partner adjustment to news that his or her spouse is homosexual or bisexual; the stages include disorientation/disbelief, facing and acknowledging reality, accepting, letting go, healing, reconfiguring and refocusing, and transforming. The client in Treyger et al. (2008)

reported that what helped the most from the approach was talking without being judged, not being given advice (which her family and friends offered plenty of), positive feedback and compliments, and scaling questions to concretely measure progress.

Solution-Focused Therapy with Men

Solution-focused therapy has also been identified as an approach that may be a particularly well-suited for working with male clients (Blundo, 2010). Specifically, Blundo describes how certain aspects of solution-based therapies correspond directly to the code of masculinity that is readily evident cross-culturally, thereby harnessing common male strengths, including:

* Stoicism: Solution-based therapies do not require expression of vulnerable emotions to be effective, which is a more comfortable process for many men.
* Self-reliance: Most men identify with being self-reliant and not needing help, which is often a barrier for coming to therapy in the first place. The collaborative, strength-based qualities of solution-based therapies honor men's desire to be self-reliant, and use this quality to help them enact their preferred solutions.
* Problem solving: Actively engaging clients in a process of identifying preferred solutions and small steps to enacting these desired outcomes engages the characteristic strength of many men: problem solving. For men, the shift offered by solution-focused therapy is that rather than try to solve the identified problem, the therapist has the client focus on solving the problem of how to enact the solution.
* Control and capability: Solution-focused techniques, such as exception questions, highlight those areas for clients where they do have some control over the problem, providing a hopeful perspective that can be motivating for men who feel powerless against their current problem or circumstance.
* Action-based: Solution-focused therapy focuses on concrete actions that clients can take outside of sessions, which fits with how many men prefer to approach challenges in their life.
* Achievement-based: Solution-focused scaling allows clients to concretely measure their progress and achievements, which is particularly motivating men whose identities are tied to feeling successful.

Research and the Evidence Base

Solution-based therapies have a steadily growing foundation of empirical support. Two meta-analyses of well-controlled clinical trial studies (Franklin, 2015; Kim, 2008; Stams et al., 2006) found that solution-focused brief therapy has modest effect sizes and typically has outcomes equivalent to those of other approaches but typically does so in less time and therefore at less cost (Gingerich et al., 2012). Similarly, a review of the effectiveness of solution-focused brief therapy provided tentative support for the approach, particularly with children and as an early intervention when problems are less severe (Bond et al., 2013). As further evidence of its growing evidence base, the Office of Juvenile Justice and Delinquency Prevention has recognized it as a promising practice, setting the stage for recognition as an evidence-based practice (Kim et al., 2010).

The majority of research has been conducted on solution-focused brief therapy, which was first described in the literature in 1986, had its first controlled study in 1993, and has had a total of 48 published studies and two meta-analytic reviews (Gingerich et al., 2012). The quality of studies is steadily improving, including randomized samples, treatment fidelity measures, and standardized outcome measures. Researchers have studied the effectiveness of solution-focused brief therapy with a wide range of clinical populations and problems, including domestic-violence offenders, couples, schizophrenics, child abuse survivors, troubled youth, school settings, parenting, alcohol, and foster care (Franklin et al., 2012). Research on the process of solution-focused brief therapy suggests that presuppositional questions, the miracle question, the first-session task, scaling questions, and solution talk have been found to accomplish their intended therapeutic effect and that the model in general engenders hope and optimism in clients (McKeel, 2012).

Currently, quantitative research in solution-focused brief therapy has focused on refining and improving clinical trial studies through the expansion of a standardized treatment manual (Trepper et al., 2012) and development of improved adherence and fidelity measures (Lehmann & Patton, 2012). In addition, process research is being done on in-session therapeutic alliance and client progress as both an outcome measure and collaborative intervention (Duncan, Miller, & Sparks, 2004; Gillaspy & Murphy, 2012; Miller et al., 2003).

Finally, of great interest in current psychotherapy research is the examination of the mechanisms of change that underlie an evidenced-based clinical approach such as solution-focused brief therapy. Laboratory experiments have provided evidence for some of the major underlying theoretical assumptions of solution-focused brief therapy; for example, that collaboration and co-construction led to significantly better outcomes in the laboratory (Bavelas, 2012). Also, microanalysis research has shown that solution-focused therapists are overwhelmingly positive in their formulations and questions as compared with client-centered and cognitive–behavioral therapists, whose formulations and questions were primarily negative (Tomori & Bavelas, 2007; Korman, Bavelas & De Jong, 2013; Jordan, Froerer, & Bavelas, 2013). It was also shown that this "positive talk" led to more positive talk, and negative talk led to more negative talk (Jordan et al., 2013). Thus, "a therapist's use of positive content seems to contribute to the co-construction of an overall positive session, whereas negative content would do the reverse" (Bavelas, 2012, p. 159). This area of research may someday refine an understanding of the exact mechanisms of change of solution-focused brief therapy and how this approach differs from other clinical models.

QUESTIONS FOR PERSONAL REFLECTION AND CLASS DISCUSSION

1. What balance of focusing on the problem versus solution makes the most sense to you?
   - How might this vary depending on the presenting problem?
   - How might this vary depending on the client?
   - How might this vary depending on the client's culture of origin?
2. Are you the type of person who tends to see the glass as half full in a given situation?
   - If so, how did you develop this skill?
   - If not, what tends to help you see the glass as half full?
   - In what situations and/or with what people are you most likely to see the glass as half full?
   - In what situations do you think there is a benefit to seeing the glass as half empty?
3. Write out the miracle question related to a current problem you are currently facing.
   - Was it difficult to imagine life without the problem?
   - Was it a challenge to describe "behaviors" that were different in positive terms?
4. Use a scaling question with a current problem. What are three small steps you can take over the next week to make small improvements?
5. What strengths does this approach have for working with clients who are marginalized because of race, ethnicity, sexual/gender orientation, economic class, or religion? What are its limitations?
6. What benefits does this approach have for working persons who have experienced sexual abuse or other forms of trauma? What are its limitations?

ONLINE RESOURCES

Institute for Solution-Focused Therapy
www.solutionfocused.net

Milton H. Erickson Foundation
www.erickson-foundation.org

Solution-Focused Brief Therapy Association
www.sfbta.org

Solution-Oriented Possibility Therapy
www.billohanlon.com

Divorce Busting
www.divorcebusting.com

European Brief Therapy Association
www.ebta.nu

Social Construction Therapy Online: Resources for collaborative, narrative and solution-focused
http://socialconstructiontherapy.com

Go to MindTap® for an eBook, videos of client sessions, activities, practice quizzes, apps, and more—all in one place. If your instructor didn't assign MindTap, you can find out more information at CengageBrain.com.

REFERENCES

*Asterisk indicates recommended introductory books.

Bavelas, J. B. (2012). Connecting the lab to the therapy room: Microanalysis, co-construction, and solution-focused brief therapy. In Cynthia Franklin, Terry S. Trepper, Wallace J. Gingerich, and Eric E. McCollum (Eds.), *Solution-focused brief therapy: A handbook of evidence-based practice* (pp. 144–164). London: Oxford University Press.

Berg, I. K. (1994). *Family based services: A solution-focused approach.* New York: Norton.

Berg, I. K., & Jaya, A. (1993). Different and same: Family therapy with Asian-American families. *Journal of Marital and Family Therapy, 19,* 31–38.

Berg, I. K., & Kelly, S. (2000). *Building solutions in child protective services.* New York: Norton.

Berg, I. K., & Miller, S. (1992). *Working with the problem drinker: A solution-focused approach.* New York: Norton.

Berg, I. K., & Reuss, N. H. (1997). *Solutions step by step: A substance abuse treatment manual.* New York: Norton.

Berg, I. K., & Steiner, T. (2003). *Children's solution work.* New York: Norton.

Berg, I. K., & Szabo, P. (2005). *Brief coaching for last solutions.* New York: Norton.

Bertolino, B. (2010). *Strength-based engagement and practice.* New York: Pearson.

Bertolino, B., & O'Hanlon, B. (1998). *Therapy with troubled teenagers: Rewriting young lives in progress.* New York: Wiley.

*Bertolino, B., & O'Hanlon, B. (2002). *Collaborative, competency-based counseling and therapy.* New York: Allyn & Bacon.

Bond, C., Woods, K., Humphrey, N., Symes, W., & Green, L. (2013). Practitioner review: The effectiveness of solution focused brief therapy with children and families: A systematic and critical evaluation of the literature from 1990–2010. *Journal of Child Psychology and Psychiatry, 54*(7), 707–723. doi:10.1111/jcpp.12058

Blundo, R. (2010). Engaging men in clinical practice: A solution-focused and strengths-based model. *Families in Society, 91*(3), 307–312.

Buxton, A. P. (2004). Paths and pitfalls: How heterosexual spouses cope when their husbands or wives come out. *Journal of Couple and Relationship Therapy, 3,* 95–109.

Chaudhry, S., & Li, C. (2011). Is solution-focused brief therapy culturally appropriate for Muslim American counselees? *Journal of Contemporary Psychotherapy, 41*(2), 109–113. doi:10.1007/s10879-010-9153-1

Corcoran, J. (2000). Solution-focused family therapy with ethnic minority clients. *Crisis Intervention & Time-Limited Treatment, 6*(1), 5–12.

*De Jong, P., & Berg, I. K. (2002). *Interviewing for solutions* (2nd ed.). New York: Brooks/Cole.

*de Shazer, S. (1985). *Keys to solution in brief therapy.* New York: Norton.

*de Shazer, S. (1988). *Clues: Investigating solutions in brief therapy.* New York: Norton.

de Shazer, S. (1994). *Words were originally magic.* New York: Norton.

*de Shazer, S., & Dolan, Y. (with H. Korman, T. Trepper, E. E. McCollum, & I. K. Berg). (2007). *More than miracles: The state of the art of solution-focused brief therapy.* New York: Haworth.

*Dolan, Y. (1991). *Resolving sexual abuse: Solution-focused therapy and Ericksonian hypnosis for survivors.* New York: Norton.

Dolan, Y. (2000). *One small step: Moving beyond trauma and therapy into a life of joy.* New York: Excel.

Dolan, Y. (2007). Tribute to Insoo Kim Berg. *Journal of Marital and Family Therapy, 33,* 129–131.

Duncan, B., Miller, S. D., & Sparks, J. A. (2004). *The heroic client: A revolutionary way to improve effectiveness through client-directed, outcome-informed therapy.* New York: Jossey-Bass.

Epstein, N. B., Curtis, D. S., Edwards, E., Young, J. L., & Zheng, L. (2014). Therapy with families in China: Cultural factors influencing the therapeutic alliance and therapy goals. *Contemporary Family Therapy: An International Journal 36*(2), 201–212. doi:10.1007/s10591-014-9302-x

Erickson, B. A., & Keeney, B. (Eds.). (2006). *Milton Erickson, M.D.: An American healer.* Sedona, AZ: Leete Island Books.

Franklin, C. (2015). An update on strengths-based, solution-focused brief therapy. *Health & Social Work, 40*(2), 73–76. doi:10.1093/hsw/hlv022

Franklin, C., Trepper, T. S., Gingerich, W. J., & McCollum, E. E. (Eds.). (2012). *Solution-focused brief therapy: A handbook of evidence-based practice.* New York: Oxford University Press.

Gillaspy, A., & Murphy, J. J. (2012). Incorporating outcome and session rating scales in solution-focused brief therapy. In C. Franklin, T. S. Trepper, W. J. Gingerich, & E. E. McCollum (Eds.). *Solution-focused brief therapy: A handbook of evidence-based practice* (pp. 73–94). New York: Oxford University Press.

Gingerich, W. J., Kim, J. S., Stams, G. J. J. M., & MacDonald, A. J. (2012). Solution-focused brief therapy outcome research. In C. Franklin, T. S. Trepper, W. J. Gingerich, & E. E. McCollum (Eds.) *Solution-focused brief therapy: A handbook of evidence-based practice* (pp. 95–111). New York: Oxford University Press.

Gingerich, W. J., & Peterson, L. T. (2013). Effectiveness of solution-focused brief therapy: A systematic qualitative review of controlled outcome studies. *Research on Social Work Practice, 23*(3), 266–283.

Haley, J. (1993). *Uncommon therapy: The psychiatric techniques of Milton H. Erikson, M.D.* New York: Norton.

Hsu, W., & Wang, C. C. (2011). Integrating Asian clients' filial piety beliefs into solution-focused brief therapy. *International Journal for the Advancement of Counselling, 33*(4), 322–334. doi:10.1007/s10447-011-9133-5

Hudson, P. O., & O'Hanlon, W. H. (1991). *Rewriting love stories: Brief marital therapy.* New York: Norton.

Jordan, S. S., Froerer, A. S., & Bavelas, J. B. (2013). Microanalysis of positive and negative content in solution-focused brief therapy and cognitive behavioral therapy expert sessions. *Journal of Systemic Therapies, 32*(3), 46–59. doi:10.1521/jsyt.2013.32.3.46

Kim, J. S. (2008). Examining the effectiveness of solution-focused brief therapy: A meta-analysis. *Research On Social Work Practice, 18*(2), 107–116. doi:10.1177/1049731507307807

Kim, J. S., & Franklin, C. (2015). Understanding emotional change in solution-focused brief therapy: Facilitating positive emotions. *Best Practices in Mental Health: An International Journal, 11*(1), 25–41.

Kim, J. S., Smock, S., Trepper, T. S, McCollum, E. E., & Franklin, C. (2010). Is solution-focused brief therapy evidence based? *Families in Society, 91,* 300–306. doi:10.1606/1044-3894.4009

Kim, J. S., Franklin, C., Zhang, Y., Liu, X., Qu, Y., & Chen, H. (2015). Solution-focused brief therapy in China:

A meta-analysis. *Journal of Ethnic & Cultural Diversity in Social Work: Innovation in Theory, Research & Practice, 24*(3), 187–201. doi:10.1080/15313204.2014.991983

Korman, H., Bavelas, J. B., & De Jong, P. (2013). Microanalysis of formulations in solution-focused brief therapy: cognitive behavioral therapy, and motivational interviewing. *Journal of Systemic Therapies, 32*(3), 31–45. doi:10.1521/jsyt.2013.32.3.31

Lankton, S. R., Lankton, C. H., & Matthews, W. J. (1991). Ericksonian family therapy. In A. S. Gurman, D. P. Kniskern (Eds.), *Handbook of family therapy*, (vol. 2, pp. 239–283). Philadelphia, PA: Brunner/Mazel.

Lee, M., & Mjelde-Mossey, L. (2004). Cultural dissonance among generations: A solution-focused approach with East Asian elders and their families. *Journal of Marital and Family Therapy, 30*(4), 497–513.

Lehmann, P., & Patton, J. D. (2012). The development of a solution-focused fidelity instrument: A pilot study. In C. Franklin, T. S. Trepper, W. J. Gingerich, & E. E. McCollum (Eds.), *Solution-focused brief therapy: A handbook of evidence-based practice* (pp. 39–54). New York: Oxford University Press.

Lipchik, E. (2002). *Beyond technique in solution-focused therapy: Working with emotions and the therapeutic relationship*. New York: Guilford.

Liu, X., Zhang, Y. P., Franklin, C., Qu, Y., Chen, H., & Kim, J. S. (2015). The practice of solution-focused brief therapy in mainland China. *Health & Social Work, 40*(2), 84–90. doi:10.1093/hsw/hlv013

McKeel, J. (2012). What works in solution-focused brief therapy: A review of change process research. In C. Franklin, T. S. Trepper, W. J. Gingerich, & E. E. McCollum (Eds.), *Solution-focused brief therapy: A handbook of evidence-based practice* (pp. 130–143). New York: Oxford University Press.

Metcalf, L. (1998). *Parenting towards solutions*. Paramus, NJ: Prentice Hall.

Metcalf, L. (2003). *Teaching towards solutions* (2nd ed.). Wales, UK: Crown House.

Metcalf, L. (2007). *Solution-focused group therapy*. New York: Free Press.

Metcalf, L. (2008). *Counseling towards solutions: A practical solution-focused program for working with students, teachers, and parents* (2nd ed.). New York: Jossey-Bass.

Meyer, D. D., & Cottone, R. R. (2013). Solution-focused therapy as a culturally acknowledging approach with American Indians. *Journal of Multicultural Counseling and Development 41*(1), 47–55. doi:10.1002/j.2161-1912.2013.00026.x

Miller, S. D., Duncan, B. L., Brown, J., Sparks, J. A., & Claud, D. A. (2003). The Outcome Rating Scale: A preliminary study of the reliability, validity, and feasibility of a brief visual analog measure. *Journal of Brief Therapy, 2,* 91–100.

Miller, S. D., Duncan, B. L., & Hubble, M. (Eds.). (1996). *Handbook of solution-focused brief therapy*. San Francisco, CA: Jossey-Bass.

Miller, S. D., Duncan, B. L., & Hubble, M. A. (1997). *Escape from Babel: Towards a unifying language for psychotherapy practice*. New York: Norton.

O'Hanlon, B. (2000). *Do one thing different: Ten simple ways to change your life*. New York: Harper.

O'Hanlon, B. (2005). *Thriving through crisis: Turn tragedy and trauma into growth and change*. New York: Penguin/Perigee.

O'Hanlon, B. (2006). *Pathways to spirituality: Connection, wholeness, and possibility for therapist and client*. New York: Norton Professional.

*O'Hanlon, B., & Beadle, S. (1999). *A guide to Possibility Land: Possibility therapy methods*. Omaha, NE: Possibility Press.

O'Hanlon, B., & Bertolino, B. (2002). *Even from a broken web: Brief and respectful solution-oriented therapy for resolving sexual abuse*. New York: Norton.

O'Hanlon, W. H., & Martin, M. (1992). *Solution-oriented hypnosis: An Ericksonian approach.* New York: Norton.

*O'Hanlon, W. H., & Davis, M. (1989). *In search of solutions: A new direction in psychotherapy.* New York: Norton.

*Selekman, M. D. (1997). *Solution-focused therapy with children: Harnessing family strengths for systemic change.* New York: Guilford.

Selekman, M. (2005). *Pathways to change: Brief therapy with difficult adolescents.* New York: Guilford.

*Selekman, M. (2006). *Working with self-harming adolescents: A collaborative, strength-oriented therapy approach.* New York: Norton.

Seligman, M. (2004). *Authentic happiness.* New York: Free Press.

Stams, G., Dekovic, M., Buist, K., & de Vries, L. (2006). Effectiviteit van oplossingsgerichte korte therapie: Een meta-analyse. *Gedragstherapie, 39*(2), 81–94.

Suitt, K. G., Franklin, C., & Kim, J. (2016). Solution-focused brief therapy with Latinos: A systematic review. *Journal of Ethnic & Cultural Diversity in Social Work: Innovation in Theory, Research & Practice, 25*(1), 50–67. doi:10.1080/15313204.2015.1131651

Tomm, K., St. George, S., Wulff, D., & Strong, T. (2014). *Patterns in interpersonal interactions: Inviting relational understandings for therapeutic change.* New York: Routledge.

Tomori, C., & Bavelas, J. B. (2007). Using microanalysis of communication to compare solution-focused and client-centered therapies. *Journal of Family Psychotherapy, 18*, 25–43.

Trepper, T. S., Dolan, Y., McCollum, E. E., & Nelson, T. (2006). Steve de Shazer and the future of Solution-Focused Therapy. *Journal of Marital and Family Therapy, 32*, 133–140.

Trepper, T. S., McCollum, E. E. de Jong, P., Korman, H., Gingerich, W. J., & Franklin, C. (2012). Solution-focused brief therapy treatment manual. In C. Franklin, T. S. Trepper, W. J. Gingerich, & E. E. McCollum (Eds.), *Solution-focused brief therapy: A handbook of evidence-based practice* (pp. 20–38). New York: Oxford University Press.

Treyger, S., Ehlers, N., Zajicek, L., & Trepper, T. (2008). Helping spouses cope with partners coming out: A solution-focused approach. *American Journal of Family Therapy, 36*(1), 30–47. doi:10.1080/01926180601057549

Walter, J. L., & Peller, J. E. (1992). *Becoming solution-focused in brief therapy.* New York: Brunner/Mazel.

Weiner-Davis, M. (1992). *Divorce busting.* New York: Summit Books.

Solution-Based Therapy Case Study: Divorce

Suzie and Jorge Nunez are seeking therapy to keep their 10-year marriage together. Suzie reports that she has "had enough" of Jorge's selfishness and lack of support. He is a manager of a local rental car agency location, and she works as a secretary for an insurance agent and is the primary caretaker of their two children, Silvia, 6, and Albert, 3. Jorge is shocked to hear that Suzie is ready to leave, as he feels he has been a good provider and treated her well. They have been arguing more and having sex less frequently over the past three years.

Based on interviews with this couple, Lilly, a solution-focused therapist, completed the following clinical documents.

SOLUTION-FOCUSED FAMILY THERAPY CASE CONCEPTUALIZATION

For use with individual, couple, or family clients.

Clinician: Lilly Ricard, MFT Trainee   **Client/Case #:** 1301   **Date:** 11/14/19

Introduction to Client & Significant Others

Identify significant persons in client's relational/family life who will be mentioned in case conceptualization:

Adults/Parents: Select identifier/abbreviation for use in rest of case conceptualization

AF1: Female Age: 32 European American Married heterosexual Occupation: receptionist for insurance agency

Other identifier: identified patient, German family background.

AM1: Male Age: 34 Hispanic/Latino Married heterosexual Occupation: manager of rental car agency

Other identifier: identified patient, Chilean American (parents immigrated)

Children/Adult Children: Select identifier/abbreviation for use in rest of case conceptualization

CF1: Female Age: 6 Multiethnic/biracial Grade: 1 School: Desert Sands Elementary
Other identifier: _____

CM1: Male Age: 3 Multiethnic/biracial Grade: Not in School School: N/A Other identifier: ____

Others: Identify all: _____

Presenting Concerns

Describe each significant person's presenting concerns:

AF1: Believes AM34 is selfish and does not support her in parenting or household tasks; does not feel emotionally supported or appreciated by him.

AM1: Believes AF32 has unrealistic expectations of him and perfectionist household standards.

CF1: N/A

CM1: N/A

Broader System: Description of problem from extended family, referring party, school, legal system, etc.:

Extended Family: AF's family views AM34 as a demanding husband; AM's family views AF32 as a demanding wife.

Friends: AF and AM generally indicate that their friends support their respective positions.

Name: _____

Background Information

Trauma/Abuse History (recent and past): <u>None reported.</u>

Substance Use/Abuse (current and past; self, family of origin, significant others): <u>None reported.</u>

Precipitating Events (recent life changes, first symptoms, stressors, etc.): <u>Although both were excited about having a second child, since his birth the couple has experienced increased tension, AF32 wants more assistance from AM34 with the children; sex and intimacy has decreased in frequency. The couple currently does not live near either set of parents, having left their families when Jorge was promoted as manager shortly after the birth of the second child.</u>

Related Historical Background (family history, related issues, previous counseling, medical/mental health history, etc.): <u>The couple met in college and married without strong parental consent on either side; both families were concerned about the cultural difference between the two. However, they had a passionate connection that made them decide to "take a chance." Suzie's family has a history of independent working women, while in Jorge's family, the women have typically stayed at home taking care of the children. No reports of prior treatment history.</u>

Preferred Solutions and Miracle Day

Describe each significant person's description of the solution or miracle day, focusing on OBSERVABLE actual behaviors (what a video camera would see) rather than what would not be happening:

AF1:   <u>AM would help her get kids ready for school, help with dinner and homework; the two would go on dates again. AM would listen to her concerns and provide emotional support.</u>

AM1:   <u>AF would wake up in good mood, greet him with a hug/kiss upon coming home; and support him when he sets limits with kids.</u>

Identifier: _____

Identifier: _____

Significance: What difference do clients say these behaviors and events make? What meanings are ascribed?

AF1:   <u>Believes these behaviors would allow her to feel less "stressed out," ultimately allowing her to be happier and more understanding during disagreements; this would also allow AF32 to feel as though AM34 sincerely cares about her welfare.</u>

AM1:   <u>Believes these behaviors would allow him to feel supported and "start the day off happy"; AM34 also feels that if AF backed him up with children that would help him feel more confident with parenting and make him want to be more involved with the family.</u>

Identifier: _____

Identifier: _____

Relational: Who is likely to notice first? What will he/she see? What difference would that make to him/her? What difference does that make for you?

Preferred Solutions and Miracle Day *(continued)*

AF1: If both of their miracle days occurred, AF believes she would notice first because she is most in tune with family. At first she says she might be suspicious of his intent, but would hope that the change would last. She reports such changes would make her feel respected and cared for; would also make her feel that he recognized the value and difficulty of "women's work."

AM1: Believes AF32 would notice that he is more involved with children and supporting her first. He reports that he would also notice her being more affectionate and that this change would make him feel like "a good husband" and that she appreciates how hard he works to support the family. He also states he would be certain that she loves him.

Identifier: _____

Identifier: _____

Exceptions and Partial Solutions

Identify as many times, places, relationships, context, etc. when the problem is less of a problem, or the solution is enacted in part or entirely. Describe these exceptions in detail, including who, where, when, what, and any other factors that might relate to the exception.

Exceptions:

1. After big fights, AM34 does more of what AF32 wants. AF32 is more affectionate when he is more involved.

2. AM34 more willing to help out with activity-based and "man-like" parenting tasks, such as teaching kids a sport, painting the baby's room, or setting up the car seats.

3. On vacation when there is less housework and child work, both feel more emotionally connected.

4. When they take the time to go on a date, they usually connect a bit more.

Solution Scaling

On a scale where 10 is the miracle day and 0 is the opposite, where are clients:

AF1: At initial interview: 2 Most recent session: 5

AM1: At initial interview: 4 Most recent session: 5

Identifier: At initial interview: _____ Most recent session: _____

Identifier: At initial interview: _____ Most recent session: _____

What does one small step on the scale look like in behavioral terms?

AF1: Believes one small step would be to have AM34 help her get the children ready for school two days a week.

AM1: Believes one small step would be to have AF32 give him a hug and kiss when he returns home from work.

Identifier: _____

Identifier: _____

Interaction Patterns

Identify one or more solution above, and describe the positive interaction pattern(s) related to the solution, including behavioral descriptions of each person's part of the pattern (e.g., showing affection/appreciating affection) or for individuals, their internal pattern (e.g., thinking positive/ trying harder).

AM34 more willing to help out in parenting tasks, ultimately allowing AF32 to feel more supported as a mother; AF32 shows affection to AM34 when he returns home from work, allowing AM34 to feel loved and appreciated by his wife.

Resources for Preferred Solutions

Personal: Describe potentially useful personal resources and qualities for enacting the preferred solution.

1. AF32 can use her organizational skills to create a list of tasks for AM34 to accomplish in his free time to help her out.

2. AM34 can help AF32 get their children ready for school in the morning since he is a "morning person" and is normally up early getting ready for work.

3. AM34 can use his management skills from work to help organize household and children's activities.

4. AF32 generally enjoys physical contact with her husband if she is not feeling stressed or resentful.

Relational and Social: Describe potentially useful relational and social resources for enacting the preferred solution.

1. AF32 would like a more egalitarian distribution of tasks in the relationship, and AM34 is not entirely opposed to that.

2. AM34 was raised with more traditional gender roles, which AF32 understands and is willing to work on dividing up household and child-rearing tasks along such lines if the overall workload is similar.

Community, Diversity, and Spiritual: Describe potentially useful resources for enacting the preferred solution:

- *Actual or potential supportive social communities, including ethnic, racial, LGBTQ, religious, gender, linguistic, local/regional, immigrant, socioeconomic, professional/job-related, etc.*
- *Spiritual beliefs and religious practices that are coping resources*

Resources for Preferred Solutions (*continued*)

1. AM34 comes from a large, Chilean family who are often available to babysit, allowing AF32 and AM34 to spend alone time together, and have a "date night."

2. AF32 and AM34 come from wealthy middle-class families that can provide additional monetary support to help pay for outside resources, if needed.

_____

_____

_____

Health and Hobbies: Describe potentially useful resources for enacting the preferred solution:

- *Healthy habits, such as exercising, eating well, regular sleep, stress-reduction strategies, etc.*
- *Hobbies, sources of fun, and nonvocational skills*

1. AF32 and AM34 used to frequently go out dancing before the birth of their children.

2. AM34 regularly plays softball on the weekends with his coworkers.

3. AF32 practices yoga "when there's time," and also meditates every morning.

_____

_____

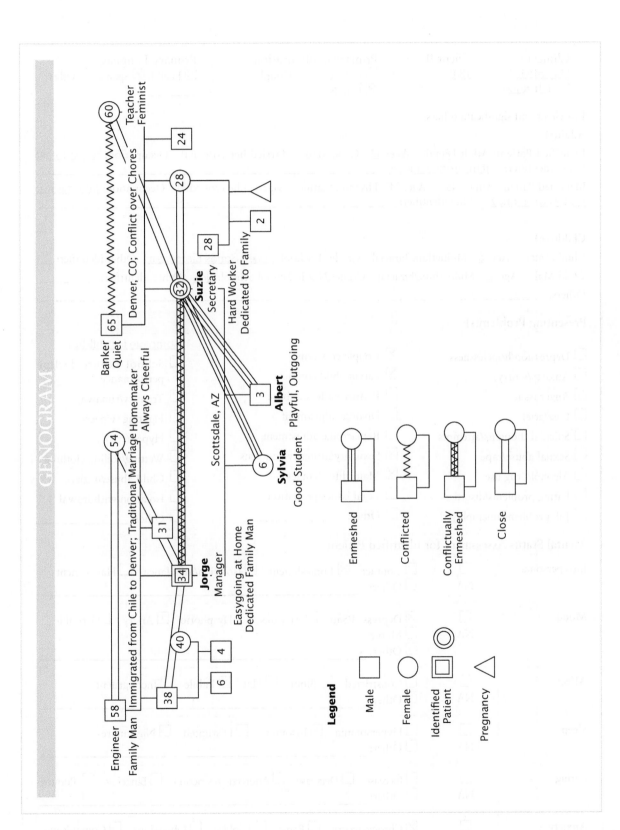

CLINICAL ASSESSMENT

Clinician: Lilly Ricard MFT Trainee	Client ID #: 1301	Primary configuration: ☐ Individual ☐ Couple ☒ Family	Primary Language: ☒ English ☒ Spanish ☐ Other: _____

List client and significant others

Adult(s)

Identified Patient: Adult Female   Age: <u>32</u>   Caucasian   Married heterosexual   Occupation: <u>receptionist</u>
Other identifier: <u>at insurance agency</u>

Identified Patient: Adult Male   Age: <u>34</u>   Hispanic/Latino   Married heterosexual   Occupation: <u>manager at rental car agency</u>   Other identifier: _____

Child(ren)

Child Female   Age: <u>6</u>   Multiethnic/biracial   Grade: 1 School: <u>Desert Sands Elementar</u>   Other identifier: ___

Child Male   Age: <u>3</u>   Multiethnic/biracial   Grade: Not in School School: <u>N/A</u>   Other identifier: _____

Others: _____

Presenting Problem(s)

☐ Depression/hopelessness   ☒ Couple concerns
☐ Anxiety/worry   ☒ Parent/child conflict
☒ Anger issues   ☐ Partner violence/abuse
☐ Loss/grief   ☐ Divorce adjustment
☐ Suicidal thoughts/attempts ☐ Remarriage adjustment
☐ Sexual abuse/rape   ☒ Sexuality/intimacy concerns
☐ Alcohol/drug use   ☒ Major life changes
☐ Eating problems/disorders   ☐ Legal issues/probation
☐ Job problems/unemployed   ☐ Other: _____

Complete for children:
☐ School failure/decline performance
☐ Truancy/runaway
☐ Fighting w/peers
☐ Hyperactivity
☐ Wetting/soiling clothing
☐ Child abuse/neglect
☐ Isolation/withdrawal
☐ Other: _____

Mental Status Assessment for Identified Patient

Interpersonal	☐ NA	☒ Conflict ☒ Enmeshment ☐ Isolation/avoidance ☐ Harassment ☐ Other: _____
Mood	☐ NA	☒ Depressed/Sad ☐ Anxious ☐ Dysphoric ☐ Angry ☐ Irritable ☐ Manic ☐ Other: _____
Affect	☐ NA	☐ Constricted ☐ Blunt ☐ Flat ☒ Labile ☐ Incongruent ☐ Other: _____
Sleep	☐ NA	☐ Hypersomnia ☒ Insomnia ☐ Disrupted ☐ Nightmares ☐ Other: _____
Eating	☐ NA	☐ Increase ☐ Decrease ☐ Anorectic restriction ☐ Bingeing ☐ Purging ☐ Other: _____
Anxiety	☐ NA	☒ Chronic worry ☐ Panic ☐ Phobias ☐ Obsessions ☐ Compulsions ☐ Other: _____

Trauma Symptoms	☐ NA	☐ Hypervigilance ☐ Flashbacks/Intrusive memories ☐ Dissociation ☐ Numbing ☐ Avoidance efforts ☐ Other: _____
Psychotic Symptoms	☐ NA	☐ Hallucinations ☐ Delusions ☐ Paranoia ☐ Loose associations ☐ Other: _____
Motor Activity/ Speech	☐ NA	☐ Low energy ☐ Hyperactive ☐ Agitated ☐ Inattentive ☐ Impulsive ☐ Pressured speech ☐ Slow speech ☐ Other: _____
Thought	☐ NA	☐ Poor concentration ☐ Denial ☒ Self-blame ☒ Other-blame ☐ Ruminative ☐ Tangential ☐ Concrete ☐ Poor insight ☐ Impaired decision making ☐ Disoriented ☐ Other: _____
Sociolegal	☐ NA	☐ Disregards rules ☐ Defiant ☐ Stealing ☐ Lying ☐ Tantrums ☐ Arrest/incarceration ☐ Initiates fights ☐ Other: _____
Other Symptoms	☒ NA	_____

Diagnosis for Identified Patient

Contextual Factors considered in making diagnosis: ☐ Age ☒ Gender ☐ Family dynamics ☒ Culture ☒ Language
☒ Religion ☐ Economic ☐ Immigration ☐ Sexual/gender orientation ☐ Trauma ☐ Dual diagnosis/comorbid ☐ Addiction ☐ Cognitive ability ☐ Other: _____

Describe impact of identified factors on diagnosis and assessment process: Couple going through difficult time adjusting to having children; each has different gender-role expectations for other based on culturally informed gender roles.

DSM-5 Level 1 Cross-Cutting Symptom Measure (optional): Elevated scores on: (free at psychiatry.org)
☐ I Depression ☒ II Anger ☐ III Mania ☒ IV Anxiety ☐ V Somatic ☐ VI Suicide ☐ VII Psychosis
☒ VIII Sleep ☐ IX Memory ☐ X Repetitive ☐ XI Dissociation ☐ XII Personality ☐ XIII Substance
☐ Not administered

DSM-5 Code	Diagnosis with Specifier *Include Z/T-Codes for Psychosocial Stressors/Issues*
1. F43.23	1. Adjustment Disorder with mixed anxiety and depressed mood
2. _____	2. _____
3. _____	3. _____
4. _____	4. _____
5. _____	5. _____

List Specific DSM-5 Criterion Met for Diagnosis
1. Stressor: Birth of second child; couple still not adjusted to change
2. Periods of sadness/hopelessness; most days
3. Periods of irritability and poor impulse control; 1–2 times per week
4. Ongoing conflict with AM
5. Ongoing worry: most days

Does not qualify for mood/anxiety disorder; no bereavement

Medical Considerations
Has patient been referred for psychiatric evaluation? ☒ Yes ☐ No
Has patient agreed with referral? ☐ Yes ☐ No ☒ NA
Psychometric instruments used for assessment: ☐ None ☒ Cross-cutting symptom inventories
☐ Other: _____
Client response to diagnosis: ☒ Agree ☐ Somewhat agree ☐ Disagree ☐ Not informed for following reason: ___

(continued)

Diagnosis for Identified Patient (*continued*)

Current Medications (psychiatric & medical) ☒ **NA**
1. ____; dose _____ mg; start date: _____
2. ____; dose _____ mg; start date: _____
3. ____; dose _____ mg; start date: _____
4. ____; dose _____ mg; start date: _____

Medical Necessity: *Check all that apply*
☐ Significant impairment   ☒ Probability of significant impairment   ☐ Probable developmental arrest
Areas of impairment:
☒ Daily activities   ☒ Social relationships   ☒ Health   ☒ Work/school   ☒ Living arrangement
☐ Other: _____

Risk and Safety Assessment for Identified Patient

Suicidality	Homicidality	Alcohol Abuse
☒ No indication/denies	☒ No indication/denies	☒ No indication/denies
☐ Active ideation	☐ Active ideation	☐ Past abuse
☐ Passive ideation	☐ Passive ideation	☐ Current; Freq/Amt: ____
☐ Intent without plan	☐ Intent without means	**Drug Use/Abuse**
☐ Intent with means	☐ Intent with means	☒ No indication/denies
☐ Ideation in past year	☐ Ideation in past year	☐ Past use
☐ Attempt in past year	☐ Violence past year	☐ Current drugs: _____
☐ Family or peer history of completed suicide	☐ History of assaulting others	Freq/Amt: _____
	☐ Cruelty to animals	☐ Family/sig. other use

Sexual & Physical Abuse and Other Risk Factors
☐ Childhood abuse history: ☐ Sexual ☐ Physical ☐ Emotional ☐ Neglect
☐ Adult with abuse/assault in adulthood: ☐ Sexual ☐ Physical ☐ Current
☐ History of perpetrating abuse: ☐ Sexual ☐ Physical ☐ Emotional
☐ Elder/dependent adult abuse/neglect
☐ History of or current issues with restrictive eating, bingeing, and/or purging
☐ Cutting or other self-harm: ☐ Current ☐ Past: Method: _____
☐ Criminal/legal history: _____
☐ Other trauma history: _____
☒ None reported

Indicators of Safety
☐ NA
☒ At least one outside support person
☒ Able to cite specific reasons to live or not harm
☐ Hopeful
☐ Willing to dispose of dangerous items
☒ Has future goals
☐ Willingness to reduce contact with people who make situation worse
☐ Willing to implement safety plan, safety interventions
☐ Developing set of alternatives to self/other harm
☐ Sustained period of safety: _____
☐ Other: _____

Elements of Safety Plan
☐ NA
☒ Verbal no harm contract
☐ Written no harm contract
☐ Emergency contact card
☐ Emergency therapist/agency number
☐ Medication management
☐ Plan for contacting friends/support persons during crisis
☐ Specific plan of where to go during crisis
☐ Specific self-calming tasks to reduce risk before reach crisis level (e.g., journaling, exercising, etc.)
☐ Specific daily/weekly activities to reduce stressors
☐ Other: _____

Legal/Ethical Action Taken: ☒ NA   ☐ Action: _____

Case Management

Collateral Contacts
- Has contact been made with treating *physicians or other professionals*: ☐ NA ☒ Yes ☐ In process. Name/Notes: _____
- If client is involved in mental health *treatment elsewhere*, has contact been made? ☒ NA ☐ Yes ☐ In process. Name/Notes: _____
- Has contact been made with *social worker*: ☒ NA ☐ Yes ☐ In process. Name/Notes: _____

Referrals
- Has client been referred for *medical assessment*: ☒ Yes ☐ No evidence for need
- Has client been referred for *social services*: ☒ NA ☐ Job/training ☐ Welfare/food/housing ☐ Victim services ☐ Legal aid ☐ Medical ☐ Other: _____
- Has client been referred for *group* or other support services: ☐ Yes: _____ ☐ In process ☒ None recommended
- Are there anticipated *forensic/legal processes* related to treatment: ☐ No ☒ Yes; describe: <u>Potential divorce</u>

Support Network
- Client social support network includes: ☒ Supportive family ☐ Supportive partner ☒ Friends ☐ Religious/spiritual organization ☐ Supportive work/social group ☐ Other: _____
- Describe anticipated effects treatment will have on others in support system (children, partner, etc.): <u>If couple issues not addressed, likely to affect children's behavior.</u>
- Is there anything else client will need to be successful? _____

Expected Outcome and Prognosis
☒ Return to normal functioning ☐ Anticipate less than normal functioning ☐ Prevent deterioration

Client Sense of Hope: <u>3</u>

Evaluation of Assessment/Client Perspective
How were assessment methods adapted to client needs, including age, culture, and other diversity issues? <u>Used tone, language comfortable for couple; allow each person to share perspective; provided opportunity for each to verbalize cultural/gender expectations.</u>
Describe actual or potential areas of client–clinician agreement/disagreement related to the above assessment: <u>Couple seem to see situation as personality rather than cultural/gender conflict.</u>

_____, _____ _____
Clinician Signature   License/Intern Status   Date

_____, _____ _____
Supervisor Signature   License   Date

TREATMENT PLAN

Clinician Name: Lilly Ricard, MFT Trainee   **Date:** 11/14/19

Case/Client: #1301   **Theory:** Solution-focused

Modalities planned: ☐ Individual Adult ☐ Individual Child ☒ Couple ☐ Family
☐ Group: _____

Recommended session frequency: ☒ Weekly ☐ Every two weeks ☐ Other: _____
Expected length of treatment: 6 months

Treatment Plan with Goals and Interventions

Early-Phase Client Goal

1. Increase activities that worked for couple during dating and "good periods in relationship" to reduce blaming/arguing.

   Measure: Able to sustain positive affect activities for period of 4 week with no more than one mild episode of arguing per week.

   a. Identify "what worked" while dating and use scaling questions to begin moving couple in this direction

   b. Formula first-session task to identify what is working

Working-Phase Client Goals

Target individual and relational dynamics using theoretical concepts.

1. Increase emotional intimacy and sexual connection between couple described in miracle question to reduce hopelessness and irritability.

   Measure: Able to sustain emotional and sexual intimacy for period of 3 ☐ wk ☒ mo with no more than two mild episodes of not talking or avoiding sex for more than 2 weeks.

   a. Use videotalk to reduce blame and increase positive affect communication and effective communication of requests.

   b. Create dedicated time for "date night" for couple to begin to reconnect.

2. Increase cooperative coparenting described in miracle question to reduce couple arguing and triangulation of children.

   Measure: Able to sustain agreed-upon division of parenting tasks for period of 3 ☐ wk ☒ mo with no more than one mild episode of arguing related to parenting per week.

   a. Use miracle question to identify expectations behaviorally, identifying cultural, gender, and family-of-origin issues related to expectations for partner's behaviors.

   b. Use scaling questions to break goals down into small, easily achieved steps that enable AM34 to more directly increase role with children and reduce AF32 triangulation of children against AM34.

3. Increase couple's agreement on each person's role in the marriage and family to reduce arguing.

   Measure: Able to sustain cooperative interactions for period of 2 ☐ wk ☒ mo with no more than 1 mild argument.

a. Use videotalk to develop behavioral description of ideal partnership.

b. Use scaling questions to help couple take small steps each week to realizing and maintaining desired relationship.

Closing-Phase Client Goals

1. Increase couple's sense of solidarity as parents and as a couple to reduce hopelessness, conflict, and irritability.

   Measure: Able to sustain positive interactions for period of 2 ☐ wk ☒ mo with no more than 2 mild episodes of conflict.

   a. Use crystal ball question to identify behavioral description of satisfying parenting and couple relationship

   b. Use scaling questions to identify small steps to move toward this goal.

Treatment Tasks

1. Develop working therapeutic relationship using theory of choice.

   Relationship-building approach/intervention:

   a. Develop collaborative relationship with all members; inspire hope and optimism, using "beginner's mind" and listening for strengths.

2. Assess individual, relational, community, and broader cultural dynamics using theory of choice.

   Assessment strategies:

   a. Use miracle question with each person to concretely and behaviorally define solutions in positive terms.

   b. Identify exceptions to conflict, times of connection, areas of life not affected by the conflict, strengths and resources, supportive relationships, and client level of motivation.

3. Identify needed referrals, crisis issues, collateral contacts, and other client needs.

   a. *Crisis assessment intervention(s):* Use time machine question to identify behavioral description of solution; use scaling questions to break down into small steps.

   b. *Referral(s):* Identify social support and childcare assistance to enable couple to focus on relationship.

Diversity Considerations

Describe specifically how treatment plan, goals, and interventions were adapted to address each area of diversity (*Note:* identify specific ethnicity, e.g., Italian American rather than white):

Age: AF and AM are similar ages and part of an American generation in which egalitarian relationships are the norm; both are also in a developmental stage in which they are working to develop stable intimate relationships. Their family is in a developmental stage that has significant physical and time demands on parents, especially for working couples.

(continued)

Diversity Considerations *(continued)*

Gender/Sexual Orientation: Gender-role expectations are a significant issue for this couple, with AF wanting more American standards of egalitarian relationships and AM wanting fair but more traditional gender roles that he witnessed growing up. However, AM is open to adopting a more American male role as long as he retains a sense of manhood that is consistent with his cultural values. AF simply wants a more equal distribution of labor, especially because she works too, and thus, she argues this is not actually a traditional relationship.

Race/Ethnicity Religion/Class/Region: AM's parents immigrated from Chili before he was born to pursue better economic opportunities. AM enjoys the freedom offered by American culture, but also has a connection to the dignity and strong family connection that he values in Chilean culture. AF shares the value of strong family connection, but does not believe that traditional Chilean male roles apply, especially because she works outside the home.

Other factors: AF has limited ability to communicate with AM's family because she is not fluent in Spanish. To maintain a standard of living that is comfortable for them, both have to work.

Evidence-Based Practice (Optional)

Summarize evidence for using this approach for this presenting concern and/or population: Solution-based therapies have a solid evidence base for working with Latino clients, including a study with Latino couples that reported positive outcomes (Suitt, Franklin, & Kim, 2016). In meta-analytic studies, solution-focused couples therapy generally has positive outcomes, but with a modest effect size (Gingerich et al., 2012).

Client Perspective (Optional)

Has treatment plan been reviewed with client: ☒ Yes ☐ No; If no, explain: _____

Describe areas of Client Agreement and Concern: Although less optimistic than AM, AF is willing to try to make the marriage work; she wants to do so for the children and because they had a good relationship in the beginning.

_____, _____   _____ _____, _____ ____
Therapist's Signature   Intern Status   Date   Supervisor's Signature   License   Date

PROGRESS NOTE

Date: 12/04/19   **Time:** 4:00 ☐ am/☒ pm   **Session Length:** ☐ 45 min ☐ 60 min ☒ Other: 50 min

Present: ☒ Adult Male ☒ Adult Female ☐ Child Male ☐ Child Female ☐ Other: _____

Billing Code: ☐ 90791 (eval) ☐ 90834 (45 min therapy) ☐ 90837 (60 min therapy) ☒ 90847 (family) ☐ Other: _____

Symptom(s)	Duration and Frequency since Last Visit	Progress
1: Conflict	2 moderate fights over past week	**No progress**
2: Irritability/ anger (both)	mild–moderate; worse on fight days	**Regressed**
3: Hopelessness (AF)	mild during fight days	**No progress**

Explanatory Notes on Symptoms: One fight related to children, one to extended family; followed typical fight pattern with slightly faster recovery. AF reports AM "slightly" more helpful with children around the house; couple had good night on "date night."

In-Session Interventions and Assigned Homework

Used scaling question to identify how to move up from a 4 to a 5 over the next week: identified specific tasks for each, and developed plan for implementing; used exception questions to identify small improvements in how couple handled arguments this week.

Client Response/Feedback

AM very responsive to compliments and exceptions; AF more hesitant to accept signs of progress, but is able to do so and reports seeing progress at home.

Plan

☒ Continue with treatment plan: plan for next session: Follow up on tasks for week; identify next small steps for change.
☐ Modify plan: _____

Next session: Date: 12/11   Time: 4:00 ☐ am/☒ pm

Crisis Issues: ☒ No indication of crisis/client denies ☐ Crisis assessed/addressed: describe below

_____

_____, _____   _____

Clinician's Signature,   License/Intern Status   Date

◇◇

(continued)

PROGRESS NOTE *(continued)*

Case Consultation/Supervision ☐ Not Applicable
Notes: Dr. Matt, Stephan, supervisor, encouraged attending to gender role inequities by incorporating the socioemotional relational therapy practices (see Chapter 3).

Collateral Contact ☒ Not Applicable

Name: _____ Date of Contact: _____ Time: ____:___ ☐ am/☐ pm
☐ Written release on file: ☐ Sent/☐ Received ☐ In court docs ☐ Other: _____

Notes: _____

_____,   _____   _____
Clinician's Signature   License/Intern Status   Date

_____,   _____   _____
Supervisor's Signature   License   Date

CHAPTER

10

Narrative and Collaborative Therapies

Learning Objectives

After reading this chapter and a few hours of focused studying, you should be able to:

- **Theory:** Describe the following elements of collaborative and narrative therapies:
  - Process of therapy
  - Therapeutic relationship
  - Case conceptualization
  - Goal setting
  - Interventions

- **Case conceptualization and treatment plan:** Complete a theory-specific case conceptualizations and treatment plans for collaborative and narrative therapies using templates that are provided.

- **Research:** Provide an overview of significant research findings for postmodern therapies.

- **Diversity:** Analyze strengths, limitations, and appropriate applications for using postmodern therapies with clients in relation to their social location/diverse identities, including but not limited to ethnic, racial, and/or sexual/gender identity diversity.

- **Cross-Theoretical Comparison:** Compare how postmodern therapies utilize interpersonal patterns (IPs) with other approaches described in this book.

This kind of listening, hearing, and responding requires that a therapist enter the therapy domain with a genuine posture and manner characterized by an openness to the other person's ideological base—his or her reality, beliefs, and experiences. This listening posture and manner involve showing respect for, having humility toward, and believing that what a client has to say is worth hearing. . . . This is best accomplished by actively interacting with and responding to what a client says by asking questions, making comments, extending ideas, wondering, and sharing private thoughts aloud. Being interested in this way helps a therapist to clarify and prevent misunderstanding of the said and learn more about the unsaid.

—Anderson, 1997, p. 153

Lay of the Land

In addition to the contemporary forms of solution-based therapies (see Chapter 9), postmodern family therapy can be broadly divided into two streams of practice:

* Narrative therapy developed by Michael White and David Epston (1990) in Australia and New Zealand
* Collaborative therapy developed by Harlene Anderson and Harry Goolishian in Texas (1988, 1992; Anderson, 1993, 1995, 1997; Goolishian & Anderson, 1987) and reflecting teams by Tom Andersen in Norway (1991, 1992)

These two approaches share many of the social constructionist premises described in Chapter 3, each being an approach to co-constructing new meanings with clients. Like solution-based therapists (see Chapter 9), postmodern therapists optimistically focus on client strengths and abilities. Despite many similarities, however, collaborative and narrative therapies differ in significant ways, most notably in their philosophical foundations, the therapist's stance, the role of interventions, and the emphasis on political issues. Broadly speaking, narrative therapists have well-defined sets of questions and strategies for helping clients enact preferred narratives, whereas collaborative therapists avoid standardized techniques and instead use postmodern and social constructionist assumptions to facilitate a unique relational and dialogical process. The following table summarizes the difference between these two therapies.

COLLABORATIVE AND NARRATIVE THERAPIES

	NARRATIVE THERAPY	COLLABORATIVE THERAPY
Primary Philosophical Foundations	Foucault's philosophical writings; critical theory; social constructionism	Postmodernism; social constructionism; hermeneutics (study of interpretation)
Therapeutic Relationship	Therapist more active: "co-editor," "co-author"	Therapist more facilitative; facilitates a dialogical process
Therapeutic Process	Structured interventions	No interventions; therapist focus is facilitating particular processes
Politics and Social Justice	Social justice issues regularly included in therapy conversations	Political issues raised tentatively for client consideration

Narrative Therapy

In a Nutshell: The Least You Need to Know

Developed by Michael White and David Epston in Australia and New Zealand, narrative therapy is based on the premise that we "story" and create the meaning of life events using available *dominant discourses*—broad societal stories, sociocultural practices, assumptions, and expectations about how we should live. People experience "problems" when their personal life does not fit with these dominant societal discourses and expectations. The process of narrative therapy involves *separating the person from the problem*, critically examining the assumptions that inform how the person evaluates himself or herself and his or her life. Through this process, clients identify alternative ways to view, act, and interact in daily life. Narrative therapists assume that all people are resourceful and have strengths, and they do not see "people" as having problems but rather see problems as being imposed upon people by unhelpful or harmful societal cultural practices.

The Juice: Significant Contributions to the Field

If you remember one thing from this chapter, it should be this:

Understanding Oppression: Dominant Versus Local Discourses

Narrative therapy is one of the few psychotherapeutic theories that integrates societal and cultural issues into its core conceptualization of how problems are formed and resolved. Narrative therapists maintain that problems do not exist separately from their sociocultural contexts, which are broadly constituted in what philosopher Michel Foucault called **dominant discourses** (Foucault, 1972, 1980; White, 1995; White & Epston, 1990). Dominant discourses are culturally generated stories about how life should go that are used to coordinate social behavior, such as how married people should act, what happiness looks like, and how to be successful. These dominant discourses organize social groups at all levels: from large cultural groups down to individual couples and families. They are described as dominant because they are so foundational to how we behave and evaluate our lives that we are rarely conscious of their impact or origins.

Foucault contrasts dominant discourses with **local discourses**, which occur in our heads, our closer relationships, and marginalized (not mainstream) communities. The "goods" and "shoulds" of local discourses are different from those of dominant discourses. A classic example is that women value relationships while men value outcome in typical work environments. Both discourses work toward a value; however, men's discourse is generally privileged over women's and is thus considered a dominant discourse, with women's discourse considered local. Narrative therapists closely attend to the fluid interactions of local and dominant discourses and how these different stories of what is "good" and valued collide in our web of social relationships, creating problems and difficulties. By attending to this level of social interaction, narrative therapists help clients become aware of how these different discourses are impacting their lives; this awareness increases clients' sense of agency in their struggles, allowing them to find ways to more successfully resolve their issues.

Rumor Has It: The People and Their Stories

Michael White

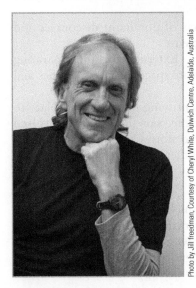

Photo by Jill Freedman, Courtesy of Cheryl White, Dulwich Centre, Adelaide, Australia

A pioneer in narrative therapy and the first to write about the process of *externalizing* problems, Michael White was based at the Dulwich Centre in Adelaide, Australia, which provides training for and publishes books and newsletters on narrative therapy. Along with David Epston, he wrote the first book on narrative therapy, *Narrative Means to Therapeutic Ends* (White & Epston, 1990). His last publication, *Maps of Narrative Practice* (White, 2007), describes his later work before his death in 2008.

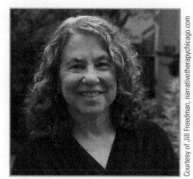

David Epston

From Auckland, New Zealand, David Epston worked closely with Michael White in developing the foundational framework for narrative therapy. His work emphasized creating unique sources of support for clients, such as writing letters to clients to solidify the emerging narratives and developing communities of concern or *leagues* (see "Leagues," below) in which clients provide support to each other.

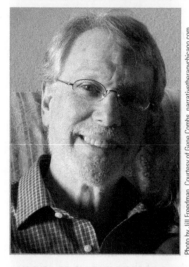

Jill Freedman and Gene Combs

Based in the United States, husband-and-wife team Jill Freedman and Gene Combs (1996) developed the narrative approach, emphasizing social construction of realities, and further developed the narrative metaphor for conceptualizing therapeutic intervention. They are the codirectors of the Evanston Family Therapy Center in Illinois.

Gerald Monk and John Winslade

After beginning their work in New Zealand, Gerald Monk and John Winslade now work in the United States and have developed narrative approaches for schools in counseling, multicultural counseling, mediation, and consultation (Monk et al., 1997; Monk, Winslade, & Sinclair, 2008; Winslade & Monk, 2000, 2007, 2008).

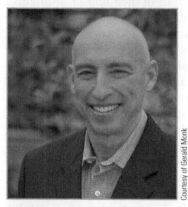

The Big Picture: Overview of Treatment

Treatment Phases

The process of narrative therapy involves helping clients find new ways to view, interact with, and respond to problems in their lives by redefining the role of those problems (White, 2007). From a narrative perspective, persons are not the problem; problems are the problem. Although there is variety of types of narrative therapy among practitioners, narrative therapy broadly involves the following phases (Freedman & Combs, 1996; White & Epston, 1990):

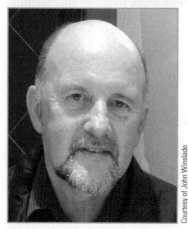

- Meeting the person: Getting to know persons as *separate* from their problems by learning about the hobbies, values, and everyday aspects of their lives
- Listening: Listening for the effects of dominant discourses and identifying times without the problems
- Separating persons from problems: Externalizing and separating persons from their problems to create space for new identities and for life stories to emerge
- Enacting preferred narratives: Identifying new ways to relate to problems that reduce their negative effects on the lives of all involved
- Solidifying: Strengthening preferred stories and identities by having them witnessed by significant others in a person's life

Use of Thickening Descriptions

The narrative therapy process is a thickening and enriching of the person's identity and life accounts rather than a "story-ectomy." Instead of replacing a problem story with a problem-free one, narrative therapists *add* new strands of identity to the problem-saturated descriptions with which clients enter therapy. In any given day, an infinite number of events can be storied into our accounts of the day and who we are. When people begin to experience problems, they tend to notice only the events that fit with the problem narrative. For example, if they are feeling hopeless, they tend to notice when things do not go their way during the day and do not give much weight to the good things that happened. Similarly, when couples start a period of fighting, they start to notice only what the other person is doing that confirms their position in the fight and ignore and/or forget other events. In narrative therapy, the therapist helps clients create more balanced, rich, and appreciative descriptions of events that will enable them to build more successful and enjoyable lives.

Making a Connection: The Therapeutic Relationship

Meeting the Person Apart from the Problem

Narrative therapists generally begin their first session with clients by meeting them "apart from the problem," that is, as everyday people (Freedman & Combs, 1996). Therapists ask questions such as the following to familiarize themselves with clients' everyday lives.

QUESTIONS FOR MEETING THE PERSON (NOT THE PROBLEM)

- What do you do for fun? Do you have hobbies?
- What do you like about living here? What don't you like?
- Can you tell me about your friends and family?
- What is important to you in life?
- What is a typical weekday like? Weekend?

The answers to these questions enable narrative therapists to know and view their clients in much the same way that clients view themselves, as everyday people.

Separating People from Problems: The Problem Is the Problem

In narrative therapy, the motto is: "The problem is the problem. The person is not the problem" (Winslade & Monk, 1999, p. 2). Once therapists have come to know the client apart from the problem and have a clear sense of who the client is as a person, they begin to "meet" the problem in much the same way, keeping their identities separate. The problem—whether depression, anxiety, marital conflict, ADHD, defiance, loneliness, or a breakup—is viewed as a separate entity or situation that is *not* inherent to the person of the client. Therapists maintain a polite, social, "getting to know you" attitude.

QUESTIONS FOR "MEETING" THE PROBLEM

- When did the problem first enter your life?
- What was going on with you then?
- What were your first impressions of the problem? How have they changed?
- How has your relationship with the problem evolved over time?
- Who else has been affected by the problem?

Narrative therapists can take an adversarial stance toward the problem (wanting to outwit, outsmart, or evict it; White, 2007) or a more compassionate stance (wanting to understand its message and concerns; Gehart & McCollum, 2007).

Optimism and Hope

Because narrative therapists view problems as problems and people as people, they have a deep, abiding optimism and hope for their clients (Monk et al., 1997; Winslade & Monk, 1999). Their hope and optimism are not sugar-coated, naive wishes but instead are derived from their understanding of how problems are formed—through language, relationship, and social discourse—and from having confidence that their approach can make a difference. Furthermore, by separating people from problems, they quickly connect with the "best" in the client, which reinforces a sense of hope and optimism.

Therapist as Co-author and Co-editor

The role of the therapist is often described as a *co-author* or *co-editor* to emphasize that the therapist and client engage in a joint process of constructing meaning (Freedman & Combs, 1996; Monk et al., 1997; White, 1995; White & Epston, 1990). Rather than attempting to offer a "better story," the therapist works alongside the client to generate a more useful narrative. Although the degree and quality of input vary greatly, narrative therapists tend to focus on the sociopolitical aspects of a client's life. Some narrative therapists maintain that therapists should take a stance on broader sociocultural issues of injustice with all clients (Zimmerman & Dickerson, 1996), but not all narrative therapists share this agenda (Monk & Gehart, 2003).

Therapist as Investigative Reporter

In his later works, White (2007) describes his relationship to problems as that of an *investigative reporter*:

> The form of inquiry that is employed during externalizing conversations can be likened to investigative reporting. The primary goal of investigative reporting is to develop an exposé on the corruption associated with abuse of power and privilege. Although investigative reporters are not politically neutral, the activities of their inquiry do not take them into the domains of problem-solving, of enacting reform, or of engaging indirect power struggles . . . their actions usually reflect a relatively "cool" engagement. (pp. 27–28)

Thus, rather than rushing in to fix problems, the therapist uses a calm but inquisitive stance to explore the origins of problems and thus to inspire clients to develop a better understanding of their larger contexts.

The Viewing: Case Conceptualization and Assessment

Problem-Saturated Stories

As clients talk, narrative therapists listen for the **problem-saturated story** (Freedman & Combs, 1996; White & Epston, 1990), the story in which the "problem" plays the leading role and the client plays a secondary role, generally that of victim. The therapist attends to how the problem affects the client at an *individual level* (health, emotions, thoughts, beliefs, identity, relationship with the divine) and at a *relational level* (with significant other, parents, friends, coworkers, teachers), as well as how it affects each of these significant others at a personal level. While the client tells the problem-saturated story, the therapist listens closely for alternative endings and subplots in which the problem is less of a problem and the person is an effective agent; these are referred to as *unique outcomes*.

Unique Outcomes and Sparkling Events

Unique outcomes (White & Epston, 1990) or **sparkling events** (Freedman & Combs, 1996) are stories or subplots in which the problem-saturated story does not play out in its typical way: the child cheerfully complies with a parent's request; a soft touch leads to a couple stopping a potential argument from erupting; a teenager decides to call a friend rather than allow herself to cut. These stories often go unnoticed because they have no dramatic ending or particularly notable outcome that warrants attention, and therefore they are not "storied" in clients' or others' minds. These unique outcomes are used to help clients create the lives they prefer and to develop a more full and accurate account of their own and others' identities.

Dominant Cultural and Gender Discourses (see also, "Juice")

As already discussed, narrative therapists listen for dominant cultural and gender themes that have informed the development and perception of a problem (Monk et al., 1997; White & Epston, 1990). The purpose of all discourses is to identify the set of "goods" and "values" that organize social interaction in a particular culture. All cultures are essentially a set of dominant discourses: social rules and values that make it possible for a group of people to interact meaningfully (see Chapter 3).

Dominant discourses are the societal stories of how life "should" happen; for example, to be a happy and good person, you should get married, get a stable, high-paying job, have kids, get a nice car, buy a house, and volunteer at your child's school. Whether you comply with this vision of happiness, rebel against it, or are not even in the game because of social or physical limitations, problems can arise in relation to it. In working with clients, narrative therapists listen closely for the dominant discourses that are most directly informing the perception of a problem. In response, they inquire about *local* or *alternative discourses*.

Local and Alternative Discourses: Attending to Client Language and Meaning

Local and alternative discourses are those that do not conform to the dominant discourse (White & Epston, 1990): couples who choose not to have children, same-sex relationships, immigrant families wanting to preserve their roots, speaking English as a second language, teen subculture in any society, and so forth. Local discourses offer a different set of "goods," "shoulds," and ethical "values" than what is portrayed in the dominant discourse. For example, teens have created a subculture with different beauty standards, sexual norms, vocabulary, and friendship rules than are found in the adult culture. The teen culture represents an alternative discourse that therapists can tap into to understand the teen's worldview and values, as well as to explore with the teen how this alternative discourse can successfully coexist with the dominant discourse. Thus, the local discourse provides a resource for generating new ways of viewing the self and for talking and interacting with others with regard to the problem.

Targeting Change: Goal Setting

Preferred Realities and Identities

As a postmodern approach, narrative therapy does not include a set of predefined goals that can be used with all clients. Instead, goal setting in narrative therapy is unique to each client. In the broadest sense, the goal of narrative therapy is to help clients enact their **preferred realities** and identities (Freedman & Combs, 1996). In most cases, enacting preferred narratives involves increasing clients' sense of *agency*, the sense that they influence the direction of their lives. When identifying preferred realities, therapists work with clients to develop thoughtfully reflected goals that consider local knowledge rather than simply adopting the values of the dominant culture. Clients often redefine their preferred reality to incorporate this local knowledge and to lessen the influence of dominant discourses. For example, a couple may come in wanting things to go back to the way they were while the couple was dating, but as they move through the therapeutic process, they realize that they want and need something different than what they had before because they are entering a new chapter in their lives as individuals and as a couple.

Thus, the key is defining the "preferred" reality and identity thoughtfully and with intention after considering the impact of dominant and local discourses as well as the meanings and impact of the proposed preferred reality. This process is often a gradual shift from "make this problem go away" to "I want to create something beautiful/meaningful/great with my/our life/lives." The therapist allows the client to take the lead in defining the preferred realities and acts as a co-editor to help the client reflect on where the idea came from and the effects it will have on the client's life.

Working-Phase Client Goals

Middle-phase goals target immediate symptoms and the presenting problem; the following are some examples:

- "Increase sense of agency in problem-resolution conversations with spouse."
- "Increase opportunities to interact with friends using 'confident, social' self."
- "Reduce number of times mother and father allow anger to take over in response to child's defiance."
- "Increase instances of defiance in response to anorexia's directions to not eat."

Late-Phase Client Goals

Late-phase goals target personal identity, relational identity, and the expanded community:

- Personal identity: "Solidify a sense of personal identity that derives self-worth from meaningful activities, relationship, and values rather than body size."
- Relational identity: "Develop a family identity narrative that allows for greater expression of differences while maintaining family's sense of closeness and loyalty."
- Expanded community: "Expand preferred 'outgoing' identity to social relationships and contexts."

The Doing: Interventions

Externalizing: Separating the Problem from the Person

The signature technique of narrative therapy, *externalizing* involves conceptually and linguistically separating the person from the problem (Freedman & Combs, 1996; White & Epston, 1990). To be successful, externalization requires a sincere belief that people are separate from their problems; thus, the *attitude* of externalization is key to its effectiveness (Freedman & Combs, 1996). More than a single-session intervention, externalization is an organic and evolving process of shifting clients' perception of their relationship to the problem: from "having" it to seeing it as outside the self. Therapists can externalize by naming the problem as an external other or by changing a descriptive adjective into a noun (e.g., from a client being depressed to having a relationship with Depression, or changing from being a conflictual couple to having a relationship with Conflict). At other times, clients respond better by talking about "sides" of themselves or a relationship: "the little girl in me who is afraid" or "the competitive side of our relationship."

For externalization to work, it cannot be forced onto the client but rather needs to emerge from the dialogue or be introduced as a possibility for how to think about the situation. In most cases, techniques such as mapping the influence of persons and problem (see "Relative Influence Questioning," below) invite a natural, comfortable process for externalizing the problem. Alternatively, therapists can ask clients if they want to refer to the problem as something separate from themselves when the conversation allows. If a client already has a name for the problem and conceptualizes the problem as a sort of external entity or very discrete part of himself or herself, the therapist needs only to build on the externalization process the client has already started.

Relative Influence Questioning: Mapping Influence of the Problem and Persons

Relative influence questioning was the first detailed method for externalization (White & Epston, 1990). Used early in therapy, it serves simultaneously as an assessment and an intervention and is composed of two parts: (a) mapping the influence of the problem and (b) mapping the influence of persons.

Mapping the Influence of the Problem

When mapping the influence of the problem, therapists inquire about how the problem has affected the lives of the client and significant others, often *expanding* the reach of the problem beyond how the client generally thinks of it; thus, it is critical that this is followed up by *mapping the influence of person* questions to ensure that the client does not feel worse afterward.

QUESTIONS FOR MAPPING THE INFLUENCE OF THE PROBLEM

How has the problem affected:

- Clients at a physical, emotional, and psychological level?
- Clients' identity stories and what they tell themselves about their worth and who they are?
- Clients' closest relationships: partner, children, parents?
- Other relationships in clients' lives: friendships, social groups, work or school colleagues, etc.?
- The health, identity, emotions, and other relationships of significant people in clients' lives (e.g., how parents may pull away from friends because they are embarrassed about a child's problem)?

Mapping the Influence of Persons

Mapping the influence of persons begins the externalization process more explicitly. This phase of questioning, which should immediately follow mapping the influence of problems, involves identifying how the person has affected the life of the problem, reversing the logic of the first series of questions.

QUESTIONS FOR MAPPING THE INFLUENCE OF PERSONS

When have the persons involved:

- Kept the Problem from affecting their mood or how they value themselves as people?
- Kept the Problem from allowing themselves to enjoy special and/or casual relationships in their lives?
- Kept the Problem from interrupting their work or school lives?
- Been able to keep the Problem from taking over when it was starting?

Try It Yourself

Find a partner and take turns mapping the influence of the problem and the influence of persons related to a current life situation. How did the first set of questions affect you? How did the second set affect you?

White and Epston (1990) report that externalization has the following beneficial effects:

- Decreases unproductive conflict and blame between family members
- Undermines sense of failure in relation to the Problem by highlighting times the persons have had influence over it
- Invites people to unite in a struggle against the Problem and reduce its influence
- Identifies new opportunities for reducing the influence of the Problem
- Encourages a lighter, less stressed approach to interacting with the Problem
- Increases interactive dialogue rather than repetitive monologue about the Problem

Externalizing Conversations: The Statement of Position Map

White (2007) describes his more recently developed process for facilitating externalizing conversations as "the statement of position map." This map includes four categories of inquiry, which are used multiple times throughout a session and across sessions to shift the client's relationship with the problem and open new possibilities for action.

Inquiry Category 1: Negotiating an Experience-Near Definition

White begins by defining the problem using the client's language (experience-near language) rather than in professional or global terms (e.g., a "diagnosis"). Thus, "feeling blue" is preferred to "depressed."

Inquiry Category 2: Mapping the Effects

As in White's early work (White & Epston, 1990), mapping the effects of problems involves identifying how the problem has affected the various domains of the client's life: home, work, school, and social contexts; relationships with family, friends, and himself or herself; and identity and future possibilities.

Inquiry Category 3: Evaluating the Effects

After identifying the effects of the problem, the therapist asks the client to evaluate these effects (White, 2007, p. 44):

- Are these activities okay with you?
- How do you feel about these developments?
- Where do you stand on these outcomes?
- Is the development positive or negative—or both, or neither, or something in between?

Inquiry Category 4: Justifying the Evaluation

In the final phase, the therapist asks about how and why clients have evaluated the situation the way they have (White, 2007, p. 48):

- Why is or isn't this okay for you?
- Why do you feel this way about this development?
- Why are you taking this stand or position on this development?

These "why" questions must be offered in a spirit of allowing clients to give voice to what is important to them rather than creating a sense of moral judgment. They should open up conversations about what motivates clients and how they want to shape their identities and futures.

Externalizing Metaphors

When externalizing using these four categories, White (2007, p. 32) employs various metaphors for relating to problems:

- Walking out on the problem
- Going on strike against the problem
- Defying the problem's requirements
- Disempowering the problem
- Educating the problem
- Escaping the problem
- Recovering or reclaiming territory from the problem
- Refusing invitations from the problem
- Disproving the problem's claims
- Resigning from the problem's service
- Stealing their lives from the problem
- Taming the problem
- Harnessing the problem
- Undermining the problem

Avoiding Totalizing and Dualistic Thinking

White (2007) avoids totalizing descriptions of the problem—the problem being all bad—because such descriptions promote dualistic, either/or thinking, which can be invalidating to the client and/or obscure the problem's broader context.

Externalizing Questions

Narrative therapists use externalizing questions to help clients build different relationships with their problems (Freedman & Combs, 1996). In most cases, these questions transform adjectives (e.g., *depressed, anxious, angry,* etc.) to nouns (e.g., *Depression, Anxiety, Anger,* etc.; capitalization is used to emphasize that the Problem is viewed as a separate entity). Externalizing questions *presume* that the persons are separate from the Problem and that they have a two-way relationship with the Problem: it affects them, and they affect it.

To experience the liberating effects of externalizing, Freedman and Combs (1996, pp. 49–50) have developed the following two sets of questions: one representing conventional therapeutic questions and the other externalizing questions. To do this exercise, choose a quality or trait that you or others find problematic, usually an adjective; substitute this for X in the questions below. Then find a noun form of that trait; substitute this for Y in the questions below. For example: X = depressed/Y = Depression; X = critical/ Y = Criticism; X = angry/Y = Anger.

CONVENTIONAL VERSUS EXTERNALIZING QUESTIONS

CONVENTIONAL QUESTIONS (INSERT PROBLEM DESCRIPTION AS ADJECTIVE FOR X)	EXTERNALIZING QUESTIONS (INSERT PROBLEM DESCRIPTION AS NOUN FOR Y)
When did you first become X?	What made you vulnerable to the Y so that it was able to dominate your life?
What are you most X about?	In what contexts is the Y most likely to take over?
What kinds of things happen that typically lead to your being X?	What kinds of things happen that typically lead to the Y taking over?

(continued)

CONVENTIONAL VERSUS EXTERNALIZING QUESTIONS (*continued*)

CONVENTIONAL QUESTIONS (INSERT PROBLEM DESCRIPTION AS *ADJECTIVE* FOR **X**)	*EXTERNALIZING QUESTIONS* (INSERT PROBLEM DESCRIPTION AS *NOUN* FOR **Y**)
When you are X, what do you do that you wouldn't do if you weren't X?	What has the Y gotten you to do that is against your better judgment?
Which of your current difficulties come from being X?	What effects does the Y have on your life and relationship?
What are the consequences for your life and relationships of being X?	How has the Y led you into the difficulties you are now experiencing?
How is your self-image different when you are X?	Does the Y blind you from noticing your resources, or can you see them through it?
If by some miracle you woke up some morning and were not X anymore, how, specifically, would your life be different?	Have there been times when you have been able to get the best of the Y? Times when the Y could have taken over but you kept it out of the picture?

Problem Deconstruction: Deconstructive Listening and Questions

Drawing from the philosophical work of Jacques Derrida, narrative therapists use **deconstructive listening** and questions to help clients trace the effects of dominant discourses and to empower clients to make more conscious choices about which discourses they allow to affect their life (Freedman & Combs, 1996). In deconstructive listening, the therapist listens for "gaps" in clients' understanding and asks them to fill in the details or has them explain the ambiguities in their stories. For example, if a client reports feeling rejected because friends did not call when they said they would, the therapist listens for the meanings that led to the sense of feeling "rejected."

Deconstructive questions help clients to further "unpack" their stories to see how they have been constructed, identifying the influence of dominant and local discourses. Typically used in externalizing conversations, these questions target problematic beliefs, practices, feelings, and attitudes by asking clients to identify the following:

- History: The *history of their relationship* with the problematic belief, practice, feeling, or attitude: "When and where did you first encounter the problem?"
- Context: The *contextual influences* on the problematic belief, practice, feeling, or attitude: "When is it most likely to be present?"
- Effects: The *effects or results* of the problematic belief, practice, feeling, or attitude: "What effects has this had on you and your relationship?"
- Interrelationships: The *interrelationship with other* beliefs, practices, feelings, or attitudes: "Are there other problems that feed this problem?"
- Strategies: *Tactics and strategies* used by the problem belief, practice, feeling, or attitude: "How does it go about influencing you?"

Mapping in Landscapes of Action and Identity or Consciousness

Based on the narrative theory of Jerome Bruner (1986), mapping the problem in the landscapes of action and identity (White, 2007) or consciousness (Freedman & Combs, 1996) is a specific technique for harnessing unique outcomes to promote desired change. Mapping in the landscapes of action, identity, and consciousness generally involves the following steps:

1. Identify a unique outcome: The therapist listens for and asks about times when the problem could have been a problem but was not.
2. Ensure that the unique outcome is preferred: Rather than assume, the therapist asks clients about whether the unique outcome is a preferred outcome: "Is this something you want to do or have happen more often?"

3. Map in landscape of action: First, the therapist begins by mapping the unique outcome in the landscape of action, identifying what actions were taken by whom in which order. The therapist does this by asking about specific details: "What did you do first? How did the other person respond? What did you do next?" The therapist carefully plots the events until there is a step-by-step picture of the actions of the client and involved others, gathering details about the following:

- Critical events
- Circumstances surrounding events
- Sequence of events
- Timing of events
- Overall plot

4. Map in the landscape of identity or consciousness: After obtaining a clear picture of what happened during the unique outcome, the therapist begins to map in the landscape of identity. This phase of mapping *thickens the plot* associated with the successful outcome, thus directly strengthening the connection of the preferred outcome with the client's personal identity. Mapping in the landscape of identity focuses on the psychological and relational implications of the unique outcomes. The following sample questions cover various areas of impact:

- "What do you believe this says about you as a person? About your relationship?"
- "What were your intentions behind these actions?"
- "What do you value most about your actions here?"
- "What, if anything, did you learn or realize from this?"
- "Does this change how you see life, God, your purpose, or your life goals?"
- "Does this affect how you see the problem?"

Intentional Versus Internal State Questions

White (2007) privileges intentional state questions (questions about a person's intentions in a given situation: "What were your intentions?") over internal state questions (questions about how a person was feeling or thinking: "What were you feeling?") because intentional state questions promote a sense of *personal agency,* whereas internal state questions can have the effect of diminishing one's sense of agency, increasing one's sense of isolation, and discouraging diversity.

Scaffolding Conversations

Drawing on Vygotsky's concept of *zones of proximal development,* White (2007) uses scaffolding conversations to move clients from that which is familiar to that which is novel. Vygotsky was a developmental psychologist who emphasized that because learning is relational, adults should structure children's learning in ways that help them interact with new information. The zone of proximal development is the distance between what the child can do independently and what the child can do in collaboration with others. **Scaffolding** is a term White developed with clients to describe five incremental movements across this zone of learning:

- Low-level distancing tasks: These tasks *characterize a unique outcome.* Because they are at a low-level distance from the client (very close to what is familiar to him or her), they encourage the client to attribute meanings to events that have previously gone unnoticed: for example, "Are there times when you don't get into an argument even though there is tension?"
- Medium-level distancing tasks: These tasks allow *unique outcomes to be taken into a chain of association.* They introduce greater "newness," encouraging more comparisons and contrasts with other unique outcomes: for example, "How was last night's 'effective problem-solving conversation' similar or different from the one you described last week?"

- Medium- to high-level distancing tasks: These tasks *reflect on a chain* of *associations*. They encourage clients to reflect on, evaluate, and learn from the differences and similarities with other tasks: for example, "Looking back over these examples of effective problem solving, is there anything that stands out as useful in preventing arguments?"
- High-level distancing tasks: These tasks promote *abstract learning and realizations*. They require clients to assume a high level of distance from their immediate experience, promoting increased abstract conceptualization of life and identity: for example, "What do these effective problem-solving conversations say about you as a person and about your relationship?"
- Very-high-level distancing tasks: These are *plans for action*. They promote high-level distancing from immediate experience to enable clients to identify ways of enacting their newly developed concepts about life and identity: for example, "Do you have ideas of how you want to translate these ideas into future action?"

Over the course of a conversation, therapists move back and forth between various levels of distancing tasks, progressively moving to higher levels of action planning.

Permission Questions

Narrative therapists use **permission questions** to emphasize the democratic nature of the therapeutic relationship and to encourage clients to maintain a clear, strong sense of agency when talking with the therapist. Put quite simply, therapists ask permission to ask a question. This goes against the prevailing assumption that therapists can ask any question they want to gather information they purportedly need to help the client. Therapists are exempt from the prevailing social norms of polite conversation topics and are free to bring up taboo subjects such as sex, past abuse, relationship problems, death, fears, and weaknesses. Many clients feel compelled to answer these questions even if they are not comfortable doing so. Narrative therapists are sensitive to the power dynamic related to taboo and difficult subjects and therefore ask for the client's permission before asking questions that are generally taboo or that the therapist anticipates will make a particular client feel uncomfortable. For example, they might say, "Would it be okay if I ask you some questions about your sex life?"

In addition, permission questions are used throughout the interview regarding *what* is being discussed and *how* to ensure that the conversation is meaningful and comfortable for the client. For example, often when starting a session the therapist may briefly outline his or her ideas for how to use the time, asking for client input and permission to continue with a particular topic or line of questioning. Similarly, when therapists find themselves asking one person more questions than the others in a family session, they pause to ask permission to continue to ensure that everyone is okay with what is going on.

Situating Comments

Like permission questions, **situating comments** are used to maintain a more democratic therapeutic relationship and to reinforce client agency by ensuring that comments from the therapist are not taken as a "higher" or "more valid" truth than the client's (Zimmerman & Dickerson, 1996). Drawing on the distinction between dominant and local discourses, narrative therapists are keenly aware that any comment made by the therapist is often considered more valid than anything the client might say. Thus, therapists *situate* their comments by revealing the source of their perspective, emphasizing that it is only one perspective among many. When the source and context of a therapist comment are revealed, a client is less likely to overprivilege the comment.

EXAMPLES OF SITUATING COMMENTS

THERAPIST COMMENT WITHOUT SITUATING	SITUATING THERAPIST COMMENT
I am noticing that you tend to . . .	Having grown up on a farm, my attention is of course drawn to . . .
Research indicates that . . .	There is one therapist who has developed a theory (or done a study) that suggests. . . . Does this sound like something that would be true for you?
I suggest that you . . .	Since you are asking me for a suggestion, I can only tell you what I think as someone who believes action is more productive than talk . . .

Narrative Reflecting Team Practices

Using Tom Andersen's collaborative practice of *reflecting teams* (see "Collaborative Therapy," below), narrative therapists have developed a similar practice that supports their work. Adapting Andersen's format, Freedman and Combs (1996) assign the team *three primary tasks:*

1. Develop a thorough understanding by closely attending to details of the story.
2. Listen for differences and events that do not fit the dominant problem-saturated narrative.
3. Notice beliefs, ideas, or contexts that support the problem-saturated descriptions.

In addition, they propose the following *guidelines* for the team:

1. During the reflecting process, the reflecting team members participate in a back-and-forth conversation rather than in a monologue.
2. Team members should not talk to each other while observing the interview.
3. Comments should be offered in a tentative manner (e.g., "perhaps," "could," "might").
4. Comments are based on what actually occurs in the room (e.g., "At one point, Mom got very quiet; I was wondering what was going on for her at that moment.").
5. When appropriate, comments are situated in the speaker's personal experience (e.g., "Having been a teacher, I may have been the only one who focused on this. . . .").
6. All family members should be responded to in some way.
7. Reflections should be kept short.

Re-Membering Conversations

White (2007) uses **re-membering conversations** to develop a multivoiced sense of personal identity that enables clients to make sense of their lives in a more coherent and orderly way. In these conversations, clients develop the sense of an identity that is grounded in *associations of life* rather than in a singular, core self. The associations of life include a "membership" of significant people and identities from the client's past, present, and projected future. In these conversations, clients are encouraged to identify who's a member, assess the influence of each member, and decide whether their membership should be upgraded, downgraded, or canceled (e.g., canceling the membership of a high school bully whose taunting still haunts the client). The process of re-membering includes the following components:

- Identifying the other person's contribution to the client's life
- Articulating how the other person may have viewed the client's identity
- Considering how the client may have affected the other person's life
- Specifying the implications for the client's identity (e.g., "I am a person who values justice")

Leagues

To solidify a new narrative and new identities, narrative therapists have created **leagues** (or clubs, associations, teams), membership in which signifies an accomplishment in a particular area. In most cases, leagues are virtual communities of concern (e.g., a Temper Tamer's Club to which a child is given a membership certificate), although some meet face to face or interact via the Internet (Anti-Anorexia/Anti-Bulimia League; see www.narrativetherapy.com).

Definitional Ceremony

Generally used toward the end of therapy to solidify the emerging preferred narrative and identity, **definitional ceremonies** involve inviting significant others to *witness* the emerging story. This ceremony has three phases:

1. The first telling: The client tells his or her life story, highlighting the emerging identity stories as the invited witnesses listen.
2. Retelling: The witnesses take turns retelling the story from their perspectives; they are prepared for the process by being asked to refrain from offering advice, making judgments, or theorizing and are asked to *situate* their comments.
3. Retelling of the retelling: The client then retells the story incorporating aspects of the witnesses' stories.

Letters and Certificates

Narrative letters are used to develop and solidify preferred narratives and identities (White & Epston, 1990). Therapists can write letters detailing a client's emerging story after a session in lieu of doing case notes (unless they work in a practice environment that requires a specific format). Narrative letters use the same techniques used in session to reinforce the emerging narrative and perform the following functions:

- Emphasize client agency: Letters highlight clients' agency in their lives, including small steps in becoming proactive.
- Take observer position: The therapist clearly takes the role of *observing* the changes the client is making, citing specific, concrete examples whenever possible.
- Highlight temporality: The time dimension is used to plot the emerging story: where clients began, where they are now, and where they are likely to go.
- Encourage polysemy: Rather than propose singular interpretations, multiple meanings are entertained and encouraged.

Letters can be used early in therapy to engage clients, during therapy to reinforce the emerging narrative and reinforce new preferred behaviors, or at the end of therapy to consolidate gains by narrating the change process.

Sample Letter

White and Epston (1990, pp. 109–110) offer numerous sample letters, such as the following:

Dear Rick and Harriet,

I'm sure that you are familiar with the fact that the best ideas have the habit of presenting themselves after the event. So it will come as no surprise to you that I often think of the most important questions after the end of an interview. . . .

Anyway, I thought I would share a couple of important questions that came to me after you left our last meeting:

Rick, how did you decline Helen's [the daughter] invitation to you to do the reasoning for her? And how do you think this could have the effect of inviting her to reason with herself? Do you think this could help her to become more responsible?

Harriet, how did you decline Helen's invitations to you to be dependable for her? And how do you think this could have the effect of inviting her to depend upon herself more? Do you think that this could have the effect of helping her to take better care of her life?

What does this decreased vulnerability to Helen's invitations to have her life for her (e.g., take responsibility for her life by making decisions, solving problems, and handling consequences) reflect in you both as people?

By the way, what ideas occurred to you after our last meeting? M.W.

Certificates

Certificates are often used with children to recognize the changes they have made and to reinforce their new "reputation" as a "temper tamer," "cooperative child," and so forth.

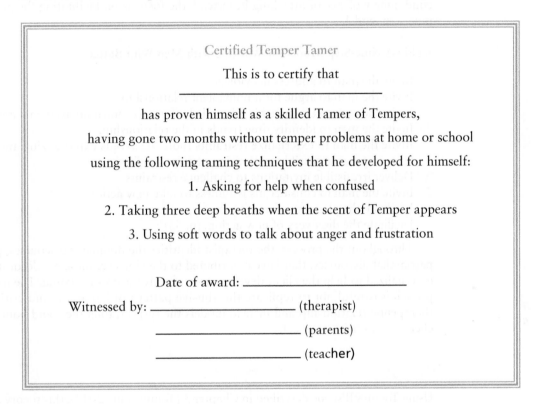

Certified Temper Tamer

This is to certify that

_____

has proven himself as a skilled Tamer of Tempers,

having gone two months without temper problems at home or school

using the following taming techniques that he developed for himself:

1. Asking for help when confused

2. Taking three deep breaths when the scent of Temper appears

3. Using soft words to talk about anger and frustration

Date of award: _____

Witnessed by: _____ (therapist)

_____ (parents)

_____ (teacher)

Interventions for Specific Problems

Children

Numerous narrative therapists have developed interventions for working with children (Freeman, Epston, & Lobovits, 1997; Smith & Nylund, 2000; Vetere & Dowling, 2005; White & Morgan, 2006). The externalization process seems to come more naturally to children, perhaps because it is reflected so often in cartoons and children's literature (e.g., the devil and angel on a cartoon character's shoulders). Externalization adapts well to play and art therapies: externalized problems (e.g., Temper, Sadness, Anger) can be portrayed in art media (drawings, clay, paintings) or acted out with puppets and dolls. In addition to externalized problems, children enjoy drawing or acting out unique outcomes and preferred narratives; this process often accelerates their adaptation of new behaviors.

Domestic Violence

Narrative therapists have developed unique and promising alternatives to the standard treatment for those who batter (Augusta-Scott & Dankwort, 2002; Jenkins, 1990). Unlike the feminist-based Duluth Model, which traces the cause of violence to men's attempts to gain power and control (Pence & Paymar, 1993; see Chapters 8 and 12), narrative approaches work from within clients' lived reality, which usually includes the experience of helplessness and powerlessness that they say leads them to try to regain control through violence (Augusta-Scott & Dankwort, 2002).

Jenkins (1990) warns therapists against accepting responsibility for the violence, which therapists inadvertently do when they challenge the man's explanations, give advice on how to stop abusive behavior, offer strong arguments against violence, or try to break down his denial, all of which are common therapist responses to violence. Instead, Jenkins uses a nine-step model that requires the *client* to take full responsibility for the violence and for ending it. Throughout this process, the therapist is supportive without condoning violence or attacking it; instead, the focus is on facilitating the process in the nine-step model.

Jenkins's Nine-Step Model for Working with Men Who Batter

1. Invite the man to address his violence.
2. Invite the man to argue for a nonviolent relationship.
3. Invite the man to examine his misguided efforts to contribute to the relationship.
4. Invite the man to identify time trends in the relationship.
5. Invite the man to externalize restraints (note: he avoids externalizing anger and violence to prevent possible minimizing of responsibility).
6. Deliver irresistible invitations to challenge restraints.
7. Invite the man to consider his readiness to take new action.
8. Facilitate the planning of new action.
9. Facilitate the discovery of new action. (p. 63)

Throughout the process, the therapist identifies the dominant discourses, particularly patriarchal discourses, that have contributed to the violence; these are deconstructed and externalized to help the client develop more effective ways of relating. The narrative approach is careful not to replicate the abusive pattern of harshness and criticism in the therapeutic relationship and instead models the respect, tolerance, and boundaries that clients are aspiring to enact.

Scope It Out: Cross-Theoretical Comparison

Using Tomm's IPscope described in Chapter 3 (Tomm et al., 2014), this theory approaches the conceptualization of systemic, interpersonal patterns as discussed below.

Theoretical Conceptualization

Narrative therapists uses a combination of pathologizing interaction patterns (PIPs), wellness interaction patterns (WIPs), and sociocultural interaction patterns (SCIPs) to conceptualize client situations. They use the following techniques to identify these IPs:

- PIPs: Externalizing; mapping the influence of the problem; statement of position map
- WIPs: Mapping the influence of persons; identifying unique outcomes and alternative narratives; externalizing questions; mapping unique outcomes in the landscapes of action and identity
- SCIPs: Identifying dominant discourses; situating comments; deconstructive listening

Goal Setting

Narrative therapists identify WIPs as the client's preferred narrative. This narrative is developed in partnership with the client to make conscious choices about how to position identity in relation to significant dominant discourses in the client's life.

Facilitating Change

Narrative therapists enact transformative interpersonal patterns (TIPs) using sets of questions designed to separate the client's identity from PIPs and problem-supporting SCIPs, such as relative influence questioning, mapping in the landscape of action and consciousness, deconstructive questioning, and scaffolding conversations. For all of these, therapists begin by exploring PIPs and SCIPs and then creating linguistic space in which the client can begin to envision and then enact WIPs.

Putting It All Together: Narrative Case Conceptualization and Treatment Plan Templates

Areas for Theory-Specific Case Conceptualization: Narrative

When conceptualizing client cases, contemporary narrative therapists typically use the following dynamics to inform their treatment plan. Go to MindTap® to access a digital version of the theory-specific case conceptualization, along with a variety of digital study tools and resources that complement this text and help you be more successful in your course and career. If your instructor didn't assign MindTap, you can find out more about it at Cengagebrain.com. You can also download the form at masteringcompetencies.com.

Meeting Persons Apart from the Problem

Describe who the person/people are apart from the problem: hobbies, interests, career, etc.

Preferred Narratives: Hopes and Aspirations for Self and Other

Describe the preferred narrative, hopes for therapy, and/or aspirations for self and other for each significant person involved in the process:

- Aspirations for self (for each person)
- Aspirations for others/relationships (for each person)

Problem-Saturated Narrative

Describe each significant person's description of the problem:

- *Extended family description(s) of problems*
- *Broader system problem descriptions:* Description of problem from referring party, teachers, relatives, legal system, etc.
- *Map the influence of the problem:* Describe how the problem is affecting the persons involved at: (a) a personal level (emotional, behavioral, identity narrative, etc.), (b) a relational level (conflicts or distance in significant relationships), and (c) in broader life circumstances (work, school, etc.).

Unique Outcomes/Sparkling Events: Influence of Persons

Describe times, contexts, relationships, etc., when the problem is less of a problem or not a problem as well as the effect of persons on the problem: What things do people do that make the problem less of a problem?

1. When is the problem less of a problem?
2. When was the problem expected but did not occur?
3. In what relationships or contexts is the problem less of a problem or not a problem?

4. What are people currently doing that keep the problem from being worse than it is or affecting more areas of life than it already does?

Based on the above, how are people most effectively influencing the problem?

Dominant Discourses and Diversity

Dominant discourses informing definition of problem:

- *Ethnic, race, class, immigration status, and religious discourses:* How do key cultural discourses inform what is perceived as a problem and the possible solutions (specify ethnicity whenever possible, e.g., Italian American rather than white)?
- *Gender and sexuality discourses:* How do the gender and sexual discourses inform what is perceived as a problem and the possible solutions? Do these intersect with ethnicity and/or religion?
- *Community, school, and extended family discourses:* How do other important community discourses inform what is perceived as a problem and the possible solutions?

Identity and Local Narratives

- *Identity narratives:* How has the problem shaped each family member's identity?
- *Local or preferred discourses:* What is the client's preferred identity narrative and/or narrative about the problem? Are there local (alternative) discourses about the problem that are preferred?

TREATMENT PLAN TEMPLATE FOR INDIVIDUAL WITH DEPRESSION/ANXIETY: NARRATIVE

You can download a blank treatment plan (with or without measures) from MindTap at www.cengagebrain.com or www.masteringcompetencies.com. The following treatment plan template can be used to help you develop individualized treatments for use with individuals with depressive or anxiety symptoms.

Narrative Treatment Plan: Client Goals with Interventions

Early-Phase Client Goals

1. Increase client's *influence over Depression* (Anxiety or crisis symptom) to reduce severity of depressed mood and anxiety.
   a. *Externalize* Depression to identify current areas of *person's influence* and possibilities for expanding this influence.
   b. *Map unique outcomes in landscapes of action and consciousness* to identify new possibilities for reducing influence of Depression on person.

Working-Phase Client Goals

1. Decrease *influence* of Depression (Anxiety) and *dominant discourses* to reduce depressed mood/anxiety.
   a. Ask *externalizing questions* to separate client from problem.
   b. *Map Depression versus unique outcomes* in landscapes of action and consciousness to separate client from Depression and strengthen alternative identity.

2. Increase sense of *agency* by developing new relationship with Depression (Anxiety) to reduce depressed mood/anxiety.
   a. Offer externalizing metaphors to define relationship with Depression (Anxiety).
   b. Use statement of position map to evaluate effects of Depression and inspire new relationship to Depression.

3. Increase actions that support *preferred identity* to reduce depressed mood/anxiety.
   a. Use scaffolding conversations to move client from contemplation to action.
   b. Use statement of position map to evaluate effects of actions and identify where and how to make adjustments.

Closing-Phase Client Goals

1. Increase and expand influence of *preferred identity* in [specify work/school, relational, and other significant areas of life] to reduce depressed mood and increase sense of wellness.
   a. Use *scaffolding conversations* to move client from contemplation to action.
   b. Use *statement of position* map to evaluate effects of actions and identify where and how to make adjustments.

2. Increase the number of relationships that support client in *preferred identity* to reduce depression and increase sense of wellness.
   a. Host *definitional ceremony* to expand network of friends and family who support client's preferred identity.
   b. Use *therapeutic letter* from therapist to document journey from being overwhelmed by Depression (Anxiety) to client being able to manage/subdue (or preferred metaphor) it.
   c. Use *narrative reflecting team* to support client in newly enacted identity.

Treatment Tasks

1. Develop working therapeutic relationship.
   a. *Meet person apart from problem*, inquiring about *identity* outside of problem.
   b. Engage client from *hopeful, optimistic* position and as *co-author/investigative reporter*.

2. Assess individual, systemic, and broader cultural dynamics.
   a. *Ask relative influence questioning to map the effects* of Depression (Anxiety) and the effects of persons on Depression; identify *unique outcomes*.
   b. Identify the *dominant discourses* that support Depression (Anxiety) and the local, alternative discourses that may be a resource in changing relationship to Depression (Anxiety).

3. Identify needed referrals, crisis issues, collateral contacts, and other client needs.
   a. *Crisis assessment intervention(s):* Address crisis issues such as self-harm, suicidal ideation, substance use, risky sexual behavior, etc.
   b. Referral(s): Connect client with resources in client's family and community that could be supportive; make collateral contacts as needed.

TREATMENT PLAN TEMPLATE FOR DISTRESSED COUPLE/FAMILY: NARRATIVE

You can download a blank treatment plan (with or without measures) from MindTap at www.cengagebrain.com or www.masteringcompetencies.com. The following treatment plan template can be used to help you develop individualized treatments for use with couples and families who report relational distress.

Narrative Treatment Plan: Client Goals with Interventions

Early-Phase Client Goals

1. Increase couple/family's *influence* over the frequency and severity of [Externalized Problem: Anger, Stress, Conflict, etc.] to reduce conflict.
   a. *Externalize* [Problem] to identify current areas of each person's influence and possibilities for expanding this influence.

b. Map *unique outcomes in landscapes of action and consciousness* to identify new possibilities for reducing influence of [Externalized Problem].

Working-Phase Client Goals

1. Decrease *influence* of [Externalized Problem] and *dominant discourses* to reduce conflict and hopelessness about the relationships.
   a. Ask *externalizing questions* to separate clients from problem.
   b. *Map Conflict versus unique outcomes* in landscapes of action and consciousness to separate clients from [Externalized Problem] and strengthen alternative identities.

2. Increase each person's sense of *agency* by developing new relationship with [Externalized Problem] to reduce conflict and increase hope.
   a. Offer externalizing metaphors to define relationship with [Externalized Problem].
   b. Use statement of position map to evaluate effects of [Externalized Problem] and inspire new relationship to it.

3. Increase actions that support *preferred relational identities* to reduce conflict.
   a. Use scaffolding conversations to move clients from contemplation to action.
   b. Use statement of position map to evaluate effects of actions and identify where and how to make adjustments.

Closing-Phase Client Goals

1. Increase and *thicken narrative of preferred couple/family identity* to reduce conflict and increase relational satisfaction.
   a. Use *scaffolding conversations* to move clients from contemplation to action.
   b. Map *unique outcomes* in landscape of action and consciousness to solidify new narrative.

2. Increase *external relationships* that support couple/family's preferred identity to reduce conflict and increase sense of cohesion.
   a. Host *definitional ceremony* to expand network of friends, family, and/or school personnel who support client's preferred identity.
   b. Write *therapeutic letter* from therapist to document journey from fighting while under the influence of [Externalized Problem] to uniting against its effects and redefining their relationship/family.
   c. Bring in *narrative reflecting team* to support couple/family in newly enacted identity.

Therapeutic Tasks

1. Develop working therapeutic relationship.
   a. *Meet persons apart from problem,* inquiring about *identities* outside of problem.
   b. Engage couple/family from *hopeful, optimistic position* and *as co-author/investigative reporter.*

2. Assess individual, systemic, and broader cultural dynamics.
   a. Ask *relative influence questioning to map the effects* of Conflict and the effects of persons on Conflict; identify *unique outcomes.*
   b. Identify the *dominant discourses* that support Conflict and the local, alternative discourses that may be a resource in changing relationship to Conflict.
   c. If possible, *externalize* a common enemy that couple/family can unite against.

3. Identify needed referrals, crisis issues, collateral contacts, and other client needs.
   a. Address crisis issues such as psychological abuse, intimate partner violence, hidden affair, self-harm, suicidal ideation, substance use, etc.
   b. *Referral(s):* Connect client with *resources* in client's *family and community* that could be supportive; make collateral contacts as needed.

Collaborative Therapy and Reflecting Teams

In a Nutshell: The Least You Need to Know

Putting postmodern, social constructionist principles into action, collaborative therapy is a two-way dialogical process in which therapists and clients co-explore and co-create new and more useful understandings related to client problems and agency. Avoiding scripted techniques, therapists focus on the *process* of therapy, on *how* the client's concerns are explored and exchanged. They listen for how clients interpret the events of their lives and then ask questions and make comments to better understand how the client's story "hangs together." These questions and comments naturally emerge from conversation as the therapist strives to understand the values and internal logic of the client's perspective—to understand the client *from within the client's worldview*. As this process unfolds, the client is naturally invited to share in the therapist's curiosity, joining the therapist in a mutual or shared inquiry—a *mutual puzzling* about how things came to be and how things might best move forward. As therapist and client engage in this *shared inquiry,* asking questions and tentatively sharing their perspectives, alternative views and future options with regard to the client's situation emerge. This process provides an opportunity for clients to see their situation differently, allowing them to make new interpretations and develop fresh ideas. Therapists do not try to control or direct the content of this meaning-making process; instead, they honor the client's ability to determine what to do with these new ideas (i.e., they honor the client's *agency*).

I am guessing this process still sounds vague, so perhaps it is best to offer an example. If a client says she is feeling "depressed," rather than hearing concrete, diagnostic information, collaborative therapists are profoundly aware of how little they know about *this* client's unique experience of depression, thus becoming sincerely curious about how the client came to this understanding of her experience. With no predetermined set of questions, the therapist asks questions that emerge from a genuine desire to better understand, such as: Does she cry often about something? About nothing? Has life gone to gray and nothing seems interesting anymore? Is her heart broken? Does she feel like a failure? There are as many unique depression stories as there are people who say they are depressed. As the therapist explores the client's view, the client is invited to join in the curiosity about her depression. Each new understanding informs alternative actions, thoughts, and feelings, thus shifting experience on multiple levels until the client has found a way to manage or resolve her initial concern.

The Juice: Significant Contributions to the Field

If you remember one thing from this chapter, it should be this:

Not Knowing and Knowing with

Perhaps one of the most frequently misunderstood concepts in collaborative therapy (Anderson, 2005), the idea of "not knowing" was first introduced by Goolishian and Anderson in 1987. At first blush, the not-knowing stance sounds contradictory: How can a paid professional like a therapist "not know"? Isn't that what they are paid for? What do you do with all that you have learned in graduate school? *Not knowing* refers to how therapists think about what they think they know and the intent with which they introduce this knowing (expertise, truths, etc.) to the client. Obviously, collaborative therapists are avoiding a particular type of knowing that Anderson calls "pre-knowing" (Anderson, 1997, 2007). In common English it's called *assuming*: believing that you can fill in the gaps or that you have enough information without sufficient evidence. Drawing from a postmodern social constructionist epistemology, collaborative therapists maintain that clients with apparently similar experiences, such as "psychosis," "mania," or "sexual abuse," have unique understandings of their situations (Anderson, 1997). Each client's understanding has evolved through conversations with significant others, acquaintances, professionals, and strangers, as well as through the larger societal discourse and stories in the media and literature. Therapists choose to *know with* and *alongside* clients as they engage in a process of better understanding clients' lives (Anderson, 1993, 2007). They view the client's knowledge to be equally as valid as their own.

This not-knowing, not-assuming stance requires the therapist to ask what, on the surface, appear to be obvious or trivial questions: "You say you are sad about the loss of your mother. Can you tell me what aspects of her loss touch you most deeply?" or "Tell me how you experience that sadness in your daily life." When clients begin to explore the ideas, experiences, and influences that led to the perception of a problem, they often hear themselves saying things they have never told anyone before. Hearing these thoughts aloud for the first time inevitably shifts their perspective of the situation, sometimes subtly and sometimes dramatically. These new perspectives inform new action and identities related to the problem (e.g., from viewing her mother as an entirely separate person, the client may shift to seeing that she is part of how her mother lives on).

Rumor Has It: The People and Their Stories

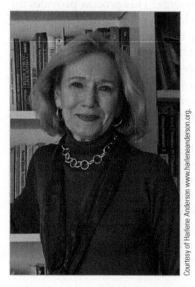

Courtesy of Harlene Anderson www.harleneanderson.org.

Harlene Anderson and Harry Goolishian

Harlene Anderson and Harry Goolishian developed collaborative therapy with their colleagues at the University of Texas Medical Branch in Galveston and later established the Houston Galveston Institute (Anderson, 1997, 2005, 2007). Their collaborative approach has roots in the early model, developed by the Galveston group, called "multiple impact therapy"; this is a multidisciplinary approach to working with hospitalized adolescents, their families, and the broader social system. Their interest in hermeneutics, social construction, postmodern assumptions, and related social and natural science theories was initially fueled by their curiosity with the ideas of the Mental Research Institute (MRI), but in their work at Galveston they began to listen differently to what clients were saying rather than trying to learn clients' language to use it as a strategic tool. They noticed that it was not the family, but rather each *member* of the family that seemed to have his or her own language, using words and phrases with unique meanings.

These interests naturally led to postmodern ideas and social construction theory and then to the work of theorists such as Ludvig Wittgenstein, Mikhail Bakhtin, Ken Gergen, and John Shotter (see Chapter 3). As a result, Anderson and Goolishian began to conceptualize their work from a postmodern perspective, focusing on the construction of meaning in relationships. They also had a mutually influencing relationship with Tom Andersen, and over the years their therapy became known as "collaborative language systems" (Anderson, 1997) and, more recently, "collaborative therapy" (Anderson & Gehart, 2007).

After Goolishian's death in 1991, Anderson and her colleagues at the Houston Galveston Institute continued developing this internationally practiced approach. Ken Gergen (see Chapter 3), Harlene Anderson, Sheila McNamee, and others joined to form the Taos Institute, an organization of collaborative practitioners working in the fields of education, business, consultation, therapy, medicine, and other disciplines. Having found that the assumptions on which collaborative therapy is based have applications beyond therapy systems, Anderson currently refers to her work as "collaborative practices."

Tom Andersen

No relation other than a close friend to Harlene Anderson (note the "e" versus the "o" in Andersen), Tom Andersen was a Norwegian psychiatrist who is best remembered for his gentle demeanor, respect for client privacy, and elegant therapeutic conceptions. Having originally studied with the Milan team using one-way mirrors, Andersen transformed the systemic practice of the observation team using postmodern sensibilities that reduced the team–client hierarchy and made the process dialogical rather than strategic. His descriptions of *inner and outer dialogues* as well as *appropriately unusual comments* provide collaborative therapists with practical concepts that can be used to facilitate therapeutic conversations without the use of technique.

Lynn Hoffman

Known for her keen theoretical insights and broad vision, Lynn Hoffman has worked closely with many of family therapy's most influential thinkers, including Virginia Satir, Jay Haley, Paul Watzlawick, Salvador Minuchin, Dick Auserwald, Gianfranco Cecchin, Luigi Boscolo, Tom Andersen, Harlene Anderson, and Peggy Penn. Her first book, *Foundations of Family Therapy* (Hoffman, 1981), provides one of the most comprehensive overviews of systemic family therapy available. She began learning about family therapy at the MRI, where she served as an editor for Satir's books. She was so inspired by these ideas that she went on to pursue a career as a social worker, training in systemic family therapies. She befriended the Milan team and, along with Peggy Penn, helped further their later development of the model (Boscolo et al., 1987). In her later years, Hoffman became increasingly attracted to postmodern, collaborative approaches (Hoffman, 1990, 1993, 2001). She has detailed her remarkable journey in *Family Therapy: An Intimate History* (Hoffman, 2001), a favorite with my students who want to learn about the theories of family therapy yet prefer a little more "juice" and excitement than is offered in a textbook such as this. Hoffman is currently exploring the notion of rhizome theory in human systems.

Peggy Penn

A former training director of the Ackerman Institute and a published poet (Penn, 2002), Peggy Penn has developed unique approaches to using writing in collaborative therapy (Penn, 2001; Penn & Frankfurt, 1994; Penn & Sheinberg, 1991). Like Hoffman, Penn began her training in systemic therapies, most notably the Milan approach (Boscolo et al., 1987), but her work evolved into a more postmodern approach. Until her death in 2012, she used various forms of writing in therapy to help clients access multiple voices and perspectives.

Jaakko Seikkula

Psychologist Jaakko Seikkula and his colleagues (Haarakangas et al., 2007) developed and researched the *open dialogue* approach to working with patients with psychotic symptoms in the Lapland region of Finland. As a result of 20 years of work, their hospital no longer has chronic cases of psychosis, and patients with psychotic symptoms need fewer medications and return to work more often. Seikkula's research provides some of the best empirical evidence for postmodern therapies (see "Clinical Spotlight," below).

Houston Galveston Institute

Originally founded by Harlene Anderson, Harry Goolishian, and their colleagues, the Houston Galveston Institute continues to be the premier training center for collaborative therapy, providing services to local child protection agencies, schools, and trauma survivors. Sue Levin currently serves as the executive director, and her research focuses on women who have been abused by their partners (Levin, 2007). Saliha Bava serves as the associate director of the institute, and her current work focuses on trauma (Bava, Levin, & Tinaz, 2002), qualitative research (Gehart, Tarragona, & Bava, 2007), and transformative performance.

Grupo Campos Elísios: Collaborative Therapy Training Center in Mexico City

Located in Mexico City and working closely with the Houston Galveston Institute, the bilingual faculty at Grupo Campos Elísios offer training in collaborative therapy and provide therapy and consultation services to local families, schools, and hospitals; the faculty and cofounders include Sylvia London, Margarita Tarragona, Irma Rodriguez-Jazcilevich, and Elena Fernandez.

The Big Picture: Overview of Treatment

Collaborative therapists do not have set stages of therapy or an outline for how to conduct a session. Instead, they use a single guiding principle: facilitate *collaborative relationships and generative, two-way dialogical conversations,* regardless of the topic and the participants. In short, they "keep the dialogue going." The key to facilitating dialogue is avoiding monologues.

Avoiding Monologues and the Therapeutic Impasse

Harry Goolishian often said that it is easier to identify what *not* to do as a therapist than what to do. Extending this logic, collaborative therapy is often easier to understand by identifying what is *not* a collaborative conversation, namely, a **monologue** (Anderson, 1997, 2007). A monologue can be a conversation with others or a silent conversation with oneself or an imagined other. In a spoken monological conversation between two people, each person is trying to sell his or her idea to the other person: a duel of realities. In such conversations, participants listen only to, or long enough to, plan their next defense—they are not trying to understand the other out of genuine curiosity or attempting to develop new understandings. In silent conversations, monologues occur when the same opinion or thought consistently occupies one's mind, leaving no room for new ones or curiosity and being closed to other thoughts.

In therapy, monological conversations lead to a **therapeutic impasse**, at which point the therapeutic discussion no longer generates useful meanings or understandings. For most, it is easy to identify monological conversations because tension develops and the conversational task becomes trying to convince the other of a particular point. Therapists may also begin to describe clients in pejorative terms, such as "resistant." When this happens—whether between therapist and client or between any two people in the room—the therapist's job is to gently shift the conversation back to a dialogical exchange of ideas. Therapists can achieve this by shifting back into a curious stance—asking to better understand the client's perspective or inquiring whether there is a particular point that the client thinks the therapist is not fully understanding. However, to reengage others in dialogue, the therapist must also be in an internal dialogical mode. In the simplest terms, a collaborative therapist's primary job is to ensure that the conversations in the room—whether between members of the client system or between the therapist and the client—do not become dueling monologues. As long as conversations are dialogical, change and transformation are inevitable.

Making a Connection: The Therapeutic Relationship

Philosophical Stance

Collaborative therapists conceptualize the therapist's position as a **philosophical stance**, a particular *way of being in relation with others.* This stance informs how therapists speak, think about, act with, and respond in session, focusing their attention on the *person* of the client and shifting attention away from roles and functions. The philosophical stance essentially encompasses a sincere embodiment of the postmodern, social constructionist ideas that inform the collaborative approach, such as viewing the client as expert and valuing the transformative process of dialogue.

Conversational Partners: "Withness"

The therapeutic relationship in collaborative therapy is best described as a conversational partnership (Anderson, 1997), a process of being *with* the client. In this way of relating, sometimes referred to as "withness" (Hoffman, 2007), the conversational partners "touch" and move one another through their mutual understandings. Withness also involves a willingness to go along for the roller-coaster ride (Anderson, 1993)—the ups and downs—of the client's transformational process, regardless of how uncomfortable, unpredictable, or scary it may be. It is a commitment to walk alongside the client, no matter where the journey leads.

Curiosity: The Art of Not Knowing

A hallmark of the collaborative therapeutic stance (Anderson, 1995, 1997), *curiosity* refers to the therapist's sincere interest in clients' unique life experiences and the meanings that are generated from these experiences. This curiosity is fueled by a *social constructionist epistemology* (assumptions about knowledge and how we know what we know; see Chapter 3), which posits that each person constructs a unique reality from the webs of relationships and conversations in which he or she is engaged. Thus, no two people experience marriage, parenting, depression, psychosis, or anxiety the same way. For example, in the case study at the end of this chapter, the therapist focuses on understanding 15-year-old Ashley's unique experience of being depressed and cutting, rather than on filling in the blanks based on research or what she has learned from other teens with this problem.

Client and Therapist Expertise

In 1992, Anderson and Goolishian radically proposed, "The client is the expert." Although sometimes misunderstood to mean that the therapist has no opinion and no role in the therapeutic process, the concept of "client as expert" means that the therapist's attention is focused on sincerely valuing clients' thoughts, ideas, and opinions. Therapists ultimately have very limited information about the fullness and complexity of clients' lives; they can never acquire the complete history and "insider" perspective that clients themselves have (Anderson, 1997). Thus, the concept of client as expert is more about respect for the client than a description of how the therapeutic process is conducted.

During the therapy session, however, therapists have a different expertise because they are responsible for ensuring that an effective and respectful dialogical conversation is conducted. They rely on the generative quality of the conversation to support client transformation rather than dictate the content, direction, or outcome of the conversation.

In broad strokes (which are always inaccurate), it may be helpful in the beginning to think of the client as holding more expertise in the area of *content* (what needs to be talked about) and the therapist as holding more expertise in the area of *process* (how things are to be talked about); however, in this collaborative process, both therapist and client have input on both content and process. If a collaborative therapist believes the client is not addressing an important area of content, the therapist will raise the issue in a nonhierarchical manner: "I know you prefer not to talk about the past, but I wonder if it might not be worthwhile to spend a little time exploring how your childhood abuse affects your marriage today." Such a comment is offered in such a way that the client feels truly free to say yes or no, and the therapist honors the client's wishes. For example, although the therapist in the case study at the end of the chapter suspects that Ashley's mother's decision to move in with her lesbian partner is affecting Ashley's reported feelings of depression, and although the therapist may invite Ashley to consider this link, he or she will not force the issue if the client does not think it is a useful line of conversation.

Conversely, the therapist is also open to client feedback about the therapeutic process, allowing clients' input on which processes work best for them, including who is in the room, the pacing, the types of homework or suggestions, the types of questions, and so forth. The therapist does not necessarily take the client's request as a dictate for how to do therapy, but thoughtfully considers the request and the need that underlies it and works to find the best possible ways to address it. This back-and-forth exchange is a sincere partnership, in which the therapist works side by side with the client to find useful ways of talking. Anderson (1997) talks about this continual openness to client feedback as "research as part of everyday practice." The therapist uses the feedback to fine-tune the therapy process, lessening the opportunity for therapeutic impasse and ensuring that therapy is tailored to each client's unique needs.

Everyday, Ordinary Language: A Democratic Relationship

Collaborative therapists listen, hear, and speak in a natural, down-to-earth way that is more congruent with the client's language and more democratic than hierarchical (Andersen, 1991; Anderson, 2007). Although they are responsible for facilitating a dialogical process that clients find useful, they do not approach the task from a position of leadership or expertise. Instead, they assume a more humble position, using everyday language, a relaxed style, and a willingness to learn that invites clients to join them in exploring how best to proceed.

Inner and Outer Talk

Tom Andersen conceptualized conversations as involving both inner and outer talk (Andersen, 2007). In a conversation, we most quickly recognize the *outer talk*, the verbal conversation between the therapy participants. Andersen also recognized that there were other dialogues going on, namely, *inner talk*, the thoughts and conversations each person has within while participating in a conversation. Thus, if a therapist is working with one client, at least three conversations are simultaneously occurring: (a) the client's inner dialogue, (b) the therapist's inner dialogue, and (c) the outer spoken dialogue. The therapist needs to allow space and time for each one of these conversations.

As Andersen (2007) pointed out, when clients are speaking, they are speaking not only to the therapist but, more importantly, *to themselves*. Often in therapy, clients are saying something aloud for the first time, and they may need time to reflect on the weight or unexpected content of what they hear themselves saying to the therapist. Andersen strongly admonished therapists to not pressure clients to share their inner dialogue, as is common in more content-based therapies. Thus, if a client does not want to speak about her sexual abuse or a difficult relationship, the therapist does not force the issue but instead leaves an open invitation for the client to speak about it when ready. Unlike most therapists, Andersen was a champion for client privacy and autonomy even in session, a reflection of his abiding faith that clients have the ability to navigate their lives in a way that works best for them.

In addition to tracking the outer dialogue with the client, Andersen encouraged therapists to track their own inner dialogues: their thoughts, feelings, and reactions to the client and the outer dialogue. The therapist's inner dialogue provides many forms of information that can facilitate the therapeutic relationship: the therapist's reaction to the client may provide information about how others are relating to the client, or it may indicate that the therapist is reacting to the client based on personal history or issues rather than professional knowledge. The therapist's inner dialogue might also include insights, ideas, or metaphors that could further the outer dialogue (Anderson, 1997). When the therapist's inner dialogue is distracting from the outer conversation—as in Anderson's notion of silent monologue—the therapist is encouraged to bring up the issue with the client if doing so furthers the dialogue in useful ways (Anderson, 1997). For example, if a client continually minimizes the role of alcohol in his stories of one-night stands and yet in each incident the therapist notices there is a clear link, the therapist can *gently* put forth this observation, while verbally and nonverbally giving permission for the client to maintain his or her opinion without feeling that the relationship is threatened (e.g., "I know from past conversations that you don't think there is a link here, but I want to say that I keep seeing a link between your nights out partying and getting into these relationships you later regret. If you do not see alcohol as the main cause, is there a minor role it might be playing?"). The key is to offer the perspective in such a way that invites curiosity rather than defensiveness.

The Viewing: Case Conceptualization and Assessment

Case conceptualization in collaborative therapy involves asking two key questions:

- *Who* is talking about the problem?
- *How* does each person who is talking about the problem define and understand the problem?

Therapists answer the first by assessing who is in the ***problem-organizing system***, or who is in conversation with whom, about what. The second question is approached using the therapist's *philosophical stance* to understand the client's worldview.

Who's Talking? Problem-Organizing, Problem-Dissolving Systems

Anderson and Goolishian (1988, 1992) initially conceptualized therapeutic systems as *linguistic systems* that organize around the identification of a problem: therapists and clients come together because someone has identified a problem, issue, or concern; the word *problem* may not always be explicitly used by the client. They referred to these systems as problem-organizing, problem-dissolving systems. They are "problem organizing" because they come into being only after someone has identified a problem. They are "problem dissolving" in that they dissolve when the participants—therapists, clients, and interested third parties—no longer have a problem to discuss. In addition, *dissolving* refers to the idea that the problem often is not "solved" in the traditional sense of finding a solution. Instead, the participants' understandings evolve through dialogue, allowing for new thoughts, feelings, and actions. In the end, the client may not feel that the problem was solved as much as it dissolved. For example, if a client initially reports feeling stressed because of a recent breakup, the problem is not solved, but rather the client comes to interpret the situation differently and therefore acts and feels differently.

Aware that all persons talking about the problem are part of the problem-organizing, problem-dissolving system, collaborative therapists ask the following questions.

QUESTIONS ABOUT THE PROBLEM

- Who is talking about the problem in session and outside of session?
- How does each define it?
- What does each think should be done about it?

Try It Yourself

Either alone on paper or with a partner in dialogue, use the above questions to assess the problem-organizing system. What similarities and differences do you notice in these multiple descriptions?

As the understanding of the problem shifts and evolves through dialogue, the therapist continually assesses who is involved in talking about it outside of the session and continually inquires about the multiple perspectives about the problem, encouraging all perspectives to be heard without trying to reconcile them or identify the "truth." Clients and therapists are most likely to generate new and more useful perspectives when they allow multiple, contradictory perspectives to constantly linger in the air. Thus, in the case study at the end of this chapter, the therapist seeks to understand not only the perspective of the identified patient, the teen, but also the perspectives of her siblings, mother, mother's girlfriend, teachers, school counselor, and friends.

Philosophical Stance: Social Constructionist Viewing

As mentioned, collaborative therapists' primary tool in therapy is not a technique or intervention but a system of viewing—their philosophical stance (Anderson, 1997). Collaborative therapists work from a social constructionist, postmodern perspective, which maintains that our realities are constructed in language and through relationships. Rather than seeing identities and meanings as fixed, social constructionism describes how we engage in a constant process of revising and reinterpreting our personal identities and social realities by the way we tell ourselves what it means to be "a good person," "happy," "successful," "cared for," "living a meaningful life," "respected," and so forth. These stories are shaped by conversations with friends, news stories, fiction pieces, and any exchange of ideas, whether in person or through media. Rather than being bent on showing how clients are "incorrect" or "off," the therapist is curious about clients and focuses on how clients construct meaning about the events in their lives.

Assessing the Client's Worldview

This curiosity means that collaborative therapists focus on better understanding clients' worldviews, their systems for interpreting life events. They do not look for "errors" or even "the source of the problem," but rather they approach clients with a gentle, nonjudging curiosity, much like a child exploring a tide pool for the first time, careful not to crush the intriguing creatures in this fascinating new world (Anderson, 1997; Hoffman, 2007). The therapist is looking for the internal logic that makes the client's world, hopes, problems, and symptoms make sense. For example, if a woman is feeling that her marriage is failing, how did she first get this idea? How did she respond? How did she make sense of her partner's changing behaviors and her own? What does she fear it says about her as a person? What does she think happened, and what does she see as the options from here? Why did her marriage work up until now, and what would it take to get it back to how it was or to make it even better? Such questions would not be in the therapist's tool bag, but rather would be responses that remain congruent with the conversation at any point. Thus, "assessment" in collaborative therapy is a continuous "co-assessment" that occurs through conversation. In the case study at the end of this chapter, the therapist asks with sincere not-knowing curiosity about how Ashley experiences and understands her feelings of sadness, how cutting "works" for her, what her mother's relationship means to her, and how she views her siblings.

Targeting Change: Goal Setting

Self-Agency

Like other postmodern approaches, collaborative therapists do not have a predefined, cookie-cutter model of health toward which they steer all clients. Instead, the overall goal is to increase clients' sense of *agency* in their lives: the sense that they are competent and able to take meaningful action. Anderson (1997) believes that agency is inherent in everyone and can only be *self-accessed,* not given by someone else, as is implied in the concept of client "empowerment"; instead collaborative therapists see their role as participating in a process that maximizes the opportunities for agency to emerge in clients.

Transformation

Rather than conceptualizing the output of therapy as change, collaborative therapists conceptualize the process as transformation, emphasizing that some "original" aspects remain, while other aspects are added or diminished. In therapy, clients' narrative of self-identity, who they tell themselves they are, is transformed through the dialogical process, opening new possibilities for meaning, relating to others, and future action. This transformational process is not controlled or directed by the therapist but emerges from within clients as they listen to themselves, the therapist, and others share their ideas, thoughts, and hopes.

The process of transformation through dialogue is inherently and inescapably *mutual*. When therapists participate in dialogical conversations, they risk being changed themselves because the same dialogical process that allows clients to change creates a context in which therapists are also transformed (Anderson, 1997). Although this transformation may not be as dramatic or immediately evident as the client's transformation, the worldview of therapists inevitably evolves and shifts as they learn from their clients about other ways to make sense of and engage life.

Setting Collaborative Goals

As the name implies, therapeutic goals are constructed collaboratively with clients using their everyday language rather than professional terms. In collaborative therapy, goals continually evolve as meanings and understandings change. The evolution of goals may be gradual (from arguing less to having more positive conversations) or dramatic (from focusing on school performance to focusing on emotionally connecting with one's parent). Therapists do not have a set of predefined goals they use with all clients. Instead, goals are negotiated with each client individually.

Examples of Working-Phase Goals That Address Presenting Problems

- Reduce arguments between couple by increasing the number of conversations where they "get" each other.
- Increase periods of "harmony" between the children.
- Increase the number of times that the child can do his or her homework without being monitored.
- Expand social network by reconnecting with old friends and family

Examples of Late-Phase Goals That Target Agency and Identity Narratives

- Increase sense of agency and assertiveness when relating to colleagues at work.
- Increase the mother's sense of agency and ability to prioritize where her time and energy go.
- Develop a family identity narrative that retains a strong sense of connection while allowing for individuality and differences of opinion.
- Develop a sense of identity that honors the difficulties of the past without living in the shadow of the past.

The Doing: Interventions and Ways of Promoting Change

Conversational Questions: Understanding from Within the Dialogue

Conversational questions are those that come naturally from within the dialogue rather than from professional theory (Anderson, 1997). They are not canned or preplanned but instead follow logically from what the client is saying and are generated from the therapist's curiosity and desire to understand more. For example, if a client describes her frustration with her husband's not helping around the house, the therapist asks questions that logically flow from the conversation in the moment, such as "What chores would you like help with? Has it always been this way?" rather than therapeutic or theoretically informed questions, such as the miracle question in solution-based therapy (see Chapter 9), externalizing questions in narrative therapy (see below), or systemic interaction questions in a systems approach (see Chapter 4).

Using the client's preferred words and expressions, therapists ask conversational questions, which help both the therapist and the client to better understand the client's situation. In research on the therapy process, clients reported that questions asked out of genuine curiosity are received quite differently than "conditional" or "loaded" questions, which are driven by a professional agenda to assess or intervene (Anderson, 1997). When the therapist in the case study at the end of this chapter asks the client to describe how and why she cuts, the therapist is genuinely curious about the meaning and reasoning Ashley attributes to her actions.

Making "Appropriately Unusual" Comments

One of the most elegant and practically useful therapeutic concepts, **appropriately unusual comments** enable therapists to offer clients reflections that make a difference. On the basis of his work with reflecting teams, Tom Andersen (1991, 1995) recommends that therapists avoid comments and questions that are "too usual" or "too unusual." Comments that are *too usual* essentially reflect the client's worldview, offering no possibility for generating new understanding or change; agreeing to or reflecting back the client's current perspective is not likely to promote change. Alternatively, comments that are *too unusual* are too different to be useful in developing new meanings. Some clients give immediate signals that a comment is too unusual by becoming "resistant," reexplaining themselves, or rejecting the comment or suggestion. Other clients give little indication in session that the comment is too unusual but afterward do not follow up on the comment and may even lose faith in the therapist and the therapy process.

Appropriately unusual comments are comments that clearly fit within the client's worldview while inviting curiosity and perhaps offering a new perspective that is easily digestible. For example, if a client comes in feeling overwhelmed with a new job that is more multifaceted than the previous job, an appropriately unusual response from the therapist might be: "It sounds like your new job may require skills in multitasking and prioritizing that weren't necessary in your old job," which speaks to the client's current experience while offering a slightly different viewpoint. Such comments capture the client's attention because they are familiar enough to be safe and viable yet different enough to offer a fresh perspective (Anderson, 1997).

Listening for the Pause

When clients hear an appropriately unusual comment, suggestion, or question, they almost always have to pause and take time to integrate the new perspective with their current perspective: in these moments it is most important for the therapist to allow the client time for inner dialogue. Sometimes a client says, "I have to think about that" or "I never thought of it that way." A client's initial response may be "I don't know," but after taking a few moments to reflect on the new idea, the client usually begins to generate a response that reflects thoughts and ideas the client never had before.

How Far to Go?

How unusual is appropriately unusual? The trick here is that each client needs a different level of unusualness; alternatively stated, each client finds a different level of difference useful for generating new ideas. I often find that when I am first working with a teen, mandated client, or someone who is unsure of therapy, appropriately unusual comments cannot include significant differences from their current worldview until they have developed greater trust in me. In addition, the more emotionally distraught clients are, the less useful they find highly unusual comments. Other clients require and prefer that the therapist deliver comments that are quite different from their own, often in a very direct manner that verges on being socially impolite. I have had clients, particularly men, say to me, "Just tell me where you think I got it wrong" or "Just tell it to me straight—don't sugarcoat it—I hate when therapists do that." Thus, "appropriately unusual" depends on the client's preferred style of communication and the quality of the therapeutic relationship. Collaborative therapists fine-tune their communication skills to deliver a range of appropriately unusual comments and carefully observe client responses to assess whether or not the comments are useful.

Mutual Puzzling Questions and Process: "Kicking Around" New Meanings

As already mentioned, the process by which collaborative therapists invite their clients to join them in becoming curious about clients' lives is referred to as **mutual puzzling** (Anderson, 1997). Anderson suggests that the therapist's curiosity becomes contagious, and clients are naturally invited into it. What begins, therefore, as the therapist's one-way inquiry shifts to a joint one. When clients join the therapist in the meaning-making process, their rate of talking may slow down, there may be more pauses in the conversation, and there is an inquisitive yet hopeful air to the conversation. Often the shift in clients is visible: their body posture softens, the head may tilt to the side, and they move more slowly or more quickly (Andersen, 2007). Mutual puzzling can occur only when therapists are successful in creating a two-way dialogical conversation in which both parties are able to sincerely take in and reflect on each other's contributions.

For example, if a client lives in daily fear of having another psychotic episode after not having had one for over 10 years and says that it is her illness that keeps her from moving forward in life, the mutual puzzling process may be sparked by a question such as: "That's interesting. You say you haven't had an episode in 10 years, so hallucinations don't seem to be plaguing you these days. But it does sound like the *worry about* hallucinations is the problem at this point. Do you think of this as part of the original problem, or is it a new problem that only developed after the first was resolved?" In this case, a new distinction is highlighted; the client is invited to "kick it around" and see what, if any, new ideas emerge and to follow where they lead. The therapist does not politely insist that worrying is the new problem, but rather listens for how the client makes sense of the comment and continues to follow the client's thinking, kicking around the next idea that evolves from the conversation. The therapist is always most curious about how the client is making sense of what is being discussed.

Being Public: Sharing One's Inner Dialogue

In **being public**, therapists share their inner dialogue potentially for two reasons: (a) to respect clients by honestly sharing their thoughts about significant issues affecting treatment and (b) to prevent monological conversation by offering their private thoughts to the dialogue (Anderson, 1997, 2005). When therapists make their perspectives publicly known, they do so tentatively and, even when discussing professional knowledge, are careful not to overshadow the client's perspective (Anderson, 2007). When therapists are open with their silent thoughts, this helps prevent them from slipping into a monological view of the client, and creates a situation in which something different may be created for the therapist as well.

Being public generally occurs in two situations: (a) in communications about professional information with clients or outside agencies or professionals (e.g., courts, psychiatrists, etc.) and (b) when the therapist has significant differences from the client in values, goals, and purposes.

Being Public with Professional Communication

Whenever collaborative therapists handle professional matters, such as making a diagnosis, speaking with a social worker, or filing a report with the court, they "make public" their thoughts, rationales, and intentions by discussing them directly with clients. Openly discussing what the therapist will reveal in an upcoming conversation with another professional and/or recapping what happened in the last conversation goes against traditional procedures, in which communications between professionals were kept confidential from the client, ostensibly because it could do "harm" to the client to know what professionals were actually thinking. The apparent "harm," however, was usually that clients would be angry.

In dramatic contrast, collaborative therapists have been pioneers in lifting the veil on dialogues between professionals, and engaging in honest, direct conversation with clients about the contents of these conversations. Such conversations are not always easy, such as when a therapist has to tell a client that she cannot recommend unification through child protective services until x, y, and z happen (typically spelled out by the social worker or court). In the past, the parent learned this in court or from a social worker; in collaborative therapy, the therapist has an upfront conversation from the beginning, clearly laying out the types of behaviors that need to be seen for the desired recommendations and then wholeheartedly and enthusiastically working with the client to reach this goal.

Most clients greatly respect the therapist's honesty and integrity and respond with increased motivation to make needed changes. They fully understand when they are not given the report they hoped for because the therapist and client have been discussing progress—or lack thereof—consistently along the way. When working with court-mandated clients, collaborative therapists St. George and Wulff (1998) have the client help write the first drafts of letters to the courts about progress, including clinical recommendations, and then use the letters to discuss the client's progress and goals.

Similarly, when working with a teen such as the one in the case study at the end of this chapter, the therapist may "make public" her concern about the teen's safety and the potential for her to injure herself more than intended, especially if the client is not highly motivated to stop cutting. When the client is invited into a discussion to address the therapist's concern about the client's safety—without having rigid requirements for the client—the client and therapist can work together to develop a plan that is meaningful to the client while also addressing the therapist's concerns about safety.

Being Public with Significant Differences in Values and Goals

The other situation in which collaborative therapists make their voice public is when there are significant differences in values or goals that make it hard for the therapist to move forward as an active participant in the conversation. For example, I recently worked with a teenager who discussed his plans to meet someone who had challenged him to a fight at a park and who had said, "Don't bring weapons or friends." The teen believed that if he didn't show up, more guys at school would gang up on him and that could lead to more events such as this. Although I saw his point, I also saw that he was at risk for seriously being hurt, a concern I decided to make "public." I invited him to explore my concerns: the guy might come with friends or weapons, there might be legal ramifications, and so forth. I offered my list of dangers from a place of serious concern without demanding a particular course of action on his part. Instead, I asked him how he would manage the dangers I saw. By the end of the conversation, we arrived at a place at which my concerns and his fears were addressed and we both felt good about his chosen course of action, namely, to avoid the park that day and to try to find out about this person's social network.

Accessing Multiple Voices in Writing

Peggy Penn and her associates (Penn, 2001; Penn & Frankfurt, 1994; Penn & Sheinberg, 1991) access multiple, alternative voices using various forms of writing (e.g., letters, poems, journals) to generate alternative perspectives and make room for silenced inner voices or the voices of significant persons not currently in the therapeutic dialogue. Penn and Frankfurt (1994) have found that "writing slows down our perceptions and reactions, making room for their thickening, their gradual layering" (p. 229). They have also found that the performative aspect, the reading aloud of letters to witnesses (the therapist, family, and others), makes things happen. Penn's writing has a different intent than writing in experiential therapies, which is meant to express repressed emotions, bring resolution to a past situation, or achieve a similar clinical aim. Instead, Penn's writing invites different voices into the conversation to generate alternative possibilities for understanding. Furthermore, writing promotes agency: "to write *gives us agency: we are not acted on by a situation, we are acting!*" (Penn, 2001, p. 49; emphasis in source). Clients may be asked to write the following:

- Letters to themselves from aspects of themselves and/or from newly emerging, future, or past selves
- Letters to themselves from significant others from the present, past, or future
- Letters to and from significant others (alive or dead) speaking from a voice or perspective that was formerly kept private
- Letters or journal entries to speak from parts of the self that are typically not expressed and/or are emerging in therapy
- Letters to the world or general audience
- Multivoiced biographies that describe the client's life from various perspectives
- Poems that express inner voices and perspectives that are not readily articulated in other ways

Try It Yourself

Pick one of the above writing exercises to explore multiple voices related to a situation.

Reflecting Teams and the Reflecting Process

Tom Andersen trained at the Milan Institute, where a small team of therapists would observe the therapist talking with families behind a one-way mirror, the preferred method for interviewing in early family therapy. Influenced by postmodern thinking as well as a gut feeling of discomfort because of the distance (Andersen, 1995), Andersen and his colleagues wanted to make the process more democratic and developed the idea of having the families listen to the team's conversation behind the mirror: thus, the reflecting team practice began. With the earliest reflecting teams, the family and team would literally switch rooms if sound could be heard in only one room, or they would turn off the lights in the family's room and turn on the lights in the team's room, reversing the one-way mirror. In later years, the team was invited to sit in the same room but separate from the family and therapist having a conversation. Over the years, the practice has developed into more of a general *process* of reflecting that is used for talking with clients, with or without a team.

The idea behind a collaborative reflecting team is to develop diverse strands of conversation so that the client can choose that which resonates and that which does not. This is in contrast to the private team conversations, which are synthesized by the team and in which the team chooses what is important for the client to hear. Collaborative reflecting teams avoid coming to agreement on any one description of what is going on with the client, allowing for multiple, contradictory perspectives to linger and promoting the development of new meanings and perspectives. Teams avoid comments that evaluate or judge the client in any way, positively or negatively.

Instead, they focus on offering what is called *reflections,* observations, questions, or comments that are clearly owned by the person making them (e.g., "As I listened, I was wondering . . . ").

General Guidelines for Reflecting Teams

Andersen (1991, 1995) provides the following guidelines for teams:

- Only use with the client's permission: The therapist should obtain the client's permission to use a team *before* the session starts. When the therapist has a strong rapport with the client and confidently explains how the reflecting process works, most clients enthusiastically agree.

- Give the client permission to listen or not to listen: Andersen gives the clients *explicit* permission to listen or not listen. I find it helpful to tell clients that they will probably hear some comments that resonate deeply and others that fit less well with their experience, and I recommend they focus on the comments that "strike a chord."

- Comment on what is seen or heard, not what is observed: Team members should comment on a specific event or statement in the conversation and then "wonder" or be "curious" about it. The wondering or curiosity statement should be appropriately unusual to help generate new perspectives.

- Talk from a questioning, speculative, and tentative perspective: Team members avoid offering opinions or interpretations and instead use "wondering" questions ("I am wondering if . . .") or offer a tentative perspective ("I am aware that I don't know enough to know the whole story, but it seems like there might be . . ."). If a team member offers a strong opinion, another team member may ask, "What did you see or hear in the conversation that made you think that?" to open the conversation up and invite multiple perspectives.

- Comment on all that you hear but not all that you see: If the family members try to cover something up, allow them the right to not talk about all that they think and feel. Andersen warned: "Don't confuse therapy with confession." Unlike in psychodynamic and humanistic traditions, Andersen explicitly stated that if a client wants to hide an emotion or not say something, the client should be free to do so. He was a rare advocate for client privacy in therapy, believing that clients will share when they are ready. If a therapist notices a client getting agitated or holding back tears, he does not comment on it, allowing the client to speak about these emotions when he or she is ready to do so.

- Separate the team and the family: The team and family can be in the same room but should not talk to each other. Andersen believed that an important psychological space is created by the physical space between the team and client and by the two not talking directly; later research studies supported his view (Sells et al., 1994). This space invites all participants to focus on their inner dialogue, more readily stimulating new thoughts and ideas.

- Listen for what is appropriately unusual: Avoid what is too usual or too unusual. To identify useful reflections, Andersen asked himself: "Is what is going on now appropriately unusual or is it too unusual?" (Andersen, 1995, p. 21).

- Ask: **"How would you like to use this session today?"** This question, although likely to be asked at the beginning of any session, is critical when a team is involved. If the client is nervous about using a reflecting team, the therapist can also add, "Are there particular topics you want to avoid with the team here?"

Try It Yourself

Next time your class watches a video or does a role-play, try adding a reflecting team to the experience.

Related Reflecting Processes

Over time, the concept of the reflecting team has developed into a number of reflecting processes:

- Multiple reflectors: A team of two to four therapists observes the therapist–client conversation, sitting in a different room using a one-way mirror (or camera) or in a separate space in the same room.
- Single reflector: If only one colleague is available, the therapist may turn and have a reflecting conversation with this one reflector while the client listens.
- No outside reflector when working with a family: When there is no outside colleague available, the therapist may choose to speak with a single family member while other family members listen.
- No outside reflector when working with an individual: When the therapist is working with an individual client, a reflective process can be created by talking about issues from the perspective of someone who is not present (e.g., a parent, friend, spouse, or famous person of significance to the client).
- With young children: When working with children, reflections can include play media. A single therapist working with an individual child can create reflecting teams using puppets or other such media (Gehart, 2007).

"As If" Reflecting

Developed by Anderson (1997), the "as if" reflecting process involves having the team members or other witnesses to the conversation speak or reflect as if they are some of the people in the problem-organized system (i.e., the people talking about the problem), which includes the client, family members, friends, bosses, teachers, school personnel, medical professionals, probation officers, and so forth. This process can be used with clients or with supervisees staffing a case.

Scope It Out: Cross-Theoretical Comparison

Using Tomm's IPscope described in Chapter 3 (Tomm et al., 2014), this theory approaches the conceptualization of systemic, interpersonal patterns as discussed below.

Theoretical Conceptualization

When facilitating dialogic conversations, collaborative therapists identify both the PIPs and healing interaction patterns (HIPs), which they do by identifying the problem-generating system (PIP) and problem-dissolving system (HIP). Often they will also explore WIPs and SCIPs as part of this process.

Goal Setting

Collaborative therapists conceptualize WIPs as identity narratives in which the client has a clear sense of agency in relation to the problem. Therapists co-construct the WIP with clients using dialogic conversation and mutual puzzling.

Facilitating Change

Collaborative therapists facilitate change through dialogic conversation, which involves both HIPs (such as dissolving the problem, appropriately unusual questions, and reflecting teams) and WIPs (mutual puzzling about what is working). The therapist sometimes introduces SCIPs by being public about the therapist's inner dialogue, other professionals, and differing values.

Putting It All Together: Collaborative Case Conceptualization and Treatment Plan Templates

Areas for Theory-Specific Case Conceptualization: Collaborative

When conceptualizing client cases, contemporary collaborative therapists typically use the following dynamics to inform their treatment plan. Go to MindTap® to access a digital version of the theory-specific case conceptualization, along with a variety of digital study tools and resources that complement this text and help you be more successful in your course and career. If your instructor didn't assign MindTap, you can find out more about it at Cengagebrain.com. You can also download the form at masteringcompetencies.com.

Problem-Organizing System: Who's Talking about the Problem?

- Client's definition of the problem
- Extended family's definition of the problem
- Broader system definition (school, work, friends, etc.)

Social Construction of the Problem

- Describe each person's significant meanings and constructions related to the problem (e.g., constructions of love, depression, duties of family members, etc.) and/or describe their worldview, inner dialogue, and/or narrative of the problem and/or their life/relational circumstances related to it

Postmodern and Cultural Discourse Conceptualization

- Dominant Discourses informing definition of problem:
  - *Ethnic, race, class, and religious discourses:* How do key cultural discourses inform what is perceived as a problem and the possible solutions (specify ethnicity when possible, e.g., Italian American rather than white)?
  - *Gender and sexuality discourses:* How do the gender and sexual discourses inform what is perceived as a problem and the possible solutions?
  - *Community, school, and extended family discourses:* How do other important community discourses inform what is perceived as a problem and the possible solutions?

Identity and Local Narratives

- *Identity Narratives:* How has the problem shaped each significant person's identity?
- *Local or Preferred Discourses:* What is the client's preferred identity narrative and/or narrative about the problem? Are there local (alternative) discourses about the problem that are preferred?

TREATMENT PLAN TEMPLATE FOR INDIVIDUAL WITH DEPRESSION/ANXIETY: COLLABORATIVE

You can download a blank treatment plan (with or without measures) from MindTap at www.cengagebrain.com or www.masteringcompetencies.com. The following treatment plan template can be used to help you develop individualized treatments for use with individuals with depressive or anxiety symptoms.

Collaborative Treatment Plan: Client Goals with Interventions

Early-Phase Client Goals

1. Increase client's sense of agency and possibilities for managing [specify crisis symptom or other issue prioritized by client] to reduce depressed mood/anxiety [or specific crisis behavior].
   a. Ask conversational questions to transform meanings associated with crisis behaviors and to identify realistic alternative responses.
   b. Invite mutual puzzling about where is the best place to start and how best to approach the identified issue.

Working-Phase Client Goals

1. Increase fluidity of the description/construction of the problem to identify new possibilities for action to reduce hopelessness.
   a. Ask appropriately unusual comments to generate new meaning.
   b. Use reflecting team/process to generate new descriptions and understandings.
   c. Suggest various written options to access multiple voices and perspectives.

2. Increase client possibilities for responding to [specify factor client identifies as related to symptoms] to reduce depression/anxiety.
   a. Invite mutual puzzling to consider alternative responses that will have more desired outcomes.
   b. Ask conversational and not-knowing questions to expand meaning and possibilities.

3. Increase effectiveness of client response to [specify factor client identifies as related to symptoms] to reduce depression/anxiety.
   a. Ask appropriately unusual questions to generate new possibilities for responding.
   b. Use reflecting team/processes to expand view of possibilities.

Closing-Phase Client Goals

1. Increase sense of personal agency in [life area related to depression/anxiety] to reduce depression and increase sense of wellness.
   a. Ask not-knowing questions to explore client construction of meaning and possibilities.
   b. Use writing to access multiple voices and perspectives.

2. Increase the number of relationships in which the client has a sense of being heard and has generative conversations to reduce depression and increase sense of wellness.
   a. Use collaborative questions to explore relational network and possibilities for supportive relationships.
   b. Invite mutual puzzling to identify how best to build relational support network.

Therapeutic Tasks

1. Develop a working therapeutic relationship. Develop a collaborative partnership with client that honors client's expertise.
   a. Use everyday, ordinary language that is comfortable for client.

2. Assess individual, systemic, and broader cultural dynamics.
   a. Identify who is talking about the problem and inquire about how each describes and constructs it.
   b. Assess client's worldview on issues related directly to the problem and other areas of significance/interest, listening for the personal meanings and interpretations that they use to construct their lived reality.

3. Identify needed referrals, crisis issues, collateral contacts, and other client needs.
   a. *Crisis assessment intervention(s):* Address crisis issues such as self-harm, suicidal ideation, substance use, risky sexual behavior, etc.
   b. *Referral(s):* Connect client with resources in client's family and community that could be supportive; make collateral contacts as needed.

TREATMENT PLAN TEMPLATE FOR DISTRESSED COUPLE/FAMILY: COLLABORATIVE

📄 You can download a blank treatment plan (with or without measures) at www.cengagebrain.com or www.masteringcompetencies.com. The following treatment plan template can be used to help you develop individualized treatments for use with couples and families who report relational distress.

Early-Phase Client Goals

1. Increase fluidity of the description/construction of the problem to identify new possibilities for action to reduce conflict.
   a. Use conversational questions to explore each person's meanings and interpretations.
   b. Ask appropriately unusual comments to generate new meaning.
   c. Use reflecting team/process to generate new descriptions and understandings

Working-Phase Client Goals

1. Increase couple/family's ability to engage in productive dialogue to handle problems in daily living to reduce conflict.
   a. Ask conversational questions to explore relational dynamics that characterize conflict interactions and explore alternative possibilities.
   b. Use mutual puzzling for how couple/family can interact in such a way that each person's perspective is included/considered.

2. Increase couple/family's ability to honor the multiple realities in the relationship to reduce conflict.
   a. Ask conversational and not-knowing questions to expand meaning and possibilities.
   b. Use reflecting team/processes to expand views of situation.

Closing-Phase Client Goals

1. Increase cohesiveness of shared relational narrative to reduce conflict and increase relational satisfaction.
   a. Ask not-knowing questions to explore client construction of meaning and possibilities.
   b. Use writing to access multiple voices and perspectives.

2. Increase each person's sense of personal agency as it relates to sustaining relationship to reduce conflict and increase sense of wellness.
   a. Offer collaborative questions to help each person story his or her contribution to improvements.
   b. Invite mutual puzzling to identify how best to build on new sense of agency

Treatment Tasks

1. Develop a working therapeutic relationship.
   a. Develop a collaborative partnership with each member of the system that honors the expertise of each.
   b. Use everyday, ordinary language that is comfortable for client.

2. Assess individual, systemic, and broader cultural dynamics.
   a. Identify who is talking about the problem (both in and out of session) and inquire about how each describes and constructs it; if two have similar definitions, look for nuanced differences.
   b. Assess each client's worldview on issues related directly to the problem and other areas of significance/interest, listening for the personal meanings and interpretations that they use to construct their lived realities.

3. Identify needed referrals, crisis issues, collateral contacts, and other client needs.
   a. Address crisis issues such as psychological abuse, intimate partner violence, hidden affair, self-harm, suicidal ideation, substance use, etc.
   b. *Referral(s):* Connect client with resources in client's family and community that could be supportive; make collateral contacts as needed.

Clinical Spotlight: Open Dialogue, an Evidence-Based Approach to Psychosis

Using the collaborative approach described by Anderson, Goolishian, and Andersen, Jaakko Seikkula (2002) and his colleagues (Haarakangas et al., 2007) in Finland developed the open dialogue approach in their work with psychosis and other severe disorders. They reported impressive outcomes in their 20 years of research, including 83% of first-episode psychosis patients returning to work and 77% with no remaining psychotic symptoms after two years of treatment. In comparison with standard treatment, the patients in open-dialogue treatment had more family meetings, fewer days of inpatient care, reduced use of medication, and a greater reduction in psychotic symptoms.

This approach uses collaborative dialogue and reflecting practices, as well as the following:

- Immediate intervention: Within 24 hours of the initial call, the person who has had a psychotic break, the significant people in his or her life, and a treatment team of several professionals (e.g., for psychosis, the team often includes a psychiatrist, psychotherapist, and nurse) meet to discuss the situation using collaborative dialogue.
- Social network and support systems: Significant persons in the client's life and other support systems are invited to participate in all phases of the process.
- Flexibility and mobility: Treatment is uniquely adapted to clients and their situations, with the treatment team sometimes meeting in the clients' homes and sometimes in a treatment setting, depending on what is most useful.
- Teamwork and responsibility: The treatment team is built on the basis of client needs; all team members are responsible for the quality of the process.
- Psychological continuity: The team members remain consistent throughout treatment regardless of the stage of treatment.
- Tolerance of uncertainty: Rather than employ set protocols, the team allows time to see how each situation will evolve and what treatment will be needed.
- Dialogue: The focus of each meeting is to establish an open dialogue that facilitates new meanings and possibilities. This process requires establishing a sense of safety for all participants to say what needs to be said.

Tapestry Weaving: Working with Diverse Populations

If you have not already noticed, more than any other approach covered in this book, postmodern therapies integrate consideration of cultural issues at the most fundamental level of their method. Therefore, many would consider them the quintessential approach for diverse populations. The broader questions of diversity and of how society, its norms, and the use of language affect individuals are the guiding premises in postmodern philosophical literature, making these therapies particularly suitable for clients from marginalized groups (for an in-depth discussion, see Monk et al., 2008). Unlike most mental health therapies, narrative therapy places societal issues of oppression at the heart of its therapeutic interventions, and many narrative therapists are active agents of social justice (Zimmerman & Dickerson, 1996). Collaborative therapy attends more to local discourses, working closely with the client and significant others to determine what the problem is (for the moment, as knowing its definition will continually evolve) and how best to resolve it. This focus on local knowledges ensures that the client's cultural values and beliefs are a central part of the therapy process. Both narrative and collaborative therapy have international roots and are practiced in numerous countries around the world. The case study that concludes this chapter uses postmodern therapy to address a teen who began cutting after her mother moved in with her girlfriend and her son.

Applications with Native American, First Nations, and Aboriginals

Narrative therapy approaches have been widely used and researched with native cultures in Canada, Australia, New Zealand, and the United States (Carey & Russell, 2011; Lee, 1997). In one study, therapists who worked with Native Americans in Wyoming identified communication and therapy practices that seemed best suited for this culture, all of which were descriptive of narrative therapy practices (Lee, 1997). Some of the observations from these therapists include:

- Subtle eye contact: Native Americans generally do not maintain sustained eye contact, and therapists should follow the client's lead.
- Active listening: Therapists should use nonverbal and verbal feedback to signal that the client's meanings are understood.
- Subtle emotional expression: Native Americans are not prone to strong, demonstrative expressions of emotions, and therapists must respect this by not pushing hard for emotional expression.
- Spirituality: Spirituality is generally highly valued by Native Americans, and therapists need to respectfully address and find ways to integrate these practices into therapeutic work.
- Self-in-relation: Native Americans are likely to construct their identity within relationships, seeing much of their identity as tied to family or the tribe.
- Home visits: Native Americans generally appreciate the therapist making home visits, and this is seen as helpful in terms of comfort, familiarity, and time flexibility.
- Gentle, reflective stance: Therapists described a therapeutic stance that was calm, reflective, nonconfrontational, and nonconflictual.
- Art, storytelling, and metaphor: The use of art, drawing, storytelling, and metaphor were found to be particularly helpful interventions.

In another study set in Manitoba, Canada, native healers and their clients were interviewed for what they believed to be helpful in changing emotions, cognitions, and behaviors (McCabe, 2007). This study included many of the above practices as well as:

- Ceremonies and rituals: Ceremony and rituals are powerful allies in the healing process and are used throughout.
- Spiritual guidance: Native Americans with traditional spiritual beliefs generally believe in a Creator spirit who provides guidance in the healing process.
- Self-acceptance: For many, themes of self-acceptance of one's identity, especially within the larger context of marginalization were particularly important to the process.
- Lessons of daily living: Identifying opportunities in daily living help to apply learning from session.
- Empathy: Expressions of empathy from the healer help in the healing process.
- Role modeling: The healer serves as a role model for the client in terms of lifestyle, behaviors, and attitudes.

Narrative therapists readily use native rituals, ceremonies, spiritual beliefs, and cultural stories to create therapeutic contexts that are respectful and responsive to the needs of native and aboriginal clients, often inviting tribal elders, leaders, and healers into the broader therapeutic dialogue. In particular, separating the person from the problem and meeting the person apart from the problem can be particularly useful. In addition, therapists can use situating and permission comments to increase the client's sense of voice and autonomy in the therapeutic relationship and to help create a more respectful healing context.

Hispanic Youth

Narrative therapy has also been used with Hispanic children and adolescents with depression, high-risk behaviors, and/or substance abuse (Malgady & Costantino, 2010). Some of their unique applications with this population include:

- Cuento therapy: Puerto Rican folktales, *cuentos,* were used to convey themes and morals to provide models for adaptive responses to problems, such as acting out, self-esteem, and anxiety. They adapted the tales to incorporate traditional Puerto Rican values as well as Anglo cultural values.
- Hero/heroine therapy: As many children were in single-parent households, the therapists had children identify male and female Puerto Rican heroes and heroines to help identify and bridge bicultural and intergenerational conflicts commonly experienced in adolescents.
- Temas storytelling therapy: Therapists selected pictures from the Thematic Apperception Tests that represented Hispanic cultural *temas,* or themes: traditional food, games, family scenes, and neighborhoods. Then the group of children was asked to develop a story with the cards. Each group member was invited to share personal experiences that related to the story the group created. The therapist reinforced adaptive, preferred narratives and helped find alternatives to maladaptive responses. Finally, the group did a dramatization of the story in class to practice preferred behaviors and responses.

Multiracial/Ethnic Individuals and Couples

The number of multiracial and multiethnic individuals and couples is growing rapidly. In the 2010 U.S. Census, nearly 6% of the population identified as multiracial and over 10% of opposite-sex households were multiracial or multiethnic, representing a 30% increase from the decade before. Several therapists have identified narrative and postmodern approaches in general as ideal for working with multiracial and multiethnic individuals (Daniel & Lee, 2014; Edwards & Pedrotti, 2004; Fukuyama, 1999; Lorick-Wilmot, 2015; Milan & Keiley, 2000; Quintana & Smith, 2012; Rockquemore & Laszloffy, 2003; Singh & Chun, 2012) and multiracial and multiethnic couples (Aniciete & Soloski, 2011; Kim, Prouty, & Roberson, 2012).

Persons and couples with mixed racial and ethnic backgrounds have unique challenges for developing their identities as individuals and/or as a couple. Most experience the negative effects of marginalization and the profoundly painful sense of not fitting in with any group or being forced to choose (Fukuyama, 1999; Gibbs, 1998; Lorick-Wilmot, 2015). Biracial youth are more likely to experience delinquency, school problems, and internalizing symptoms (Milan & Keiley, 2000), and biracial marriages are more likely to end in divorce (Kim et al., 2012). However, numerous therapists have found that narrative therapy can be especially effective for helping clients to relate to their racial and cultural identity narratives in ways that create agency and new possibilities. Narrative practices that identify dominant discourses and their effects on the clients and their relationships enable clients to more consciously choose which elements of these discourses they want to embrace and which they want to revise or not use at all.

Whether working with individuals or couples, narrative practitioners use similar techniques to help clients restory their multiracial and/or multiethnic identities and relationships:

Identifying Racial and Cultural and Related Gender Discourses

Therapists can begin by having clients identify relevant racial and cultural identity discourses and the associated gender-role discourses (Aniciete & Soloski, 2011; Edwards & Pedrotti, 2004; Kim et al., 2012; Milan & Keiley, 2000). When exploring multiple cultures, identifying whether they are collectivist or individualist can help identify predictable areas of conflict, especially for couples; individualistic cultures tend to value independence and individual needs at the expense of the relationship or others, whereas collectivist cultures expect sacrificing personal needs for the relationship. Within these cultural discourses are gendered discourses that define how men and women should behave and define themselves, with women typically expected to sacrifice more for relationships and assert fewer personal needs. However, women living in contexts in which alternative discourses for female identity are part of the dominant culture often gravitate toward these local possibilities rather than that of their culture of origin. Similarly, biracial individuals often experience pressure from family, peer groups, or community members to choose to identify more with one race or another (Gibbs, 1998; Lorick-Wilmot, 2015).

Externalizing Conversations

Narrative practitioners use externalizing conversations to help individuals and couples begin to separate their identities from influential discourses and allow them to develop curiosity and new perspectives (Aniciete & Soloski, 2011; Kim et al., 2012; Rockquemore & Laszloffy, 2003). When working with multiethnic and multicultural clients, therapists can externalize to help them develop a new stance in relation to the dominant discourses:

- If we were to imagine the story of who your race/culture says you should be, what would it say? How much of it do you agree with? Disagree with? What are you ambivalent about?
- When you define and evaluate yourself [or relationship] using the values and expectations of [name dominant cultural, racial, or gender discourse], what story do you tell yourself? What behaviors, emotions, and thoughts does this story inform? Is there a person or group who uses this discourse to evaluate you?
- How do these discourses fit with your preferred self-narrative? What elements fit well? Which do not?
- Is there anyone or anything else that offers an alternative story about how you can define yourself? Do you know of anyone who has successfully resisted and not gone along with elements of these discourses?

Re-authoring Conversations

Re-authoring conversations are used to help clients develop preferred identity and relational narratives (Aniciete & Soloski, 2011; Ash, 2015; Kim et al., 2012; Milan & Keiley, 2000). Therapists can do this by identifying unique outcomes that represent clients' preferred identities—whether in their own lives or in the lives of others—and mapping these in the landscapes of action and consciousness.

- You said you feel "most you" when you are with your best friend. Can you describe what behaviors are associated with this "most you" way of being? When you feel "most you," what do you like about yourself? How do you see yourself differently? Is there evidence to support this version of you?
- When you feel harmony in your relationship, what are the two of you doing differently? During these moments what do you tell yourself about who you are, who your partner is, and what your relationship is? What beliefs support this way of viewing you, your partner, and the relationship? Is there any evidence in other areas of your relationship that support these views?
- If you could pick and choose from these various cultural discourses to create your own unique identity (for self or relationship), which elements would be most important to keep? Why? Which would you be less likely to keep? Why?
- Reflecting teams can also be effective in helping multiracial individuals, couples, and families find new ways to restory their identities and experiences.

Remembering Practices

Remembering practices are used to solidify the new identity narratives, typically by expanding the scope of the narrative to other aspects of life and/or the number of persons who contribute and/or relate to the new narrative (Aniciete & Soloski, 2011; Kim et al., 2012). Some options include:

- Can you identify an important role model or figure in your life and describe yourself as you imagine this person sees you? How has this person contributed to your life? What implications does this person have for how you want to define and identify yourself going forward?
- Definitional ceremonies in which significant others are invited to witness the retelling of an individual or couple's identity narrative can be helpful to make the preferred identity public and therefore easier to maintain going forward.
- For couples: what do you most appreciate about your partner's racial/cultural background? Why? In which ways does that connect with your own set of values?

Cultural Genogram

Although the genogram is not a typical narrative tool, some narrative therapists have used it when working with multicultural couples and families to facilitate discussion of the multiple cultural discourses that are shaping the relationship (Milan & Keiley, 2000). They recommend including the following information on the cultural genogram: identities of individuals, coping strategies, and child-rearing practices; strengths; and marginalization experiences. These genograms can be particularly helpful in families in which one person identifies as "white" and has not reflected much on the cultural values that have shaped his/her family in the past and are shaping expectations in the current relationships.

Sexual and Gender Identity Diversity

Postmodern therapies are often the theory of choice for working with lesbian, gay, bisexual, transgender, and questioning (LGBTQ) clients because they help deconstruct the heterosexist discourses that are often the source of the greatest suffering in LGBTQ clients. When working with LGBTQ clients, most therapists recommend an advocacy stance with expertise in the subject matter rather than a strict not-knowing stance (Aducci & Baptist, 2011; Perez, 1996). In addition, many LGBTQ clients benefit from therapeutic conversations that help them construct positive labels and identity narratives for themselves and their relationships (Perez, 1996). Furthermore, it is important for therapists to identify how much of the presenting problem is due directly to a client's sexual identity versus more general life or relationship circumstances (Aducci & Baptist, 2011).

Narrative therapists have developed a specific approach that can be used with LGBTQ clients struggling with dissonance between heterosexual dominant discourses and their own lived experience. Yarhouse (2008) describes *narrative sexual identity therapy* as a middle ground to *gay-affirmative therapy* on one hand, which affirms the inherent goodness of identifying as LGBTQ, and *reorientation therapy* on the other, a highly controversial approach (so much so it essentially banned in California for minors due to its potential to do significant harm) designed to help clients change their sexual orientation to heterosexual. In contrast, narrative sexual identity therapy, which is based on narrative therapy principles, helps clients seek to live their lives in *congruence* between their personal beliefs and behaviors, a process that focuses on deconstructing dominant discourses that constrain and confuse clients' sexual identity. Designed to help clients struggling with their sexual identity, this approach is particularly relevant for clients from religious and cultural backgrounds that have strong antigay messages.

Drawing from standard narrative therapy practices, the therapist helps clients identify the problem narrative and then identify potential counternarratives that are more congruent with the client's lived experience and values. In this approach, the client determines what values and intentions he or she wants to define his or her life. The approach has six general steps or phases, which are of course fluid, but can nonetheless be helpful to therapists in conceptualizing treatment.

1. Client presents sexual identity concern: Initially, a client presents with concerns about sexual identity. These concerns may be related to external (e.g., religious, cultural, or family) or internal voices (e.g., personal values) that believe their lived experience of sexual attraction is somehow wrong, immoral, or otherwise problematic.

2. Map dominant narratives: The next step is to explore the dominant discourse, its origin and specific nuanced meanings. Questions therapists can ask to map the dominant discourse include:
   - What were some of the messages you received growing up about identifying as gay? (Yarhouse, 2008, p. 205)
   - How was the message communicated to you that feelings toward the same sex meant you were gay? (Yarhouse, 2008, p. 205)
   - How did you respond to these views of same-sex attraction?

3. Identify preferred narratives: In the next phase, clients reflect on their own personal lived experience of same-sex attraction. Most often the metaphor used to describe this is "*discovery*": discovering a preexisting fact about their true selves. In other cases, the metaphor is more one of "integration": integrating their experience of same-sex attraction with their other aspects of their identity. The metaphor of integration is more common when a person chooses not to assume a gay identity but instead chooses to integrate only certain elements.

4. Recognize exceptions/emerging counternarrative: Next, the therapist helps clients identify exceptions to the dominant discourses to create space for a counternarrative to emerge. Questions therapists can use to facilitate this process include:
   - In what ways are you understanding your sexual identity differently than when you first thought of yourself? (Yarhouse, 2008, p. 206)
   - Have you had experiences that call into question the meaning of same-sex attraction that you learned when you were young?
   - In what ways have your personal experiences of same-sex attraction contrasted to messages you have heard about what gay people are like?

5. Highlight identity-congruent attributes, activities, and resources: As the counternarrative emerges, the therapist listens for and highlights personal attributes, activities, and resources that are congruent with the client's preferred identity.
   - In what ways would you like to challenge some of the messages you received about your sexual identity? (Yarhouse, 2008, p. 207)
   - In what ways are you already living in accordance—even in small measure—with your preferred values and identity?
   - What type of relationships, activities, or communities might further provide support for your preferred identity and values?

6. Resolution/Congruence: Finally, clients are able to live according to their preferred sexual identity, one that is congruent with their lived experience, spiritual beliefs, and cultural values. Questions that therapists can use to facilitate this process include:
   - In the course of the next few months or so, what do you see as the relationship between your sexual identity and your religious or spiritual identity? (Yarhouse, 2008, p. 208)
   - Can you share a little of the way you would like to describe your sexual identity in the year to come? (Yarhouse, 2008, p. 208)

Research and the Evidence Base
Research on Postmodern Therapies

Consistent with their philosophical underpinnings, narrative and collaborative therapists have conducted more qualitative than quantitative investigations about their approaches to therapy (Anderson, 1997; Gehart et al., 2007). Qualitative research on postmodern therapies has focused on clients' lived experiences of therapy and its effects on their lives, emphasizing the clients' experience over researcher-defined measures of successful therapy (Andersen, 1997; Gehart & Lyle, 1999; Levitt & Rennie, 2004; London et al., 1999). A notable exception, Finnish psychiatrist Jaakko Seikkula (2002) and his team (Haarakangas et al., 2007) have used qualitative and quantitative methods to study their open-dialogue approach to working with psychosis and other severe diagnoses for over 20 years, generating significant evidence for their model's effectiveness (see "Clinical Spotlight," above). They report that they have nearly eradicated chronic cases of psychosis, with most clients returning to normal functioning within two years; their work is an exemplary, evidence-based approach for recovery-oriented approaches to treating severe mental health issues (see "Recovery in Mental Health Movement" in Chapter 12).

Outcome research on narrative therapy has increased in recent years. For example, Lopes and colleagues have conducted a clinical trial comparing narrative and cognitive–behavioral therapies for treating depression, including a follow up at 31 months; both in the initial and follow-up studies, the two approaches were similarly effective (Lopes et al., 2014; Lopes Goncalves, Machado, Sinai, Bento, Salgado, 2014). Similarly, another study from Australia examined the effectiveness of narrative therapy for treating major depressive disorder and found that its effects were comparable to those of other approaches, with 74% of clients achieving reliable improvement (Vromans & Schweitzer, 2011). In another Australian study, women with eating disorder and depressive issues engaged in a 10-week narrative therapy group that resulted in reduced self-criticism and changes in daily practices/activities (Weber, Davis, & McPhie, 2006). Additional studies have found that narrative groups for children significantly reduce symptoms for those diagnosed with attention-deficit disorder (Looyeh, Kamali, & Shafieian, 2012) and social phobia (Looyeh et al., 2014).

Narrative therapists are also beginning to conduct process research to identify which elements are most significant for promoting change. In one study, researchers found that unique outcomes that specifically enable clients to reconceptualize their problems and foster new experiences are correlated with positive outcomes (Matos et al., 2009). In another study, researchers found that clients diagnosed with depression who were more ambivalent toward change and returned to the problem narrative in later phases of therapy were less likely to make progress in therapy.

Neurobiology of Narrative

The assumptions and premises of postmodern therapy are also receiving support from an unexpected area: psychiatry, more specifically interpersonal neurobiology (Beaudoin, & Zimmerman, 2011; Gehart, 2012; Siegel, 2012). Like postmodern therapists, Siegel (2012) proposes that storytelling is how humans make sense of life:

> We are storytelling creatures, and stories are the social glue that binds us to one another. Understanding the structure and function of narrative is therapy a part of understanding what it means to be human. (pp. 31–32)

Siegel describes how in childhood, humans are born into a story, take on cultural meaning, and then in adolescence and adulthood continue to reshape these meanings, thus evolving human culture. These narratives constrain or expand a person's options for responding to life. Siegel suggests that *reflection*—a detached examination of these narratives—enables clients to liberate themselves from these limiting stories of who they are and what their life is; this same process is emphasized in postmodern therapies.

In describing how people change, Siegel (2012) emphasizes the importance of bottom-up processing, as compared with top-down processing. *Bottom-up processing* refers to processing experience using the bottom three layers of the prefrontal cortex to generate new understandings, categories, and stories for what is happening. In contrast, *top-down processing* involves using the top three layers of the prefrontal cortex to categorize lived experience with preexisting categories. Both forms of processing are important, but most people who feel "stuck" related to a problem are stuck in top-down processing, unable to change how they see their situation or possibilities for changing it. The *not-knowing* position of postmodern therapists is an excellent approach for facilitating bottom-up processing: in fact, the entire collaborative therapy process can be viewed as an approach for expanding bottom-up processing (Gehart, 2012).

In addition, Siegel (2012) describes trauma resolution as a process of creating an integrative narrative, similar to thickening the plot in narrative therapy. Traumatic experiences overwhelm the hippocampus and explicit (narrative) memory not encoded with implicit memory, as happens in nontraumatic situations. Thus, traumatic memories are encoded primarily as implicit memories, which do not have a sensation of being from the past and are often experienced as fragmented auditory, visual, and sensual experiences that are occurring in the here and now (i.e., flashbacks). These fragmented memories create chaotic and rigid patterns that impair the brain's ability to enter into healthy integrated neural states. Siegel suggests that the treatment for trauma essentially involves pulling the implicit memories together into a coherent narrative, which is most easily achieved by entering into "interpersonal attunement" with a therapist. He proposes that when two minds become entrained, in sync, the client can "borrow" the therapist's neural integrated state to help cope with the traumatic memories long enough to put them into a coherent narrative. Through this process of recreating an integrated explicit narrative of the trauma, the client is then able to recall the trauma while remaining in an integrated neural state (i.e., not have symptoms when recalling the trauma).

Finally, Beaudoin and Zimmerman (2011) note that the postmodern techniques that help clients "give voice" to their lived experience and put into words things that have never been said before help move clients from their anxiety-focused limbic system to the more calm and reason-focused prefrontal cortex. By labeling and giving voice to their stress-based experiences, clients are able to reduce the firing of the limbic system, allowing them to make more conscious choices and responses. Furthermore, therapeutic conversations about preferred realities strengthen neural connections that support clients' preferred identities and associated behaviors. In particular, *affect-infused descriptions* of preferred realities help solidify new identity narratives, which are predominantly associated with the right brain hemisphere; such affect-infused descriptions include not only emotion but also sensory experiences, such as imagery, scent, and tactile experiences.

QUESTIONS FOR PERSONAL REFLECTION AND CLASS DISCUSSION

1. In what ways does the co-construction of reality seem to make sense to you? In what ways does it not?

2. Identify one dominant discourse that is affecting your life in a negative way.
   • Where were you first exposed to this discourse?
   • How does it affect your view of yourself?
   • What helps you to resist defining yourself by this discourse?

3. Describe a moment in your life when you felt marginalized, invisible, or oppressed.
   • How did this experience affect how you saw yourself? Does it still affect you today?
   • How did this experience affect how you saw others involved?

4. Describe the effect of gender discourses on you and your relationships.
   • In what ways do you live in accordance to these? What are the effects of doing so?
   • In what ways do you not follow these? What are the effects of not doing so?
   • How do these gender discourses affect your relationships?

5. Does the idea of "client expertise" make sense to you? Why or why not?

6. Describe a time when a person made a comment that was:
   • Too unusual. How did you respond?
   • Too usual. How did you respond?
   • Appropriate unusual. How did you respond?

ONLINE RESOURCES

Collaborative Websites

Harlene Anderson

www.harleneanderson.org

Houston Galveston Institute: Collaborative Therapy

www.talkhgi.org

Taos Institute: Collaborative Practices in Therapy, Consultation, Education, Business

www.taosinstitute.net

Grupo Campos Elíseos: Collaborative Therapy, Mexico City

www.grupocamposeliseos.com

Social Construction Therapy Online: Resources for collaborative, narrative and solution-focused

http://socialconstructiontherapy.com

Narrative Websites

Anti-Anorexia/Anti-Bulimia League

http://www.narrativeapproaches .com/?page_id=42

Dulwich Centre: Michael White's Narrative Therapy

www.dulwichcenter.com

Evanston Family Therapy Center: Freedman and Combs' Narrative Therapy

www.narrativetherapychicago.com

The Institute of Narrative Therapy: United Kingdom

http://www.theinstituteofnarrativetherapy .com/papersandresources.html

Narrative Approaches: Lobovits, Freeman, and Epston

www.narrativeapproaches.com

Narrative Practices Adelaide

http://narrativepractices.com.au

Yaletown Family Therapy: Narrative Therapy, Canada

www.yaletownfamilytherapy.com

Open Dialogue

MindFreedom/Finland Open Dialogue: Finland

http://www.mindfreedom.org /kb/mental-health-alternatives /finland-open-dialogue

Institute for Dialogic Practice: United States

http://www.dialogicpractice.net

Open Dialogue: United Kingdom http://opendialogueapproach.co.uk

A collection of resources on Open Dialogue and Open Dialogue practices

http://willhall.net/opendialogue

Journals

International Journal of Collaborative Practices

https://collaborative-practices.com

Narrative Works Journal

http://w3.stu.ca/stu/sites/cirn/current _issue.aspx

Journal of Systemic Therapies

http://www.guilford.com/journals /Journal-of-Systemic-Therapies /Jim-Duvall,-MEd,-RSW/11954396

Go to MindTap® for an eBook, videos of client sessions, activities, digital forms, practice quizzes, apps, and more—all in one place. If your instructor didn't assign MindTap, you can find out more information at CengageBrain.com.

REFERENCES

*Asterisk indicates recommended introductory readings.

Aducci, C. J., & Baptist, J. A. (2011). A collaborative-affirmative approach to supervisory practice. *Journal of Feminist Family Therapy: An* *International Forum, 23*(2), 88–102. doi:10.1080/08952833.2011.574536

*Andersen, T. (1991). *The reflecting team: Dialogues and dialogues about the dialogues.* New York: Norton.

Andersen, T. (1992). Relationship, language and pre-understanding in the reflecting process. *Australian and New Zealand Journal of Family Therapy, 13*(2), 87–91.

Andersen, T. (1995). Reflecting processes; acts of informing and forming: You can borrow my eyes, but you must not take them away from me! In S. Friedman (Ed.), *The reflecting team in action: Collaborative practice in family therapy* (pp. 11–37). New York: Guilford.

Andersen, T. (1997). Researching client–therapist relationships: A collaborative study for informing therapy. *Journal of Systemic Therapies, 16*(2), 125–133.

*Andersen, T. (2007). Human participating: Human "being" is the step for human "becoming" in the next step. In H. Anderson & D. Gehart (Eds.), *Collaborative therapy: Relationships and conversations that make a difference* (pp. 81–97). New York: Brunner/Routledge.

Anderson, H. (1993). On a roller coaster: A collaborative language systems approach to therapy. In S. Friedman (Ed.), *The new language of change* (pp. 323–344). New York: Guilford.

Anderson, H. (1995). Collaborative language systems: Toward a postmodern therapy. In R. Mikesell, D. D. Lusterman, & S. McDaniel (Eds.), *Family psychology and systems therapy* (pp. 27–44). Washington, DC: American Psychological Association.

*Anderson, H. (1997). *Conversations, language, and possibilities: A postmodern approach to therapy.* New York: Basic Books.

Anderson, H. (2005). Myths about "not knowing." *Family Process, 44,* 497–504.

Anderson, H. (2007). Historical influences. In H. Anderson & D. Gehart (Eds.), *Collaborative therapy: Relationships and conversations that make a difference* (pp. 21–31). New York: Brunner/Routledge.

*Anderson, H., & Gehart, D. (2007). *Collaborative therapy: Relationships and conversations that make a difference.* New York: Brunner/Routledge.

Anderson, H., & Goolishian, H. (1988). Human systems as linguistic systems: Preliminary and evolving ideas about the implications for clinical theory. *Family Process, 27,* 157–163.

*Anderson, H., & Goolishian, H. (1992). The client is the expert: A not-knowing approach to therapy. In S. McNamee & K. J. Gergen (Eds.), *Therapy as social construction* (pp. 25–39). Newbury Park, CA: Sage.

Aniciete, D., & Soloski, K. L. (2011). The social construction of marriage and a narrative approach to treatment of intra-relationship diversity. *Journal of Feminist Family Therapy: An International Forum, 23*(2), 103–126. doi:10.1080/08952833.2011.576233

Ash, A. (2015). Fragmented but unbroken: Forming a Black White biracial identity in the South. In S. D. Hancock, A. Allen, C. W. Lewis, S. D. Hancock, A. Allen, & C. W. Lewis (Eds.), *Auto-ethnography as a lighthouse: Illuminating race, research, and the politics of schooling* (pp. 103–125). Charlotte, NC: IAP Information Age.

Augusta-Scott, T., & Dankwort, J. (2002). Partner abuse group intervention: Lessons from education and narrative therapy approaches. *Journal of Interpersonal Violence, 17,* 783–805.

Bava, S., Levin, S., & Tinaz, D. (2002). A polyvocal response to trauma in a postmodern learning community. *Journal of Systematic Therapies, 21*(2), 104–113.

Beaudoin, M. N., & Zimmerman, J. (2011). Narrative therapy and interpersonal neurobiology: Revisiting classic practices, developing new emphases. *Journal of Systemic Therapies, 30,* 1–13.

Boscolo, L., Cecchin, G., Hoffman, L., & Penn, P. (1987). *Milan systemic family therapy.* New York: Basic Books.

Bruner, J. (1986). *Actual minds, possible worlds.* Cambridge, MA: Harvard University Press.

Carey, M., & Russell, S. (2011). Pedagogy shaped by culture: Teaching narrative approaches to Australian Aboriginal health workers. *Journal of Systemic Therapies, 30*(3), 26–41. doi:10.1521/jsyt.2011.30.3.26

Daniel, G. R., & Lee, A. M. (2014). Competing narratives: Race and multiraciality in the Brazilian racial order. In R. C. King-O'Riain, S. Small, M. Mahtani, M. Song, P. Spickard, & R. C. (Eds.), *Global mixed race* (pp. 91–118). New York: New York University Press.

Edwards, L. M., & Pedrotti, J. T. (2004). Utilizing strengths of our cultures: Therapy with biracial women and girls. *Women and Therapy, 27,* 33–43.

Foucault, M. (1972). *The archeology of knowledge* (A. Sheridan-Smith, trans.). New York: Harper & Row.

Foucault, M. (1980). *Power/knowledge: Selected interviews and other writings.* New York: Pantheon Books.

*Freedman, J., & Combs, G. (1996). *Narrative therapy: The social construction of preferred realities.* New York: Norton.

*Freeman, J., Epston, D., & Lobovits, D. (1997). *Playful approaches to serious problems.* New York: Norton.

Fukuyama, M. A. (1999). Personal narrative: Growing up biracial. *Journal of Counseling & Development, 77*(1), 12–14. doi:10.1002/j.1556-6676.1999.tb02404.x

Gehart, D. (2007). Creating space for children's voices: A collaborative and playful approach to working with children and families. In H. Anderson & D. Gehart (Eds.), *Collaborative therapy: Relationships and conversations that make a difference* (pp. 183–197). New York: Brunner/Routledge.

Gehart, D. (2012). *Mindfulness and acceptance in couple and family therapy.* New York: Springer.

Gehart, D. R., & Lyle, R. R. (1999). Client and therapist perspectives of change in collaborative language systems: An interpretive ethnography. *Journal of Systemic Therapy, 18*(4), 78–97.

Gehart, D., & McCollum, E. (2007). Engaging suffering: Towards a mindful re-visioning of marriage and family therapy practice. *Journal of Marital and Family Therapy, 33,* 214–226.

Gehart, D., Tarragona, M., & Bava, S. (2007). A collaborative approach to inquiry. In H. Anderson & D. Gehart (Eds.), *Collaborative therapy: Relationships and conversations that make a difference* (pp. 367–390). New York: Brunner/Routledge.

Gibbs, J. T. (1998). Biracial adolescents. In J. T. Gibbs, L. N. Huang & Associates (Eds.), *Children of color: Psychological interventions with culturally diverse youth* (pp. 305–332). San Francisco, CA: Jossey-Bass.

Goolishian, H., & Anderson, H. (1987). Language systems and therapy: An evolving idea. *Psychotherapy, 24*(3S), 529–538.

Haarakangas, K., Seikkula, J., Alakare, B., & Aaltonen, J. (2007). Open dialogue: An approach to psychotherapeutic treatment of psychosis in Northern Finland. In H. Anderson & D. Gehart (Eds.), *Collaborative therapy: Relationships and conversations that make a difference* (pp. 221–233). New York: Brunner/Routledge.

*Hoffman, L. (1981). *Foundations of family therapy: A conceptual framework for systems change.* New York: Basic Books.

Hoffman, L. (1990). Constructing realities: An art of lenses. *Family Process, 29,* 1–12.

Hoffman, L. (1993). *Exchanging voices: A collaborative approach to family therapy.* London: Karnac Books.

*Hoffman, L. (2001). *Family therapy: An intimate history.* New York: Norton.

Hoffman, L. (2007). The art of "withness": A bright new edge. In H. Anderson & D. Gehart (Eds.), *Collaborative therapy: Relationships and conversations that make a difference* (pp. 63–79). New York: Brunner/Routledge.

Jenkins, A. (1990). *Invitations to responsibility: The therapeutic engagement of men who are violent and abusive.* Adelaide, Australia: Dulwich Centre.

Kim, H., Prouty, A. M., & Roberson, P. E. (2012). Narrative therapy with intercultural couples: A case study. *Journal of Family Psychotherapy, 23*(4), 273–286. doi:10.1080/08975353.2012.735591

Lee, S. (1997). Communication styles of Wind River Native American clients and the therapeutic approaches of their clinicians. *Smith College*

Studies in Social Work, 68(1), 57–81. doi: 10.1080/00377319709517516

Levin, S. (2007). Hearing the unheard: Advice to professionals from women who have been battered. In H. Anderson & D. Gehart (Eds.), *Collaborative therapy: Relationships and conversations that make a difference* (pp. 109–128). New York: Brunner/Routledge.

Levitt, H., & Rennie, D. L. (2004). Narrative activity: Clients' and therapists' intentions in the process of narration. In L. Angus & J. McLeod (Eds.), *The handbook of narrative and psychotherapy: Practice, theory, and research* (pp. 299–313). Thousand Oaks, CA: Sage.

London, S., Ruiz, G., Gargollo, M., & M. C. (1999). Clients' voices: A collection of clients' accounts. *Journal of Systemic Therapies, 17*(4), 61–71.

Looyeh, M., Kamali, K., Ghasemi, A., & Tonawanik, P. (2014). Treating social phobia in children through group narrative therapy. *Arts in Psychotherapy, 41*(1), 16–20.

Looyeh, M., Kamali, K., & Shafieian, R. (2012). An exploratory study of the effectiveness of group narrative therapy on the school behavior of girls with attention-deficit/hyperactivity symptoms. *Archives of Psychiatric Nursing, 26*(5), 404–410.

Lopes, R., Gonçalves, M., Fassnacht, D., Machado, P., & Sousa, I. (2014). Long-term effects of psychotherapy on moderate depression: A comparative study of narrative therapy and cognitive-behavioral therapy. *Journal of Affective Disorders, 167,* 64–73.

Lopes, R. T., Gonçalves, M. M., Machado, P. P., Sinai, D., Bento, T., & Salgado, J. (2014). Narrative therapy vs. cognitive-behavioral therapy for moderate depression: Empirical evidence from a controlled clinical trial. *Psychotherapy Research, 24*(6), 662–674. doi:10.1080/10503307.2013.874052 (requested)

Lorick-Wilmot, Y. S. (2015). Narrating negotiations of racial-ethnic identity and belonging among second-generation Black Caribbean immigrants in the United States. In L. Way (Ed.), *Representations of internarrative identity* (pp. 93–114). New York: Palgrave Macmillan.

Malgady, R. G., & Costantino, G. (2010). Treating Hispanic children and adolescents using narrative therapy. In J. R. Weisz & A. E. Kazdin (Eds.), *Evidence-based psychotherapies for children and adolescents* (2nd ed.) (pp. 391–400). New York: Guilford.

Matos, M., Santos, A., Gonçalves, M., & Martins, C. (2009). Innovative moments and change in narrative therapy. *Psychotherapy Research, 19*(1), 68–80. doi:10.1080/10503300802430657

McCabe, G. H. (2007). The healing path: A culture and community-derived indigenous therapy model. *Psychotherapy: Theory, Research, Practice, Training, 44*(2), 148–160. doi:10.1037/0033-3204.44.2.148

Milan, S., & Keiley, M. K. (2000). Biracial youth and families in therapy: Issues and interventions. *Journal of Marital and Family Therapy, 26,* 305–315.

Monk, G., & Gehart, D. R. (2003). Conversational partner or socio-political activist: Distinguishing the position of the therapist in collaborative and narrative therapies. *Family Process, 42,* 19–30.

Monk, G., Winslade, J., Crocket, K., & Epston, D. (1997). *Narrative therapy in practice: The archaeology of hope.* San Francisco, CA: Jossey-Bass.

Monk, G., Winslade, J., & Sinclair, S. (2008). *New horizons in multicultural counseling.* Thousand Oaks, CA: Sage.

Pence, E., & Paymar, M. (1993). *Education groups for men who batter: The Duluth Model.* New York: Springer.

Penn, P. (2001). Chronic illness: Trauma, language, and writing: Breaking the silence. *Family Process, 40,* 33–52.

Penn, P. (2002). *So close.* Fort Lee, NJ: Cavankerry.

Penn, P., & Frankfurt, M. (1994). Creating a participant text: Writing, multiple voices, narrative multiplicity. *Family Process, 33,* 217–231.

Penn, P., & Sheinberg, M. (1991). Stories and conversations. *Journal of Systemic Therapies, 10*(3–4), 30–37.

Perez, P. J. (1996). Tailoring a collaborative, constructionist approach for the treatment of same-sex couples. *Family Journal, 4*(1), 73–81. doi:10.1177/1066480796041016

Quintana, S. M., & Smith, A. V. (2012). African American children's racial identifications and identity: Development of racial narratives. In J. M. Sullivan & A. M. Esmail (Eds.), *African American identity: Racial and cultural dimensions of the Black experience* (pp. 289–313). Lanham, MD: Lexington Books/Rowman & Littlefield.

Rockquemore, K. A., & Laszloffy, T. A. (2003). Multiple realities: A relational narrative approach in therapy with Black-White mixed-raced clients. *Family Relations, 52,* 119–128.

Seikkula, J. (2002). Open dialogues with good and poor outcomes for psychotic crises: Examples from families with violence. *Journal of Marital and Family Therapy, 28*(3), 263–274.

Sells, S., Smith, T., Coe, M., & Yoshioka, M. (1994). An ethnography of couple and therapist experiences in reflecting team practice. *Journal of Marital and Family Therapy, 20,* 247–266.

Siegel, D. (2012). *Pocket guide to interpersonal neurobiology.* New York: Norton.

Singh, A. A., & Chun, K. S. (2012). Multiracial/multiethnic queer and transgender clients: Intersections of identity and resilience. In S. H. Dworkin & M. Pope (Eds.), *Casebook for counseling lesbian, gay, bisexual, and transgendered persons and their families* (pp. 197–209). Alexandria, VA: American Counseling Association.

Smith, C., & Nylund, D. (2000). *Narrative therapy with children and adolescents.* New York: Guilford.

St. George, S., & Wulff, D. (1998). Integrating the client's voice within case reports. *Journal of Systemic Therapies, 17*(4), 3–13.

Tomm, K., St. George, S., Wulff, D., & Strong, T. (2014). *Patterns in interpersonal interactions: Inviting relational understandings for therapeutic change.* New York: Routledge.

Vetere, A., & Dowling, E. (2005). *Narrative therapies with children and their families: A practitioner's guide to concepts and approaches.* New York: Routledge.

Vromans, L. P., & Schweitzer, R. D. (2011). Narrative therapy for adults with major depressive disorder: Improved symptom and interpersonal outcomes. *Psychotherapy Research, 21*(1), 4–15. doi:10.1080/10503301003591792

Weber, M., Davis, K., & McPhie, L. (2006). Narrative therapy, eating disorders and groups: Enhancing outcomes in rural NSW. *Australian Social Work, 59*(4), 391–405. doi: 10.1080/03124070600985970

White, M. (1995). *Re-authoring lives: Interviews and essays.* Adelaide, Australia: Dulwich Centre.

*White, M. (2007). *Maps of narrative practice.* New York: Norton.

*White, M., & Epston, D. (1990). *Narrative means to therapeutic ends.* New York: Norton.

White, M., & Morgan, A. (2006). *Narrative therapy with children and their families.* Adelaide, Australia: Dulwich Centre.

Winslade, J., & Monk, G. (1999). *Narrative counseling in schools: Powerful and brief.* Thousand Oaks, CA: Corwin.

Winslade, J., & Monk, G. (2000). *Narrative mediation.* San Francisco, CA: Jossey-Bass.

Winslade, J., & Monk, G. (2007). *Narrative counseling in schools: Powerful and brief* (2nd ed.). Thousand Oaks, CA: Corwin.

Winslade, J., & Monk, G. (2008). *Practicing narrative mediation: Loosening the grip of conflict.* San Francisco, CA: Jossey-Bass.

Yarhouse, M. A. (2008). Narrative sexual identity therapy. *American Journal of Family Therapy, 36*(3), 196–210. doi: 10.1080/01926180701236498

Zimmerman, J. L., & Dickerson, V. C. (1996). *If problems talked: Narrative therapy in action.* New York: Guilford.

Postmodern Case Study: Self-Harm, Depression, Lesbian Blended Family

Christie and Suzanne bring Christie's 15-year-old daughter, Ashley, in for therapy because Ashley has become increasingly depressed and has begun cutting to relieve pain. Ashley has always been a "sensitive" child and has had a difficult time finding a place in high school. Suzanne and her eight-year-old son, Matt, moved in a little over a year ago, and they report that the transition has generally gone well. Ashley also has a half-brother from her father's second marriage, although they live five hours away and she visits only during the holidays. Ashley says she is "cool" with her mother's relationship with another woman and that she is "okay" with how often she sees her dad. Both Christie and her mother (Ashley's grandmother) have been treated for depression. In addition, Christie was sexually abused by her cousin while young. Ashley's greatest passion is her art and writing music.

After meeting with the family, a narrative family therapist developed the following case conceptualization.

POSTMODERN THERAPY CASE CONCEPTUALIZATION
For use with individual, couple, or family clients.

Date: 10/4/19   Clinician: Roxana Gilbert   Client/Case #: 1420

Introduction to Client & Significant Others
List all significant others for client.

Adults/Parents: Select identifier/abbreviation for use in rest of case conceptualization

AF1: Female Age: 47 European American Married gay/lesbian/bisexual Occupation: High school music teacher Other: recently married AF40; German American

AF2: Female Age: 40 European American Married gay/lesbian/bisexual Occupation: book-keeper Other: recently married AF47; Irish American

Children/Adult Children: Select identifier/abbreviation for use in rest of case conceptualization

CF1: Child Female Age: 15 European American Grade: 10 School: Sun Valley High School
Other: AF47's daughter, artistic and musically talented; German/Italian American

CM1: Child Male Age: 8 European American Grade: 3 School: Green Meadows Elementary School Other: AF 40's son, enjoys sports; Irish American

Others: AM, CF15's father: high school math teacher, remarried with one child from second marriage.

Meeting Persons Apart from Problem
Describe who the person/people are apart from the problem: hobbies, interests, career, etc.:

AF47: Caring/involved mother; musically talented (violin, voice, piano, guitar); enjoys career as music teacher; strong sense of spirituality.

AF40: Reliable; easy for both children to talk to; organized; structured person; enjoys bookkeeping; strong connection to local lesbian community.

CF15: Intelligent, artistic, and musically talented (piano, singing); makes good choices; diligent student. Has a supportive best friend; English teacher provides mentoring.

CM8: Enjoys sports: soccer, baseball, and basket ball; cooperative at school.

Preferred Narratives: Hopes and Aspirations for Self and Other
Describe the preferred narrative, hopes for therapy, and/or aspirations for self and other for each significant person involved in the process:

AF47: Aspirations for Self: Hopes to be able to better support CF15; to be a better parent for her; to help her learn how to navigate social pressures and discrimination.

Aspirations for Others/Relationship: Hopes CF15 starts to make a place for herself in the new school; build a group of friends; use music to help find peace when she needs it.

(continued)

Preferred Narratives: Hopes and Aspirations for Self and Other (*continued*)

AF40:   Aspirations for Self: <u>Wants to be able to be a good stepparent to CF15; be her confidante if CF does not want to talk to mother.</u>

Aspirations for Others/Relationship: <u>Create a strong and happy family where everyone feels carefed for, protected, and safe to be themselves.</u>

CF15:   Aspirations for Self: <u>Find a way to enjoy high school, probably have more friends; get into a better band; go out and do more things with friends; keep up grades; go to music academy.</u>

Aspirations for Others/Relationship: <u>Does not want AF47 or AF40 to feel guilty about the move or how others treat her. Wants to be able to talk about anything with them and to have their guidance as she goes through high school.</u>

CM8:   Aspirations for Self: <u>Wants to be a top soccer player and get good grades.</u>

Aspirations for Others/Relationship: <u>Wants to be able to do more with CF15; wants the family to have fun and play board games once per week.</u>

Problem Saturated Narrative

Describe each person's significant meanings and constructions related to the problem (e.g., constructions of love, depression, duties of family members, etc.) and/or describe their worldview, inner dialogue, and/or narrative of the problem and/or their life/relational circumstances related to it:

Adult Female: <u>AF47: Sees CF15's depression as related to being shy and sensitive at a big high school; she relates to her and her mother's depression and sexual abuse at age six.</u>

Adult Female: <u>AF40: Worries that CF15's depression is related to her not accepting her and her mother's relationship; she feels guilt but is also frustrated with AF47 for not considering this as a factor.</u>

Child Female: <u>CF15: Believes her depression stems from not having friends at school; feeling out of place at home and at school.</u>

Child Male: <u>CM8: Is not quite sure why CF15 cries, but hopes it is not because of him.</u>

Broader System: Description of problem from extended family, referring party, school, legal system, etc.: <u>Extended Family: CF15's father (AM): Has not been made aware of her depression and cutting but believes it is "unhealthy" for her mother to be living with another woman with CF15.</u>

<u>English teacher: CF15's mentor: Believes CF15 is just a thoughtful young woman who is "too mature" for high school. CF15's Best friend: Believes CF15 needs more friends at high school.</u>

Background Information

Trauma/Abuse History (recent and past): CF15 was sexually abused by her cousin at age 6 (one incident); the father of that cousin sexually abused her mother when they were children. CF15 was treated for the abuse at that time.

Substance Use/Abuse (current and past; self, family of origin, significant others): None reported.

Precipitating Events (recent life changes, first symptoms, stressors, etc.): AF40 and CM8 moved in together 15 months ago; CF15 began high school a year and half ago, leaving her best friend from middle school who went to another high school. She takes art and works on the sets for plays. She has made a couple of friends at school, but she is closest to her old best friend, whom she sees on weekends. She had a crush on a guy at school in the fall, and he is now dating someone else. She often spends lunch and Friday night alone.

Related Historical Background (family history, related issues, previous counseling, medical/mental health history, etc.): CF15 has lived with her mother since her parents' divorce when she was 3 years old. Her mother reports that she was an easy child to raise; CF15's father moved away and she has visited him most holidays. AF47 started dating women 7 years ago and has been with AF40 for 3 years now.

Social Location and Dominant Discourses

Dominant Discourses informing definition of problem:

- **Ethnic, Race, Class, and Religious Discourses:** *How do key cultural discourses inform what is perceived as a problem and the possible solutions (specify ethnicity when possible, e.g., Italian American rather than white)?* AF47 seems to embrace self-sufficient and "tough it out" values from her German American background; she does not shy away from problems and prefers to deal with them directly. AF40 seems to draw upon similar values from her Irish American background and is comfortable "being different" and does not shy from problems. All members, including CF15, seem to have a bit of stoicism that can lead to depression.

- **Gender and Sexuality Discourses:** *How do the gender and sexual discourses inform what is perceived as a problem and the possible solutions?* _____

- **Community, School, and Extended Family Discourses:** *How do other important community discourses inform what is perceived as a problem and the possible solutions?* As she prefers to socialize one-on-one, she has had difficulty finding a place.

Unique Outcomes and Influence of Persons

Describe times, contexts, relationships, etc., when the problem is less of a problem or not a problem as well as the effect of persons on the problem: what things do people do that make the problem less of a problem?

(continued)

Unique Outcomes and Influence of Persons *(continued)*

1. When is problem less of problem? CF15 is less depressed when mother spends time with her or family does art together; after CF talks with her English teacher about what is going on; when with best friend.

2. When was the problem expected but did not occur? Family vacation; when working on school play.

3. In what relationships or contexts is the problem less of a problem or not a problem? When CF15 hangs out with best friend; when AF47 and AF40 spend time with other same-sex parents and families.

4. What are people currently doing that keep the problem from being worse than it is or affecting more areas of life than it already does? Spending time together; listening to one another; AF47 trying to do more fun things together; CF15 seeing best friend and being part of theater at school.

Based on the above, how are people most effectively influencing the problem?

1. Staying connected and talking regularly in their family relationship.

2. Connecting with families having similar challenges.

3. CF15 spending time with friends; connecting with teacher/mentor; becoming involved with theater and other structured school activities that enable her to meaningfully interact with peers at school.

Identity and Local Narratives

Identity Narratives: How has the problem shaped each significant person's identity? Since entering high school and having AF40 move in, CF15 is feeling increasing marginalized in all social worlds: "it's like there is no place for me anywhere." "No one wants me." AF47 feels like she is finally coming out and expressing her true self and that it is hurting her child.

Local or Preferred Discourses: What is the client's preferred identity narrative and/or narrative about the problem? Are there local (alternative) discourses about the problem that are preferred? AF47 describes CF15 as "mature for her age" and not fitting in because she is not "shallow" and "judgmental" like other kids. AF47 has always seen CF15 more as a peer than child. The family feels most supported when around other same-sex couples and their families.

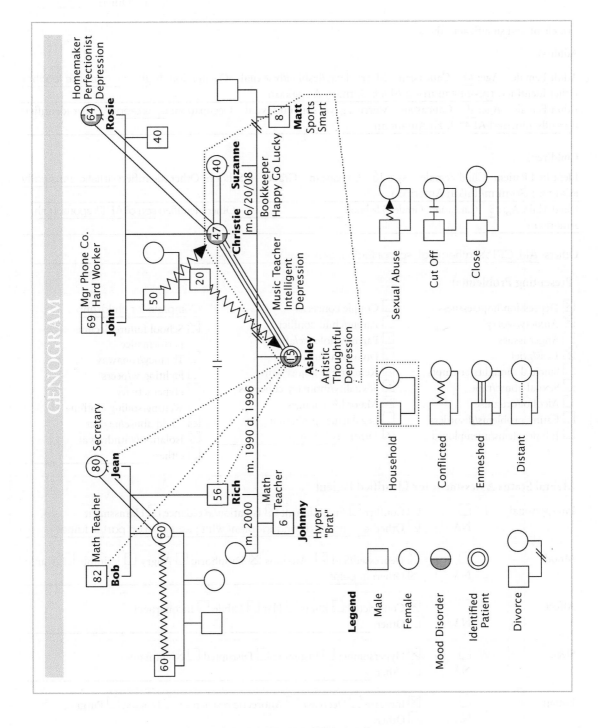

GENOGRAM

Legend

- Male ☐
- Female ○
- Mood Disorder ◑
- Identified Patient ◎
- Divorce

Household
Conflicted
Enmeshed
Distant

Sexual Abuse
Cut Off
Close

CLINICAL ASSESSMENT

Clinician: Roxana Gilbert	Client ID #: 1420	Primary configuration: ☒ Individual ☐ Couple ☒ Family	Primary Language: ☒ English ☐ Spanish ☐ Other: _____

List client and significant others

Adult(s)

Adult Female   Age: 47   Caucasian   Married gay/lesbian/bisexual   Occupation: high school music teacher
Other identifier: recently married AF40; German American

Adult Female   Age: 40   Caucasian   Married gay/lesbian/bisexual   Occupation: bookkeeper Other identifier:
recently married AF47; Irish American

Child(ren)

Identified Patient: Child Female   Age: 15   Caucasian   Grade: 10 School: Other identifier: artistic; musically
talented; German/Italian American

Child Male Age: 8   Caucasian Grade: 3 School: _____   Other identifier: son of AF40; sports; Irish
American

Others: AM; CF15's father; high school math teacher

Presenting Problem(s)

☒ Depression/hopelessness
☒ Anxiety/worry
☐ Anger issues
☒ Loss/grief
☐ Suicidal thoughts/attempts
☐ Sexual abuse/rape
☐ Alcohol/drug use
☐ Eating problems/disorders
☐ Job problems/unemployed

☐ Couple concerns
☐ Parent/child conflict
☐ Partner violence/abuse
☐ Divorce adjustment
☒ Remarriage adjustment
☐ Sexuality/intimacy concerns
☒ Major life changes
☐ Legal issues/probation
☒ Other: self-harm

Complete for children:
☒ School failure/decline
  performance
☐ Truancy/runaway
☐ Fighting w/peers
☐ Hyperactivity
☐ Wetting/soiling clothing
☒ Child abuse/neglect
☒ Isolation/withdrawal
☐ Other: _____

Mental Status Assessment for Identified Patient

Interpersonal	☐ NA	☐ Conflict ☐ Enmeshment ☒ Isolation/avoidance ☐ Harassment ☒ Other: emotional disengagement with peers and on part of father
Mood	☐ NA	☒ Depressed/Sad ☒ Anxious ☒ Dysphoric ☐ Angry ☐ Irritable ☐ Manic ☒ Other: hopeless
Affect	☐ NA	☒ Constricted ☐ Blunt ☐ Flat ☐ Labile ☐ Incongruent ☐ Other: _____
Sleep	☐ NA	☒ Hypersomnia ☐ Insomnia ☐ Disrupted ☐ Nightmares ☐ Other: _____
Eating	☐ NA	☒ Increase ☐ Decrease ☐ Anorectic restriction ☐ Binging ☐ Purging ☐ Other: _____
Anxiety	☐ NA	☒ Chronic worry ☐ Panic ☐ Phobias ☐ Obsessions ☐ Compulsions ☐ Other: _____

Trauma symptoms	☐ NA	☐ Hypervigilance ☐ Flashbacks/Intrusive memories ☒ Dissociation ☐ Numbing ☐ Avoidance efforts ☐ Other: _____
Psychotic symptoms	☒ NA	☐ Hallucinations ☐ Delusions ☐ Paranoia ☐ Loose associations ☐ Other: _____
Motor activity/Speech	☐ NA	☒ Low energy ☐ Hyperactive ☐ Agitated ☐ Inattentive ☐ Impulsive ☐ Pressured speech ☐ Slow speech ☐ Other: _____
Thought	☐ NA	☒ Poor concentration ☐ Denial ☒ Self-blame ☐ Other-blame ☒ Ruminative ☐ Tangential ☐ Concrete Poor insight ☐ Impaired decision making ☐ Disoriented ☐ Other: _____
Sociolegal	☒ NA	☐ Disregards rules ☐ Defiant ☐ Stealing ☐ Lying ☐ Tantrums ☐ Arrest/incarceration ☒ Initiates fights ☐ Other: _____
Other symptoms	☒ NA	_____

Diagnosis for Identified Patient

Contextual Factors considered in making diagnosis: ☒ Age ☒ Gender ☒ Family dynamics ☐ Culture ☐ Language ☐ Religion ☐ Economic ☐ Immigration ☒ Sexual/gender orientation ☒ Trauma ☐ Dual diagnosis/comorbid ☐ Addiction ☐ Cognitive ability ☐ Other: _____

Describe impact of identified factors on diagnosis and assessment process: Used age-appropriate language; considered gender and recent family changes, including mother's change in sexual orientation, when diagnosing mood and adjustment.

DSM-5 Level 1 Cross-Cutting Symptom Measure (optional): Elevated scores on: (free at psychiatry.org) ☒ I Depression ☐ II Anger ☐ III Mania ☐ IV Anxiety ☐ V Somatic ☐ VI Suicide ☐ VII Psychosis ☐ VIII Sleep ☐ IX Memory ☐ X Repetitive ☒ XI Dissociation ☐ XII Personality ☐ XIII Substance ☐ Not administered

DSM-5 Code	**Diagnosis with Specifier** *Include Z/T-Codes for Psychosocial Stressors/Issues*
1. F33.1	1. Major depressive disorder, recurrent, moderate
2. T74.22XA	2. Sexual abuse of child
3. Z62.820	3. Parent–child relational problem
4. Z91.5	4. Personal history of self-harm
5. Z60.4	5. Social exclusion or rejection

List Specific DSM-5 Criterion Met for Diagnosis

1. Depressed mood, most days, past 6 months

2. Loss of interest in pleasurable activities, most days

3. Hypersomnia, esp on weekends

4. Feelings of worthlessness, most days

5. Lack of concentration, esp at school

6. No manic or mixed episodes; most recent episode 6 months

(continued)

Diagnosis for Identified Patient *(continued)*

Medical Considerations

Has patient been referred for psychiatric evaluation? ☒ Yes ☐ No

Has patient agreed with referral? ☒ Yes ☐ No ☐ NA

Psychometric instruments used for assessment: ☒ None ☐ Cross-cutting symptom inventories
☐ Other: _____

Client response to diagnosis: ☒ Agree ☐ Somewhat agree ☐ Disagree ☐ Not informed for following reason: _____

Current Medications (psychiatric & medical) ☐ NA

1. Zoloft ; dose 50 mg; start date: 10/4/08
2. _____ ; dose _____ mg; start date: _____
3. _____ ; dose _____ mg; start date: _____
4. _____ ; dose _____ mg; start date: _____

Medical Necessity: *Check all that apply*

☒ Significant impairment ☒ Probability of significant impairment ☒ Probable developmental arrest

Areas of impairment:

☒ Daily activities ☒ Social relationships ☒ Health ☒ Work/school ☐ Living arrangement
☐ Other: _____

Risk and Safety Assessment for Identified Patient

Suicidality
☐ No indication/denies
☐ Active ideation
☒ Passive ideation
☐ Intent without plan
☐ Intent with means
☐ Ideation in past year
☐ Attempt in past year
☐ Family or peer history of completed suicide

Homicidality
☒ No indication/denies
☐ Active ideation
☐ Passive ideation
☐ Intent without means
☐ Intent with means
☐ Ideation in past year
☐ Violence past year
☐ History of assaulting others
☐ Cruelty to animals

Alcohol Abuse
☒ No indication/denies
☐ Past abuse
☐ Current; freq/amt: _____

Drug Use/Abuse
☒ No indication/denies
☐ Past use
☐ Current drugs: _____
   Freq/Amt: _____
☐ Family/sig.other use

Sexual & Physical Abuse and Other Risk Factors
☒ Childhood abuse history: ☒ Sexual ☐ Physical ☐ Emotional ☐ Neglect
☐ Adult with abuse/assault in adulthood: ☐ Sexual ☐ Physical ☐ Current
☐ History of perpetrating abuse: ☐ Sexual ☐ Physical ☐ Emotional
☐ Elder/dependent adult abuse/neglect
☐ History of or current issues with restrictive eating, bingeing, and/or purging
☒ Cutting or other self-harm: ☒ Current ☐ Past: Method: razor
☐ Criminal/legal history: _____
☐ Other trauma history: _____
☐ None reported

Indicators of Safety
☐ NA
☒ At least one outside support person
☒ Able to cite specific reasons to live or not harm
☐ Hopeful
☒ Willing to dispose of dangerous items
☒ Has future goals
☐ Willingness to reduce contact with people who make situation worse
☒ Willing to implement safety plan, safety interventions
☐ Developing set of alternatives to self/other harm
☒ Sustained period of safety: 1 month
☐ Other: _____

Elements of Safety Plan

☐ NA
☒ Verbal no harm contract
☒ Written no harm contract
☒ Emergency contact card
☒ Emergency therapist/agency number
☒ Medication management:

☒ Plan for contacting friends/support persons during crisis
☐ Specific plan of where to go during crisis
☐ Specific self-calming tasks to reduce risk before reach crisis level (e.g., journaling, exercising, etc.)
☒ Specific daily/weekly activities to reduce stressors
☐ Other: _____

Legal/Ethical Action Taken: ☐ NA ☒ Action: Report past abuse to CPS; Riley West, 4:00 pm 10/4/08

Case Management

Collateral Contacts

- Has contact been made with treating *physicians or other professionals:* ☐ NA ☒ Yes ☐ In process. Name/Notes: : Susan Roth, School Counselor

- If client is involved in mental health *treatment elsewhere,* has contact been made? ☒ NA ☐ Yes ☐ In process. Name/Notes: _____

- Has contact been made with *social worker:* ☐ NA ☒ Yes ☐ In process. Name/Notes: Social Worker: Riley West

Referrals

- Has client been referred for *medical assessment:* ☒ Yes ☐ No evidence for need
- Has client been referred for *social services:* ☐ NA ☐ Job/training ☐ Welfare/food/housing ☒ Victim services ☐ Legal aid ☐ Medical ☐ Other: _____
- Has client been referred for *group* or other support services: ☒ Yes: School group ☐ In process ☐ None recommended
- Are there anticipated *forensic/legal processes* related to treatment: ☒ No ☐ Yes; describe: _____

Support Network

- Client social support network includes: ☒ Supportive family ☐ Supportive partner ☒ Friends ☐ Religious/spiritual organization ☐ Supportive work/social group ☐ Other: _____
- Describe anticipated effects treatment will have on others in support system (children, partner, etc.): Mother struggling with guilt for not protecting daughter better and for burdens her life choices have placed on her daughter.
- Is there anything else client will need to be successful? Mother may need individual therapy; will want to work with school counselor.

Expected Outcome and Prognosis

☒ Return to normal functioning ☐ Anticipate less than normal functioning ☐ Prevent deterioration

Client Sense of Hope: 5 out of 10

Evaluation of Assessment/Client Perspective

How were assessment methods adapted to client needs, including age, culture, and other diversity issues?
Used age- and gender-appropriate language; created sense of safety, esp. reabuse assessment.
Respectfully addressed sexual orientation of mother; used humor to connect with CF.
Describe actual or potential areas of client–clinician agreement/disagreement related to the above assessment:
AF47 wanted CF on medication because she found it helpful for herself and because CF is now cutting. No areas of identified disagreement.

_____ , _____   _____
Clinician Signature   License/Intern Status   Date

_____ , _____   _____
Supervisor Signature   License   Date

TREATMENT PLAN

Date: 10/4/19   **Case/Client #:** 1420

Clinician Name: Roxana Gilbert   **Theory:** Therapy

Modalities planned: ☐ Individual Adult ☒ Individual Child ☐ Couple ☒ Family ☐ Group:
Recommended session frequency: ☒ Weekly ☐ Every two weeks ☐ Other: _____
Expected length of treatment: 8 months

Treatment Plan with Goals and Interventions

Early-Phase Client Goal

1. Increase CF15's sense of influence over Depression and her ability to manage her feelings and emotions to reduce cutting.

   Measure: Able to sustain safety for period of 4 ☒ wk ☐ mo with no more than 0 mild episodes of cutting.

   a. Develop safety plan using scaling for safety; involve CF15 and AF47 in identifying level 7 and alternative plan.

   b. Map influence of problem and person's with family to increase sense of influence and identify specific things that already are helping.

Working-Phase Client Goals

1. Increase CF15's sense of belonging at home and school to reduce social withdrawal and feelings of loneliness.

   Measure: Able to sustain sense of belonging for period of 8 ☐ wk ☒ mo with no more than 2 mild episodes of withdrawal.

   a. Map problem and unique outcomes in landscapes of action and consciousness to CF15 to view her connections with friends in new ways and identify potential action steps.

   b. Scaffolding questions to help CF15 and family move from contemplation to action.

2. Increase CF's sense of agency related to past abuse and restory identity narrative related to abuse to reduce depressed mood, anxiety, and hopelessness.

   Measure: Able to sustain agency for period of 2 ☐ wk ☒ mo with no more than 1 mild episode of depressed mood.

   a. Externalize effects of abuse by mapping influence of problem and persons, highlighting any and all acts of resistance to abuse on her part or the part of her family to increase sense of agency and reduce sense of victimization.

   b. Map unique outcomes related to abuse in landscape of action and consciousness, emphasizing new identity that is emerging and using witnessing ceremony, letter writing and other options for solidifying new identity.

Closing-Phase Client Goals

1. Expand and thicken narrative of CF15's preferred individual identity especially the theme of "belonging" to reduce social isolation.

Measure: Able to sustain behaviors associated with preferred identity for period of 2 ☐ wk ☒ mo with no more than 1 mild episode of social isolation.

  a. Scaffolding conversations to move CF15 from contemplation to action related to integrating into new school and enacting preferred identity.

  b. Map unique outcomes in landscape of action and consciousness to solidify new identity narrative and identify specific actions associated with this identity.

  c. Definitional ceremony and narrative letter from therapist to solidify new identity in larger community of support.

2. Increase external relationships that support family's preferred identity to reduce sense of marginalization.

Measure: Able to sustain preferred family identity and expanded support network for period of 2 ☐ wk ☒ mo with no more than 1 mild episode of isolation.

  a. Scaffolding conversations to help family move from contemplate to specific actions to create the support network and connections they desire.

  b. Definitional ceremony to expand network of friends, family, and/or school personnel who support client's preferred identity.

  c. Narrative reflecting team to support couple/family in newly enacted identity.

Treatment Tasks

1. Develop working therapeutic relationship using theory of choice.
  a. *Meet persons apart from problem,* inquiring about *identities* outside of problem.
  b. Engage couple/family from *hopeful, optimistic position,* and *as co-author/investigative reporter.*

2. Assess individual, relational, community, and broader cultural dynamics using theory of choice.

  a. Use relative influence questioning to map the effects of depression and the effects of persons on depression; identify unique outcomes.

  b. Identify the dominant discourses that support depression, especially those related to same-sex relationships, and the local, alternative discourses that may be a resource in changing relationship to depression.

3. Identify needed referrals, crisis issues, collateral contacts, and other client needs.

  a. *Crisis assessment intervention(s):* Discuss and complete safety plan related to cutting using scaling for safety (see Chapter 12); report past abuse to child protective services; contact school counselor to discuss concerns.

  b. *Referral(s):* Discuss referral to pediatrician for medication evaluation; school-based support groups for CF; community-based support for family.

Diversity Considerations

Describe specifically how treatment plan, goals, and interventions were adapted to address each area of diversity (*Note:* Identify specific ethnicity, e.g., Italian American rather than white):

Age: Adjust relationship-building, assessment, and interventions to be age-appropriate for CF15 and CM8 so that they can feel part of process. Greater use of humor and art.

(continued)

Diversity Considerations (*continued*)

Gender/Sexual Orientation: Assessed family's sense of marginalization as same-sex couple with children and considered how this may be impacting CF's current sense of isolation at school. Helped family to connect with supportive community to reduce sense of isolation. Also, explored CF's gender identity as a young female and compared to gender identities of both mothers.

Race/Ethnicity Religion/Class/Region: Both AF47 and AF40 have European American immigrant backgrounds, including German and Irish. These cultures tend to be more stoic when handling stress and examined if this was true of their families of origin and if that relates to current situation.

Other factors: CF's father has minimal contact with her; identified how she stories this and how it may affect current depression.

Evidence-Based Practice (Optional)

Summarize evidence for using this approach for this presenting concern and/or population: Several studies and streams of research support using narrative therapy to treat depression and related issues. An Australian study which examined the effectiveness of narrative therapy for treating major depressive disorder found that narrative therapy is comparable to other approaches (Vromans & Schweitzer, 2011). Another Australian study that treated women with eating disorders and depression issues with narrative therapy resulted in reduced self-criticism and changes in daily activities (Weber et al., 2006). Process research on narrative therapy indicates that unique outcomes that specifically enable clients to reconceptualize their problems and foster new experiences are correlated with positive outcomes (Matos et al., 2009). Renowned author and psychiatrist Daniel Siegel describes a human's conception of their problems and potentials for change occur through story-telling, reflection, bottom-up processing, and creating an integrative narrative, all of which are utilized in postmodern therapies (Beaudoin & Zimmerman, 2011; Gehart, 2012; Siegel, 2012).

Client Perspective (Optional)

Has treatment plan been reviewed with client: ☒ Yes ☐ No; If no, explain: _____

Describe areas of Client Agreement and Concern: Clients want to start with family for the first few weeks and later move to a mix of individual sessions with CF and family sessions.

_____, _____   _____ _____, _____   _____

Therapist's Signature   Intern Status   Date   Supervisor's Signature   License   Date

PROGRESS NOTE

Date: 10/11/19 **Time:** 1:00 ☐ am/☒ pm   **Session Length:** ☐ 45 min. ☐ 60 min. ☒ Other: 50 minutes

Present: ☐ Adult Male ☒ Adult Female ☐ Child Male ☒ Child Female ☐ Other: _____

Billing Code: ☐ 90791 (eval) ☐ 90834 (45 min therapy) ☐ 90837 (60 min therapy) ☒ 90847 (family) ☐ Other: _____

Symptom(s)	Duration and Frequency Since Last Visit	Progress
1: Cutting	Scratch arm (no blood) 1x	**Progressing**
2: Depressed mood	Mild, most days	**Progressing**
3: Withdrawal	Moderate, most days	**Progressing**

Explanatory Notes on Symptoms: CF reported greater hope after first session last week; did not "cut" because of safety plan but did scratch. Reports continued depressed mood but slightly more hopeful; continued hypersomnia and social withdrawal, although reports feeling more connected to AF47 after last session. Report saw psychiatrist and has begun taking Zoloft, 50 mg.

In-Session Interventions and Assigned Homework

Developed detailed safety plan using scaling for safety; identified signals at 7 and strategies to manage mood at this point: call friend, talk with mom, play music, go for run. CF generated own plan easily and was open with AF47, who was supportive.

Client Response/Feedback

CF appeared motivated to change behavior and although hesitant when describing what she actually feels became more animated when identifying how to stop downward spiral.

Plan

☒ Continue with treatment plan: plan for next session: Follow up on safety plan; collaboratively identify next goals/ steps.
☐ Modify plan: _____

Next session: Date: 10/18 Time: 2:00 ☐ am/☒ pm

Crisis Issues: ☐ No indication of crisis/client denies ☒ Crisis assessed/addressed: describe below

Denies cutting (no evidence) but admits to scratching without drawing blood; developed safety plan and CF readily agreed to plan and was willing to include AF47.

_____, _____ _____
Clinician's Signature   License/Intern Status   Date

(continued)

PROGRESS NOTE *(continued)*

Case Consultation/Supervision ☐ Not Applicable

Notes: Supervisor went over safety plan.

Collateral Contact ☐ Not Applicable

Name: Dr. Jessic Erker Date of Contact: 10/12 Time: 5:00 ☐ am/☒ pm ☒ Written release on file:
☒ Sent/☐ Received ☐ In court docs ☐ Other: _____

Notes: Consult with psychiatrist on medication, diagnosis, and safety plan.

_____ , _____   _____
Clinician's Signature   License/Intern Status   Date

_____ , _____   _____
Supervisor's Signature   License   Date

PART III

Clinical Case Documentation

11

Case Conceptualization

Learning Objectives

After reading this chapter and a few hours of focused studying, you should be able to:

- Describe the purpose of case conceptualization.

- Complete a cross-theoretical systemic case conceptualization using the form provided.

Step 1: Mapping the Territory

There are few moments as exciting or neurosis-inducing in a therapist's training as "the first session": seeing your first client and losing your therapeutic "virginity," so to speak. We know the questions that follow: "Was it good for you?" "Did I get it right?" "Was I okay?" Before the session, there are other predictable questions: "What do I say?" "What do I do?" "What if I can't remember X?" Although logical, these questions can cause a new therapist to quickly become lost and off course. That is why the first step in therapy is to map the territory. To develop a good map, therapists need to master the art of *viewing*, which in a talking profession like therapy refers to knowing where to focus your attention while listening.

The heart of therapy—the seeming brilliance of a great therapist—has always been in the viewing. The most useful question for new therapists to ask their supervisors is: *What should I be noticing and listening for when I talk with this client?* Thankfully, this is much easier than trying to memorize what to say. The apparent magic that distinguishes master therapists from average therapists and average therapists from the average person lies in what someone attends to when another is speaking. Essentially, the better you get at knowing how to focus your viewing, the better therapist you will be. I believe it is a skill that great therapists continually develop and refine over the course of their careers—so don't plan on mastering it anytime soon.

Case conceptualization is the technical term for the therapeutic art of viewing. Although it is also sometimes called *assessment,* this is a tricky term because it can refer to two different therapeutic tasks: a case conceptualization approach to assessing individual and family dynamics (covered in this chapter) or a diagnostic approach to assessing symptomatology (covered in Chapter 12 on clinical assessment). To reduce confusion, I refer to a theory-informed assessment as *case conceptualization* and to a diagnostic assessment as *clinical assessment.*

Theories provide therapists with unique lenses through which to view clients' problems. Like a detailed map, they place problems in a broader and more comprehensive context that allows therapists to see how pieces fit together and that provides clues to the best path out of a tangled situation.

Case Conceptualization and the Art of Viewing

Case conceptualization enables therapists to generate new perspectives that facilitate being helpful to clients. For example, Ron and Dawn have been arguing for months. They seek out a therapist hoping that somehow, some way, the therapist can help them resolve their differences. When they enter therapy, each is thinking: "I hope the therapist can help my spouse see what he/she is doing wrong and encourage him/her to fix it. I know I have problems too, but I am sure that as soon as my spouse changes, it will be easy for me to change." They have told this and less benevolent versions of their stories to their family and friends, yet no one has been able to help either Ron or Suzie make meaningful changes. So what makes the therapist different from the family, friends, and hairdressers who listen to this story? Does the therapist have special knowledge that will allow him or her to provide the "answer" to the couple's problem? Or does the therapist simply serve as a socially sanctioned referee to this dispute? Or does the therapist do something more?

Although some therapists define themselves as "educators" or "mediators," most define their roles as promoting change through a transformational interpersonal process that is far more nuanced than education or mediation. Therapists differ from friends, educators, and mediators in their ability to view the situation in new and useful ways. From these new perspectives, possibilities for intervention emerge that did not arise in any of the previous conversations between the partners or with their family and friends.

Overview of Cross-Theoretical Case Conceptualization

As therapists become more experienced, case conceptualization takes place primarily in their heads—while clients are talking. It happens so fast that often therapists have difficulty retracing their steps. However, new therapists must take things more slowly. Similar to learning a new dance step, the new move needs to be broken down into small pieces with specific instructions for where the hands and feet go; with practice, the dancer is able to put the pieces together more quickly and smoothly until it becomes "natural." That is what we are going to do here with case conceptualization.

In each of the theory chapters, you were introduced to theory-specific case conceptualization. In this chapter, you are introduced to a comprehensive cross-theoretical case conceptualization. This comprehensive approach is good for learning theories and seeing how they interconnect. I have found it particularly useful for self-supervision whenever you feel stuck or lost with a case. Sometimes seeing through multiple theoretical lenses helps to identify a dynamic you have missed when using just one theory. Warning: this form takes longer to complete than you might initially imagine. So, let's start with identifying the components of a systemic case conceptualization:

1. Introduction to Client and Significant Others
2. Presenting Concerns
3. Background Information

4. Client/Family Strengths and Social Location
5. Family Structure
6. Interactional Patterns
7. Intergenerational and Attachment Patterns
8. Solution-Based Assessment
9. Postmodern: Social Location and Dominant Discourses
10. Client Perspectives

The complete form for case conceptualization is available on MindTap® (see Cengagebrain .com) or you can download the form at masteringcompetencies.com. The rest of this chapter describes how to complete the form. An example of completed form is at the end of the chapter based on the case study in Chapter 4.

Introduction to Client and Significant Others

Case conceptualization starts by identifying: (a) who the client is (individual, couple, or family) and (b) the most salient demographic features that relate to treatment. Common demographic information includes the following:

- Gender: Female, Male, Trans-female, Trans-male, Other
- Age
- Race and Ethnicity: Try to be as specific as possible for ethnicity; instead of white, Caucasian, Hispanic, or Latino, try to specify ethnicity.
- Sexual orientation
- Current occupation/work status or grade in school
- Any other useful identifier, such extracurricular activities for children.

I use a combination of abbreviations that make it easy to track family members using confidential notation:

AF = Adult female
AM = Adult male
CF = Child female
CM = Child male

To distinguish members in large families and same-sex couples, I add the age after each abbreviation (AF36, CM8). This can also be particularly helpful to a supervisor or instructor to follow your notes.

Presenting Concerns

The presenting concern is a description of how all parties involved are defining the problem: client, family, friends, school, workplace, legal system, and society. Often new—and even some experienced therapists—assume that this description is a straightforward and clear-cut matter. It can be, but it is usually surprisingly complex. Collaborative therapists (Anderson, 1997; Anderson & Gehart, 2006) developed a unique means of conceptualizing the presenting problem in their collaborative language systems approach, also referred to as collaborative therapy (see Chapter 10). This postmodern approach maintains that each person who is talking about the problem is part of the problem-generating system, the set of relationships that produced the perspective or idea that there is a problem. Each person involved has a different definition of the problem; sometimes the difference is slight and sometimes it is stark. For example, when parents bring a child to therapy, the mother, father, siblings, grandparents, teachers, school counselors, doctors, and friends have different ideas of what the problem actually is. The mother may think it is a medical problem, such as attention-deficit/hyperactivity disorder (ADHD); the father may believe it is related to his wife's permissiveness; the teacher may say it is poor parenting; and the child may think there really is no problem.

PRESENTING CONCERN(S)

Describe each significant person's description of the problem:

Identifier: _____

Identifier: _____

Identifier: _____

Identifier: _____

Additional: _____ *Broader System: Description of problem from extended family, referring party, school, legal system, etc.:*

Extended Family: _____

Name: _____

Name: _____

Historically, therapists moved rapidly to define the problem according to their theoretical worldview—either a formal diagnosis (ADHD, depression, etc.) or another mental health category (such as parenting style, defense mechanism, family dynamics, etc.)—with little reflection on the contradictory opinions and descriptions of the various people involved. Although this may be practical at one level, the more therapists can remain open to the family's alternative descriptions of the problem, the more they can remain adaptable and creative. They can maintain stronger rapport with each person involved, honoring each person's perspective and referring to it throughout treatment. Furthermore, being mindful of the multiple problem definitions gives the therapist greater maneuverability when treatment stagnates or conditions do not improve.

A description of the presenting problem should include the following:

1. The reason(s) each client states he or she is seeking counseling or has been referred
2. Any information from the referring agent (teacher, doctor, psychiatrist, etc.) and his or her description of the problem
3. A brief history of the problem and family (if applicable)
4. Descriptions of the attempted solutions and the outcome of these attempts
5. Any other problem-related information that may be relevant to the situation

Background Information

Obtaining background information about the problem is the next step. Traditionally, therapists have included information such as the following:

- History of trauma and abuse, including sexual abuse, physical violence, assaults, discrimination, harassment, stalking, national disasters, etc.
- Substance use and abuse, current or past
- Precipitating events: recent events that may be related to the problem, occurrence of first symptoms, recent stressors, etc.
- Related historical background, such as health situation and medications, previous counseling, medical issues, etc.

BACKGROUND INFORMATION

Trauma/Abuse History (recent and past): _____

_____

Substance Use/Abuse (current and past; self, family of origin, significant others): _____

_____

Precipitating Events (recent life changes, first symptoms, stressors, etc.): _____

_____

Related Historical Background (family history, related issues, previous counseling, medical/mental health history, etc.): _____

_____

Often, this background information is considered the "facts" of the case. However, as family therapists have historically cautioned, how we describe the facts makes all the difference (Anderson, 1997; O'Hanlon & Weiner-Davis, 1989; Watzlawick, Weakland, & Fisch, 1974). For example, saying that the client "recently won a state-level academic decathlon" and saying that "her mother recently divorced her alcoholic father" paints two very different pictures of the same client for you as therapist and for anyone else who reads the assessment. Therefore, although this may seem like the "factual" part of the report in which you as a professional are not imposing any bias, in fact, therapists impose bias by their subtle choice of words, their ordering of information, and their emphasis on particular details.

Based on research about the importance of the therapeutic relationship and of hope (Lambert & Ogles, 2004; Miller, Duncan, & Hubble, 1997), I recommend that therapists write the background section so that they and anyone reading the report, potentially including the client, will have a positive impression of the client and hope for the client's recovery; these two factors affect the outcome of treatment.

Client/Family Strengths and Social Location

Client strengths and resources should be the first thing assessed. This is a lesson I learned the hard way. When I began teaching systemic assessment, I put the client strength section at the end because it is more clearly associated with solution-based and postmodern approaches (see Chapters 9 and 10; Anderson, 1997; de Shazer, 1988; White & Epston, 1990), which were historically developed later. What I discovered is that after reading about the presenting problem, history, and problematic family dynamics, I was often feeling quite hopeless about the case. However, often upon reading the strengths section at the end, I would immediately perk up and find myself having hope, deep respect, and even excitement about the clients and their future. I have since decided to start by assessing strengths; I believe it puts the therapist in a more resourceful mind-set, whether working from either a systemic or postmodern perspective.

Emerging research supports the importance of identifying client strengths and resources. Researchers who developed the *common factors model* (discussed in Chapter 2; Lambert & Ogles, 2004; Miller et al., 1997) estimate that 40% of outcomes can be attributed to client factors, such as severity of symptoms, access to resources, and support system; the remaining factors include the therapeutic relationship (30%), therapist interventions (15%), and the client's sense of hope (15%). Assessing for resources leverages client factors (40%), strengthens the therapeutic relationship (30%), and instills hope (15%), thus drawing on three of the four common factors. Thus, the benefit of assessing strengths is hard to overestimate.

STRENGTHS AND SOCIAL LOCATION

Strengths and Resources:

Personal: _____

Relational/Social: _____

Spiritual: _____

Based on the client's social location—age, gender race, ethnicity, sexual orientation, gender identity, social class, religion, geographic region, language, family configuration, abilities, etc.—identify potential resources and challenges:

Unique Resources: _____

Potential Challenges: _____

To conceptualize a full spectrum of client strengths and resources, therapists can include strengths at several levels:

1. Personal/individual strengths
2. Relational/social strengths and resources
3. Spiritual resources

Personal or Individual Strengths

When assessing for personal or individual strengths and resources, the therapist can begin by reviewing two general categories of strengths: abilities and personal qualities.

Abilities

Where and how are clients functioning in daily life? How do they get to sessions? Are they able to maintain a job, a hobby, or a relationship? Do they have (or have they had in the past) any special talents? If you look, you will always find a wide range of abilities with even the most "dysfunctional" of clients, especially if you consider the past as well as the present and future.

Naming their abilities can increase clients' sense of hope and confidence to address the problem at hand. I find this especially helpful with children. If a child is having academic problems, the family, teachers, and child may not notice that the child is excelling in an extracurricular activity such as karate, soccer, or piano. Often noticing these areas of accomplishment makes it easier for all involved to find hope for improving the situation.

Identifying abilities may also give clients or therapists creative ideas about how to solve a current problem. For example, I worked with a recovering alcoholic who hated the idea of writing but often spoke of how music inspired her. By drawing on this strength, we developed the idea of creating a special "sobriety mix" of favorite songs to help maintain sobriety and prevent relapse, an activity that had deep significance and inspiration for her.

Personal Qualities

Ironically, the best place to find personal qualities is within the presenting problem or complaint. What brings clients to see a therapist is usually the flip side of a strength. For example, if a person complains about worrying too much, that person is equally likely to be a diligent and productive worker. Persons who argue with a spouse or child are more likely to speak up for themselves and are generally invested in the relationship in which they are arguing. In virtually all cases, the knife cuts both ways: each liability contains within it a strength in another context. Conversely, a strength in one context is often a problem in another. The following is a list of common problems and their related strengths.

PROBLEMS AND RELATED STRENGTHS

PROBLEM	POSSIBLE ASSOCIATED STRENGTH
Depression	• Is aware of what others think and feel • Is connected to others and/or desires connection • Has dreams and hopes • Has had the courage to take action to realize dreams • Has a realistic assessment of self/others (according to recent research; Seligman, 2004)
Anxiety	• Pays attention to details • Desires to perform well • Is careful and thoughtful about actions • Is able to plan for the future and anticipate potential obstacles
Arguing	• Stands up for self and/or beliefs • Fights injustice • Wants the relationship to work • Has hope for better things for others/self
Anger	• Is in touch with feelings and thoughts • Stands up against injustice • Believes in fairness • Is able to sense his/her boundaries and when they are crossed
Overwhelmed	• Is concerned about others' needs • Is thoughtful • Is able to see the big picture • Sets goals and pursues them

Try It Yourself

With a partner or on your own, identify a personal quality that is a problem in one area of your life. Next, identify another context in which that same quality is a form of strength.

Identifying strengths relies heavily on the therapist's viewing skills. A skilled therapist is able to see the strengths that are the flip side of the presenting problem while still remaining aware of the problem.

Relational or Social Strengths and Resources

Family, friends, professionals, teachers, coworkers, bosses, neighbors, church members, salespeople, and numerous others in a person's life can be part of a social support network that helps the client in physical, emotional, and spiritual ways:

• Physical support includes people who may help with running errands, picking up the children, or doing tasks around the house.
• Emotional support may take the form of listening to or helping to resolve relational problems.
• Community support includes friendships and acceptance provided by any community and is almost always there in some form for a person who may be feeling marginalized because of culture, sexual orientation, language, religion, or similar factors. These communities are critical for coping with the stress of marginalization.

Simply naming, recognizing, and appreciating that there is support can immediately increase a client's sense of hope and reduce feelings of loneliness.

Spiritual Resources

Increasingly, family therapists are becoming aware of how clients' spiritual resources can be used to address their problems (Walsh, 2003). For this reason, therapists should become familiar with the major religious traditions in their community, such as Protestantism, Catholicism, Judaism, Islam, New Age religions, and Native American practices.

Spirituality can be defined as how a person conceptualizes his or her relationship to the universe, life, or God (or however he or she constructs that which is larger than the self). Everyone has some form of spirituality, or a belief in how the universe operates (see Bateson, 1972, 1979/2002; Gergen, 1999).

SPIRITUALITY

The rules of "how life should go" always inform: (a) what the person perceives to be a problem, (b) how a person feels about it, and (c) what that person believes can "realistically" be done about it—all of which a therapist needs to know to develop an effective therapeutic plan.

Questions for Assessing Spirituality

A therapist can use some of the following questions to assess a client's spirituality, whether traditional or nontraditional:

- Do you believe there is a god or some form of intelligence that organizes the universe? If so, over what types of things does that being or force have control?

- If there is not a god, by what rules does the universe operate? Why do things happen? Or is life entirely random?

- What is the purpose and/or meaning of human existence? How does this understanding inform how a person should approach life?

- Is there any reason to be kind to others? To oneself?

- What is the ideal versus the realistic way to approach life?

- Why do "bad" things happen to "good" people?

- Do you believe things happen for a reason? If so, what reason?

- Do you belong to a religious community or spiritual circle of friends that provides spiritual support, inspiration, and/or guidance in some way?

With the answers to these questions, therapists can create a map of the client's world that they can use to develop conversations and interventions that are deeply meaningful and a good "fit" for the client. An accurate understanding of a client's "map of life" reveals what logic and actions will motivate the client to make changes, providing therapists with invaluable resources. Often many clients from traditional religious backgrounds and New Age groups believe that "things happen for a reason." These clients can use this one belief to radically and quickly transform how they feel, think, and respond to difficult situations. For example, a recent client of mine who was feeling depressed after being unexpectedly fired experienced a rapid improvement in mood when she began to see the situation as a sign from the divine that she needed to pursue an old career dream she had been putting off for years; this belief allowed her to mobilize her energy and hope to start moving in a positive direction.

Social Location: Resources and Limitations

In addition to client and family strengths, all clients bring with them certain resources and limitations from their experiences of diversity, including race, ethnicity, age, gender, sexual orientation, gender orientation, socioeconomic status, educational level, abilities, religion, language, etc. Thus, therapists can assess for these too.

Common resources due to diversity include:

- Strong support network of people who understand client's situation
- Sense of community and connection
- Sense of purpose and direction
- Resources for solving problems
- Beliefs that provide comfort
- Connections with persons outside of immediate network
- Access to social services

Common limitations include:

- Isolation, difficulty meeting others
- Experiences of harassment and discrimination
- Difficulty finding opportunities
- Difficulty communicating with institutions
- Difficulty accessing social services
- Lack of sufficient financial resources, housing, legal representation, etc.

Family Structure

This assessment can be used with individuals, couples, or families. The approach presented here draws from the major theories in family therapy. Consistent with both systemic (earlier forms of family therapy) and postmodern (later forms of family therapy) practices, it uses multiple descriptors to generate a complete, "both/and" perspective (Keeney, 1983) and a rich, multivoiced depiction of the problem (Anderson, 1997).

FAMILY STRUCTURE

Family Life-Cycle Stage (Check all that apply)

☐ Single adult ☐ Committed Couple ☐ Family with Young Children ☐ Family with Adolescent Children ☐ Divorce ☐ Blended Family ☐ Launching Children ☐ Later Life

Describe struggles with mastering developmental tasks in one or more of these stages: _____

_____

_____

Typical style for regulating closeness and distance in couple/family: _____

_____

_____

Boundaries with/between

Primary couple (A_/A_): ☐ Enmeshed ☐ Clear ☐ Disengaged ☐ NA Description/ example: _____

_____

Parent A_ & Children: ☐ Enmeshed ☐ Clear ☐ Disengaged ☐ NA Description/ example: _____

_____

Parent A_ & Children: ☐ Enmeshed ☐ Clear ☐ Disengaged ☐ NA Description/
example: _____
_____

Siblings: ☐ Enmeshed ☐ Clear ☐ Disengaged ☐ NA Description/example:
_____
_____

Extended Family: ☐ Enmeshed ☐ Clear ☐ Disengaged ☐ NA Description/
example: _____
_____

Friends/Colleagues/Other:☐Enmeshed☐Clear☐Disengaged☐NADescription
/example: _____
_____

Triangles/Coalitions
☐ Cross-generational coalitions: Describe: _____
☐ Other coalitions: _____

Hierarchy Between Parents and Children ☐ *NA*
AF/AM: ☐ Effective ☐ Insufficient (permissive) ☐ Excessive (authoritarian)
☐ Inconsistent
AM/AF: ☐ Effective ☐ Insufficient (permissive) ☐ Excessive (authoritarian)
☐ Inconsistent

Description/Example to illustrate: _____
_____

Complementary Patterns Between _____ and _____:
☐ Pursuer/distancer ☐ Overfunctioner/underfunctioner ☐ Emotional/logical
☐ Good/bad parent
☐ Other: _____; Example: _____

Family Life-Cycle Stage

Assessment of the family structure often begins by identifying the client or family's stage in the family life cycle. Each stage of the life cycle involves different developmental tasks, often requiring rebalancing independence and interdependence (Carter & McGoldrick, 1999). For example, the stage of single adult involves high levels of independence, while the committed-couple stage requires greater degrees of interdependence, and the stage of families with young children requires even greater degrees of interdependence. Often the presenting problem is closely linked to the changes required as a person transitions from one stage to the next. In the case of divorced or blended families, a person may actually be experiencing challenges related to more than one stage; an example is raising a teen while trying to form a committed partnership, which creates even more complex developmental challenges. The stages are:

- Leaving home, the single adult: Accepting emotional and financial responsibility for oneself

- Committed relationship: Committing to a new system; realigning boundaries with family and friends
- Families with young children: Adjusting marriage to make space for children; joining in child-rearing tasks; realigning boundaries with parents and grandparents
- Families with adolescent children: Adjusting parental boundaries to increase freedom and responsibility for adolescents; refocusing on marriage and career life
- Divorce: Interruption to the family life cycle, typically requiring most members to increase their sense of independence, with parents also developing a new form of interdependence (i.e., coparenting without being a couple).
- Blended families: Typically involves a complex balance of independence and interdependence that requires two or more family systems to be entwined, often at different stages of the family life cycle. Explicit discussion of needs for interdependence and interdependence is helpful to navigate this challenging transition, which typically takes several years (Visher & Visher, 1979).
- Launching children: Renegotiating the marital subsystem; developing adult-to-adult relationships with children; coping with aging parents
- Family in later life: Accepting the shift of generational roles; coping with loss of abilities; middle generation takes more central role; creating space for wisdom of the elderly

Boundaries: Regulating Closeness and Distance

Most commonly associated with structural family therapy (see Chapter 5), *boundaries* are the rules for negotiating interpersonal closeness and distance (Minuchin, 1974). Boundaries exist *internally* within the family and *externally* with those outside the nuclear family. These rules are generally unspoken and unfold as two people interact over time, each defining when, where, and how he or she prefers to relate to the other. With couples, these rules are often highly complex and difficult to track. Boundaries can be clear, diffuse, or rigid; all boundaries are strongly influenced by culture.

- Clear boundaries and cultural variance: Clear boundaries refer to a range of possible ways that couples and families can negotiate a healthy balance between closeness (weness) and separation (individuality). Cultural factors shape how much closeness or separation is preferred. Collectivist cultures tend toward greater degrees of closeness, whereas individualistic cultures tend to value greater independence. The best way to determine whether boundaries are clear is to determine whether symptoms have developed in the individual, couple, or family. If symptoms have developed, boundaries are probably too diffuse or too rigid. Most people who come in for therapy have reached a point at which boundaries that may have worked in one context are no longer working, often because of shifting needs in the family life cycle. For relationships to weather the test of time, couples and families must constantly renegotiate their boundaries (rules for relating) to adjust to each person's evolving needs. The more flexible couples are in negotiating these rules, the more successful they will be in adjusting to life's transitions and setbacks.
- Diffuse boundaries and enmeshed relationships: When couples or families begin to overvalue togetherness at the expense of respecting each other's individuality, their boundaries become *diffuse* and the relationship becomes *enmeshed*. (*Note:* Technically, boundaries are not enmeshed; they are diffuse.) In these relationships, one or more parties may feel that they are being suffocated, that they lack freedom, or that they are not cared for enough. Often people in these relationships feel threatened whenever the other disagrees or does not affirm them, resulting in an intense tug-of-war to convince the other to agree with them. Couples with diffuse boundaries may also have diffuse boundaries with their children, families of origin, and/ or friends, with the result that these outside others become overly involved in one

or both of the partners' lives (e.g., parents, friends, or children become involved in couple's arguments).

• Rigid boundaries and disengaged relationships: When couples or families privilege independence over togetherness, their boundaries can become *rigid* and the relationship *disengaged*. In these relationships, a person may not allow the other to influence them, often values a career or external interest more than the relationship, and frequently has minimal emotional connection. Such couples may have a pattern of keeping others at a distance or compensate by having diffuse boundaries with children, friends, family, or an outside love interest (e.g., an emotional or physical affair). Rigid boundaries are often difficult to accurately assess; their key indicator is whether they are creating problems individually or for the partnership/ family.

QUESTIONS FOR ASSESSING BOUNDARIES

The following are sample questions to think about while working with an individual, couple, or family to assess boundaries:

Assessing Boundaries in Couple Relationships

• Does the couple have clear boundaries that are distinct from their parenting and family-of-origin relationships?
• Does the couple spend time alone not talking about the children?
• Does the couple report an active sex and romantic life?
• Does the couple still feel a sense of connection apart from being parents?

Assessing Boundaries in Couple, Family, and Social Relationships

• Does one or more persons experience anxiety or frustration when there is a difference of opinion?
• Is one hurt or angry if another has a different opinion or perspective on a problem?
• Do they use "we" or "I" more often when speaking? Is there a balance?
• Does each person have a set of personal friends and activities separate from the family and partnership?
• How much energy goes into the couple/family versus outside relationships?
• What gets priority in each person's schedules? Children? Work? Personal activities? Couple time? Friends?

Triangles and Coalitions

Problem systems are identified in most systemic family therapy approaches. Triangles (Kerr & Bowen, 1988), covert coalitions (Minuchin & Fishman, 1981), and cross-generational coalitions (Minuchin & Fishman, 1981) all refer to a similar process: tension between two people is resolved by drawing in a third person (or a fourth, a "tetrad"; Whitaker & Keith, 1981) to stabilize the original dyad. Many therapists include inanimate objects or other processes as potential "thirds" in the triangulation process. In this situation, some*thing* else is used to manage the tension in the dyad, such as drinking, drug use, work, or hobbies, which are used to help one or both partners soothe their internal stress at the expense of the relationship.

Therapists assess for triangles and problematic subsystems in several ways:

- Clients overtly describe another party as playing a role in their tension; in these cases, the clients are aware of the process at some level.
- When clients describe the problem or conflict situation, another person plays the role of confidant or takes the side of one of the partners (e.g., one person has a friend or another family member who takes his or her side against the other).
- After being unable to have a need met in the primary dyad, a person finds what he or she is not getting in another person (e.g., a mother seeks emotional closeness from a child rather than from a husband).
- When therapy is inexplicably "stuck," there is often a triangle at work that distracts one or both parties from resolving critical issues (e.g., an affair, substance abuse, a friend who undermines agreements made in therapy, etc.).

Identifying triangles early in the assessment process enables therapists to intervene more successfully and quickly in a complex set of family dynamics.

Hierarchy between Child and Parents

A key area in assessing parent and child relationships is hierarchy, a structural family concept (see Chapter 5). When assessing parental hierarchy, therapists must ask themselves: Is the parent–child hierarchy developmentally and culturally appropriate? If the hierarchy is appropriate, the child usually has few behavioral problems. If the child is exhibiting symptoms or there are problems in the parent–child relationship, there is usually some problem in the hierarchical structure: either an excessive (authoritarian) or insufficient (permissive) parental hierarchy given the family's current sociocultural context(s). Immigrant families, because they usually have two different sets of cultural norms for parental hierarchy (the traditional and the current cultural context), have difficulty finding a balance between authoritarian and permissive hierarchies.

Assessing hierarchy is critical because it tells the therapist where and how to intervene. If therapists assess only the symptoms, they may make inappropriate interventions. For example, though children diagnosed with ADHD have similar symptoms—hyperactivity, defiance, failing to follow through on parents' requests—these same symptoms can occur in two dramatically different family structures: either too much or too little parental hierarchy. When the parental hierarchy is too rigid, the therapist works with the parents to develop a stronger personal relationship with the child and to set developmentally and culturally appropriate expectations. If there is not enough parental hierarchy, the therapist helps parents to be more consistent with consequences and to set limits and rules. Thus, the same set of symptoms can require very different interventions.

When conceptualizing parental hierarchy, it can also be helpful to consider the balance of roles within the parental system. Raser (1999) describes the parenting relationship as comprising *business roles* (setting rules, socializing) and *personal roles* (warmth, fun, caring, play); the former correlates most often with an effective hierarchy and the latter with secure attachment (see "Attachment Patterns," below). Typically, a parent is better at one than the other, which often leads to problematic polarization between the parents. Ideally, both parents are able to balance *within themselves* the business and personal sides of parenting, and both parents can then set an effective hierarchy as well as maintain a close emotional bond. Assessing just this single dimension can provide therapists with a razor-sharp focus for treatment, often resulting in rapid improvements.

Complementary Patterns

Complementary patterns characterize most relationships to a certain degree, especially long-term committed relationships. *Complementary* in this case refers to each person taking on opposite or complementary roles, which range from functional to problematic. For example, a complementary relationship of introvert and extrovert can exist in a balanced and well-functioning relationship as well as in an out-of-balance, problematic relationship; the difference is in the rigidity of the pattern. Classic examples of complementary roles that often become problematic include pursuer/distancer, emotional/logical, overfunctioner/underfunctioner, friendly parent/strict parent, and so forth. Gottman (1999) indicated that the female–pursue (demand) and male–withdraw pattern existed to some extent in the majority of marriages he studied. However, in distressed marriages, this pattern becomes exaggerated and begins to be viewed as innate personality traits. Assessing for these patterns can help therapists intervene in couples' interactions. In most cases, couples readily identify their complementary roles in their complaints about the relationship: "He's too strict with the kids"; "She always emotionally overreacts"; "I have to do it all the time"; "She never wants sex." These broad, sweeping descriptions of the other suggest a likely problematic complementary pattern.

Interaction Patterns

One of the hallmarks of family therapy is the ability to assess the family's interaction patterns with regard to the presenting problem. In all honesty, I prefer to do this *before* assessing family structure; but most of my students seem to prefer this order as they find structure a bit easier. You should feel free to do it in whichever order works for you.

INTERACTIONAL PATTERNS

Primary Pathologizing Interpersonal Pattern (PIPs; A ⇆ B): Describe dynamic of primary PIP:

☐ Pursuing/Distancing ☐ Criticizing/Defending ☐ Controlling/Resisting
☐ Other: _____

Problem Interaction Pattern (A ⇆ B):

Start of tension: _____

Conflict/symptom escalation: _____

Return to "normal"/homeostasis: _____

Hypothesized homeostatic function of presenting problem: How might the symptom serve to maintain connection, create independence/distance, establish influence, reestablish connection, or otherwise help organize the family?

_____
_____

This ability to assess interaction patterns is central to the Mental Research Institute (MRI) approach (see Chapter 4; Watzlawick et al., 1974), strategic therapy (Haley, 1976), and the Milan approach (see Chapter 4; Selvini Palazzoli et al., 1978) and is featured prominently in Satir's communication approach (see Chapter 6; Satir et al., 1991) and Whitaker's symbolic–experiential therapy (see Chapter 6; Whitaker & Bumberry, 1988). In interactional assessment, the therapist traces reciprocal relational patterns: how person A responds to person B and vice versa. Because more than one person may be involved (persons C, D, E, etc.) in families or larger groups, patterns can become quite complex. Whether the client reports an individual symptom or relational problem, the therapist addresses the fact that the behavior is always embedded within larger systems and that the symptoms help maintain the system's homeostasis or sense of normalcy (even if the behavior is not considered normal by the members of the system). I find it most helpful to think of tracing the problem interaction through three basic phases, which can vary significantly from problem to problem.

THREE PHASES OF PROBLEM INTERACTION PATTERN

- *Start of tension*: What are the behaviors that signal a rise in tension or the start of the problem? How do things unfold from here? How does each person respond and react to the rise in tension?
- *Conflict/symptom escalation*: What happens when the problem fully emerges (it may be a conflict for a family or a depressive episode for an individual)? The focus here is on the behavioral actions and responses of each person involved, even in cases of "individual" problems, such as anxiety, depression, or psychosis.
- *Return to "normal"/homeostasis*: Often the most enlightening part, the interaction cycle is finally traced back to "normal" or homeostasis. What does each person do to get back to the sense of "normal"?

A therapist can assess these patterns using a series of questions, first by identifying the emergence of the problem and then by tracing each person's emotional and/or behavioral responses to others until "normalcy" or homeostasis is achieved again. The process looks something like this.

ASSESSING INTERACTION PATTERNS

Client describes how the problem begins:

Example: Mother gets a call from the school saying her son is failing a class.

The therapist inquires about the mother's next actions and the son's response:

Example: Mother lectures son and sets an extensive punishment; the child argues and says she is being unfair. Mother says, "Wait until I tell your dad."

The therapist continues to trace this exchange in terms of how each responded to the other until they return to normal:

Example: Mother responds to son's accusations of her being unfair by adding more consequences and punishments.

The therapist also inquires about how significant others in the family system respond to the problem situation:

Example: How did the father participate? What does the younger sister do while this is going on? What effects does this have in the marital relationship?

The therapist continues assessing the interaction pattern until it is clear that the entire family has returned to a sense of "normalcy."

Systemic Hypothesis

After assessing family structure and interaction patterns, therapists develop a working hypothesis about the problem, a potential role the symptom may be playing in maintaining the family homeostasis (see Chapter 4; Selvini Palazzoli et al., 1978). A classic example is that a child's symptom (e.g., tantrums, running away, school failure, eating disorder): (a) creates a common problem that forces the couple to cooperate, work together, and stay together and/or (b) distracts one or more parents from an ailing marriage. Obviously, a child is rarely thinking, "Gee, I think I'll act out to keep Mom and Dad together," and a parent isn't thinking, "I'll just obsessively overfocus on the children to distract me from my pathetic marriage." Instead, the symptoms naturally emerge to fill "gaps" or systemic needs to maintain a sense of balance without anyone consciously cooking up a plan.

The following strategies may be used for developing hypotheses:

- Client language and metaphors: The MRI team often described the entire homeostatic pattern using client language (Watzlawick et al., 1974). For example, if the family members were sports enthusiasts, they would describe the interaction pattern using the metaphor of a game in which person A has to play defense (withdraw) when person B plays offense (pursues).
- Positive connotation: The Milan team made it a rule to emphasize the positive and helpful effects of the symptom in the family (Selvini Palazzoli et al., 1978). For example, the therapist would praise a child who was sacrificing personal success to give his mother someone to care for so she felt useful.
- Love and power: Strategic therapists developed hypotheses around love and power. For example, they might hypothesize that the seemingly helpless person's role (e.g., as depressed, compliant, sexually uninterested) had the hidden dimension of giving the person power (through influencing others' behavior) that she could not acquire by other means.

Intergenerational and Attachment Patterns

Assessing for intergenerational patterns is easiest when using a genogram (McGoldrick, Gerson, & Petry, 2008), which provides a visual map of these patterns. Traditionally an intergenerational assessment instrument (see Chapter 7; McGoldrick et al., 2008), genograms have also been adapted for use with other models (Hardy & Laszloffy, 1995; Kuehl, 1995; Rubalcava & Waldman, 2004) and are regularly used by all therapists to conceptualize family dynamics.

Therapists can create comprehensive genograms, which map numerous intergenerational patterns, or problem-specific genograms, which focus on patterns related to the presenting problem and how family members have dealt with similar problems across generations (e.g., how other couples have dealt with marital tension). See McGoldrick et al. (2008) for comprehensive instructions on using a genogram. The following figure depicts the symbols family therapists commonly use to create a genogram.

In addition, the following patterns and information are frequently included in genograms:

- Family strengths and resources
- Substance and alcohol abuse and dependence
- Sexual, physical, and emotional abuse
- Personal qualities and/or family roles; complementary roles (e.g., black sheep, rebellious one, overachiever/underachiever, etc.)
- Physical and mental health issues (e.g., diabetes, cancer, depression, psychosis, etc.)
- Historical incidents of the presenting problem, either with the same people or how other generations and family members have managed this problem

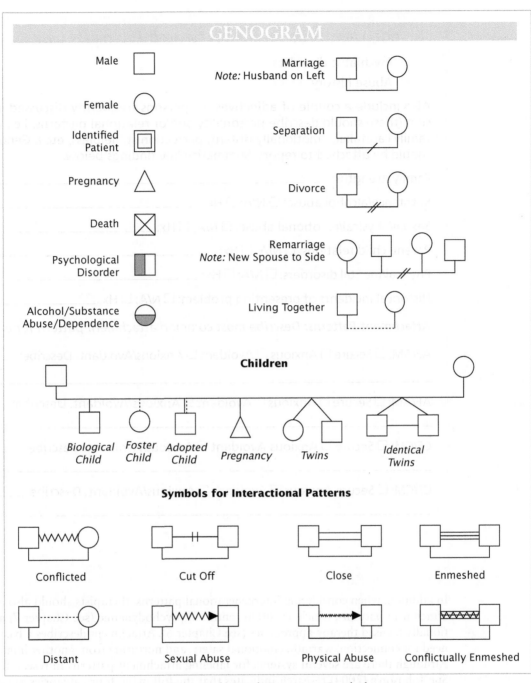

Commonly Used Genogram Symbols

INTERGENERATIONAL AND ATTACHMENT PATTERNS

Construct a family genogram and include all relevant information including:

- Ages, birth/death dates
- Names
- Relational patterns
- Occupations
- Medical history

(continued)

INTERGENERATIONAL AND ATTACHMENT PATTERNS (*continued*)

- Psychiatric disorders
- Abuse history

Also include a couple of adjectives for persons frequently discussed in session (these should describe personality and/or relational patterns, i.e., quiet, family caretaker, emotionally distant, perfectionist, helpless, etc.). Genogram should be attached to report. Summarize key findings below.

Family strengths: _____

Substance/alcohol abuse: ☐ N/A; ☐ Hx: _____

Sexual/physical/emotional abuse: ☐ N/A; ☐ Hx: _____

Parent–child relations: ☐ N/A; ☐ Hx: _____

Physical/mental disorders: ☐ N/A; ☐ Hx: _____

Historical incidents of presenting problem: ☐ N/A; ☐ Hx: _____

Attachment Patterns: Describe most common attachment pattern for each

AF/AM: ☐ Secure ☐ Anxious ☐ Avoidant ☐ Anxious/Avoidant. Describe: _____

_____

AF/AM: ☐ Secure ☐ Anxious ☐ Avoidant ☐ Anxious/Avoidant. Describe: _____

_____

CF/CM: ☐ Secure ☐ Anxious Avoidant ☐ Anxious/Avoidant. Describe: _____

_____

CF/CM: ☐ Secure Anxious ☐ Avoidant ☐ Anxious/Avoidant. Describe: _____

_____

Attachment Patterns

In addition, when considering intergenerational patterns, therapists should also assess for attachment patterns, which are often central in psychodynamic (see Chapter 7) and emotionally focused therapy approaches (see Chapter 6). Attachment describes a basic human need for connection, warmth, emotional safety, and nurturing from another human being. Although there are several systems for labeling attachment patterns in research settings, Sue Johnson's (2004) research indicates that the following four categories are generally sufficient for couple and family therapy:

- Secure: When attachment needs are not met, the person is still generally able to maintain a sufficient level of coping and is able to pursue reconnection in constructive ways.
- Anxious and hyperactive: When attachment needs are not met, the person becomes anxious and clingy, relentlessly pursues connection, and may become aggressive, blaming, and critical.
- Avoidance: When attachment needs are not met, the person suppresses attachment needs and instead focuses on tasks or other distractions.
- Combination anxious and avoidant: In this style, when attachment needs are not met, the person pursues closeness and then avoids it once offered; this is often associated with a trauma history.

Solution-Based Assessment

SOLUTION-BASED ASSESSMENT

Attempted Solutions that DIDN'T work:

1. _____

2. _____

3. _____

Exceptions and Unique Outcomes (Solutions that DID work): Times, places, relationships, contexts, etc. when problem is less of a problem; behaviors that seem to make things even slightly better:

1. _____

2. _____

3. _____

Answer to the Miracle Question: If the problem were to be resolved overnight, what would client be doing differently the next day? (Describe in terms of doing X rather than not doing Y).

1. _____

2. _____

3. _____

Previous Solutions That Did Not Work

When assessing solutions, therapists need to assess two kinds: those that have worked and those that have not. The MRI group (Watzlawick et al., 1974) and cognitive–behavioral therapists (Baucom & Epstein, 1990) are best known for assessing what has not worked, although they use these in different ways when they intervene. With most clients, it is generally easy to assess failed previous solutions.

QUESTIONS FOR ASSESSING SOLUTIONS THAT DID NOT WORK

The therapist may begin by asking a straightforward question:

> *What have you tried to solve this problem?*

Most clients respond with a list of things that have not worked. If they need more prompting therapists may ask:

> *I am guessing you have tried to solve this problem (address this issue) on your own and that some things were not as successful as you had hoped. What have you tried that did not work?*

Exceptions and Unique Outcomes: Previous Solutions That Did Work

Solution-focused therapists (de Shazer, 1988; O'Hanlon & Weiner-Davis, 1989) assess for previous solutions that *did* work, a process that is similar to identifying *unique outcomes* to the dominant problem story in narrative therapy (Freedman & Combs, 1996; White & Epston, 1990). Assessing previous solutions and unique outcomes is difficult because most clients are less aware of when the problem is not a problem and how they have kept things from getting worse. Some of the questions therapists ask are the following:

QUESTIONS FOR ASSESSING SOLUTIONS AND UNIQUE OUTCOMES

- What keeps this problem from being worse than it is right now?
- Is there any solution you have tried that worked for a while? Or made things slightly better?
- Are there times or places when the problem is less of a problem or not a problem?
- Have you ever been able to respond to the problem so that it is less of a problem or less severe?
- Does this problem occur in all places with all people, or is it better in certain contexts?

These questions generally require more thought and reflection from the client and more follow-up questions from the therapist. Their answers often provide invaluable clues about how best to proceed and intervene in therapy.

Answer to the Miracle Question

Solution-based therapists use the miracle question (de Shazer, 1988) and similar questions—crystal ball questions (de Shazer, 1985), magic wand questions (Selekman, 1997), and time machine questions (Bertolino & O'Hanlon, 2002)—to assess the client's preferred solution or outcome (see Chapter 9 for a detailed discussion of exactly how to ask this question successfully—it's harder than you'd think). The answers to these questions are often very helpful in setting goals for treatment.

THE MIRACLE QUESTION

"Imagine that you go home tonight and during the middle of the night a miracle happens: all the problems you came here to resolve are miraculously resolved. However, when you wake up, you have no idea a miracle has occurred. What are some of the first things you would notice that would be different? What are some of the first clues that a miracle has occurred?"

The therapist then helps the client generate a behavioral description of what the client would be *doing*. Often this requires gently asking follow-up questions when clients describe what they or others would *not* be doing or what they would be feeling. Instead, the therapist tries to get a clear video-like picture of what the clients are actually doing in their miracle scenario. These are then used to create specific goals for therapy.

Postmodern: Social Location and Dominant Discourses

Narratives and social discourses outline the broader contexts in which the client's problem occurs. They can be divided into dominant discourses, identity narratives, and local and preferred discourses.

POSTMODERN: SOCIAL LOCATION AND DOMINANT DISCOURSES

Dominant discourses informing definition of problem:

Cultural, ethnic, socioeconomic status, religious etc.: How do key cultural discourses inform what is perceived as a problem and the possible solutions?

_____

_____

Gender, sexual orientation, etc.: How do the gender/sexual discourses inform what is perceived as a problem and the possible solutions? _____

_____

Contextual, family, community, school, and other social discourses: How do other important discourses inform what is perceived as a problem and the possible solutions? _____

_____

_____

Identity/self-narratives: How has the problem shaped each family member's identity?:_____

_____

_____

Local or preferred discourses: What is the client's preferred identity narrative and/or narrative about the problem? Are there local (alternative) discourses about the problem that are preferred?: _____

_____

_____

Dominant Discourses

Assessing the *dominant social discourses* in which a client's problems are embedded often creates a new and broader perspective on a client's situation (Freedman & Combs, 1996; White & Epston, 1990). I find that this broader perspective frequently helps me feel more freedom and possibility, increasing my emotional attunement to clients and allowing me to be more creative in my work. For example, when I view a client's reported "anxiety" as part of a larger discourse in which the client feel powerless, such as being gay or lesbian, I begin to see the anxiety as part of this larger social dance. I also see how it is possible for this person to give less "faith," weight, or credence to the dominant discourse and generate new stories about what is "normal" sexual behavior and what is not. By discussing the difficulty in concretely defining what is normal sexual behavior and what is not, the client and I can begin to explore the truths that this person has experienced. We join in an exploratory process that offers new ways for the client to understand the anxiety as well as his/her identity.

Common dominant discourses or broader narratives that inform clients' lives include the following:

- Culture, race, ethnicity, class, immigration, religion
- Gender identity and sexual orientation
- Community, school, and professional cultures
- Wealth, poverty, power, fame
- Small-town, urban, regional discourses
- Health, illness, body image, etc.

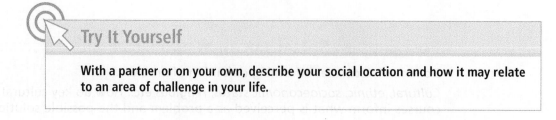

Try It Yourself

With a partner or on your own, describe your social location and how it may relate to an area of challenge in your life.

Identity Narratives

When clients come for therapy, the problem discourse has usually become a significant part of their *identity narrative,* the story they tell themselves about who they are. For example, a child having problems in school may begin to think, "I am stupid"; his mother may be feeling, "I have failed as a mother" because of her child's academic performance. Obviously, these negative sweeping judgments of a person's value or ability need to be addressed in therapy. Assessing them early in the process helps the therapist understand how to engage and motivate each person.

Client Perspectives

Finally, therapists should reflect on areas of client agreement and disagreement with a case conceptualization. Although it is often not clinically appropriate to hand the entire case conceptualization over to a client, discussing the key findings is. Which descriptions seem accurate from the client's perspective? Which do not? Would the client be surprised to hear any of this? If there is a significant disagreement between the client's and therapist's perspective, the therapist needs to consider how he/she will navigate this difference and remain open to the possibility that the assessment is not accurate.

CLIENT PERSPECTIVES

Areas of agreement: Based on what the clients have said, what parts of the above assessment do they agree with or are likely to agree with? _____

_____

Areas of disagreement: What parts do they disagree with or are likely to disagree with? Why? _____

_____

How do you plan to respectfully work with areas of potential disagreement?

_____

_____

Considering the client perspective is particularly important when the client differs from the therapist in age, cultural background, gender, sexual orientation, or socioeconomic status, in which case the therapist may be less likely to fully understand the client's context. Conversely, many therapists have even more trouble with clients who are similar to them because they assume they know more than they do or that they already know the answer to the situation. Whether clients are similar or different, therapists need to carefully consider their perspectives when conceptualizing treatment.

Case Conceptualization, Diversity, and Sameness

Just in case you were beginning to feel that you finally understood something about case conceptualization, let me throw a wrench or two into the mix: diversity and sameness. The problem with case conceptualization and assessments in general is that, unfortunately, there are no objective standards against which a person can be measured for "clear boundaries," "healthy hierarchies," or "clear communication." Healthy, emotionally engaged boundaries look quite different in a Mexican American family and an Asian American family. In fact, problematic boundaries in a Mexican American family (e.g., cool, disengaged) may look *more like* healthy boundaries (e.g., quietly respectful) than problem boundaries (e.g., overly involved) in Asian American families. Thus, therapists cannot rely simply on objective descriptions of behavior in assessment. They must also consider the broader culture norms, which may include more than one set of ethnic norms as well as local neighborhood cultures, school contexts, sexual orientation subcultures, religious communities, and so forth. Although you will undoubtedly take a course on cultural issues and will read that professional codes of ethics require respecting diversity, it takes working with a diverse range of families and a willingness to learn from them to cultivate a meaningful sense of cultural sensitivity. I believe this to be a lifelong journey.

Ironically, I have found that new therapists in training today sometimes have the most difficulty accepting diversity in clients from within their *same* culture of origin. The more similar clients are to us, the more we expect them to share our values and behavioral norms and the lower our tolerance of difference. For example, middle-class Caucasian therapists often expect middle-class Caucasian clients to have particular values regarding emotional expression, marital arrangements, extended family, and parent–child relationships and may be quick to encourage particular systems of values—namely, their own. Thus, whether working with someone very similar to or very different from yourself, you need to *slowly* assess and evaluate, always considering clients' broader sociocultural context and norms. Therapists who excel in conceptualization and assessment approach these tasks with profound humility and a continual willingness to learn.

ONLINE RESOURCES

Genoware, Inc.: Genogram Maker

www.genogram.org

Go to MindTap® for an eBook, videos of client sessions, activities, digital forms, practice quizzes, apps, and more—all in one place. If your instructor didn't assign MindTap, you can find out more information at CengageBrain.com.

REFERENCES

Anderson, H. (1997). *Conversations, language, and possibilities.* New York: Basic.

Anderson, H., & Gehart, D. R. (Eds.). (2006). *Collaborative therapy: Relationships and conversations that make a difference.* New York: Brunner-Routledge.

Bateson, G. (1972). *Steps to an ecology of mind.* New York: Ballantine.

Bateson, G. (1979/2002). *Mind and nature: A necessary unity.* Cresskill, NJ: Hampton.

Baucom, D. H., & Epstein, N. (1990). *Cognitive-behavioral marital therapy.* New York: Brunner/Mazel.

Bertolino, B., & O'Hanlon, B. (2002). *Collaborative, competency-based counseling and therapy.* New York: Allyn & Bacon.

Carter, B., & McGoldrick, M. (1999). *The expanded family life cycle: Individuals, families, and social perspectives* (3rd ed.). New York: Allyn & Bacon.

de Shazer, S. (1985). *Keys to solution in brief therapy.* New York: Norton.

de Shazer, S. (1988). *Clues: Investigating solutions in brief therapy.* New York: Norton.

Freedman, J., & Combs, G. (1996). *Narrative therapy: The social construction of preferred realities.* New York: Norton.

Gergen, K. J. (1999). *An invitation to social construction.* Thousand Oaks, CA: Sage.

Gottman, J. M. (1999). *The marriage clinic: A scientifically based marital therapy.* New York: Norton.

Haley, J. (1976). *Problem-solving therapy: New strategies for effective family therapy.* San Francisco, CA: Jossey-Bass.

Hardy, K. V., & Laszloffy, T. A. (1995). The cultural genogram: Key to training culturally competent family therapists. *Journal of Marital and Family Therapy, 21,* 227–237.

Johnson, S. M. (2004). *The practice of emotionally focused marital therapy: Creating connection* (2nd ed.). New York: Brunner/Routledge.

Keeney, B. P. (1983). *Aesthetics of change.* New York: Guilford.

Kerr, M., & Bowen, M. (1988). *Family evaluation.* New York: Norton.

Kuehl, B. P. (1995). The solution-oriented genogram: A collaborative approach. *Journal of Marital and Family Therapy, 21,* 239–250.

Lambert, M. J., & Ogles, B. M. (2004). The efficacy and effectiveness of psychotherapy. In M. J. Lambert (Ed.), *Bergin and Garfield's handbook of psychotherapy and behavior change* (5th ed., pp. 139–193). New York: Wiley.

McGoldrick, M., Gerson, R., & Petry, S. (2008). *Genograms: Assessment and intervention* (3rd ed.). New York: Norton.

Miller, S. D., Duncan, B. L., & Hubble, M. (1997). *Escape from Babel: Toward a unifying language for psychotherapy practice.* New York: Norton.

Minuchin, S. (1974). *Families and family therapy.* Cambridge, MA: Harvard University Press.

Minuchin, S., & Fishman, H. C. (1981). *Family therapy techniques.* Cambridge, MA: Harvard University Press.

O'Hanlon, W. H., & Weiner-Davis, M. (1989). *In search of solutions: A new direction in psychotherapy.* New York: Norton.

Raser, J. (1999). *Raising children you can live with: A guide for frustrated parents* (2nd ed.). Houston, TX: Bayou.

Rubalcava, L. A., & Waldman, K. M. (2004). Working with intercultural couples: An intersubjective-constructivist perspective. *Progress in Self Psychology, 20,* 127–149.

Satir, V., Banmen, J., Gerber, J., & Gomori, M. (1991). *The Satir model: Family therapy and beyond.* Palo Alto, CA: Science and Behavior Books.

Selekman, M. D. (1997). *Solution-focused therapy with children: Harnessing family strengths for systemic change.* New York: Guilford.

Seligman, M. (2004). *Authentic happiness: Using the new positive psychology to realize your potential for lasting fulfillment.* New York: Free Press.

Selvini Palazzoli, M., Boscolo, L., Cecchin, G., & Prata, G. (1978). *Paradox and counterparadox.* New York: Aronson.

Visher, E., & Visher, J. (1979). *Stepfamilies: A guide to working with stepparents and stepchildren.* New York: Brunner/Mazel.

Walsh, F. (Ed.). (2003). *Spiritual resources in family therapy.* New York: Guilford.

Watzlawick, P., Weakland, J., & Fisch, R. (1974). *Change: Principles of problem formation and problem resolution.* New York: Norton.

Whitaker, C. A., & Bumberry, W. M. (1988). *Dancing with the family: A symbolic experiential approach.* New York: Brunner/Mazel.

Whitaker, C. A., & Keith, D. V. (1981). Symbolic-experiential family therapy. In A. S. Gurman & D. P. Kniskern (Eds.), *Handbook of family therapy* (pp. 187–224). New York: Brunner/Mazel.

White, M., & Epston, D. (1990). *Narrative means to therapeutic ends.* New York: Norton.

CROSS-THEORETICAL SYSTEMIC CASE CONCEPTUALIZATION

For use with individual, couple, or family clients.

Date: 6/19/16   **Clinician:** Maria Sanchez, MFT Trainee   **Client/Case #:** 4001

Introduction to Client & Significant Others

Identify significant persons in client's relational/family life who will be mentioned in case conceptualization:

Adults/Parents: Select identifier/abbreviation for use in rest of case conceptualization

AF1: Female Age: 36   Hispanic/Latino   Married heterosexual   Occupation: Department store clerk

   Other: Catholic

AM1: Male Age: 34   Hispanic/Latino   Married heterosexual   Occupation: Insurance Agent Other:

   Son of Immigrants from Mexico, Catholic

Children/Adult Children: Select identifier/abbreviation for use in rest of case conceptualization

CF1: Female Age: 16   Hispanic/Latino Grade: 10 School: Green Field Highschool Other identifier:

   Active in multiple school activites, including music and soccer

CM1: Male Age: 14   Hispanic/Latino Grade: 8 School: Valley Middle School Other identifier: Honor

   Student

Others: Identify all:

Presenting Concerns

Describe each significant person's description of the problem, focusing on OBSERVABLE behaviors:

AF1:   Couple separated six months ago due to AM34's affair; AF36's family is very disapproving but
AF36 refuses to stay together; primary concern is CF16's recent alcohol/drug use.

AM1:   Fell in love with another woman; feels bad about effects on family but is not sure what else to
do; primary concern is the children and CF16's drug use.

CF1:   Angry about parent's likely divorce; feels father abandoned family; sees "partying" as normal
and feels that she is entitled because of the stress her parents caused her.

CM1:   Sees father as weak for affair and frustrated with mother's anxiety over religious issues. Disappointed in parents but copes by staying focused on school.

Broader System: Description of problem from extended family, referring party, school, legal system, etc.:
Extended Family: AF Family of Origin: Views divorce from religious perspective and believes couples
should work things out. AM Family of Origin: Understanding of divorce given the distant marriage that
AM34 parents had.

Mrs.Gomez: School Counselor: Concerned that CF16 is starting down dangerous path in reaction to
parents' separation.

Name:

Background Information

Trauma/Abuse History (recent and past): AF reports one incident of sexual abuse as child (7 yr) by neighbor; AM report that in the early years of his youth, his family was very poor, often not having housing or enough to eat.

Substance Use/Abuse (current and past; self, family of origin, significant others): AM34's father was an alcoholic, as is his brother, which has resulted in numerous distant relationships in his family. The parents are concerned that CF16 may develop substance abuse issues that run on AM34's side of the family. CF16 regularly partakes in alcohol and pot but has only tried the harder drugs a couple of times. Since the separation, CF16 started hanging out for longer hours with friends, getting connected with a crowd that regularly uses alcohol and pot and has periodic access to heroin and methamphetamines.

Precipitating Events (recent life changes, first symptoms, stressors, etc.): Six months prior, the CF16 and CM14 were both excelling academically and socially, and they report things at home were relatively calm. However, six months ago, AF36 discovered AM34 was having an affair; AM34 refused to end it. AF36 asked him to leave and she stayed in the home with the children. They have filed for divorce but are not actively moving the process along. Both children were very surprised and disappointed in father. Parents bickered frequently but seemed to be committed to the relationship. Since the separation, CM14 has been quieter than usual, focusing on his studies. Neither of the children is enthusiastic about seeing their father, often choosing to go with friends or engaging in school activities during their scheduled visits.

Related Historical Background (family history, related issues, previous counseling, medical/mental health history, etc.): The couple had sought marital counseling two years prior for their arguing; things improved for awhile but later returned to about the same level of conflict. AF36 comes from a very religious family, her oldest brother is a Catholic priest and her younger brother is cut off from the family because he is in a same-sex relationship.

Strengths and Social Location

Strengths and Resources:

Personal: CF16 is an active, socially skilled, intelligent young woman; she excels at most everything she attempts; CM14 is in honors classes and is a dedicated student with goals of becoming a doctor; AF36 has strong family and friend relationships that has kept her going during this difficult time; AM34 has proven himself to be a dedicated father even after his kids have been rejecting him; he understands their anger and is willing to work for their forgiveness.

Relational/Social: The children have strong support networks that are helping them through this difficult time: CF16's school counselor is aware of what is going on. AF36's sister has helped with child care. AM34's new girlfriend supports him and has stayed out of the family dynamics.

Spiritual: AF36 has a strong faith that she turns to for inspiration during this difficult time; AM34 also has a sense that "things happen for a reason," which he finds consoling.

Based on the client's social location—age, gender race, ethnicity, sexual orientation, gender identity, social class, religion, geographic region, language, family configuration, abilities, etc.— identify potential resources and challenges:

Unique Resources: AF has strong familial support even though they do not agree with her actions entirely; AF has strong religious faith and community that she finds very helpful; parents have overall been successful in handling cross-generational differences in terms of acculturation.

Potential Limitations: When AF contemplates divorce, she must consider religious, cultural, and family values and balance them with asserting her personal needs. Heavy drinking is part of family's culture, making it harder for CF16 to reflect on her use.

Family Structure

☐ Single Adult
☐ Committed Couple
☐ Family with Young Children
☒ Family with Adolescent Children
☒ Divorce
☐ Blended Family
☐ Launching Children
☐ Later Life

Describe struggles with mastering developmental tasks in one or more of these stages: Couple has had difficulty maintaining couple connection since having children. AF36 feels as though she has had primary responsibility for raising the children, AM34 feeling disconnected from family life.

Boundaries with/between:

Primary couple ☒ Enmeshed ☐ Clear ☐ Disengaged ☐ NA Example: Historically en-meshed, the couple's boundary definition has only gotten more confusing with the separation, each hav-ing a more difficult time allowing the other to have unique opinions and feelings, especially about the children. Most every interaction is charged with over-personalization

AF & Children ☒ Enmeshed ☐ Clear ☐ Disengaged ☐ NA Example: AF36 can be highly reactive when kids do not follow rules and has taken CF16's drug use very personally.

AM & Children ☐ Enmeshed ☐ Clear ☒ Disengaged ☐ NA Example: AM34 has always been a more detached father figure, which is even more exaggerated since the separation.

Siblings ☐ Enmeshed ☒ Clear ☐ Disengaged ☐ NA Example: _____

Extended Family ☒ Enmeshed ☐ Clear ☐ Disengaged ☐ NA Example: Extended family very involved in separation.

Friends/Peers/Others ☒ Enmeshed ☐ Clear ☐ Disengaged ☐ NA Example: AM has left family for lover; he does not balance time with her and children.

(continued)

Family Structure (*continued*)

Triangles/Coalitions:

☒ Cross-generational coalitions: Describe: AF36, CF16, and CM14 have united against AM34

because of the affair, CF16 and CM14 hold AM34 responsible for parents' separation

☐ Other coalitions: _____

Hierarchy between Parents and Children: ☐ NA

Select: ☐ Effective ☒ Insufficient (permissive) ☐ Excessive (authoritarian) ☐ Inconsistent

Select: ☐ Effective ☐ Insufficient (permissive) ☒ Excessive (authoritarian) ☐ Inconsistent

Description/Example to illustrate hierarchy: AF36 has tended to be a lenient parent with moderate

effectiveness. AM34 has always left the majority of daily parenting to AF36, but when he does discipline,

he is very directive, wanting the kids to "shape up" quickly.

Complementary Patterns between AF and AM:
☒ Pursuer/distancer
☐ Over/underfunctioner
☐ Emotional/logical
☒ Good/bad parent
☐ Other: _____

Example of pattern: Historically, AF36 pursued AM34 for connection and engagement, similar dynamic

during separation. In addition, due to the affair, AF plays the role of "good parent" and AM "bad parent."

Interactional Patterns

Primary Pathologizing Interpersonal Pattern (PIPs; A ⇆ B): *Describe dynamic of primary PIP:*
☐ Pursuing/Distancing ☐ Criticizing/Defending ☒ Controlling/Resisting ☐ Other:_____
Describe Start of Tension: CF 16 gets caught drinking.

Describe Conflict/Symptom Escalation: AF36 begins yelling and lecturing and sets a harsh punish-

ment for which she does not follow through. When AM34 hears about what happens the next day, he

tries having a long talk with CF16 about her choices, focusing on the detrimental effects on her future

and ignoring her emotional reasons for "escaping."

Describe Return to "Normal"/Homeostasis: After a day or two of distance, AF softens and reconnects

with CF; within a couple of weeks the pattern repeats.

What is the metacommunication in this interaction? The metacommunication seems to be about

power and control: CF16's behavior communicates wanting more independence and separation on one

level, while the parents are also trying to assert their power and influence.

Intergenerational & Attachment Patterns

Construct a family genogram and include all relevant information including:
- Names, ages, and birth/death dates
- Relational patterns
- Occupations
- Psychiatric disorders and alcohol/substance abuse
- Abuse history
- Personality adjectives

Genogram should be attached to report. Summarize key findings below:

Substance/Alcohol Abuse: ☐ NA ☒ History: <u>AM34's father and brother</u> <u>abuse alcohol; CF has poten-</u> <u>tial to develop same problem</u>

Sexual/Physical/Emotional Abuse: ☒ NA ☐ History: _____

Parent/Child Relations: ☐ NA ☒ History: _____

Physical/Mental Disorders: ☐ NA ☒ History: _____

History Related to Presenting Problem: ☐ NA ☒ History: _____

Describe family strengths, such as the capacity to self-regulate and to effectively manage stress: AF36 has strong religious tradition, which helps to stabilize her and the family.

Describe typical attachment behavior when person does not feel secure in relationships.

AF: ☒ Anxious ☐ Avoidant ☐ Anxious/Avoidant. Frequency: <u>Select</u> Describe: <u>Pursue husband,</u> and often tried to use verbal attack to reengage him; she also pursues children when they distance themselves.

AF: ☐ Anxious ☒ Avoidant ☐ Anxious/Avoidant. Frequency: <u>Select</u> Describe: <u>Distancer in mar-</u> riage; using affair to "solve" marital problems.

CF: ☒ Anxious ☐ Avoidant ☐ Anxious/Avoidant. Frequency: <u>Select</u> Describe: <u>When feels unsafe,</u> generally pursues connection, often through conflict or approval from friends.

CM: ☐ Anxious ☒ Avoidant ☐ Anxious/Avoidant. Frequency: <u>Select</u> Describe: <u>Generally avoids</u> conflict; tries to be perfect to avoid criticism.

Additional: _____

Solution-Based Assessment

Attempted Solutions that DIDN'T work:

1. Parents lecturing CF16 has not reduced her drinking and drug use.

2. AF36 setting harsh but unenforced consequences not working; stalling on moving forward with the divorce may not be as effective as hoped.

Exceptions and Unique Outcomes (Solutions that DID work): Times, places, relationships, contexts, etc., when problem is less of a problem; behaviors that seem to make things even slightly better:

1. CF16 reports choosing to not continue using harder drugs because she is afraid of them; although her grades have dropped, she is still passing; she has retained some friends who support healthier choices.

2. CF16 reports using less the weekend the family went out of town.

Miracle Question/Answer: If the problem were to be resolved overnight, what would client be doing differently the next day? (Describe in terms of doing X rather than not doing Y):

1. AF and AM would wake up in the same house, happy to be together (AF and kids).

2. CF would have new group of friends; more freedom if able to prove making good decisions re: substances (parents; CF somewhat agree).

3. CF and CM would both be getting good grades, involved in school activities, and the family would have more fun family adventures.

(continued)

Postmodern: Social Location and Dominant Discourses

Describe the client(s) overall social location (the groups a person belongs to based on diversity factors) and influential dominant discourses related to presenting concerns:

- *Ethnic, Race, Class, Immigration Status, and Religious Discourses: How do key cultural inform client identity(ies) and what is perceived as the problem and possible solutions (specify ethnicity, e.g., Italian American rather than white or Caucasian)?* AF36's cultural, religious, and family background reinforce the idea that divorce is a sin, which is creating significant internal struggle for her because a part of her believes it is unwise to remain in a relationship with a man who will not leave his mistress. This view seems to increase the stress of the potential divorce for all family members, possibly informing CF16's acting out and CM14's withdrawal.

- *Gender and Sexuality Discourses: How do gender and sexuality discourses inform identity(ies) and what is perceived as a problem and the possible solutions? Do these intersect with ethnicity and/or religion?* Although AF36 maintains many traditional Mexican views on family and even her role as a wife and mother, she also holds modern American views on women's rights in relationships, especially with regard to accepting her husband's affair.

- *Community, School, Work, and/or Extended Family Discourses: How do other important community discourses inform identity(ies) and what is perceived as a problem and the possible solutions?* CF16 is now hanging around with a "party" crowd, which is shifting how she defines herself and her family.

- *Identity Narratives: How has the problem shaped each significant person's identity?* AF36 feels extremely conflicted between her traditional cultural and religious values and her modern gender identity; AM34 reports some guilt but a stronger pull to do what is true in his heart—he appears to be trying to reclaim an emotional side of himself that he has not frequently acted upon; CF16 reports feeling a sense of power and freedom with her new party lifestyle that separates her from the chaos at home; CM14 is focusing all of his energy into his studies but slowly losing connection with friends and family.

Client Perspectives (Optional)

Areas of Agreement: Based on what the client(s) has(ve) said, what parts of the above assessment do they agree with or are likely to agree with? Role of AF36 family, family dynamics

Areas of Disagreement: What parts do they disagree with or are likely to disagree with? Why? Depiction of CM14 potentially having problems down the road because they view him as the "star" right now.

How do you plan to respectfully work with areas of potential disagreement? Tentatively raise issues related to CM14 functioning, perhaps after CF16 has shown initial improvements

12

Clinical Assessment

Learning Objectives

After reading this chapter and a few hours of focused studying, you should be able to:

- Identify the purpose of as well as potential risks associated with diagnostic assessment.

- Describe social justice and gender issues related to mental health diagnosis.

- Articulate at least one clinical assessment approach that is consistent with family therapy theories.

- Complete a clinical assessment using the forms provided.

- Outline the major innovations and changes in the DSM-5.

Step 2: Identifying Oases and Obstacles

After completing a case conceptualization (see Chapter 11), you have a good sense of the "big picture" as it relates to the client and the problem and are probably feeling ready to set out on your therapeutic journey. But before you do, there is another type of assessment that will help you avoid obstacles and identify rest stops: clinical assessment. Clinical assessment focuses more on the psychological and health dynamics of clients, allowing you to have a better sense of how to more effectively partner with them as you start off on your journey. Although often assessment may not turn up information that causes you to radically shift direction from your case conceptualization, sometimes it does—and when it does, you will be very glad you spent the time to ask.

Clinical Assessment and Diagnosis

Mental health professionals from all disciplines—psychology, psychiatry, psychiatric nursing, counseling, family therapy, and social work—share a common set of standards related to clinical assessment:

- Monitoring for client safety
- Monitoring for medical and psychiatric conditions that warrant medical attention outside the therapist's scope of practice
- Performing a **mental status exam** and making a **mental health diagnosis**
- Case management, including referrals to necessary social services

Although these basic skills are required of all mental health practitioners, therapists generally have significant freedom in choosing *how* they perform these tasks: through structured or unstructured interview methods, written or verbal assessments, or standardized or original instruments. The best method depends on the clinical setting and client characteristics. Although considered standard practice, therapists should be mindful that clinical assessment and diagnosis have both benefits and potential liabilities.

Purpose of Clinical Assessment and Diagnosis

Clinical assessment and mental health diagnosis serve several practical purposes. They can help therapists: (a) coordinate care with other professions, (b) decide how best to keep clients and the public safe, (c) determine the need for referrals and additional services, and (d) identify potential courses of treatment. Diagnostic language provides a relatively simple way for a wide range of medical and mental health professionals to serve the same client—if we all had different systems of identifying problems, coordinating care would be far more challenging. In addition, certain diagnoses are known to be correlated with particular crisis issues, such as depression and suicide and self-harm; thus, diagnosis can help clinicians remember to screen for potential crises and assist clients in seeking more appropriate resources. Furthermore, certain diagnoses have a well-established research base that helps the clinician identify a preferred treatment method, such as behavioral interventions for phobias.

Moreover, some clients find that having a diagnosis is helpful, even liberating. For example, many survivors of sexual abuse are relieved to hear that the symptoms they are experiencing—hypervigilance, nightmares, and flashbacks—are part of a larger syndrome, post-traumatic stress disorder, and that this condition has a good prognosis. Similarly, depending on their view of mental health diagnosis, some clients with whom I have worked report feeling relief when they learn that they (or their partner) meet the criteria for major depressive disorder, a condition that is less severe or humiliating than they feared (such as "lazy," "uncaring," "out of love," or "really crazy").

In addition to potential clinical benefits, there are some practical benefits for researchers and third-party payers. An inspiring example, because researchers around the globe have been able to collectively study the diagnoses of "autism" and "Asperger's syndrome," they have been able to move forward a focused research agenda that has dramatically changed our understanding of and the prognosis for these disorders (American Psychiatric Association [APA], 2013). Without an agreed-upon set of diagnostic definitions and criteria, researchers would have had no way to coordinate their efforts in order to better the lives of children and families struggling with these issues. In a similar fashion, having agreed-upon descriptions and criteria for mental health concerns makes it possible for third-party payers to reimburse persons diagnosed with a particular condition, enabling mental health services to be paid through health insurance and similar mechanisms. Although not everyone may agree that it is ultimately desirable to have insurance involved in mental health treatment, it is a reality for many who need services, and most clients of average or lower financial means would have much greater difficulty utilizing services without the help of insurance.

Diagnosis and Our Inescapable Cultural Lenses

Each therapist views a client through a unique lens. As a therapist, your lens is your personal culture, values, history, beliefs, and norms. These things generally make us who we are and they cannot be cast aside by simply telling yourself to be "neutral." In addition, systemic therapists remind us that we are part of the system we are trying to observe, thus significantly influencing the behavior of the observed (Keeney, 1983). Think about it: the last time you were in a doctor's office describing your medical problem, were you your "normal self"? Most of us significantly alter how we speak and act when working with a professional, making it more difficult for the professional to get an accurate read of what is happening. In addition, any words the therapist uses to describe the client, comes from the *therapist's* worldview, not the client's. Therapist's descriptions of clients reveal more about the therapist than the client: clinical assessment reveals what the therapist and the broader mental health culture values as "good," "healthy," and "valuable" enough to focus on.

Postmodern philosophers are keenly aware of the intersubjectivity that occurs in therapeutic relationships. Two "horizons of meaning" or worldviews meet when therapist and client talk (Gadamer, 1975). Because therapists cannot step out of their cultures, beliefs, personalities, histories, or theoretical training in order to be neutral and unbiased, therapists must always interpret the client from where they are standing, their particular horizon of meaning. For example, a Latina therapist who grew up in a well-to-do suburb will have a different interpretation of an urban teen's story than a Latina whose parents were migrant farm labors, with neither being necessarily more accurate than the other. The "nearness" of the suburban therapist does not ensure greater accuracy because the therapist may have *more* biases from repeat encounters with this type of client; the rural therapist may be more objective or more biased, depending on how aware the therapist is of his or her horizon of meaning and its effects on viewing the client. Thus, therapists' ability to become aware of their lenses (horizon for making meaning and interpreting others) increases their ability to see the other person more clearly and with less unreflected bias. When beginning their journey, all therapists have limited awareness of the lenses through which they view others. Part of the goal of training is to help therapists to be aware of the lenses through which they view their clients.

At the same time, however, professional training provides therapists with an entirely new set of lenses in the form of theories of health and normalcy. These can also be problematic, especially when working with people who are inherently different from the norm, such as cultural, sexual, or other minority clients. Mental health practitioners use the *Diagnostic and Statistical Manual* (DSM; APA, 2013). Statistics are based on *norms,* making it difficult to accurately apply DSM criteria to those whose demographics vary significantly from the norm. Clinical assessment is one of the most dangerous places for therapists to practice if they are not clearly aware of their personal biases, because there is little feedback if one gets off course.

For example, when you try using a counseling technique that is not appropriate for a client, it is often immediately obvious because the client will refuse to participate or in some way signal that he or she does not like the idea—the major exception to this is a client who wants to please the therapist. Similarly, if one's case conceptualization is incorrect, the client will not progress and/or new information will come to light that helps the therapist refine the conceptualization as part of the hypothesizing process itself; case conceptualization is by nature a process of hypothesizing, gathering feedback from the family through interactions, then refining the hypothesis based on this information. However, when doing clinical assessment, it is easier to get off course.

The medical model that informs DSM diagnosis is based on the concept that the professional has access to a more precise truth; thus, the therapist is less likely to continually question and refine diagnoses and mental status reports (Anderson, 1997). The model is predicated on the assumption that it is easy to distinguish between normal and abnormal behaviors, which is more difficult in the psychological than in the physical realm. For example, behaviors such as drinking, talking, emoting, eating, worrying, or seeing ghosts have different meanings and norms depending on one's family, culture, social class, etc.

Thus, although it *appears* that we begin with a clear set of norms for mental health, when a therapist begins to fully attend to the broader social context of the client, it becomes much less clear where normal ends and abnormal begins. In fact, some argue that because the concept of "mental illness" lacks any reliable corollary measurement of health, it is more of a socially constructed myth than factual science (Hansen, 2003). Furthermore, just because medications can ameliorate psychiatric symptoms, this validates only the drugs' effectiveness, not the particular diagnostic categories. Thus, therapists must cautiously and thoughtfully approach diagnosis, especially with diverse clients.

Diagnosis and Gender

Although the authors of the DSM tried to reduced gender bias while developing the most recent edition (APA, 2013), historically, the enterprise of psychiatric diagnosis is frequently criticized for pathologizing feminine traits and behaviors while failing to develop diagnoses for issues more likely to affect men (Eriksen & Kress, 2008). Feminists argue that diagnoses such as nymphomania, hysteria, neurasthenia, erotomania, kleptomania, and masochism have served to unnecessarily pathologize and subordinate women (Eriksen & Kress, 2008). In particular, personality diagnoses, such as borderline, dependent, and histrionic, can be understood as an exaggeration of otherwise socially promoted female qualities. Furthermore, several studies have shown that women who enter treatment are more likely to be characterized as "unhealthy" by professionals simply because they exhibit typical female qualities, such as greater emotional expression, less independence, and less goal-directed activity and are more easily influenced by others (Eriksen & Kress, 2008). Thus, therapists need to carefully attend to gender bias when making diagnoses, carefully considering whether female clients are being overpathologized. Conversely, some argue that men may be underdiagnosed, especially if they are reticent to talk about emotions, and are therefore potentially undertreated.

Social Justice and the Cultural Case Formulation

As part of an attempt to address the cultural bias of the DSM, the most recent edition includes a cultural formulation and cultural interview protocol to assist clinicians in considering cultural and diversity issues when conducting a clinical assessment and making a diagnosis (APA, 2013; see "Cultural Formulation and Assessment," below). In particular, therapists committed to social justice may find this interview useful in their work. Similar to case conceptualization, discussed in Chapter 11, *cultural formulation* invites clinicians to take a step back and learn from clients about how their problems (or apparent problems) are understood within their cultural context as well as consider relevant sociopolitical and social justice issues. In situations in which they are ostracized, marginalized, or abused, most people act and behave in ways that may appear odd or pathological because of the inherent trauma, stigma, and social pressures. For example, in some cases, people *are* out to get your client—the client isn't paranoid and actually needs assistance with ensuring personal safety. In other cases, what may look like paranoia, depression, or anxiety may actually be best understood as post-traumatic stress disorder, which may be due to abuse or maltreatment related to cultural and social differences. Thus, therapists need to perform a broad, socially aware assessment of their clients to ensure accurate and appropriate diagnoses. Building on the cultural formulation in the DSM-IV (APA, 2000), the DSM-5 (APA, 2013) includes a revised outline for cultural formulation as well as an interview guide, complete with sample prompts and questions to be used in session to gather cultural information (see "Cultural Formulation and Assessment," below; APA, 2013, pp. 752–775).

Try It Yourself

With a partner, share your thoughts on psychiatric diagnosis and how a person's social location may affect this process.

Mental Health Diagnosis in Family Therapy

Systemic Perspectives on Diagnosis

From a systemic perspective, a diagnosis describes the behaviors that a person has adopted to maintain balance in his or her current web of relationships; given a different set of circumstances, it is possible and even likely that the person will have a different set of behaviors, thoughts, and feelings. Thus, a diagnosis is not viewed as an illness or an inherently individual phenomenon, as it is in the traditional medical model. This does not mean that neurological changes have not occurred or that medication is unnecessary. Physiology interacts with the environment in an interdependent, mutually reinforcing system: when depression is part of maintaining a system's balance, the depressed person is likely to develop physiological symptoms of depression.

Postmodern Perspectives on Diagnosis

Postmodern therapists are skeptical of diagnoses because these become labels that clients use to inform their identity, often silencing their strengths, resiliencies, and capabilities (Gergen, Anderson, & Hoffman, 1996). Once they are given a diagnostic label, clients tend to interpret future behaviors and events through this lens, creating a self-fulfilling prophecy. For example, when a child is diagnosed with ADHD, parents, teachers, and the child tend to develop telescopic vision, focusing their attention on the child's hyperactivity and attention deficit and missing exceptions to the label as well as other elements of the child's identity, such as the fact that the child mentors a younger sibling, has a musical talent, or cares about the family.

A General Family Therapy Approach to Diagnosis

Although some differences exist between postmodern and systemic perspectives on mental health diagnosis, there is general agreement that diagnosis can focus on what is *least* likely to help the therapist effectively treat the client. When therapists focus on psychiatric symptoms and codes of classifications, they are less likely to bring about change using the models that are most closely associated with family therapy. However, this does not mean that family therapists should avoid diagnosis and the medical model altogether. Instead, they should find the proper place for diagnosis, which family therapists would say is "one voice among many."

Whether working from a systemic or a postmodern approach, most family therapists value multiple descriptions of problems. For example, in Milan and Mental Research Institute (MRI) systemic approaches, each family member's description of the problem is used to construct the hypotheses about the family dynamics (Selvini Palazzoli et al., 1978; Watzlawick, Weakland, & Fisch, 1974). Similarly, in collaborative therapy, multiple, contradictory descriptions of the problem are allowed to coexist to encourage the generation of new possibilities and understandings (Anderson, 1997). Thus, each description of the problem is considered one of many possible "truths" that depend on webs of relationships and social discourse; it does not stand on its own. For example, even though a person may meet the diagnostic criteria for major depressive disorder at a given time based on one or more persons' description of the problem, this diagnosis does not carry the same fixed or essential truth that it would in traditional psychiatry. Instead, family therapists recognize that the symptoms, feelings, and behaviors that qualify a person for this diagnosis are subject to change based on the meanings generated by the person's relationships.

The importance of the diagnosis also varies from client to client rather than always being considered more important than other perspectives. Diagnosis is one voice in the conversation, a description that clients and therapists are free to question, try on, and refine. Therapists, outside professionals, or clients may introduce medical studies and knowledge into the conversation, but they never use medical knowledge to silence the voices or ignore the unique experiences of clients or therapists that may or may not be in alignment with this particular form of knowledge. In some cases, the diagnosis that fits early in treatment rapidly loses its meaning. At other times, clients use diagnostic descriptions to move forward with their goals, hopes, and dreams. The therapist's task is to be flexible in allowing a wide range of possible in-session uses for diagnosis with each client rather than insisting on the same diagnostic label based on the therapist's philosophy.

Contemporary Issues in Diagnosis

Dimensional Assessment: The Future of Diagnosis

In 2013, the American Psychiatric Association released the DSM-5, which represents the most significant change to mental health diagnosis in over 30 years. Some of the more noteworthy changes in this manual include the removal of the five-axis diagnosis system, reorganization of the chapters, and inclusion of new assessment measures (APA, 2013). However, the most significant changes associated with this version are arguably at a more fundamental and philosophical level: the DSM-5 represents the initial efforts to shift away from identifying discrete categories of mental disorders, for which there is less supportive evidence, and a move toward a dimensional approach to diagnosis that recognizes the heterogeneity of symptoms within and across disorders (APA, 2013). For example, the new DSM conceptualizes substance use problems along a spectrum of mild to severe rather than two discrete categories of abuse and dependence, for which only arbitrary distinctions could be made. Although there is insufficient science to propose alternative definitions for most disorders at this time, the new structure of the manual is designed to serve as a bridge between the historic categorical approach to diagnosis to the more likely future version with a dimensional approach, which will better account for the wide variation and forms that mental health disorders can take.

Toward this end, the National Institute of Mental Health will focus future research on Research Domain Criteria (RDoC), a project designed to "transform [mental health] diagnosis by incorporating genetics, imaging, cognitive science, and other levels of information to lay the foundation for a new classification system" (Insel, 2013, para. 3). Future federally funded research will focus more on general domains of symptoms and functioning than on specific diagnoses, as it has in the past. Thus, future research may include all clients in a mood disorder clinic rather than exclude participants who don't meet strict diagnosis criteria. The overarching goal will be to develop a system of mental health diagnosis that more accurately captures the complexity of human psychological functioning. These potential changes would begin to address some of the concerns raised by humanistic, systemic, and postmodern critics about the effects of labeling on a person's identity and the therapist process.

The Recovery Model and Diagnosis

At the same time that psychiatrists and researchers are reconceptualizing the future direction of mental health diagnosis, consumer movements related to mental health treatment have become formally recognized and mainstreamed. An international movement, the Recovery Model is quickly reshaping how government-funded agencies view diagnosis and mental illness (Davidson et al., 2008; Fisher & Chamberlin, 2004; Onken et al., 2007; Repper & Perkins, 2006). With its origins in consumer self-help in the 1930s, the Recovery Movement captured the attention of rehabilitation and substance abuse professionals in the 1990s and mental health policy makers since 2000, having been formally adopted by most first-world countries. In the United States, the 2002 New Freedom Commission on Mental Health proposed transforming the national mental health system using a paradigm of recovery, and in 2004 the Department of Health and Human Services launched a nationwide recovery campaign (Fisher & Chamberlin, 2004; U.S. Department of Health and Human Services, 2004).

Emerging research findings have led to wide adoption of the recovery movement. In the 1990s, the World Health Organization (WHO) released research findings from a cross-national study on recovery from severe mental illness that revealed surprising results: 28% of patients diagnosed with severe mental illness (e.g., schizophrenia, bipolar disorder, etc.) make a full recovery and 52% reported a social recovery (e.g., able to return to work, satisfying family relationships, etc.; Ralph, 2000). Similarly, the Open Dialogue approach to treating clients with psychotic symptoms, a collaborative therapy approach that shares principles similar to those of the Recovery Model, has even more impressive outcomes: 83% of first-episode psychosis patients return to work and 77% have no remaining psychotic symptoms after two years of treatment (Haarakangas et al., 2007; Seikkula, 2002). These findings do not fit with medical model assumptions about severe mental illness—assumptions that the genetic and biological predispositions precluded meaningful recovery (Ramon, Healy, & Renouf, 2007). Thus, the Recovery Model is about helping clients lead rich, meaningful lives rather than simply reducing symptoms related to a mental health diagnosis; this perspective resonates with the field of mental health and its historically uneasy relationship with the medical model and its emphasis on pathology.

The Department of Health and Human Services (2004) defines mental health recovery as "a journey of healing and transformation enabling a person with a mental health problem to live a meaningful life in a community of his or her choice while striving to achieve his or her full potential" (p. 2). The recovery model uses a social model of disability rather than a medical model; thus, it deemphasizes diagnostic labeling and emphasizes psychosocial functioning, an emphasis that is the hallmark of family approaches. The "National Consensus Statement on Mental Health Recovery" includes "10 Fundamental Components of Recovery" (U.S. Department of Health and Human Services, 2004):

COMPONENTS OF MENTAL HEALTH RECOVERY-ORIENTED CARE

- **Self-direction:** Consumers (clients) exercise choice over their path to recovery/treatment.
- **Individualized/person-centered:** Paths to recovery are individualized based a person's unique strengths, resiliencies, preferences, experiences, and cultural background.
- **Empowerment:** Consumers have the authority to choose from a range of options and participate in decision making; professional relationships encourage decision making and assertiveness.
- **Holistic:** Recovery encompasses all aspects of life: mind, body, spirit, and community.
- **Nonlinear:** Recovery is not a step-by-step process but rather an ongoing process that includes growth and setbacks.
- **Strengths-based:** Recovery focuses on valuing and building upon strengths, resiliencies, and abilities.
- **Peer support:** Consumers are encouraged to engage with other consumers in pursuing recovery.
- **Respect:** For recovery to occur, consumers need to experience respect from professionals, their communities, and other systems.
- **Responsibility:** Consumers are personally responsible for their recovery and self-care.
- **Hope:** Recovery requires a belief in the self and a willingness to persevere through difficulty.

These elements play leading roles in many family therapy theories, most notably approaches such as systemic–structural (e.g., holistic view; see Chapters 4 and 5), humanistic (e.g., hope, respect, and responsibility; see Chapter 6), solution-based therapy (e.g., emphasis on client strengths, empowerment, and hope; see Chapter 9), and postmodern (e.g., views "client as the expert"; people as separate from problems; dealing with social stigma, peer support, etc.; see Chapter 10). The Recovery Movement's approach to harnessing client strengths to help them fashion meaningful lives while reducing the expert role of the therapist fits with many approaches to working with clients diagnosed with severe mental illness. Although diagnosis still has its place, both family therapy models and the Recovery Model share the premise that diagnosis is not the most beneficial driving force of treatment, as it is in the medical model. Instead the client's motivation for a quality life directs the course of treatment.

Therapists can draw from numerous approaches to facilitate mental health recovery (Gehart, 2012a). For example, using principles from narrative therapy (see Chapter 10), a therapist could help clients restory their identity narratives related to their diagnoses:

- How has being diagnosed with mental illness changed how you see yourself, your role in relationships, and/or your role in society? Where did you get these ideas? Do you think they are fair and accurate?
- Do you think being diagnosed with XXX changes your value as a person? Why or why not? How? Where did these ideas come from?
- How did you define yourself before the [diagnosis or symptoms] began? How did you develop these ideas about who you were? Did others see you this way? Do you think this depiction is still true today in some ways?
- Do you believe that you can still lead a meaningful life with the symptoms you are experiencing? If not, where did you get this idea? If so, how can you make this happen? (Gehart, 2012b, p. 451).

Try It Yourself

With a partner or on your own, share your perspective on the concept of recovery and severe mental illness. Do you know anyone who has struggled with recovering from a chronic mental health condition, such as schizophrenia, bipolar disorder, or persistent depression?

Parity and Nonparity Diagnoses

A seemingly minor development in the field of mental health that will significantly shape the future of the field, certain mental health disorders have recently been deemed to be "equal" to physical health conditions in laws regulating insurance reimbursement. The Paul Wellstone and Pete Domenici Mental Health Parity and Addiction Equity Act was passed as part of the Economic Stabilization Act of 2008. This act requires that insurance companies reimburse for mental health and substance abuse disorders the same as for any other physiological disorders, thereby requiring insurance companies to cover mental health issues as part of their health plans. Prior to the bill's passage, only approximately 30 states had mental health parity laws.

State mental health parity laws, which tend to be more comprehensive than the federal act passed in 2008, often distinguish between parity and nonparity diagnoses. When a client is diagnosed with a *parity* mental health diagnosis, insurance plans must reimburse the same as they would for physiological disorders, which most critically implies that the number of sessions cannot be artificially limited as was previously the practice with HMO-type plans and co-pays must be the same as those for physiological disorders.

Parity diagnoses typically include severe mental health disorders and must be the *primary diagnosis* (first one listed) in order for insurance co-pays and reimbursement policies to apply. Parity diagnoses typically include:

- Anorexia and bulimia
- Bipolar disorder
- Major depressive disorder
- Obsessive–compulsive disorder (OCD)
- Panic disorder
- Pervasive-developmental disorder
- Schizoaffective disorder
- Schizophrenia
- Any mental health disorder in children (including Adjustment Disorders)

Introduction to the DSM-5

Even if you are of the generation that was never trained using the DSM-IV, you are guaranteed to encounter client files, supervisors, billing systems, and other texts that refer to it. So, this following section is designed to help both Generation-IV and Generation-5 therapists successfully engage with the core features of the DSM-5 and its most critical cross-diagnosis changes.

Title of the DSM-5

One of the first changes a seasoned clinician may notice is the shortened title: *DSM-5* (note that using a hyphen is the correct format). The APA decided to stop using the Roman numeral system (DSM-V is considered incorrect) and switch to Arabic numerals to more easily allow for multiple text revisions in the years ahead. Digital technologies will enable updated publication of a DSM-5.1 and DSM-5.2, etc. Given expected changes, such as new diagnosis codes with the *International Statistical Classification of Diseases and Related Health Problems,* 11th ed. (ICD-11) due out in 2018 (see "Diagnostic Codes and the ICD" below), more frequent text revisions may be particularly important in the future.

Manual Structure

Unlike the DSM-IV, there are three major sections of the DSM-5 in addition to the appendices:

- Section I: DSM-5 Basics
  - History of the manual
  - Use of the manual and cautionary statements
  - Definition of a mental disorder
- Section II: Diagnostic Criteria and Codes
  - 20 chapters that describe recognized disorders
- Section III: Emerging measures and models
  - Emerging assessment measures
  - Cultural formulation
  - Alternative DSM-5 model for personality disorders
  - Conditions for further study
- Appendices
  - Highlights of changes
  - Glossaries of technical terms and cultural concepts of distress
  - Various listings of the disorders and codes

Organization of Diagnostic Chapters

For those familiar with the DSM-IV, one of the most notable changes in the DSM-5 is the reorganization of chapters in the new Section II. The chapters have been reorganized to more closely group disorders by known etiologies, underlying vulnerabilities, symptom characteristics, and shared environmental factors. The intention behind this reorganization is to facilitate more comprehensive diagnostic and treatment approaches as well as facilitate research across related disorders (APA, 2013).

Of particular note, the DSM-IV chapter "Disorders Usually Diagnosed in Infancy, Childhood, and Adolescents" was removed, and these disorders have been placed in other chapters based on common causes. Each DSM-5 chapter is organized developmentally, with those occurring in childhood toward the front of the chapter and those associated with later life toward the end. In addition, the 20 diagnostic chapters are broadly organized with *internalizing disorders* (those with mostly emotional and cognitive symptoms that occur within the person) first and *externalizing disorders* (those with more behavioral and external symptoms) second.

DSM-5 Chapters Describing Mental Health Disorders (Section II)

1. Neurodevelopmental Disorders
2. Schizophrenia Spectrum and Other Psychotic Disorders
3. Bipolar and Related Disorders
4. Depressive Disorders
5. Anxiety Disorders
6. Obsessive–Compulsive and Related Disorders
7. Trauma- and Stressor-Related Disorders
8. Dissociative Disorders
9. Somatic Symptom Disorders
10. Feeding and Eating Disorders
11. Elimination Disorders
12. Sleep–Wake Disorders
13. Sexual Dysfunctions
14. Gender Dysphoria
15. Disruptive, Impulse Control and Conduct Disorders
16. Substance Use and Addictive Disorders
17. Neurocognitive Disorders
18. Personality Disorders
19. Paraphilic Disorders
20. Other Conditions that May be the Focus of Clinical Attention (V/Z codes)

Note: Similar to the DSM-IV, the DSM-5 does not include chapter numbers; the above numbers are added to facilitate learning and answer the burning question: how many chapters is that?

Diagnostic Codes and the ICD

The diagnostic coding system in the DSM-5 is derived from another set of diagnostic codes, those published in the ICD. Published by the WHO, the ICD is the most widely used set of diagnostic codes, and like DSM, it attempts to statistically classify health disorders. It is used internationally by virtually all physical health practitioners and is used in most other countries for mental health diagnosis as well. The codes in the DSM-IV correlated to the ICD-9 (the ninth edition). These same five-digit codes are included in the DSM-5 as the first code you will see. In October 2015, the United States finally adopted ICD-10 codes, which have been used in other countries since 1994 (the ICD-10 was released by WHO in 1990). The delayed implementation of ICD-10 codes in the United States was due to the bureaucratic complexity and expense of the task in such a large health care system.

The ICD-10 codes are alphanumeric codes that are included in the DSM-5 in parentheses and in gray text next to the old ICD-9 codes.

To complicate matters further, during the revision of the DSM-5, the WHO worked with the APA to correlate DSM-5 and ICD-11 codes and criteria for mental illness. The ICD-11 is due out in 2018, however, it may be awhile until the ICD-11 codes are implemented in the United States. The ICD-11 codes are expected to be longer alphanumeric codes than those in the ICD-10 to allow for a greater number of diagnostic codes, which is a significant issue for the medical health professions.

	ICD-9	ICD-10
Diagnostic Code Format	###.##	A##.#
Sample Diagnosis: Major Depression, Recurrent, Severe	296.33	F33.2
Sample Diagnosis: Disruption of Family by Separation or Divorce	V61.03	Z63.5

New Diagnosis Format

The five-axis system used in the DSM-IV was removed from the DSM-5 and a nonaxial (i.e., single-line) system is used instead (APA, 2013). The nonaxial diagnosis approach was identified as an option in the DSM-IV, text revision (DSM-IV-TR), however, most clinicians and third-party payers used the five-axis approach. In the nonaxial system, diagnoses from the former Axis I (mental health diagnosis), Axis II (personality disorders and mental retardation), and Axis III (physical health issues affecting mental health) are simply listed out, generally on a single line or set of lines. In addition, former Axis IV issues (psychosocial and environmental problems that may affect diagnosis, treatment, and prognosis) are recorded similarly to other diagnoses using ICD-9 "V codes" or ICD-10 "Z codes." The former Axis V (global assessment of functioning [GAF] score) has been removed. Although no required replacement for the GAF was identified, the WHODAS (WHO Disability Assessment Schedule) is included in Section III of the DSM-5 as an optional global measure of disability (APA, 2013). As in the former diagnosis system, the principal diagnosis or reason for visit should be listed first.

Quick Review: DSM-IV Five-Axis Diagnosis Format

For those unfamiliar with the five-axis system, it is reviewed here. You will find it referred to both in professional literature and client files for years to come.

DSM-IV FIVE-AXIS DIAGNOSIS FORMAT

- **Axis I:** Clinical disorders that are the focus of treatment, including developmental and learning disorders; primary reason for visit listed first.
- **Axis II:** Underlying or pervasive conditions, including personality disorders, defensive mechanisms, and mental retardation.
- **Axis III:** Medical conditions and disorders
- **Axis IV:** Psychosocial stressors and environmental conditions that may be contributing to condition and/or its treatment, such as:
  - problems with the primary support system (family, partner, etc.)
  - economic or housing problems

(continued)

DSM-IV FIVE-AXIS DIAGNOSIS FORMAT (*CONTINUED*)

- problems accessing health care
- legal situations
- social, school, and/or occupational issues
- **Axis V:** GAF score: a score from 0 to 100 indicating level of functioning.

  - **70 and above:** Indicates adaptive coping, with higher scores indicating greater mental health
  - **60–69:** Mild symptoms (Most third-party payers require a client's level of functioning be 69 or below to be a reimbursable medical expense.)
  - **50–59:** Moderate symptoms
  - **40–49:** Severe systems
  - **39 and below:** Significant impairment that generally requires hospitalization and intensive treatment.

DSM-5 EQUIVALENTS TO DSM-IV FORMAT

DSM-IV FIVE-AXIS SYSTEM	DSM-5 EQUIVALENT
Axis I: Mental Health Disorders	Record on diagnosis line (primary reason for visit listed first)
Axis II: Personality Disorders and Mental Retardation	Record on diagnosis line (primary reason for visit listed first)
Axis III: General Medical Conditions	Record on diagnosis line (especially those important to understanding mental disorder)
Axis IV: Psychosocial and Environmental Problems	Record on diagnosis line using V, Z, or T codes from chapter on "Other Conditions that May be the Focus of Clinical Attention"
Axis V: Global Assessment of Functioning	Optional use of WHODAS scale

The formatting for a DSM-5 diagnosis is simpler than that for the former five-axis diagnosis. In most cases, third-party payers, such as insurance companies, will provide several numbered lines; these do not correlate to axes but rather are a prompt to write one diagnosis per line. The diagnostic code generally goes first and then the name of the diagnosis followed by any specifiers (see "Subtypes and Specifiers," below).

INSURANCE COMPANY/THIRD PARTY PROMPT:

Diagnosis(ses)

1. _____
2. _____
3. _____
4. _____

The diagnosis is written as follows:

DSM-5 DIAGNOSIS FORMAT SAMPLE (ICD-10 CODES)

1. <u>F33.1 Major depressive disorder, recurrent, moderate, with mild anxious distress</u>
2. <u>F43.10 Post-traumatic stress disorder, with delayed onset</u>
3. <u>Z59.1 Inadequate housing</u>
4. <u>Z59.5 Extreme poverty</u>

Subtypes and Specifiers

The DSM-5 includes several new subtypes and specifiers. Subtypes identify mutually exclusive subgroups within the diagnostic category, whereas specifiers are more general. All subtypes are diagnosis-specific and many are described below with individual diagnoses. Similarly, many specifiers are used with only specific diagnoses; however, several new specifiers are used across several or all diagnoses in the manual. These specifiers are used to note information about a person's condition that may be useful for treatment decisions, often alerting clinicians to additional symptoms or qualities of symptoms that need specific attention in treatment planning. When adding a specifier, the diagnostic code does not change; however, the specifier is written *after* the name of the diagnosis on the diagnosis line (see diagnosis examples above).

Cross-Diagnostic Specifiers

- With catatonia (for neurodevelopmental, psychotic, mood, etc.)
- With anxious distress (depression and bipolar disorders; see example above)
- With panic attacks (all disorders)
- With poor insight (OCD and certain anxiety disorders)
- With mixed features (bipolar and mood disorders)
- In remission or partial remission

In addition, many of the specific diagnoses have new specifiers, such as "with limited prosocial emotions" for conduct disorder (APA, 2013). The new manual clearly lists these condition-specific specifiers after a diagnostic criterion in bold text, making it easy to identify and include the specifiers.

Dimensional Assessment

As mentioned above, emerging research supports a more dimensional approach (variation of intensity on a given symptom or dimension) to mental health diagnosis in contrast to its historical categorical approach (APA, 2013; Narrow et al., 2013). Current research is not sufficiently developed to warrant a radical reorganization of the manual using a dimensional approach; however, in the years ahead, the DSM is likely to move in this direction. Nonetheless, the current DSM takes steps toward the dimensional approach by organizing chapters by etiology and by separating internalizing from externalizing disorders (APA, 2013). In addition, certain diagnoses for which there was sufficient evidence to support the change, dimensional assessments—such as mild, moderate, and severe—were introduced rather than retaining separate and discrete categories to indicate levels of severity. Among the diagnosis that use dimensional assessment in the DSM-5 are:

- Schizophrenia (pen-and-paper assessment available for free download)
- Depression (pen-and-paper assessment available for free download)
- Separation anxiety disorder (pen-and-paper assessment available for free download)
- Specific phobia (pen-and-paper assessment available for free download)
- Social anxiety disorder (pen-and-paper assessment available for free download)

- Panic disorder (pen-and-paper assessment available for free download)
- Agoraphobia (pen-and-paper assessment available for free download)
- Generalized anxiety disorder (pen-and-paper assessment available for free download)
- Post-traumatic stress disorder (pen-and-paper assessment available for free download)
- Acute stress disorder (pen-and-paper assessment available for free download)
- Dissociative symptoms (pen-and-paper assessment available for free download)
- Intellectual disability
- Sexual disorders
- Substance abuse
- Anxious distress specifier

These dimensional assessments are intended to help clinicians assess severity and simplify tracking progress during treatment.

NOS versus NEC Diagnosis

Because of their overuse and lack of clinical utility, the NOS (Not Otherwise Specified) diagnoses of the DSM-IV have been replaced in the DSM-5 with Not-Elsewhere-Classified (NEC) diagnoses, which may be an "other specified disorder" or an "unspecified disorder."

Other Specified Disorder

The other specified disorder allows the clinician to document the specific reason a particular client does not meet the criteria for a specific diagnosis (APA, 2013). This is done by recording the name of the diagnostic category followed by the specific reason the person does not meet the criteria. The text lists common examples of how to write the "other specified" diagnosis for a given diagnosis. For example, in the chapter on depression, three examples of "other specified" are given:

- Recurrent brief depression
- Short-duration depressive episode (4 to 13 days)
- Depressive episode with insufficient symptoms (APA, 2013, p. 183)

Thus, if a client has depressive symptoms for several weeks but does not meet the diagnostic threshold the diagnosis would read: "311. Other specified depressive disorder, depressive episode with insufficient symptoms."

Unspecified Disorders

When the clinician cannot or chooses not to specify the characteristics of the disorder, then the "unspecified disorder" can be used. This is used when a client experiences significant clinical distress but does not meet the criteria for the disorder. This can be used when there is insufficient information, such as that from emergency departments, to make a full diagnosis. Example: "311. Unspecified depressive disorder."

WHODAS 2.0

Another assessment measure that may be used as part of the clinical assessment is the World Health Organization Disability Assessment Schedule 2.0 (WHODAS 2.0; APA, 2013). The most likely replacement for the former Axis V, this measure is 36-item, self-administered test for adults to assess disability across six domains of functioning: communication, getting around, self-care, getting along with people, life activities, and participation in society. The instrument can be scored in two ways:

- *Simple scoring* involves simply adding up points without weighting individual items; this type of scoring can be done by hand.
- *Complex scoring* involves weighting scores based on multiple levels of difficulty for each item. This method requires a computer program from the WHO website, which can convert the score to a 100-point scale, with 100 being full disability.

The instrument is available on the APA resources for the DSM-5, and the adult version is published in the text.

Cultural Formulation and Assessment

As mentioned above, when working with diverse clients, best practices include conducting a **cultural formulation** interview to identify specific cultural issues that may be affecting the presentation and significance of symptoms (APA, 2013). Building on the cultural formulation in the DSM-IV, the DSM-5 includes a revised outline for cultural formulation as well as an interview guide, complete with sample prompts and questions to be used in session to gather cultural information (APA, 2013, pp. 752–775).

The elements of the cultural formulation include:

* Cultural identity of the individual: Involves identifying important racial, ethnic, and cultural reference groups as well as other clinically relevant aspects of identity, such as religious affiliation, socioeconomic status, sexual orientation, and migrant status.
* Cultural conceptualization of distress: Requires outlining the cultural constructs and significance of presenting symptoms.
* Psychosocial stressors and cultural features of vulnerability and resilience: Entails identifying specific stressors and supports related to cultural factors, including the role of religion, family, and social networks.
* Cultural features of the relationship between the individual and the clinician: Requires identifying the cultural, linguistic, and social status issues that may impede communication, therapeutic relationship, diagnosis, and treatment.
* Overall cultural assessment: Involves a summary of the key findings and implications of salient issues for diagnosis and treatment.

Conducting a Clinical Assessment
Diagnostic Interview and Mental Status Exam

In formal clinical environments, therapists are usually asked to conduct a structured diagnostic interview with clients, most frequently called a Mental Status Exam (MSE). Based on the medical model, these exams often involve a more hierarchical, detached therapeutic relationship than that found in most family therapies. If the therapist does not help contextualize the MSE questions that typically come early in the process from the process of therapy, clients may be confused when the therapist shifts to a more empathetic or egalitarian stance. Ideally, family therapists develop strategies for conducting a mental status exam that preserve the type of therapeutic alliance they intend to use throughout treatment.

COMMON ELEMENTS OF STANDARD MENTAL STATUS EXAM (MSE)

Assessed through Observations

* **Appearance:** Observations of client's overall appearance: age, weight, height, grooming, and manner of dress
* **Attitude:** Observations of client's attitude toward the interviewer: cooperative, uncooperative, hostile, guarded, suspicious, or regressed
* **Affect:** Observations of the client's outer expression of emotion: congruent, incongruent, flat, labile, etc.
* **Motor activity:** Observations of client behavior, such as eye contact, gait, tics, tremors, repetitive movements, hyperactivity, or other qualities of movement

(continued)

COMMON ELEMENTS OF STANDARD MENTAL STATUS EXAM (MSE) (CONTINUED)

- **Speech:** Observations of the client's manner of speech: speed, volume, rate, spontaneity, etc.

Assessed with Questions and Observations

- **Mood:** The client's *reported* emotional state, such as euthymic, dysphoric, euphoric, angry, anxious.
  - How have you been feeling recently: Irritable? Elated? Sad? Hopeless? Angry?
  - How often? How long do these emotions last? What situations seem to trigger these moods?
  - What do you think about when you are sad/angry?
- **Sleeping and eating**
  - Have there been any changes in your sleep recently (or since symptoms started)?
  - Have there been any changes in your eating recently (or since symptoms started)?
  - Describe your eating and sleeping habits.
- **Anxiety and trauma**
  - Do you worry a lot? Would your friends say you worry too much?
  - Have you ever had a panic or anxiety attack and felt like you might die?
  - Are there thoughts or images you have a hard time getting out of your head?
  - Do you find yourself repetitively doing the same thing, knowing it does not make sense?
  - Do you ever feel detached from people around you?
- **Psychotic symptoms:** Client reports of unusual sensory experiences, such as hallucinations, illusions, or depersonalization
  - Do you ever see, hear, small, taste, or feel things that others do not experience?
  - Do you have beliefs or knowledge that others do not seem to share?
- **Thought:** Describe thought patterns, concentrations, insight and judgment
  - Are you able to concentrate easily at work/school?
  - What do you think is causing your problems?
  - How would you describe your role in this situation?
  - When you are very upset, do you ever make bad decisions that you later regret?

Mental Status Exam in Couple and Family Therapy

Numerous case conceptualization techniques from family therapy methods lend themselves to clinical assessment while still preserving a strong therapeutic alliance characterized by nonjudgment and empathy. Therapists may choose to use one of these methods rather than the more traditional—and arguably less friendly—set of MSE questions. Broadly speaking, there are two approaches to clinical assessment: systemic and postmodern.

Systemic Approach to the MSE

A systemic approach to assessing a client's mental status and making a diagnosis uses a combination of two common systemic techniques: (a) problem interaction assessment (Watzlawick et al., 1974) and (b) circular questions (Selvini Palazzoli et al., 1978).

As introduced in Chapter 4, *systemic problem assessment* involves tracing interactions from initial homeostasis to escalation of symptoms (the positive feedback loop) until the system returns to normal or homeostasis. When using this assessment for mental status, the therapist should select a time when the presenting symptom occurs. This assessment describes the following:

1. The initial homeostasis (what was going on before the problem/symptom occurred)
2. The trigger that started an escalation in the system
3. The first person's behavioral response/symptom
4. The second (and additional) person's behavioral response to the first person
5. The first person's response to the second person
6. The back-and-forth interactions that occur between people until the symptoms dissipate and some sort of "normalcy" or "homeostasis" is restored

Therapists can use variants on *circular questions* to inquire about each person's symptoms at each stage of the cycle:

SYSTEMIC CLINICAL ASSESSMENT QUESTIONS

- Describe your mood during each phase of the cycle of events. Describe the mood of others during each phase. How do these compare?

- Does this cycle affect your sleeping or eating patterns? How does this compare to "normal" times?

- During this cycle, do you experience any unusual thoughts or experiences, such as feeling a sense of panic, seeing things other people do not, feeling disconnected from yourself or the situation, or engaging in repetitive behaviors or thoughts? Do these sorts of things happen outside the problem cycle of events?

- Do you ever use alcohol, drugs, or other things to help manage your feelings when things feel out of control? Does anyone else?

- At any time do you have thoughts of hurting yourself or others? Have you had these thoughts in the past? Are these feelings stronger or weaker during the escalation of events?

- Have you ever inflicted physical pain on yourself to manage emotions? Have you thought about it? When are these thoughts the strongest? The weakest?

- Have you or anyone else involved in this cycle used physical violence or emotional abuse? Is it worse or better during the problem cycle you describe?

- Did you experience any childhood abuse: sexual, physical, emotional, or neglect? Do you think these experiences are affecting the current problem cycle of behaviors?

- Have you experienced physical or sexual assault or abuse as an adult? Do you think these experiences are affecting the current problem cycle of behaviors?

- Are there any medical or physical issues that might be affecting the problem cycle you describe?

Postmodern Approach to the MSE

A mental status exam from a postmodern perspective involves honoring a client's description and perception of the problem. Narrative therapists can easily adapt the technique of mapping the influence of problems and persons (White & Epston, 1990; see Chapter 10) to collect information for a mental status exam and make a diagnosis. Mapping the influence of the problem involves the following:

1. Mapping the effect of the problem on persons in the areas of individual, relational, social, and spiritual functioning
2. Mapping the effect of persons on problems in the areas of individual, relational, social, and spiritual functioning

Therapists can ask the following questions to gather the information necessary for a diagnosis:

POSTMODERN APPROACH TO CLINICAL ASSESSMENT

Mapping the Effects of the Problem

- How does the problem affect you and others who are involved? Are there changes in:
  - Mood
  - Eating and sleeping
  - Feelings of panic, worry, or obsessive thinking
  - Seeing or hearing what others do not
  - Drinking or drug use
  - Thoughts of harming oneself or others
  - Cutting or other self-harming behaviors
  - Violent behaviors by self or others
- Is there a history of sexual, physical, or emotional abuse in childhood or adulthood that may be affecting the situation?
- How does the problem affect your relationships at home, work, school, extended family, or social circle?
- How does the problem affect your participation in social activities?
- How does the problem affect your spiritual life or beliefs?

Mapping the Effects of Persons

- How have you been able to affect the life of the problem—keeping the things you just mentioned from getting worse?
- Are there times when you were able to not allow the problem to completely change your mood, thoughts, eating, sleeping, drinking, or other areas of functioning?
- Are there times when you were able to protect your relationships from being influenced by the problem?
- Are there times when you were able to continue with your normal social life despite the problem?
- Are there ways you have been able to maintain your sense of spirituality with the problem present?

Cross-Cutting Symptom Measures

A significant addition to the manual, the DSM-5 includes a set of cross-cutting symptom measures that are free to clinicians to facilitate the diagnostic process. These measures are designed to enable clinicians to efficiently identify key symptoms that may occur across various diagnoses (thus, "cross cutting"). These measures are divided into a two-tier system: Level 1 is a broad assessment for identifying potential areas of concern, and Level 2 is used to assess in greater detail areas of functioning identified in the Level 1 measure. These are ideal for newer therapists who are learning diagnosis, as well as for seasoned clinicians who want to ensure that their practice remains on the cutting edge.

A single, short assessment measure, the Level 1 Cross-Cutting Measure is initially given to clients at the beginning of treatment to determine whether further assessment is needed in a given area. The adult version has 23 items and measures 13 domains of functioning; the child version has 25 items and measures 12 domains of functioning. The assessment asks clients if "during the past two (2) weeks, how much (or how often) have you [or your child, on the child measure] been bothered by the following problems?" (APA, 2013, p. 738). Each of the 23 to 25 questions addresses basic areas of functioning, such as "little interest or pleasure in doing things," "feeling down, depressed, or hopeless," or "thoughts of actually hurting yourself" (APA, 2013, p. 738).

Level 1 Domains for Adults:

- Somatic symptoms
- Sleep problems
- Inattention (not on adult)
- Depression
- Anger
- Irritability (not on adult)
- Mania
- Anxiety
- Psychosis
- Repetitive thoughts and behaviors
- Substance use
- Suicidal ideation/attempts

Level 1 Domains for Children

- Somatic symptoms
- Sleep problems
- Inattention (not on adult)
- Depression
- Anger
- Irritability (not on adult)
- Mania
- Anxiety
- Psychosis
- Repetitive thoughts and behaviors
- Substance use
- Suicidal ideation/attempts

Level 2 Assessments

If a client scores at or above the specific cutoff in a given domain, then a Level 2 Cross-Cutting Symptom Measure is given (except for Suicidal ideation, psychosis, memory, dissociation, or personality functioning, which do not have Level 2 measures). A child-specific cross-cutting symptom measure is available for children 6 to 17; these are completed by a parent or guardian. These measures are available for free download on the APA-hosted websites (www.psychiatry.org/dsm5 and www.dsm5.org).

Symptom Severity Scales

In field trials, practitioners had significant variance when rating severity of symptoms; so now the DSM-5 includes severity scales that can be used to determine whether symptoms are mild, moderate, or severe when making a diagnosis. The severity scale for psychosis is in the book, and similar severity scales are available online (www.dsm5.org) for other disorders, including:

- Depression
- Separation anxiety disorder
- Specific phobia
- Social anxiety disorder
- Panic disorder
- Agoraphobia
- Generalized anxiety disorder
- Post-traumatic stress disorder
- Acute stress disorder
- Dissociative symptoms
- Psychosis

Early Development and Home Background

Another useful diagnostic measure that was released as part of the DSM-5, is the Early Development and Home Background Form; parents should complete one, as should the clinician. This form is designed for use with children, and covers key diagnostic information to help when making a diagnosis for a child. The topics covered include:

- Early development events: pregnancy, birth, major milestones
- Early communication development: Speech and communication milestones
- Home environment: Living situations, hospitalizations, persons in the home, quality of home life, etc.

Other Possible Assessment Instruments

In addition to the Cross-Cutting Symptom Inventories, therapists have numerous other assessment measures available to assist in making a diagnosis. The ones primarily used for diagnostic screening are discussed here.

Measures for Broad Range of Symptoms

The Outcome Questionnaire and Symptom Checklist are discussed in more detail in Chapter 14 as options for measuring client progress in therapy.

- Outcome Questionnaire: The Outcome Questionnaire comes in adult and youth versions with 10-, 30-, and 45-item versions; the longer versions provide more detailed assessments of mental health symptoms. Because of its brevity, it is popular in outpatient settings. More information can be found at www.oqmeasures.com.
- Symptom Checklist 90: The Symptom Checklist is a 90-item test that assesses for mental health symptoms and their intensity (mild, moderate, severe). It is designed for individuals 13 years and older and requires 12 to 15 minutes to complete. More information can be found at www.pearsonassessments.com
- Minnesota Multiphasic Personality Inventory (MMPI-2): The MMPI is the most frequently used clinical assessment instrument for diagnosing moderate to severe pathology. It contains 567 true–false items and takes one to two hours to complete; there are adult and adolescent versions. The MMPI is most frequently used in hospital settings and forensic psychology. More information can be found at www.pearsonassessments.com.

Measures for Specific Symptoms/Syndromes

- Beck Depression Inventory (BDI) and related inventories: The BDI is a 21-item self-assessment inventory that assesses a client's level of depression for people 13 years of age or older. Because it is quick and easy to administer, it is one of the more frequently used tests. Beck also has several other similar inventories for assessing anxiety, suicidality, hopelessness, and obsessive–compulsiveness. More information can be found at www.harcourtassessment.com.

- Michigan Alcoholic Screening Test (MAST): The MAST is a 22-item self-report instrument to screen for problem drinking. Much like the Beck, the instrument is quick and easy to administer. The test is available for free download on numerous websites (simply search for "Michigan Alcoholic Screening Test").
- Trauma Symptom Inventory (TSI-2): A broad measure, the TSI is used to help assess post-traumatic stress and related trauma symptoms, such as those related to abuse, domestic violence, war, car accidents, mass casualty events, and medical trauma.

Making a Diagnosis

The initial process of making a diagnosis should include ruling out key factors that might better explain some or all of the symptoms:

- Rule out substance misuse: Substance, including alcohol, misuse can often cause or exacerbate symptoms that appear to be another syndrome, such as depression. Because many clients do not reveal their substance use issues, therapists should ask both verbally and in writing about the client's pattern of substance use. In addition, therapists should listen for clues in client stories that might indicate a substance misuse problem (e.g., frequent stories about partying with friends) as well as look for visible signs of substance misuse.
- Rule out medications and medical conditions: Therapists should rule out medications and medication conditions that might be the cause of symptoms, such as low thyroid functioning affecting mood. A list of common drug interactions is in "Medical Considerations and Medication," below.
- Trauma: Past or recent trauma often present as another mood and anxiety disorder. Assessing for childhood and adult trauma can help clinicians correctly identify the source of symptoms.

After all the interviewing, test taking, and ruling out key issues, a diagnosis is ultimately made using your best clinical judgment. Therapists need to take time to weigh the various forms of information on hand—client report, therapist observation, family dynamics, gender and cultural factors, and inventory scores—to arrive at the most accurate diagnosis. In some cases, cultural factors, such as not losing face, may require reinterpreting the scores on a symptom inventory. In other situations, family dynamics may be the better explanation for a client's concern. Making a diagnosis also requires considering ethical issues, such as the effect of labeling and its potential consequences for clients. At the end of the day, therapists use their best judgment, knowing they may need to revise a diagnosis as new information emerges.

Documenting Clinical Assessment

You can download a copy of this form with MindTap® (see Cengagebrain.com) or you can download the form at masteringcompetencies.com. This text includes a clinical assessment form with elements common to most outpatient clinical assessments: client identifiers, presenting problem, mental status, diagnosis (including medication information), risk assessment, case management (including prognosis), and evaluation of assessment. Although the clinical assessment you may find at your agency probably looks different, it most likely has the same basic information.

Identifying Information

Generally, a client number is used instead of a name to maximize client confidentiality. Abbreviations are used to refer to the client and significant others:

> AF: Adult Female
> AM: Adult Male
> CF: Child Female
> CM: Child Male

These abbreviations can be followed by each person's age. Other important identifiers are profession or grade in school, ethnicities, and languages spoken. These provide a basic introduction to the client.

Presenting Problem

Presenting problems include what clients identify as the initial problems when they enter therapy, including the primary reason they are seeking treatment (e.g., a child's behavior problem) as well as secondary issues they may mention more casually (e.g., marital tension). The list of presenting problems provides a quick overview of the client's and/or family's current difficulties.

Mental Status Exam

Based on your findings from the MSE interview, cross-cutting symptom measures, and any other diagnostic assessments used, a written MSE is typically included to support diagnoses. The final section of this chapter defines the common terms used in a mental status exam. The diagnosis(ses) should be clearly supported by the symptoms in the mental status section of the clinical assessment. For example, if you check the "depressed" mood box, there should be some diagnosis that accounts for this in some way.

Diagnosis

Contextual Factors

Before making a diagnosis, therapists should consider contextual factors, such as age, ethnicity, family dynamics, language, religion, economic issues, sexual orientation, trauma history, addictions, and cognitive ability. For example, often a woman from a culture that values emotional expression and who has a history of trauma will present with histrionic features that are more a function of cultural communication than an actual personality disorder; these symptoms generally dissipate as trauma is treated. Taking such issues into consideration improves the accuracy of diagnosis.

Making a Diagnosis

When making a diagnosis, clinicians consult the DSM; each diagnosis requires that a certain number of criteria be met, and these criteria should be reflected in the MSE. In addition, medical causes, trauma, and substance abuse should be ruled out. Depending on the diagnosis, therapists may want to make a referral for an evaluation for medication; diagnoses with symptoms that typically warrant referral include depression, anxiety, mania, psychosis, trauma, disordered eating, alcohol and substance abuse, and sleep disorders.

Medical Considerations and Medication

Medical Considerations

A clinical assessment report typically includes a section in which therapists document the need for medical or psychiatric referrals as well as listing current medications.

Medications

Therapists should list both psychotropic and other prescribed medications. In some cases, a client's mental health may be affected by medication interactions or side effects. Some suspected interactions and/or side effects therapists should consider include:

- Corticosteroids, such as hydrocortisone, may contribute to mood swings.
- Antidepressants may contribute to mania in clients who have bipolar disorder.
- Certain antibiotics may contribute to mania or depression.
- Birth control pills and rings may contribute to depression.
- Beta-blockers used for heart issues may contribute to depression.
- Statins, used to lower cholesterol or protect against artery disease, may contribute to depression.
- Barbiturates and benzodiazepines (e.g., Xanax) used to treat anxiety might contribute to depression.
- Opioids (e.g., OxyContin) used to treat pain can contribute to depression.
- Amphetamine, corticosteroid, or marijuana may cause paranoia.
- Antidepressant, antihypertensive (for high blood pressure), and hormone treatments may affect sexual desire.

Medical Necessity

Most third-party payers require that therapists document that the condition meets the criteria for medical necessity and that there is significant impairment in functioning, a high probability of significant impairment, and/or probable developmental arrest in children. Areas of impairment may include the following:

- Daily activities (e.g., getting out of bed, feeding self, chores)
- Social relationships (e.g., maintaining satisfying marriage, friendships)
- Health (e.g., maintaining physical health)
- Work and school (e.g., able to maintain employment, complete school tasks)
- Living arrangement (e.g., having a place to live)

Risk Management

Therapists also assess for crisis and danger in clinical assessment, including a client's potential for suicide, homicide, substance abuse (past, present, or by others), and sexual or physical abuse history. If a client has any indicators of potential problems in these areas, therapists should assess for indicators of safety, generate a safety plan, and document the legal actions taken.

Suicidality and Homicidality

Clients who present with depression and hostility for others should be assessed for suicidal and/or homicidal intentions. Each state has different laws governing when and how therapists can take action to protect clients, the public, and property from danger. In most states, they must take some form of action to protect clients who have a clear plan and intent for killing themselves or others; when there is no clear plan or intent, therapists are still ethically bound to create safety plans in case the situation escalates. The following are various indicators of degrees of danger:

- No indication: No verbal, nonverbal, or situational indications of danger.
- Denial: Client was asked and denies suicidal and/or homicidal intent.
- Passive ideation: Client "would like to be dead" or "have the other person gone" but denies any plan or willingness to kill self or another.
- Active ideation: Client thinks about killing self or others.
- Attempt: Client has attempted to kill self or another at any point—a significant risk factor.
- Family history: A family history of suicide is another significant risk factor.

Substance Abuse

The therapist can use pen-and-paper tests such as the MAST (see discussion above) as well as verbal and written self-reports to assess for alcohol and substance abuse. Because often these issues are not fully revealed early in treatment, therapists should routinely and frequently inquire about substance and alcohol use throughout treatment, especially when they see lack of progress.

Child Abuse

Four types of child abuse are generally outlined in state child abuse laws:

- Sexual abuse: Inappropriate sexual contact with a minor by an adult or another minor; may or may not be consensual (defined by state laws).
- Physical abuse: Hitting, beating, kicking, or otherwise inflicting bodily harm by hand, with an object, and/or other means (e.g., locking child in enclosed space); includes most forms of spanking in many states.
- Emotional abuse: Inflicting severe psychological harm, such as fear of death, physical intimidation, and intense rejection and disapproval.
- Neglect: Failing to provide for basic physical needs, such as sufficient food, clothing, shelter, and medicine.

In most states, all forms of child abuse except emotional abuse legally require reporting child abuse to state authorities (e.g., child protective services, sheriff, police).

Elder and Dependent Adult Abuse

Most states have laws for reporting elder and dependent adult abuse and neglect, which includes the categories for child abuse as well as *financial abuse:* illegal or unauthorized use of a person's property, money, or pension.

Other Risk Factors

- Anorexia, bulimia, and other eating disorders: Eating disorders are some of the most dangerous mental health disorders; anorexia is frequently cited as having the highest fatality rate of any mental health diagnosis. These disorders almost always require coordinated care with a medical professional.
- Cutting and self-harm: Cutting, burning, and other forms of self-harm are used to cope with emotional pain; therapists need to interview clients to determine whether there is suicidal intent or if the self-harm is intended for another purpose, such as relieving emotional pain.
- Criminal or legal history: Criminal or legal history is helpful in assessing the potential for harm and danger.

Safety and Safety Planning

Indicators of Safety

In addition to assessing for danger, therapists should assess for the potential for safety: What factors are in place to keep the client safe? The balance of these two potentials helps therapists determine the overall level of crisis. The following indicators suggest safety:

- At least one outside support person
- Is able to cite reasons to live and/or not harm others (e.g., "I couldn't do it because of my kids")
- Hope; goals for future
- Is willing to dispose of dangerous items (e.g., gun)
- Agrees to reduce contact with people who make the situation worse
- Agrees to safety plan and develops an alternative to harming self or other

Safety Plans

Safety plans should be developed for any situation in which potential risk is identified, such as passive suicidal ideation, history of cutting, and history of abuse. These plans should be tailored to each client's individual needs using combinations of the following components as well as unique elements for each client:

Safety Plan Components

- Verbal or written agreement or contract to not harm themselves or others
- A card with emergency contact numbers for local hotlines, supportive friends, therapist's emergency contact number, etc.
- Working with medical professionals who prescribe medication to reduce crisis potential
- Specific action plan with regard to whom to call and what to do if a crisis arises
- Identifying tasks to calm self, such as journaling and exercising, at low levels of pre-crisis stress
- Specific daily or weekly activities to reduce overall level of stress and triggers for crisis

Scaling for Safety

I have developed scaling for safety, a variation of solution-oriented scaling questions (O'Hanlon & Weiner-Davis, 1989), to help stabilize crisis situations with clients who are dealing with severe depression, suicidal ideation, cutting, eating disorders, substance abuse, and violence. Using a white board, I have clients define both emotionally and behaviorally a "1" when things are good, a "5" when things are neutral or okay, and a "10" for the crisis point of a dangerous activity. I then have them describe emotions and behaviors for each point on the scale (or if there is limited time, from 5 to 9), looking for the point at which they are relatively able to take action, generally a 7. Then we develop a realistic safety plan for what to do when they reach a 7, detailing what the clients will do, whom they will call, and so forth. If clients still engage in the dangerous behavior after the plan is in place, the plan should be revised to take action at a lower level on the scale. For most clients, this is specific and realistic enough to prevent them from getting close to the crisis behavior.

The following form can be used for this technique:

SCALING FOR SAFETY FORM		
	BEHAVIORS AND ACTIONS	**THOUGHTS AND FEELINGS**
10: Crisis/Dangerous Act Occurs		
9		
8		
7		
6		
5: Doing/Feeling Okay		
4		
3		
2		
1: Feeling Great		
• Number at which I feel I still have enough control to easily enact safety plan: _____ • Top 5 warning signs that I have hit #_____. • 5 things I can do when I hit #_____.		

> **Try It Yourself**
>
> With a partner or on your own, identify a behavior you would like to stop and use the scaling for safety format to help identify some options for stopping.

Commitment to Treatment

In cases involving suicide, Rudd, Mandrusiak, and Joiner (2006) recommend obtaining a commitment-to-treatment agreement rather than a no-harm contract, which, although standard practice, has no empirical support. In a no-harm contract, clients agree not to harm themselves and to contact emergency services when they feel in danger of doing so. In contrast, a commitment to treatment is an agreement between the client and therapist in which the client agrees to commit to the treatment process. The commitment involves three elements:

1. The commitment identifies the roles, obligations, and expectations of both the therapist and the client in treatment.
2. The client promises to communicate openly about all aspects of treatment, including suicidal thoughts and plans.
3. The client promises to use agreed-upon emergency resources during a crisis that might threaten the client's ability to fulfill his or her commitment to treatment (e.g., a crisis during which the client contemplates suicide).

Rudd et al. (2006) believe that obtaining a commitment to treatment provides a more useful clinical intervention than a no-harm contract because it is a more hopeful and therapeutically useful framework for both client and therapist, clearly outlining each person's responsibilities and encouraging open communication. Rather than emphasizing *not* committing suicide, the focus is on *committing* to meaningfully participate in psychotherapy treatment.

Case Management

Case management is a collaborative process of working with clients to develop a comprehensive plan of care that takes into account the resources and services necessary to ensure a successful treatment outcome. Therapists rendering mental health services must develop treatment plans (see Chapter 13) that detail how they plan to address the client's presenting problems as part of standard practice. In addition, they need to "think outside of the therapy room" to coordinate care with other professionals, advocate for clients, and help clients identify and access necessary resources.

Common Case Management Activities

- Contacting and coordinating care with client's social workers
- Referring client for a medical assessment to rule out medical causes and/or exacerbating conditions
- Referring client for a psychiatric evaluation for diagnosis and/or prescription for psychotropic medication
- Contacting treating physician regarding mental health treatment
- Referring client for social services such as job training, welfare, housing, victim services, and legal assistance
- Referring client for legal and/or forensic services (e.g., custody evaluations)
- Referring client for group counseling and/or psychoeducational classes (e.g., parenting classes)

- Helping client connect with new or existing social supports, such as religious groups, friends, and family
- Considering the effects of treatment on significant others in the system (e.g., the effect on the family of treating substance dependence)
- Identifying any unique needs the client has to be successful (e.g., transportation, safe place to exercise, a computer)

Evaluation of Assessment

The final section of the clinical assessment encourages therapists to reflect on how they have adapted the assessment to fit the client's unique needs, including diversity factors, effects of treatment on the family system, and areas of client–therapist agreement and disagreement. Considering these factors helps therapists develop a plan that is likely to succeed and also helps identify potential pitfalls.

Communicating with Other Professionals

DSM-ese

Perhaps one of family therapy's earliest contribution to the field of mental health is the concept of learning to speak your client's language. Rooted in communications theory, family therapists from the beginning have emphasized the importance of delivering messages in a way that the audience can receive it. Originally, this insight was applied to clients and later to help therapists work with diverse clients from different backgrounds, age groups, and social classes. As the field has become more integrated into formalized mental health services, it has become increasingly important to learn how to speak with other medical and mental health practitioners. Therefore, family therapists must learn to speak the language of other professionals to effectively work with the larger system that is involved with the client's care.

When speaking to medical doctors and psychiatrists involved in a patient's care, therapists need to speak their language, or "DSM-ese," even if this is not the language they used to conceptualize the case. It is much like learning to speak a foreign language. In the beginning, therapists must clumsily translate from one language to another in their heads. With time and practice, they learn to actually think in the foreign language and speak more fluidly and eloquently, expressing more and more complex ideas. As with any foreign language, it often helps to "go abroad" and spend time living in an environment where the language is spoken: inpatient, intensive outpatient, county mental health, and similar settings.

DSM-ese is a technical language whose preferred vocabulary is found in its dictionary, the DSM-IV-TR. It is not hard to learn but can seem too dry and boring for most therapists. If you like the warm, fuzzy feel, you will need to shift gears to get into the mood, which should remind you of your math and science classes more than English and history. To speed up the process of learning how to speak DSM-ese, just memorize the following four principles:

1. **Use DSM symptom language:** Rather than use vernacular descriptions of client symptoms, DSM-ese describes the symptoms that are the foundation for making diagnoses:
   - Panic attack (rather than "nervous breakdown")
   - Depressed mood (rather than "feeling down")
   - Irritability (rather than "feeling upset")
2. **Use behavioral descriptions:** When symptoms can be described in more detail using behavioral description, the behavioral description should be added.
   - Yells at partner (rather than "gets angry")
   - Loss of interest in hobbies (rather than "doesn't care anymore")
   - Loses focus on homework after 15 minutes (rather than "doesn't pay attention")

3. **Include duration of symptoms**
   - Depressed mood for three months
   - Hypomanic episode for three days
   - Auditory hallucinations reported since age 14
4. **Include frequency of symptoms**
   - Tantrums three to four times per week for past year
   - Violent outburst every one to two months for past three years
   - Bingeing and vomiting two times per week for past six months

By simply using symptom and behavioral descriptors with frequency and duration, therapists can quickly achieve fluency in DSM-ese and improve their communication with other professionals. The following comprehensive list of the symptoms and mental status terms provides a good starting place for learning the language of clinical assessment.

Mental Status Terms

Interpersonal Issues

- *Conflict:* Frequent arguments and conflict with one or more person.
- *Enmeshment:* Boundaries with one or more persons are diffuse, not allowing for significant sense of independence (e.g., needing the other to always agree to feel okay; unable to tolerate differences with significant others; feelings easily hurt and/or easily feels rejected).
- *Isolation/avoidance:* Avoids social contact to manage difficult feelings; reports actively isolating self or feeling isolated; reports few social contacts.
- *Emotional disengagement:* Clients are in a relationship but lack meaningful emotional connection with one or more significant persons in their life.

Common Mood Descriptors

- *Mood versus affect:* Mood is how a person reports feeling inside; affect is the outer expression of emotion.
- *Depressed:* Feeling of sadness and unhappiness; "blue," "down."
- *Hopeless:* Feeling as though there is no possibility of a good future.
- *Fearful:* Concerns about a specific negative event happening.
- *Anxiety:* Generalized worry about unspecified or vague negative events happening.
- *Angry:* Feeling indignant or wronged about a specific happening.
- *Irritability:* Generalized feelings of anger or upset without a specific object of anger; angry reactions are easily triggered.
- *Manic:* Unusually energetic feelings of elation, euphoria, or irritability.

Common Affect Descriptors

- *Constricted or restricted:* Emotional expression is restrained but emotions are evident.
- *Blunt or blunted:* Emotional expression is severely restrained; little emotional reactivity.
- *Flat:* Associated with psychosis and severe pathology; emotional expression is virtually nonexistent.
- *Labile:* Mood vacillates frequently, rapidly, and abruptly.
- *Dramatic:* Expression of emotion is generally overdramatized.

Common Sleep Descriptors

- *Hypersomnia:* Sleeping more than usual.
- *Insomnia:* Unable to get usual amounts of sleep because of difficulty falling or staying asleep.
- *Disrupted sleep:* Sleep disturbed by nightmares, night terrors, or other issues.
- *Nightmares:* Dreams that frighten the dreamer; occur during rapid-eye-movement (REM) sleep.

- *Night terrors:* A general sense of panic or terror is experienced while sleeping without dream content; the sleeper generally cannot be roused during night terrors, although he or she may scream or act panicked; occur in slow-wave sleep, not REM.

Common Eating Descriptors

- *Anorectic restriction:* Restrictive eating that characterizes anorexia.
- *Bingeing:* Episodes of uncontrolled overeating.
- *Purging:* Following a binge episode, an attempt to rid body of food by vomiting, over-exercising, fasting, or abusing laxatives.
- *Body image distortion:* Image of body, particularly related to weight, is grossly inconsistent with others' perception and medical weight norms.

Common Anxiety Descriptors

- *Anxiety:* Anticipation of danger, problems, or misfortune that creates uneasiness, tension, and/or somatic symptoms.
- *Chronic worry:* A specific form of anxiety that involves dwelling on anticipated problems.
- *Panic attacks:* Discrete periods of intense anxiety or terror that may be characterized by shortness of breath, pounding heart, sense of losing control, or sense of doom; may be unexpected or situationally bound.
- *Dissociation:* Disruption in integration of consciousness, memory, identity, and/or perception; may come on suddenly or gradually.
- *Phobias:* Persistent, irrational fears of specific objects or situations.
- *Obsessions:* Intrusive and recurrent thoughts, impulses, or images that cause marked distress.
- *Compulsions:* Repetitive behaviors or mental acts (counting, praying, etc.) that one is driven to perform to reduce some form of distress; generally the act is not realistically related to the distress.

Common Psychotic Descriptors

- *Hallucinations:* Sensory perceptions (sight, sound, touch, smell, or taste) that have no external stimuli; perceptions are experienced as real.
- *Delusions:* False beliefs based on an incorrect inference about external reality that is rigidly maintained despite substantial evidence to the contrary. May be bizarre (considered logically and/or culturally implausible) or nonbizarre.
- *Paranoia:* Suspicion that one is being harassed or persecuted with little corroborating evidence; less severe than delusion.
- *Loose associations:* Thought disorder characterized by frequent derailment from topic of conversation, jumping from thought to thought often triggered by a "loose" connection to a word or phrase.

Common Motor Activity Descriptors

- *Low energy:* Little movement or energy behind movement.
- *Restless:* Excessive movement associated with emotional or physical discomfort.
- *Agitated:* Excessive activity associated with inner tension or frustration.
- *Hyperactive:* Excessive motor activity, such as fidgeting or moving about; not necessarily associated with tension or discomfort.

Common Thought Descriptors

- *Poor concentration or attention:* Unable to sustain the attention expected for the developmental level.

- *Denial:* Unable or refuses to acknowledge clearly evident problems that most others in the situation identify as problems.
- *Self-blame:* Tendency to blame self for things that are outside of personal control and/or that others hold greater responsibility for.
- *Other-blame:* Tendency to blame others for things that are primarily a personal responsibility.
- *Insightful:* Able to articulate insight into personal behaviors and emotions even if unable to behave consistently with insight.
- *Poor insight:* Unusually great difficulty identifying one's own thoughts, feelings, and motivations.
- *Impaired decision making:* Pattern of making decisions that result in negative consequences for self and others.
- *Tangential:* Tendency to make comments that move conversation away from original topic to a tangentially or loosely related topic; typically done when discussing a difficult subject.

QUESTIONS FOR PERSONAL REFLECTION AND CLASS DISCUSSION

1. Describe the benefits and risks to diagnosis that you believe to be most critical.
2. What potential improvements and limitations do you see with dimensional assessment?
3. Describe the benefits and risks of the recovery in mental health movement.
4. Describe what you might do to preserve a strong therapeutic relationship with clients when conducting a mental status exam.
5. Describe your concerns about how culture, social class, immigration status, and sexual orientation/identity might impact the diagnosis process? What suggestions do you have for addressing this issues?
6. Describe the move toward dimensional assessment and away from discrete disorders in mental health. What benefits or problems do you see?
7. How comfortable do you anticipated you will be discussing suicidal thoughts, sexual abuse, and substance use with clients? How can you develop greater confidence with these topics?

ONLINE RESOURCES

Official DSM-5 website with access to Cross-Cutting Measures, WHODAS 2.0, and cultural assessment as well as Fact Sheets for specific disorders, and videos on the changes.

www.psychiatry.org/dsm5

Originally serving as the site to solicit public feedback on the DSM-5, this site documents the development of the DSM-5, including monographs, conference proceedings, and related reference lists, and also includes many of resources on the sister site: psychiatry.org/dsm5, including the online measures for download.

www.dsm5.org

Beck Depression Inventory (BDI) and related inventories

www.pearsonassessments.com

Michigan Alcoholic Screening Test (MAST)

Available at several sites for free download: Google "Michigan Alcoholic Screening Test"

Minnesota Multiphasic Personality Inventory (MMPI-2)

www.pearsonassessments.com

National Consensus Statement on Recovery: U.S. Department of Health and Human Services

www.mentalhealth.samhsa.gov/publications /allpubs/sma05-4129

Outcome Questionnaire

More information at **www.oqmeasures .com**

Symptom Checklist 90

www.pearsonassessments.com

Go to MindTap® for an eBook, videos of client sessions, activities, digital forms,

practice quizzes, apps, and more—all in one place. If your instructor didn't assign MindTap, you can find out more information at CengageBrain.com.

REFERENCES

American Psychiatric Association. (2000). *Diagnostic and statistical manual for mental disorders* (4th ed., text rev.). Washington, DC: Author.

American Psychiatric Association. (2013). *Diagnostic and statistical manual for mental disorders* (5th ed.). Washington DC: Author.

Anderson, H. (1997). *Conversations, language, and possibilities.* New York: Basic Books.

Davidson, L., Tondora, J., O'Connell, M. J., Lawless, M. S., & Rowe, M. (2009). *A practical guide to recovery-oriented practice: Tools for transforming mental health care.* New York: Oxford University Press.

Eriksen, K., & Kress, V. E. (2008). Gender and diagnosis: Struggles and suggestions for counselors. *Journal of Counseling and Development, 86,* 152–161.

Fisher, D. B., & Chamberlin, J. (2004, March). *Consumer-directed transformation to a recovery-based mental health system.* Retrieved from www.mentalhealth.samhsa.gov/publications/allpubs/NMH05-0193/default.asp.

Gadamer, H. (1975). *Truth and method.* New York: Seabury.

Gehart, D. (2012a). The mental health recovery movement and family therapy, part I: Consumer-lead reform of services to persons diagnosed with severe mental illness. *Journal of Marital and Family Therapy, 38,* 429–442.

Gehart, D. (2012b). The mental health recovery movement and family therapy, part II: A collaborative, appreciative approach for supporting mental health recovery. *Journal of Marital and Family Therapy, 38,* 443–457.

Gergen, K., Anderson, H., & Hoffman, L. (1996). Is diagnosis a disaster? A constructionist trialogue. In F. Kaslow (Ed.), *Relational diagnosis.* New York: Wiley.

Haarakangas, K., Seikkula, J., Alakare, B., & Aaltonen, J. (2007). Open Dialogue: An approach to psychotherapeutic treatment of psychosis in Northern Finland. In H. Anderson & D. Gehart (Eds.), *Collaborative therapy: Relationships and conversations that make a difference* (pp. 221–233). New York: Brunner/Routledge.

Hansen, J. T. (2003). Including diagnosis training in counseling curricula: Implications for professional identity development. *Counselor Education and Supervision, 43*(2), 96–107. doi:10.1002/j.1556-6978.2003.tb01834.x

Insel, T. (2013, April). *Director's blog: Transforming diagnosis.* Retrieved from http://www.nimh.nih.gov/about/director/2013/transforming-diagnosis.shtml.

Keeney, B. P. (1983). *Aesthetics of change.* New York: Guilford.

Narrow, W. E., Clarke, D. E., Kuramoto, S. J., Kraemer, H. C., Kupfer, D. J., Greiner, L., & Regier, D. A. (2013). DSM-5 field trials in the United States and Canada, part III: Development and reliability testing of a cross-cutting symptom assessment for DSM-5. *American Journal of Psychiatry, 170*(1), 71–82. doi: 10.1176/appi.ajp.2012.12071000

O'Hanlon, W. H., & Weiner-Davis, M. (1989). *In search of solutions: A new direction in psychotherapy.* New York: Norton.

Onken, S. J., Craig, C., Ridgway, P., Ralph, R. O., & Cook, J. A. (2007). An analysis of the definitions and elements of recovery: A review of the literature. *Psychiatric Rehabilitation Journal, 31,* 9–22.

Ralph, R. (2000). *Review of the recovery literature: Synthesis of a sample recovery literature 2000.* National Association for State Mental Health Program

Directors. Retrieved from www.bbs. ca.gov/pdf/mhsa/resource/recovery /recovery_oriented_resources.pdf.

Ramon, S., Healy, B., & Renouf, N. (2007). Recovery from mental illness as an emergent concept and practice. *Australia and the UK International Journal of Social Psychiatry, 53*(2), 108–122.

Repper, J., & Perkins, R. (2006). *Social inclusion and recovery: A model for mental health practice.* Oxford, UK: Bailliere Tindall.

Rudd, M. D., Mandrusiak, M., & Joiner, T. E., Jr. (2006). The case against no-suicide contracts: Commitment to Treatment Statement as a practice alternative. *Journal of Clinical Psychology in Session, 62,* 243–251.

Seikkula, J. (2002). Open dialogues with good and poor outcomes for psychotic crises: Examples from families with violence. *Journal of Marital and Family Therapy, 28*(3), 263–274.

Selvini Palazzoli, M., Boscolo, L., Cecchin, G., & Prata, G. (1978). *Paradox and counterparadox.* New York: Aronson.

U.S. Department of Health and Human Services. (2004). *National consensus statement on mental health recovery.* Retrieved from www.mentalhealth. samhsa.gov/publications/allpubs /sma05-4129.

Watzlawick, P., Weakland, J., & Fisch, R. (1974). *Change: Principles of problem formation and problem resolution.* New York: Norton.

White, M., & Epston, D. (1990). *Narrative means to therapeutic ends.* New York: Norton.

CLINICAL ASSESSMENT

Clinician:	Client ID #:	Primary configuration: ☐ Individual ☐ Couple ☐ Family	Primary Language: ☐ English ☐ Spanish ☐ Other: _____

List client and significant others

Adult(s)

Select Gender Age: ____ Select Ethnicity Select Relational Status Occupation: ____ Other identifier: ____

Select Gender Age: ____ Select Ethnicity Select Relational Status Occupation: ____ Other identifier: ____

Child(ren)

Select Gender Age: _____ Select Ethnicity Grade: Select Grade School: _____ Other identifier: _____

Select Gender Age: _____ Select Ethnicity Grade: Select Grade School: _____ Other identifier: _____

Others: _____

Presenting Problem(s)

☐ Depression/hopelessness
☐ Anxiety/worry
☐ Anger issues
☐ Loss/grief
☐ Suicidal thoughts/attempts
☐ Sexual abuse/rape
☐ Alcohol/drug use
☐ Eating problems/disorders
☐ Job problems/unemployed

☐ Couple concerns
☐ Parent/child conflict
☐ Partner violence/abuse
☐ Divorce adjustment
☐ Remarriage adjustment
☐ Sexuality/intimacy concerns
☐ Major life changes
☐ Legal issues/probation
☐ Other: _____

Complete for children:
☐ School failure/decline performance
☐ Truancy/runaway
☐ Fighting w/peers
☐ Hyperactivity
☐ Wetting/soiling clothing
☐ Child abuse/neglect
☐ Isolation/withdrawal
☐ Other: _____

Mental Status Assessment for Identified Patient

Interpersonal	☐ NA	☐ Conflict ☐ Enmeshment ☐ Isolation/avoidance ☐ Harassment ☐ Other: _____
Mood	☐ NA	☐ Depressed/Sad ☐ Anxious ☐ Dysphoric ☐ Angry ☐ Irritable ☐ Manic ☐ Other: _____
Affect	☐ NA	☐ Constricted ☐ Blunt ☐ Flat ☐ Labile ☐ Incongruent ☐ Other: _____
Sleep	☐ NA	☐ Hypersomnia ☐ Insomnia ☐ Disrupted ☐ Nightmares ☐ Other: _____
Eating	☐ NA	☐ Increase ☐ Decrease ☐ Anorectic restriction ☐ Binging ☐ Purging ☐ Other: _____
Anxiety	☐ NA	☐ Chronic worry ☐ Panic ☐ Phobias ☐ Obsessions ☐ Compulsions ☐ Other: _____
Trauma symptoms	☐ NA	☐ Hypervigilance ☐ Flashbacks/Intrusive memories ☐ Dissociation ☐ Numbing ☐ Avoidance efforts ☐ Other: _____

(continued)

Mental Status Assessment for Identified Patient (*continued*)

Psychotic symptoms	☐ NA	☐ Hallucinations ☐ Delusions ☐ Paranoia ☐ Loose associations ☐ Other: _____
Motor activity/speech	☐ NA	☐ Low energy ☐ Hyperactive ☐ Agitated ☐ Inattentive ☐ Impulsive ☐ Pressured speech ☐ Slow speech ☐ Other: _____
Thought	☐ NA	☐ Poor concentration ☐ Denial ☐ Self-blame ☐ Other-blame ☐ Ruminative ☐ Tangential ☐ Concrete ☐ Poor insight ☐ Impaired decision making ☐ Disoriented ☐ Other: _____
Sociolegal	☐ NA	☐ Disregards rules ☐ Defiant ☐ Stealing ☐ Lying ☐ Tantrums ☐ Arrest/incarceration ☐ Initiates fights ☐ Other: _____
Other symptoms	☐ NA	_____

Diagnosis for Identified Patient

Contextual Factors considered in making diagnosis: ☐ Age ☐ Gender ☐ Race/Ethnicity ☐ Language ☐ Religion ☐ Social class ☐ Immigration ☐ Sexual/gender orientation ☐ Cognitive ability ☐ Other: _____

Describe impact of identified factors on diagnosis and assessment process: _____

DSM-5 Level 1 Cross-Cutting Symptom Measure (optional): Elevated scores on: (free at psychiatry.org)

☐ I Depression ☐ II Anger ☐ III Mania ☐ IV Anxiety ☐ V Somatic ☐ VI Suicide VII ☐ Psychosis ☐ VIII Sleep ☐ IX Memory ☐ X Repetitive ☐ XI Dissociation ☐ XII Personality ☐ XIII Substance ☐ Not administered

DSM-5 Code	Diagnosis with Specifier *Include Z/T-Codes for Psychosocial Stressors/Issues*
1. _____ 2. _____ 3. _____ 4. _____ 5. _____	1. _____ 2. _____ 3. _____ 4. _____ 5. _____

List Specific DSM-5 Criterion Met for Diagnosis

1. _____
2. _____
3. _____
4. _____
5. _____

Medical Considerations

Has patient been referred for psychiatric evaluation? ☐ Yes ☐ No

Has patient agreed with referral? ☐ Yes ☐ No ☐ NA

Psychometric instruments used for assessment: ☐ None ☐ Cross-cutting symptom inventories ☐ Other: _____

Client response to diagnosis: ☐ Agree ☐ Somewhat agree ☐ Disagree ☐ Not informed for following reason: _____

Diagnosis for Identified Patient (*continued*)

Current Medications (psychiatric & medical) ☐ NA

1. _____ ; dose _____ mg; start date: _____
2. _____ ; dose _____ mg; start date: _____
3. _____ ; dose _____ mg; start date: _____
4. _____ ; dose _____ mg; start date: _____

Medical Necessity: *Check all that apply*

☐ Significant impairment ☐ Probability of significant impairment ☐ Probable developmental arrest

Areas of impairment:

☐ Daily activities ☐ Social relationships ☐ Health ☐ Work/school ☐ Living arrangement
☐ Other: _____

Risk and Safety Assessment for Identified Patient

Suicidality
☐ No indication/denies
☐ Active ideation
☐ Passive ideation
☐ Intent without plan
☐ Intent with means
☐ Ideation in past year
☐ Attempt in past year
☐ Family or peer history of completed suicide

Homicidality
☐ No indication/denies
☐ Active ideation
☐ Passive ideation
☐ Intent without means
☐ Intent with means
☐ Ideation in past year
☐ Violence past year
☐ History of assaulting others
☐ Cruelty to animals

Alcohol Abuse
☐ No indication/denies
☐ Past abuse
☐ Current; Freq/Amt: _____

Drug Use/Abuse
☐ No indication/denies
☐ Past use
☐ Current drugs: _____
   Freq/Amt: _____
☐ Family/sig.other use

Sexual & Physical Abuse and Other Risk Factors

☐ Childhood abuse history: ☐ Sexual ☐ Physical ☐ Emotional ☐ Neglect
☐ Adult with abuse/assault in adulthood: ☐ Sexual ☐ Physical ☐ Current
☐ History of perpetrating abuse: ☐ Sexual ☐ Physical ☐ Emotional
☐ Elder/dependent adult abuse/neglect
☐ History of or current issues with restrictive eating, binging, and/or purging
☐ Cutting or other self-harm: ☐ Current ☐ Past: Method: _____
☐ Criminal/legal history: _____
☐ Other trauma history: _____
☐ None reported

Indicators of Safety

☐ NA
☐ At least one outside support person
☐ Able to cite specific reasons to live or not harm
☐ Hopeful
☐ Willing to dispose of dangerous items
☐ Has future goals

☐ Willingness to reduce contact with people who make situation worse
☐ Willing to implement safety plan, safety interventions
☐ Developing set of alternatives to self/other harm
☐ Sustained period of safety: _____
☐ Other: _____

(continued)

Risk and Safety Assessment for Identified Patient (*continued*)

Elements of Safety Plan

☐ NA
☐ Verbal no harm contract
☐ Written no harm contract
☐ Emergency contact card
☐ Emergency therapist/agency number
☐ Medication management:

☐ Plan for contacting friends/support persons during crisis
☐ Specific plan of where to go during crisis
☐ Specific self-calming tasks to reduce risk before reach crisis level (e.g., journaling, exercising, etc.)
☐ Specific daily/weekly activities to reduce stressors
☐ Other: _____

Legal/Ethical Action Taken: ☐ NA ☐ Action: _____

Case Management

Collateral Contacts

- Has contact been made with treating *physicians or other professionals:* ☐ NA ☐ Yes ☐ In process. Name/Notes: _____

- If client is involved in mental health *treatment elsewhere,* has contact been made? ☐ NA ☐ Yes ☐ In process. Name/Notes: _____

- Has contact been made with *social worker:* ☐ NA ☐ Yes ☐ In process. Name/Notes: _____

Referrals

- Has client been referred for *medical assessment:* ☐ Yes ☐ No evidence for need
- Has client been referred for *social services:* ☐ NA ☐ Job/training ☐ Welfare/Food/Housing ☐ Victim services ☐ Legal aid ☐ Medical ☐ Other: _____

- Has client been referred for *group* or other support services: ☐ Yes: _____ ☐ In process ☐ None recommended
- Are there anticipated *forensic/legal* processes related to treatment: ☐ No ☐ Yes; describe: _____

Support Network

- Client social support network includes: ☐ Supportive family ☐ Supportive partner ☐ Friends ☐ Religious/spiritual organization ☐ Supportive work/social group ☐ Other: _____
- Describe anticipated effects treatment will have on others in support system (Children, partner, etc.): _____

- Is there anything else client will need to be successful? _____

Expected Outcome and Prognosis

☐ Return to normal functioning ☐ Anticipate less than normal functioning ☐ Prevent deterioration
Client Sense of Hope: Select _____

Evaluation of Assessment/Client Perspective
How were assessment methods adapted to client needs, including age, culture, and other diversity issues? _____

Describe actual or potential areas of client–clinician agreement/disagreement related to the above assessment: _____

_____ , _____ _____
Clinician Signature   License/Intern Status   Date

_____ , _____ _____
Supervisor   License   Date

Treatment Planning

Treatment + Plan = ?

It was the first day at my new training site, one of the best in town. During the orientation, my supervisor went over the clinical paperwork that we would need to complete: intake forms, assessments, and **treatment plans**. Although I had learned about gathering intake and assessment information in my diagnosis class, I had never actually seen a treatment plan. Using sophisticated etymological skills that all graduate students rely on—treatment + plan—I deduced that this document would somehow describe my plans for how to treat the client. But how?

Like many interns, I was too embarrassed to ask and kept my ignorance quiet. I decided that if I could find a sample, I could probably fake it and not have to risk looking ignorant in the eyes of my well-respected supervisor. Thankfully, I was assigned cases handled by previous interns that included this oh-so-mysterious document. So, I gathered up as many files as I could and found an uncomfortable, well-worn seat in a poorly lit corner assigned to interns and tried to crack the code. *That* is how I learned to do treatment plans: secretly and shamefully. Thankfully, because you have this book in your hands, you have the opportunity to learn this once secret art with more dignity—and without a backache.

Just in case you missed it, the moral of the above story is to talk with your supervisors—no matter how brilliant they may appear—and do not be afraid to ask what seems like a silly question. Trust me, the chair was not the hardest part of learning treatment planning on my own.

Step 3: Selecting a Path

After completing your case conceptualization and clinical assessment, you are ready to develop a plan for addressing the problems you have identified in these other two documents. Treatment plans are fun: they are filled with hopes and dreams. In creating them, you have tremendous freedom, but you also have the burden of responsibility. Because numerous good plans can be developed for any one client, you may choose which theory and techniques are the best fit for a specific client, a specific problem, and a particular therapist–client relationship. As the therapist, you are responsible for shepherding an effective process and selecting a plan that is most likely to help the client; this plan should be based on clinical experience, current research, and standards of practice.

A Brief History of Mental Health Treatment Planning

The history of treatment planning in the field of marriage and family therapy is relatively short. The original theorists did not talk or write about treatment planning; in fact, if you search the literature you will find no form that would be accepted for payment by a managed-care company or county mental health agency. If the approved approach to treatment planning did not come from the field of family therapy or even mental health more broadly, where did it come from? The short answer: the medical field.

Symptom-Based Treatment Plans

The type of treatment planning that most marriage and family therapists must complete to receive third-party payment and to maintain standard practice of care in the 21st century is derived from the medical model. Jongsma and his colleagues (Dattilio & Jongsma, 2000; Jongsma, Peterson, & Bruce, 2006; Jongsma, Peterson, McInnis, & Bruce et al., 2006; O'Leary, Heyman, & Jongsma, 1998) have developed the most extensive models. Called *symptom-based treatment plans,* these documents focus solely on clients' medical symptoms. Most publications on treatment planning use a similar symptom-based model (Johnson, 2004; Wiger, 2005). But although these plans are relevant to those in the medical community, they do not help therapists conceptualize treatment in the most useful ways.

For example, if a parent brings a child who is having tantrums to therapy and the therapist develops a plan around the presenting problem (e.g., "reduce child's tantrums to less than one per week") and proceeds to deal directly with the tantrums without thoroughly conceptualizing the case, treatment is unlikely to be successful. A systemic assessment will typically reveal that marital and/or parenting issues are contributing to the presenting problem, and couples therapy that targets tension in the marriage may actually be the best way to reduce the child's tantrums. The danger of symptom-based treatment planning is that the therapist will underutilize theory, focus on symptoms, and forget to assess the larger picture. Arguably, a good therapist would not do this; however, today's workplace realities—including: (a) heavy caseloads, (b) pressure to complete diagnosis and treatment plans by the end of the first session, and (c) highly structured paperwork and payment systems—all make it hard for a therapist to do a good job. Symptom-based treatment planning, although convenient, may not be the best choice for today's practice environments.

Theory-Based Treatment Plans

Theory-based treatment planning, described by Gehart and Tuttle (2003), uses theory to create more clinically relevant treatment plans than the symptom model offers. Berman (1997) developed a similar approach for traditional psychotherapies. Both models include goals that are informed by clinical theories. However, I found that new trainees confuse theory-based goals and interventions because they use the same language. Furthermore, it is difficult for most students to address diagnostic issues and clinical symptoms in these theory-based plans because the language of these two systems is radically different. The solution was to develop a new, "both/and" model, called the "clinical treatment plan," that draws from the best of theory-based and symptom-based treatment plans and adds elements of measurability.

Clinical Treatment Plans

Clinical treatment plans provide a straightforward, comprehensive overview of treatment. They include the following parts:

- Introduction: Identifies the theory, modalities, session frequency, and expected length of treatment.
- Treatment plan with goals and interventions: The main body of the treatment plan is a set of goals with interventions; outside the classroom, this is what a treatment plan typically looks like. The goals specify what dynamics are going to change. *Change* is the operative word: goals typically start with "increase" or "decrease" to clarify what is going to change. Interventions describe what interventions are going to be used to achieve that change. So, "reducing enmeshment" is a goal and "enactment" is the intervention.
- Treatment tasks: In the treatment tasks, you identify how you are going to use your theory to: (a) create a therapeutic relationship, (b) develop a case conceptualization using a specific theory, and (c) identify crises and referrals.
- Diversity considerations: The section on diversity considerations encourages you to consider how age, gender, race, ethnicity, social class, and other aspects of the client's social location are taken into consideration when developing the treatment plan.
- Evidence-based practice: The optional (unless your professor or supervisor requires it) evidence-based practice section invites you to review the "evidence-based practice" section of Chapter 2 and the related professional literature and describe the match between the presenting problem, theory, and clients' social location factors.
- Client perspective: Describes areas of client agreement and concern with the outlined plan.

The basic template looks like this:

TREATMENT PLAN

Date: _____   Case/Client #: _____

Clinician Name: _____   Theory: _____

Modalities planned: ☐ Individual Adult ☐ Individual Child ☐ Couple ☐ Family ☐ Group: _____
Recommended session frequency: ☐ Weekly ☐ Every 2 weeks ☐ Other: _____
Expected length of treatment: __ months

Treatment Plan with Goals and Interventions

Early-Phase Client Goal: Manage crisis; reduce distressing symptoms.

1. Select Goal Type <u>personal/relational dynamic from theory</u> to reduce <u>symptom.</u>

   Measure: Able to sustain _____ for a period of _____.
   Interventions:
   a. _____
   b. _____

Working-Phase Client Goals: Target individual and relational dynamics using theoretical concepts.

1. Select Goal Type <u>personal/relational dynamic from theory</u> to reduce <u>symptom.</u>

   Measure: Able to sustain _____ for a period of _____.
   Interventions:
   a. _____
   b. _____

2. Select Goal Type <u>personal/relational dynamic from theory</u> to reduce <u>symptom.</u>

   Measure: Able to sustain _____ for a period of _____.
   Interventions:
   a. _____
   b. _____

3. Select Goal Type <u>personal/relational dynamic from theory</u> to reduce <u>symptom.</u>

   Measure: Able to sustain _____ for a period of _____.
   Interventions:
   a. _____
   b. _____

Closing-Phase Client Goals: Long-term goals or goals set by theory's definition of health.

1. Select Goal Type <u>personal/relational dynamic from theory</u> to reduce <u>symptom.</u>

   Measure: Able to sustain _____ for a period of _____.
   Interventions:
   a. _____
   b. _____

2. Select Goal Type <u>personal/relational dynamic from theory</u> to reduce <u>symptom</u> _____.

   Measure: Able to sustain _____ for a period of _____.
   Interventions:
   a. _____
   b. _____

Treatment Tasks

1. Develop working therapeutic relationship using theory of choice:

   Relationship building approach/intervention:
   a. _____

2. Case conceptualization of individual, relational, and community dynamics using theory of choice.

   Strategies and techniques:
   a. _____
   b. _____

3. Identify needed referrals, crisis issues, collateral contacts, and other client needs.

    a. *Crisis assessment intervention(s):* _____

    b. *Referral(s):* _____

Diversity Considerations

Describe how treatment plan, goals, and interventions were adapted to address each area of diversity:

Age: *Include developmental tasks, cognitive ability, family life cycle, generational differences, etc.:*

Gender: *Include specific gender-role identity (e.g., working mother, traditional male, male–female transsexual, etc.), sexual orientation, ethnically based gender roles, etc.:*

Race/Ethnicity/Religion/Class/Region: *Include race, ethnicity (i.e., Italian American rather than white), immigration status, religious beliefs, socioeconomic status, and geographic region:*

Other factors: *Identify any other significant diversity considerations, such as school, work, community etc.:*

Evidence-Based Practice (Optional)

Summarize evidence for using this approach for this presenting concern and/or population: _____

Client Perspective (Optional)

Has treatment plan been reviewed with client: ☐ Yes ☐ No; If no, explain: _____

Describe areas of Client Agreement and Concern: _____

_____, _____ _____ _____, _____ _____

Therapist's Signature   Intern Status   Date   Supervisor's Signature   License   Date

📑 You can download this form from www.cengagebrain.com and www.masteringcompetencies.com.

Writing Useful Client Goals

I am going to tell you the truth: writing good client goals is a difficult task. The trick is that they can be written only after one has done a thorough case conceptualization and clinical assessment.

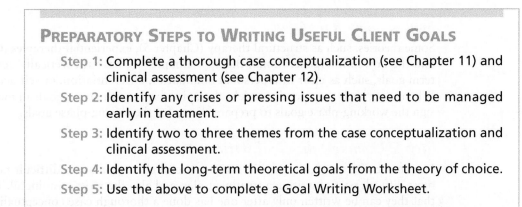

PREPARATORY STEPS TO WRITING USEFUL CLIENT GOALS

Step 1: Complete a thorough case conceptualization (see Chapter 11) and clinical assessment (see Chapter 12).

Step 2: Identify any crises or pressing issues that need to be managed early in treatment.

Step 3: Identify two to three themes from the case conceptualization and clinical assessment.

Step 4: Identify the long-term theoretical goals from the theory of choice.

Step 5: Use the above to complete a Goal Writing Worksheet.

The Basic Steps

Step 1: Case Conceptualization and Clinical Assessment

Therapists should use the forms in Chapters 11 and 12 to conduct a thorough conceptualization and assessment. The case conceptualization is the most important and difficult step, and the one most new therapists would prefer to skip. Why? It requires significant reflective and critical thinking; it is *not* formulaic. It will take some time to apply theoretical concepts to your client's actual situation. You will struggle. It most often will *not* be as clear as in the textbook (painful truth: nothing in life is). But in that struggle, you will actually learn how to use theory. You will become a competent therapist. The clinical assessment is generally a bit more straightforward. So set aside a lot of time to do these two steps, and know that it is well worth the effort—you have officially begun your license exam preparation. Whatever you master now, you will not need to pay to learn once you are out of school.

Step 2: Crises or Pressing Issues

In the clinical assessment, the therapist should have identified crisis issues such as the following:

- Suicidal or homicidal threats
- Potential, current, or past child, dependent adult, or elder abuse
- Current or past domestic or social violence
- Alcohol or substance abuse issues
- Need for an evaluation for medication or other medical issues that could impact treatment
- Eating disorders, self-mutilation, or other danger symptoms that need immediate attention
- Severe depressive, psychotic, or panic episodes or other serious symptoms that need to be stabilized for outpatient treatment

If any of these issues have been identified, they should be addressed in the "Early-Stage Client Goal" section; if not, the therapist can include an early-stage goal that relates to the presenting problem.

Step 3: Themes from the Case Conceptualization and Clinical Assessment

After completing these two assessments, the therapist steps back and asks the following questions:

- What two to three key patterns emerged in the case conceptualization?
- How do these fit with the clinical assessment?
- What theory do I want to use, and how would it describe these key themes?

Step 4: Long-Term Goals

Some theories, such as structural therapy (Chapter 5), experiential therapies (Chapter 6), and the Bowen intergenerational therapy (Chapter 7), have theoretically defined long-term goals, such as clear interpersonal boundaries, differentiation, or self-actualization. When using such therapeutic models, therapists begin with larger goals in mind and design the working-phase goals to prepare clients for the closing-phase goals.

Step 5: Complete the Goal Writing Worksheet

I am not going to sugarcoat this: writing useful client goals is a difficult task; it's *the* most difficult part of writing a treatment plan and also the most meaningful. The trick is that they can be written only after one has done a thorough case conceptualization and clinical assessment. The following Goal Writing Worksheet will help you link together the following:

- Client's reported problem
- Problematic relational dynamic identified in the case conceptualization
- Psychiatric or relational symptoms (from clinical assessment)

I promise you—in any given situation, you should be able to find two to four core dynamics that line up all three of these. Sometimes it takes awhile, but when you get it, everything else is easy.

GOAL WRITING WORKSHEET

Presenting problem: These are used to help identify problem *dynamics*.

What does the client say is the problem(s)? Use the client's words and phrases as much as possible.

1. _____
2. _____
3. _____

Dynamic: These are used to write your *goals*. Develop a case conceptualization based on "The Viewing: Case Conceptualization" section of each theory chapter. Identify two to four of the most salient problematic relational dynamics or discourses from the case conceptualization; these are the dynamics that are most likely to be contributing to the client's presenting problem. In some cases, you will see that certain dynamics overlap or are related; in these situations, try to summarize these overlapping dynamics into one point below.

1. _____
2. _____
3. _____

Symptoms: Identify two to four of the most salient psychological symptoms or issues from the clinical assessment (e.g., depression, anxiety, substance use, conflict with loved ones, isolation, loss of interest, hallucinations, etc.). List these below.

1. _____
2. _____
3. _____

Put It All Together

This keeps you honest: Do all the pieces fit together?

PRESENTING PROBLEM	DYNAMIC	SYMPTOM
1.		
2.		
3.		

Note: If for any reason you have symptoms that don't seem to be related to the dynamics you chose, review your case conceptualization again. The pieces should fit together.

(continued)

> ## GOAL WRITING WORKSHEET (*CONTINUED*)
>
> **Evidence-Base Practice** (Optional): Helps you determine theory and technique.
> Use PsychInfo or a similar search engine to do a review of the research literature related to: (a) the client's presenting problem, (b) diagnosis, (c) personal demographics/diversity factors, and/or (e) your intended therapy approach. Describe the key interventions, techniques, or guidelines below.
>
> 1. _____
> 2. _____
> 3. _____
>
> Based on the most salient dynamics and evidence-base as well as your client's needs, which theory and/or techniques do you plan to use with this case? ____

The Goal-Writing Process

If you have completed the above steps, writing the goal becomes much easier. However, there are no clear rules for every situation because each client is unique. However, goal writing has three basic components:

> ## GUIDELINES FOR WRITING USEFUL GOALS
>
> 1. **Start with a key concept or assessment area from the theory of choice:** Start with "increase" or "decrease," followed by a description using language from the chosen theory about what is going to change (this comes from the case conceptualization).
>
> 2. **Link to symptoms:** Describe what symptoms will be addressed by changing the personal or relational dynamic (this comes from the clinical assessment).
>
> 3. **Use the client's name:** Using a name (or equivalent confidential notation) ensures that it is a unique goal rather than a formulaic one.
>
> ### Anatomy of a Client Goal
>
> "Increase/Decrease" + [individual/relational dynamic] + "to reduce/increase" + [symptom/behavior]
>
> Part A   Part B

Part A of the figure gives the therapist a clear focus of treatment that fits with the theory of choice. Part B clearly links the changes in symptoms to the focus of treatment stated in A. Examples:

* *Increase* effectiveness of parental hierarchy between AF and CF *to reduce* frequency of CF's tantrums per week (structural therapy)
* *Reduce and interrupt* pursuer/distancer pattern between AF and AM *to reduce* AF's sense of hopelessness and AM's irritability (systemic therapy)
* *Increase* frequency of social interaction and reengagement in music and sports hobbies *to increase* periods of positive mood (solution-focused therapy)

Each part has a different function. Part A is most useful to therapists for conceptualizing treatment; Part B is most useful to third-party payers, who require a medical model assessment. When therapists write goals that address both A and B, they allow themselves maximum freedom and flexibility to work in their preferred way while also answering the needs of third-party payers.

Writing Measurable Goals

Most third-party payers require goals to be "measurable," meaning that somehow, the client and therapist will know when the goal is achieved. Starting the goal with "increase/decrease" helps in this effort. In addition, some third parties want therapists to specify exactly what the criterion will be to determine if the goal has been met. To meet this requirement, you may use the following:

Measure: Able to sustain ___ for a period of ___ ☐ weeks ☐ months.
Examples:

* Able to sustain <u>positive mood</u> for a period of 2 ☐ weeks ☐ months.
* Able to sustain <u>positive relational interactions</u> for a period of 2 ☐ weeks ☐ months.
* Able to sustain <u>sobriety</u> for a period of 6 ☐ weeks ☐ months.
* Able to sustain <u>C grade point average</u> for a period of 4 ☐ weeks ☐ months.

Early-Phase Client Goals

During the initial phase of therapy—in most cases, the first one to three sessions—client goals generally involve stabilizing crisis symptoms, such as suicidal and homicidal thinking, severe depressive or panic episodes, and poor eating and sleeping patterns; managing child, dependent adult, and elder abuse issues; addressing substance and alcohol abuse issues; and stopping self-harming behaviors, such as cutting.

In addition to stabilizing crisis issues, some theories have specific clinical goals that should be addressed in the initial phases. For example, solution-based therapists begin working on clinical symptoms in the first session by setting small, measurable goals toward desired behaviors as well as by increasing clients' level of hope (O'Hanlon & Weiner-Davis, 1989).

Working-Phase Client Goals

Working-phase goals address the dynamics that create and/or sustain the symptoms and problems for which clients came to therapy. These are the goals that most interest third-party payers. The secret to writing good working-phase goals is framing them in the theoretical language used for conceptualization and then linking this language to the psychiatric symptoms. Using theoretical language enables therapists to document a coherent treatment using their preferred language of conceptualization rather than language that is geared to those who prescribe medication.

For example, when a client is diagnosed with depression, many therapists include a goal such as "reduce depressed mood." Let's not kid ourselves: a person does not need a master's degree and thousands of hours of training to come up with such a goal. This medical-model, symptom-based goal does not provide clues as to what the therapist will actually do. Furthermore, all documentation for the case will need to monitor the client's level of depression each week. In contrast, a clinical client goal should address the theoretical conceptualization that will guide the reduction of depression. For example:

* Structural therapy: Reduce enmeshment with children and increase parental hierarchy to reduce episodes of depressed mood.
* Satir's communication approach: Reduce placating behaviors in marriage and at work to increase congruent communication and positive mood.

• Narrative therapy: Reduce influence of family and societal evaluations of self-worth to increase sense of autonomy and reduce depressed mood.

Each of these goals addresses a client's depressed mood and provides a clear clinical conceptualization and sense of direction, being much more useful to therapists than the medical goal of "reduce depressed mood."

Closing-Phase Client Goals

Closing-phase client goals address: (a) larger, more global issues that clients bring to therapy and/or (b) move the client toward greater "health" as defined by the therapist's theoretical perspective. As an example of the former type, clients may present with one issue, perhaps marital discord, and then later in therapy want to address their parenting issues. Similarly, often clients may present with depression or anxiety and in the later phase want to address relationship issues or an unresolved issue with their family of origin. A couple may present with several pressing issues, such as conflict and sexual concerns, to be treated in the working phase, and in the later phase they may want to examine more global issues, such as redefining their identities and relational agreements.

The second type of client goal is driven by the therapist's agenda. Some approaches, such as Bowen intergenerational, humanistic, and structural therapies, have clearly defined theories of health toward which therapists work. Other approaches, such as systemic and solution-focused therapies, have less clearly defined long-term goals and theories. Closing-phase goals often include an agenda item that clients may not have verbalized. For example, differentiation, a long-term goal that is embedded in the theory of Bowenian intergenerational therapy, is too theoretical for clients to present.

Try It Yourself

With a partner or on your own, try to write a goal using your preferred theory for an actual client or a client you saw in a video recently.

Writing Useful Interventions

The final element of treatment plans is including interventions to support each therapeutic task or client goal. Once treatment has been conceptualized and therapeutic tasks and client goals have been identified, identifying useful interventions is generally quite easy. The interventions should come from the therapist's chosen theory and be specific to the client. The following points are guidelines for writing interventions:

GUIDELINES FOR WRITING INTERVENTIONS

• **Use specific interventions from chosen theory:** Interventions should be clearly derived from the theory used to conceptualize therapeutic tasks and client goals. If an intervention from another theory is integrated, the modifications should be clearly spelled out. For example, genograms can be adapted to solution-focused therapy. (Kuehl, 1995)

• **Make interventions specific to client:** Use confidential notation (e.g., AF for adult female and AM for adult male) to make the goal as specific

> and clear as possible: for example, "Sculpt AF's pattern of pursuing and AM's tendency to withdraw."
> - **Include exact language when possible:** Whenever possible, therapists should use the exact question or language they will use to deliver the intervention; for example, "On a scale of 1 to 10, how would you rate your current level of satisfaction in the marriage?"

Writing Useful Therapeutic Tasks

The therapeutic tasks are, for lack of a better word, the *training wheels,* of the plan, meaning these are included primarily to help newer therapists fully conceptualize their tasks early in their careers (although most older folks also benefit from a reminder of basic competencies). However, these will typically not be included in plans you send to insurance companies or third-party payers. That said, they are an excellent thing to have documented if there are ever any legal or ethical questions about your performance.

As I believe in truth in advertising, therapeutic tasks are generally the easiest part of the treatment plan to develop because they are the most formulaic. Each theory has its own language and interventions for describing how to approach treatment tasks, such as creating a therapeutic relationship, and a good plan should reflect these differences. For example, a Bowen intergenerational therapist focuses on remaining nonreactive to clients, whereas a therapist using experiential family therapy has a more emotionally engaged approach to creating a therapeutic relationship. There are three essential treatment tasks:

- Establish a therapeutic relationship
- Case conceptualization of individual, family, and social dynamics
- Crisis management and referrals

The treatment plan templates in chapters on specific theories provide excellent examples for how to do this for each approach (and, yes, you can copy these almost verbatim—at least in my class).

Social Location and Diversity Considerations

In this section of the plan, you are asked to identify how you modified your plan—including choice of theory, goals, interventions, and treatment tasks—to account for client social location and diversity issues, such as ethnicity, race, sexual orientation, gender orientation, religion, language, ability, age, gender, etc. The form includes four broad areas of social location, and all four areas should be considered for all clients. Here are some examples:

- Age: Include developmental tasks, cognitive ability, family life cycle, generational differences, etc.:
  - Use of humor with teens
  - Use of play and age-appropriate explanations with children
  - Menopause with women
  - Acculturation differences between generations
  - Family life-cycle transitions such as launching children, transition to school, etc.
- Gender/sexual orientation and identity: Include specific gender-role identity (e.g., working mother, traditional male, male–female transsexual, etc.), sexual orientation, ethnically based gender roles, etc.:
  - Use of humor with men

- Women's sources of identity, such as working mother
- Addressing gender power issues
- Assessing family-of-choice with gay, lesbian, bisexual, or transgendered clients
- Accounting for the stress of marginalization and discrimination in assessment with gay, lesbian, bisexual, or transgendered clients

- Race/ethnicity/religion/class/region: Include race, ethnicity (i.e., Italian American rather than white), immigration status, religious beliefs, socioeconomic status, and geographic region:
  - More formal, respectful relational style with immigrants or clients from ethnic backgrounds that prefer such relations with professionals (*respecto* with Latino clients)
  - Use of *personalismo* with Hispanic/Latino clients
  - Including spirituality and religious beliefs and resources
  - Including more extended family or tribe members with clients who come from backgrounds where the extended family/tribal system is the primary system
  - Using interventions, assessments, and questions that enable Asian clients to avoid losing face
  - Use of present-focused, problem-focused approaches with clients who do not value exploring the past
  - Including culturally appropriate resources and persons in therapy
  - Accounting for the stress of marginalization and discrimination in assessment
  - Adjusting interventions based on client's level of education and/or professional status
  - Adjusting goals or interventions based on geographic region, such as rural, Midwest, Southwest, etc.
- Other factors: Identify any other significant diversity considerations, such as school, work, community etc.
  - School culture for children and teens
  - Work or professional culture, such as entertainment industry

Try It Yourself

With a partner or on your own, identify some considerations that a therapist should have in mind when working with you based on your social location (e.g., age, gender, ethnicity, education, class, etc). Which of these considerations are most likely to have a negative impact on you if the therapist missed it?

Evidence-Based Practice

In this section, you can summarize the research that supports your treatment plan. You can find this evidence in several places, including:

- Chapter 2 of this text, which reviews multiple forms of evidence in the field of family therapy
- The "research and evidence-base" section in each of the theory chapters in Part II of this text
- Your own research, such as a PsychInfo search

The case studies at the end of each theory chapter in the book have examples of how to complete this section.

Client Perspectives

Finally, therapists need to ask themselves, or better yet, their clients, "What do my clients think of this plan?"

- Are these the things the client wants to change?
- Are these interventions and activities that my client would be willing to try?
- Do the goals and interventions "fit" with my client's personality, cultural background, age, gender, values, educational level, cognitive level, and lifestyle?
- Are there areas where the client and I have different ideas about what might be the source of the problem?
- Will we be starting where my client wants to start or where there is the most immediate distress?
- Does the plan make sense to my client?

Considering the client's perspective is crucial to designing an effective plan. Therapists should discuss the plan directly with clients and ensure that there is a shared understanding about the goals, strategies for change, and outcomes. Many agencies have moved to having clients sign the treatment plan to ensure agreement. However, to avoid overwhelming the client with too much jargon, the therapist should probably include only the client goals from the treatment plan.

Do Plans Make a Difference?

Of course, therapy rarely goes according to plan. Life happens; new problems arise; original problems lose their importance; new stressors change the playing field. But that does not make plans useless. Treatment plans:

- Help therapists think through which dynamics need to be changed and how.
- Provide therapists with a clear understanding of the client situation so that they can quickly and skillfully address new crisis issues or stressors.
- Give therapists a sense of confidence and clarity of thought that make it easier to respond to new issues.
- Ground therapists in their theory and in their understanding of how their theory relates to clinical symptoms.

All this is to say, do not be surprised when therapy does not go according to plan; instead, expect it. And know that the time you took to create a treatment plan makes you much better able to respond to the unplanned.

QUESTIONS FOR PERSONAL REFLECTION AND CLASS DISCUSSION

1. How do you think a treatment plan will be helpful to you? In what ways may it not be as helpful as you would hope as a new clinician?
2. If a client comes in and continually talks about something other than what you have on your treatment plan, how would you handle this? What might make you stick to your plan? What might make you revise your plan?
3. Which part of the plan seems most daunting to you? Which seems easiest?
4. After watching a video in class or movie at home, try to write a treatment plan based on the problems presented.
5. Describe a situation in which you imagine the treatment plan would need to adjusted for the following reason:
   - For client age?
   - For client gender?

- For client ethnicity?
- For client religion?
- For client sexual orientation or gender identification?
- For client's educational level?
- For clients' social class?
- Ethnic differences between therapist and client?
- Gender differences between therapist and client?

ONLINE RESOURCES

Symptom-Based Treatment Planners from Dr. Arthur Jongsma

www.jongsma.com

Go to MindTap® for an eBook, videos of client sessions, activities, digital forms, practice quizzes, apps, and more—all in one place. If your instructor didn't assign MindTap, you can find out more information at CengageBrain.com.

REFERENCES

Berman, P. S. (1997). *Case conceptualization and treatment planning.* Thousand Oaks, CA: Sage.

Dattilio, F. M., & Jongsma, A. E. (2000). *The family therapy treatment planner.* New York: Wiley.

Gehart, D. R., & Tuttle, A. R. (2003). *Theory-based treatment planning for marriage and family therapists: Integrating theory and practice.* Pacific Grove, CA: Brooks/Cole.

Johnson, S. L. (2004). *Therapist's guide to clinical intervention: The 1-2-3's of treatment planning* (2nd ed.). San Diego, CA: Academic.

Jongsma, A. E., Peterson, L. M., & Bruce, T. J. (2006). *The complete adult psychotherapy treatment planner* (4th ed.). New York: Wiley.

Jongsma, A. E., Peterson, L. M., McInnis, W. P., & Bruce, T. J. (2006). *The child psychotherapy treatment planner* (4th ed.). New York: Wiley.

Kuehl, B. P. (1995). The solution-oriented genogram: A collaborative approach. *Journal of Marital and Family Therapy, 21,* 239–250.

O'Hanlon, W. H., & Weiner-Davis, M. (1989). *In search of solutions: A new direction in psychotherapy.* New York: Norton.

O'Leary, K. D., Heyman, R. E., & Jongsma, A. E. (1998). *The couples psychotherapy treatment planner.* New York: Wiley.

Wiger, D. E. (2005). *The psychotherapy documentation primer* (2nd ed.). New York: Wiley.

CHAPTER
14

Evaluating Progress in Therapy

Learning Objectives

After reading this chapter and a few hours of focused studying, you should be able to:

- Identify brief, practical ways to measure client change in family therapy.

- Describe nonstandardized measures of client progress.

- Outline several possible procedures that can be used to measure client progress, including symptom inventories as well as couple and family measures.

Step 4: Evaluating Progress

Critics tease therapists on numerous fronts: we make people lie on couches; repeatedly ask, "How does that make you feel?"; encourage omphaloskepsis (the technical term for navel gazing); and often lead crazier lives than our clients. There may or may not be much truth in any of these accusations. But there is one question that therapists need to take seriously: Do I make a difference?

Increasingly, insurance companies, state legislators, and other third-party payers are asking therapists to evaluate progress (Lambert & Hawkins, 2004). This is a daunting task, especially when compared to evaluation in other medical professions. It is relatively easy to determine whether a surgery was successful, physical therapy made a difference, or a medication is working: these are physical things that can be measured with a fair degree of reliability. But when therapists are asked to measure whether depression is getting better, anxiety has decreased or a person is worrying less, measurement becomes trickier. If we could x-ray a person's mind or psyche and get an objective measure of levels of mood, that might help. If we could control for all the factors that contribute to a person's feelings and behaviors—including relationship ups and downs, work stress, news headlines, physical illness, and weather—that would also give us a clearer sense of whether or not we are helping. If we could factor out the biases of our own personalities, histories, and moods, that might also give us a clearer picture. Because these factors are difficult to pinpoint, therapists need to be creative and thoughtful when measuring progress.

Because of the subtlety of what is being measured, assessing client progress—the fourth step of competent therapy—requires strategy and thought. Therapists have two general options for measuring progress: (a) nonstandardized measures, the client's and therapist's subjective reports of progress; and (b) standardized measures, which track specific psychological variables.

Nonstandardized Evaluations

Nonstandardized evaluations of progress are simply verbal or written descriptions by either the client or the therapist. In either case, the evaluation should be included in the written documentation for the client (his or her "file"). Increasingly, third-party payers require client evaluations of their progress in addition to therapist descriptions. Many insurance companies have shifted from having therapists complete treatment plans to having clients complete progress checklists to assess whether therapy is warranted and effective. Although some research suggests that clients' assessment of their level of functioning is useful, such self-reports are generally considered less reliable than standardized measures.

Pros and Cons

Nonstandardized evaluations have both advantages and disadvantages.

Advantages of Nonstandardized Evaluations
- Financial costs are minimal.
- They can be done every session.
- Including client and therapist perspectives creates greater validity.
- They are easily adapted for diverse clients
- When used weekly, they provide feedback on what is not working so that the therapist can adjust the treatment plan.

Disadvantages of Nonstandardized Evaluations
- They are not as reliable or valid as standardized measures.
- They are difficult to use with children if parents are not there to help provide information (although this is an even bigger problem with standardized instruments).
- They are more difficult to use with persons with severe pathology and/or with those who are unable to accurately recall events between sessions.
- With certain couples or families, data should be collected on paper to get assessments that are not influenced by the comments of other members.

Strategies for Nonstandardized Assessment

There are several easy ways to gather information for nonstandardized assessment:

* Ask clients to assess their progress since the last meeting. Ask about changes in specific symptoms or progress toward goals (how often were you depressed, how often did you have a panic attack, how often did you binge?).
* Ask clients to rate their own change using solution-focused scaling questions (see Chapter 9; Berg & de Shazer, 1993).

Therapists can document both the clients' and their own assessment of progress: (a) in a narrative style (using phrases or sentences) or (b) by using a scale.

Examples of Narrative Descriptions

* Client reports an increase in depressive episodes over the week (five out of seven days).
* Clients report a decrease in conflict over the week; only one major argument.
* Client reports no change in difficulty sleeping in past week (one to two hours to fall asleep).

Example of Scaling

Solution-Focused Scaling:
This week = _____ (with 1 = Worst things have been 1 and 10 = Goal achieved)
This week: Start of treatment": _____ (with 1 = Worst things have been and 10 = Goals achieved).

Standardized Evaluations

Standardized measures of progress are generally considered more accurate than nonstandardized measures. These evaluations involve pen-and-paper or electronic questionnaires that are completed by clients and/or significant others. They have been tested for reliability and validity and allow therapists to more carefully track changes and compare a single client with a group norm, which is most meaningful when the client is similar to a comparable group (e.g., in level of functioning, culture, age).

The common problem with these evaluations is that each person has unique frames of reference and situations that make it difficult to interpret the scores. In general, the more diverse the clientele, the more difficult it is to accurately interpret scores. For example, I once had a trainee work with a Chinese immigrant (sessions were in Mandarin), and she used a standardized instrument to collect initial symptoms and symptoms at the end of the semester three months later. Although the client appeared to have made significant progress, the instrument indicated that she had gotten *worse*. When the student followed up with the client about whether things were significantly worse, the client stated that she had minimized the reporting of symptoms initially because she did not trust the therapist and was uncomfortable admitting to certain problems. After she had developed a good rapport with the therapist, she felt free to more accurately answer the questions, which is consistent with her cultural value of saving face. The moral of the story is that standardized forms work only if clients are able to "play by the rules" by answering questions the way the authors intended. Clearly, therapists need to proceed with caution when trying to interpret standardized forms, and they must talk with clients when the results are unexpected.

Pros and Cons

As with nonstandardized evaluations, standardized measures have both advantages and disadvantages.

Advantages of Standardized Evaluations

- They are considered more reliable and valid.
- The therapist is better able to make cross-client comparisons.
- The therapist is better able to make comparisons across time.
- They can be used to document the therapist's effectiveness.

Disadvantages of Standardized Evaluations

- Almost all standardized forms must be purchased; some require a fee for each administration of the instrument, which can quickly become expensive.
- They may require more therapist time and/or equipment and resources (e.g., computers, copiers).
- They require more client time, and clients may be reluctant to give this time without a motivating explanation.
- Not all measures are standardized for diverse populations and/or available in the client's primary language.

Effects on the Therapeutic Relationship

Using questionnaires always impacts the therapeutic relationship because it places the therapist above the client in hierarchical position. Therefore, therapists need to be thoughtful about how they present formal assessments and help clients make sense of the therapeutic relationship when they do use these measures.

Real-World Options for Standardized Evaluations of Progress

In the ideal world (or obsessive–compulsive fantasy, depending on your perspective) described by academics, theoreticians, and researchers, therapists would have clients complete the most reliable and valid assessments at regular intervals over the course of therapy. This is great in theory—that is, until you factor in that reliability and validity are generally correlated with the *length* of the instrument (Lambert & Hawkins, 2004; Miller et al., 2003), and for those who work in typical clinical settings—community agencies and private practices—the reality is that neither clients nor clinicians are enthusiastic about completing lengthy questionnaires. Short and sweet is the reality with most clients and therapists. Thankfully, therapists have an increasing number of shorter options.

Guidelines for Using Standardized Measures in Everyday Practice

The following are guidelines for using standardized measures in everyday practice:

- First session: Because there is evidence that most change occurs early in therapy, the initial measures of symptoms and functioning should occur in the first session (Lambert & Hawkins, 2004).
- Five minutes or less: Lambert and Hawkins (2004) recommend that instruments take no longer than five minutes to complete.

- Regular (weekly or monthly) intervals: Although pretest and posttest measures are straightforward in research studies, defining "post" in real-world practice is difficult because clients may drop out rather than announce their intention to end treatment—and they rarely agree to return to complete the posttest. Therefore, therapists should develop a regular interval for measuring client progress in clinical settings. Depending on the instrument and setting, weekly, monthly, or quarterly evaluations may be appropriate.
- Before the session: It does not take much time to learn that asking clients to complete a questionnaire before the session is generally much more successful than afterward, when clients are often in a rush to leave. When used before, questionnaires help develop an agenda for the session.
- Framing the measurement: If the therapist conveys the message that the measurement is helpful to treatment, most clients will be willing to spend five minutes to improve their treatment outcomes. Lambert and Hawkins (2004) recommend comparing it to a medical doctor getting blood pressure or vital signs at the beginning of each visit: this information helps the doctor or therapist be more useful to the client.

Ultrabrief Measures

Marriage and family therapists have several options for measuring both clinical and relational functioning with instruments that are *ultrabrief,* requiring as little as 1 minute to complete, or *brief,* requiring less than 10 minutes to complete. Ultrabrief measures include the Outcome Rating Scale (ORS) and the Session Rating Scale (SRS); these have been gaining in popularity because of their cost-effectiveness, brevity, simple administration, and clinical relevance (Campbell & Hemsley, 2009).

Outcome Rating Scale (ORS)

Miller et al. (2003) developed the ORS as an ultrabrief version of the Outcome Questionnaire (OQ; discussed under "Brief Measures," below) in response to client and therapist complaints that even 45 questions were too much. It was designed by clinicians for clinicians and is the most clinician-friendly of the outcome measures. The ORS is composed of only four visual analog scales that take less than a minute to complete, making it ideal for weekly use and highly economical: it is free via the Internet, with photocopying the only cost. The scale measures four areas of functioning:

- **Individually** (personal well-being)
- **Interpersonally** (family and close relationships)
- **Socially** (work, school, friendship)
- **Overall** (general sense of well-being)

Two versions for children are also available: the Child Outcome Rating Scale, which includes a scale similar to that of the adult version, and the Young Child Outcome Rating Scale, which uses happy, neutral, and unhappy faces to measure how the child is feeling (Duncan et al., 2003). Scoring is simple: a ruler is used to measure how far on the 10-cm scale the client scored, and cutoff scores are used to address potential problems.

The ORS has high internal consistency (0.93) and test–retest reliability (0.84) and moderate concurrent validity with the Outcome Questionnaire 45.2, which is a longer and more established instrument OQ-45.2 (0.59; Miller et al., 2003). Given its ultrabrief format, it is not as sensitive as other outcome measures, such as the OQ-45.2, but it is sensitive enough to measure change in clinical settings, which is the primary aim of the everyday practitioner. The ORS's greatest strength is its feasibility for regular and consistent use in real-world practice settings. When therapists were trained in using either the ORS or OQ-45.2 for outcome measures, 86% were still using the ORS after one year, as compared with only 25% still using the 45-item OQ-45.2 (Miller et al., 2003), a dramatic difference.

Outcome Rating Scale (ORS)

Name _____ Age (Yrs):____
ID# _____ Sex: M / F
Session # ____ Date: _____

Looking back over the last week, including today, help us understand how you have been feeling by rating how well you have been doing in the following areas of your life, where marks to the left represent low levels and marks to the right indicate high levels.

Individually:
(Personal well-being)

I----Examination Copy Only----I

Interpersonally:
(Family, close relationships)

I----Examination Copy Only----I

Socially:
(Work, School, Friendships)

I----Examination Copy Only----I

Overall:
(General sense of well-being)

I----Examination Copy Only----I

Institute for the Study of Therapeutic Change
_____
www.talkingcure.com

© 2000, Scott D. Miller and Barry L. Duncan

Session Rating Scale (SRS)

Also developed by Duncan et al. (2003), the SRS, Version 3.0 (SRS V3.0), is typically used with the ORS. Whereas the ORS is given at the beginning of the session, the SRS is used at the end of the session to measure the therapeutic alliance, which is consistently found to be one of the best predictors of positive outcome (Orlinsky, Rønnestad, & Willutzki, 2004). Client ratings of alliance are better predictors of outcome than therapist ratings of alliance (Batchelor & Horvath, 1999). In a study conducted by Whipple et al. (2003), therapists who had access to both alliance and outcome information were twice as likely to achieve clinically significant change as those who did not.

Like the ORS, the SRS consists of only four analog scales:

* Relationship: Does the client feel heard, understood, and respected?
* Goals and topics: Does the client feel that the session focused on what he or she wanted to work on?
* Approach or method: Was the therapist's approach a good fit?
* Overall: Was the session helpful ("right") for the client?

As with the ORS, two versions for children are also available: the Child Session Rating Scale (CSRS), which includes a scale similar to that of the adult version, and the Young Child Session Rating Scale (YCSRS), which uses happy, neutral, and unhappy faces to measure how the child is feeling (Duncan et al., 2003). Scoring is simple: a ruler is used to measure how far on the 10-cm scale the client scored, and cutoff scores are used to address potential problems. Research has identified a very high cutoff score for this instrument, meaning that when clients start indicating that there are minor problems with alliance, therapists need to swiftly address these issues to ensure a positive outcome. This scale can be particularly helpful for newer therapists who want to create a strong alliance.

The SRS has good internal consistency (0.88) and a test–retest reliability of 0.64, which is comparable to other alliance measures (Duncan et al., 2003). The concurrent validity of the measure when compared to similar measures is 0.48, providing evidence that a similar construct is being measured. The greatest strength of the SRS, as of the ORS, is its feasibility and user-friendliness. It is used by 96% of clinicians who are introduced to it, as compared with only 29% of clinicians using the 12-item Working Alliance Inventory.

Try It Yourself

Make a copy of the SRS and ORS and complete one based on a therapy session you once experienced as well as your current functioning this week.

Brief Measures

Brief measures are assessment instruments that require less than 10 minutes to complete. Two of the more common ones are the Outcome Questionnaire (OQ) and the Symptom Check List (SCL).

Outcome Questionnaire (OQ-45.2)

The Outcome Questionnaire (OQ-45.2) was designed to measure outcome in clinical settings (Lambert et al., 1996). The questionnaire has a total of 45 items, takes less than five minutes to complete, and includes three subscales:

1. Symptom Distress (clinical, mental health symptoms)
2. Interpersonal Relationships
3. Social Role Performance

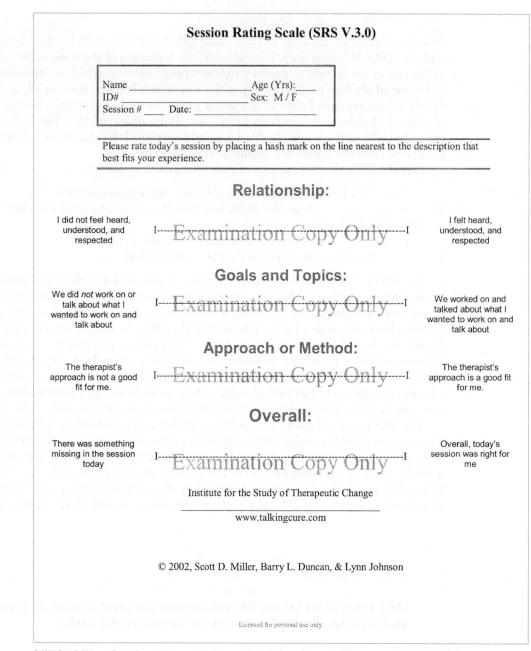

Session Rating Scale (SRS V.3.0)

Name _____ Age (Yrs): _____
ID# _____ Sex: M / F
Session # ____ Date: _____

Please rate today's session by placing a hash mark on the line nearest to the description that best fits your experience.

Relationship:

I did not feel heard, understood, and respected   I-----Examination Copy Only-----I   I felt heard, understood, and respected

Goals and Topics:

We did *not* work on or talk about what I wanted to work on and talk about   I-----Examination Copy Only-----I   We worked on and talked about what I wanted to work on and talk about

Approach or Method:

The therapist's approach is not a good fit for me.   I-----Examination Copy Only-----I   The therapist's approach is a good fit for me.

Overall:

There was something missing in the session today   I-----Examination Copy Only-----I   Overall, today's session was right for me

Institute for the Study of Therapeutic Change

www.talkingcure.com

© 2002, Scott D. Miller, Barry L. Duncan, & Lynn Johnson

There is also a youth version, the Youth Outcome Questionnaire (YOQ), which can be completed by parents, and a Youth Outcome Questionnaire Self-Report (YOQ-SR) for youth from 12 to 18. Briefer, single-scale (only a global score), 30-item versions are available for the OQ and YOQ, and a 10-item version is also available for the OQ. These measures are affordable and easy to administer, score, and interpret, with the briefer versions being more practical for frequent measurement.

The OQ-45.2 has good test–retest reliability (0.66–0.86) and internal consistency (0.7–0.9; Lambert & Hawkins, 2004). One minor weakness is that the subscales are highly correlated with one another, meaning that they may not be measuring unique constructs. Most of the research on its validity and reliability has been conducted on the summary score, and clinicians are encouraged to use this as the primary measure of progress (Lambert & Hawkins, 2004). The following are some sample questions used on this questionnaire:

SAMPLE QUESTIONS FROM THE OUTCOME QUESTIONNAIRE

	NEVER	RARELY	SOMETIMES	FREQUENTLY	ALMOST ALWAYS
1. I get along well with others.	☐	☐	☐	☐	☐
2. I tire quickly	☐	☐	☐	☐	☐
3. I feel no interest in things.	☐	☐	☐	☐	☐
4. I feel stressed at work/school	☐	☐	☐	☐	☐
5. I blame myself for things.	☐	☐	☐	☐	☐
6. I feel irritated.	☐	☐	☐	☐	☐
18. I feel lonely.	☐	☐	☐	☐	☐
19. I have frequent arguments.	☐	☐	☐	☐	☐
20. I feel loved and wanted.	☐	☐	☐	☐	☐
21. I enjoy my spare time.	☐	☐	☐	☐	☐
22. I have difficulty concentrating.	☐	☐	☐	☐	☐
23. I feel hopeless about the future.	☐	☐	☐	☐	☐
24. I like myself	☐	☐	☐	☐	☐

Developed by Michael J. Lambert, Ph.D. and Gary M. Burlingame, Ph.D. For more information, contact OQ Measures LLC © Copyright, 2005.

Symptom Check List (SCL-90-R) and Brief Symptom Inventory (BSI)

The Symptom Check List is a 90-item test that assesses for mental health symptoms and their intensity (mild, moderate, severe). It is designed for individuals 13 years or older and requires 12 to 15 minutes to complete. The Brief Symptom Inventory (BSI) is based on the SCL but is, as the name indicates, briefer. The BSI has 53 items, is designed for individuals 13 years or older, and takes 8 to 10 minutes to complete. Both measures have nine symptom subscales and three global indices:

Subscales
- Somatization
- Obsessive–compulsive
- Interpersonal sensitivity
- Depression
- Anxiety
- Hostility
- Phobic anxiety
- Paranoid ideation
- Psychoticism

Global Indexes
- Global Severity Index: overall psychological distress
- Positive Symptom Distress Index (PSDI): intensity of symptoms
- Positive Symptom Total (PST): number of self-reported symptoms

Ultrabrief 6- and 10-item versions that correlate to the overall distress scores have also been developed (Rosen et al., 2000), and are more feasible options for everyday practice. The SCL-90-R has good test–retest validity, ranging from 0.63 to 0.86 for online versions and 0.68 to 0.84 for pen-and-paper versions (Derogatis & Fitzpatrick, 2004; Vallejo et al., 2007). The internal consistency coefficients are also good, ranging from 0.70 to 0.90.

Cross-Cutting Symptom Measures

Described in detail in Chapter 12, therapists can use the DSM cross-cutting symptom measures to assess whether there has been a change in symptoms. As these are newer measures, less research has been done using them as progress or outcome measures, but in initial reliability test–retest studies, the measures had good to excellent reliability, especially for the adult scales (Narrow et al., 2013).

Couple Measures

Dyadic Adjustment Scale

One of the most widely used couples inventories, the Dyadic Adjustment Scale is often used to measure progress with couples; it is a 32-item self-report instrument that requires 5 to 10 minutes to complete (Anderson et al., 2014). The scale is designed to measure the quality of the relationship and is commonly used to measure overall satisfaction; it is available for free download.

Locke–Wallace Marital Adjustment Test

Originally developed in 1959, the Locke–Wallace Marital Adjustment Test is a brief 15-item scale that measures overall marital adjustment. Also free to clinicians, this measure provides a simple method for measuring each party's marital adjustment (Freeston & Pléchaty, 1997).

Marital Satisfaction Inventory

The Marital Satisfaction Inventory, Revised (MSI_R) is a more extensive couple inventory that includes 150 true/false items and can be used clinically to quickly identify the focus of treatment. The instrument includes the following areas of couple functioning:

- Affective communication
- Role orientation
- Problem-solving communication
- Aggression
- Family history of distress
- Time together
- Dissatisfaction with children
- Disagreement about finances
- Conflict over child rearing
- Sexual dissatisfaction
- Global distress

Family Measures

Systemic Assessment of the Family Environment

One of the briefest family measures, the Systemic Assessment of the Family Environment (SAFE) is a 21-item scale that measures organizational structure and interactional processes over three generations. Therapists can use this to help design treatment and measure improvements.

Family Assessment Measure

The Family Assessment Measure III (FAM-III) is a comprehensive measure that provides a detailed assessment of all areas of family functioning: family, couple, and individual functioning. The assessment process involves multiple raters, including preadolescents, adolescents as well as adults. The scales for this measure include task accomplishment, communication/affective expression, role performance, affective involvement, control and values/norms.

Family Adaptability and Cohesion Evaluation Scale

The Family Adaptability and Cohesion Evaluation Scale (FACES-IV) is based on the Circumplex Model of Marital and Family Systems, which proposes that the balance of cohesion and flexibility are the two primary factors for conceptualizing relational functioning (Olson, 2011). This measure can be used with couples or families to measure enmeshment, disengagement, balance cohesion, chaos, balanced flexibility, and rigidity.

Final Thoughts on Outcome

Therapists are assessing client progress more closely and more precisely than in the past. Although assessment involves additional paperwork, expense, and time, numerous quick and effective options are available that integrate easily into today's practice environment. Therapist attitude is critical to the success and usefulness of an assessment instrument. If therapists believe in it, they communicate this to clients and the assessments become a unique resource for helping clients achieve their goals. Furthermore, many clients welcome standardized measures as a means of making sense of their struggle, validating their concerns, and measuring progress. In the years ahead, therapists are likely to integrate more measures of progress and outcome and use it to inform treatment.

QUESTIONS FOR PERSONAL REFLECTION AND CLASS DISCUSSION

1. What potential benefits and problems do you see with trying to measure client progress?
2. If you could choose, would you want to use standardized measures with clients? Why or why not?
3. Do you think measures would be most helpful with individuals, couples, or adults? Why?
4. If you received a low rating on the SRS, how might you discuss the issue in the next session with your client?
5. Research on the SRS indicates that if clients do not score their therapist highly, the possibility of positive outcomes is significantly less. Why do you think this is?

ONLINE RESOURCES

DSM-5 Cross-Cutting Measures
Inventories

www.psychiatry.org/dsm5

Dyadic Adjustment Scale

https://www.mhs.com/product.aspx?gr
=cli&prod=das&id=overview

Family Adaptability and Cohesion
Scale

http://www.facesiv.com/studies
/family_scales.html

Family Assessment Measures

http://www.mhs.com/product.aspx?gr=ed
u&id=overview&prod=famiii

Marital Satisfaction Inventory

http://www.wpspublish.com/store/p/2870
/marital-satisfaction-inventory-revised-msi-r

Outcome Rating Scale and Session Rating Scale

scottdmiller.com or heartandsoulofchange.com (free downloads)

Outcome Questionnaire 45

www.oqmeasures.com (for purchase)

Symptom Checklist 90

www.pearsonassessments.com/tests/scl90r.htm (for purchase)

Go to MindTap® for an eBook, videos of client sessions, activities, digital forms, practice quizzes, apps, and more—all in one place. If your instructor didn't assign MindTap, you can find out more information at CengageBrain.com.

REFERENCES

Anderson, S. R., Tambling, R. B., Huff, S. C., Heafner, J., Johnson, L. N., & Ketring, S. A. (2014). The development of a reliable change index and cutoff for the Revised Dyadic Adjustment Scale. *Journal of Marital and Family Therapy, 40*(4), 525–534. doi:10.1111/jmft.12095

Batchelor, A., & Horvath, A. (1999). The therapeutic relationship. In M. A. Hubble, B. L. Duncan, & S. D. Miller (Eds.), *The heart and soul of change* (pp. 133–178). Washington, DC: APA.

Berg, I., & de Shazer, S. (1993). Making numbers talk: Language in therapy. In S. Friedman (Ed.), *The new language of change: Constructive collaborative in psychotherapy.* New York: Guilford.

Campbell, A., & Hemsley, S. (2009). Outcome Rating Scale and Session Rating Scale in psychological practice: Clinical utility of ultra-brief measures. *Clinical Psychologist, 13*(1), 1–9. doi:10.1080/13284200802676391

Derogatis, L. R., & Fitzpatrick, M. (2004). The SCL-90-R, the Brief Symptom Inventory, and the BSI-81. In M. E. Murish (Ed.), *The use of psychological testing for treatment planning and outcome.* New York: Routledge.

Duncan, B. L., Miller, S. D., Sparks, J. A., Claud, D. A., Reynolds, L. R., Brown, J., & Johnson, L. D. (2003). Session Rating Scale: Preliminary psychometrics of a "working" alliance scale. *Journal of Brief Therapy, 3,* 3–12.

Freeston, M. H., & Pléchaty, M. (1997). Reconsiderations of the Locke-Wallace Marital Adjustment Test: Is it still relevant for the 1990s? *Psychological Reports, 81*(2), 419–434. doi:10.2466/PR0.81.6.419-434

Lambert, M. J., Hansen, N. B., Umphress, V. J., Lunnen, K., Okiishi, J., Burlingame, G. M., Huefner, J. C., & Reisinger, C. W. (1996). *Administration and scoring manual for the Outcome Questionnaire (OQ-45.2).* Wilmington, DE: American Professional Credentialing Services.

Lambert, M. J., & Hawkins, E. J. (2004). Measuring outcome in professional practice: Considerations in selecting and using brief outcome instruments. *Professional Psychology: Research and Practice, 35,* 492–499.

Miller, S. D., Duncan, B. L., Brown, J., Sparks, J. A., & Claud, D. A. (2003). The Outcome Rating Scale: A preliminary study of the reliability, validity, and feasibility of a brief visual analog measure. *Journal of Brief Therapy, 2,* 91–100.

Narrow, W. E., Clarke, D. E., Kuramoto, S. J., Kraemer, H. C., Kupfer, D. J., Greiner, L., & Regier, D. A. (2013). DSM-5 field trials in the United States and Canada, part III: Development and reliability testing of a cross-cutting symptom assessment for DSM-5. *American Journal of Psychiatry, 170*(1), 71–82. doi:10.1176/appi.ajp.2012.12071000

Olson, D. (2011). FACES IV and the circumplex model: Validation study. *Journal of Marital and Family Therapy, 37*(1), 64–80.

Orlinsky, D. E., Rønnestad, M. H., & Willutzki, U. (2004). Fifty years of process-outcome research: Continuity and change. In M. J. Lambert (Ed.), *Bergin and Garfield's handbook of psychotherapy and behavior change* (5th ed., pp. 307–393). New York: Wiley.

Rosen, C. S., Drescher, K. D., Moos, R. H., Finney, J. W., Murphy, R. T., & Gusman, F. (2000). Six- and ten-item indexes of psychological distress based on the Symptom Checklist-90. *Assessment, 7,* 103–111.

Vallejo, M. A., Jordán, C. M., Díaz, M. I., Comeche, M. I., & Ortega, J. (2007). Psychological assessment via the Internet: A reliability and validity study of online (vs paper-and-pencil) versions of the General Health Questionnaire-28 (GHQ-28) and the Symptoms Check-List-90-Revised (SCL-90-R). *Journal of Medical Internet Research, 10,* 2.

Whipple, J. L., Lambert, M. J., Vermeersch, D. A., Smart, D. W., Nielsen, S. L., & Hawkins, E. J. (2003). Improving the effects of psychotherapy: The use of early identification of treatment and problem strategies in routine practice. *Journal of Counseling Psychology, 50,* 59–68.

Document It: Progress Notes

Learning Objectives

After reading this chapter and a few hours of focused studying, you should be able to:

- Complete a progress note using the form provided.

- Define the difference between progress and process notes and know the legal implications of each.

- Outline the required elements of a HIPAA-compliant progress note.

Step 5: Documenting It: A Profession behind Closed Doors

Here's a fact that frightens many: the majority of therapists practicing today have never had another professional observe them conducting a session with a live, in-the-flesh client (Jordan, 1999). Rather than live supervision, what usually happens is case consultation, meaning that therapists report to their supervisor what was said, what happened, and what they did (Jordan, 1999). The more that interested outsiders—especially third-party payers—learn about how therapists are trained, the more they start to wonder what goes on behind closed doors. As health costs keep rising, third-party payers increasingly demand to know what therapists are doing and whether it makes a difference.

Thankfully, rather than bugging our offices or hiring spies, third-party payers have decided that the most practical means of tracking what happens in closed therapy sessions is to require therapists to leave a detailed paper trail in the form of case or progress notes, which is the final step to competent therapy. Progress notes are therapists' primary means of showing that they are rendering professional care that conforms to legal and ethical guidelines. Unless they're written down, the therapist's opinion, supervisor's judgment, and even the client's enthusiastic exclamation that "that was a helpful session" do not mean much to third-party payers. The information documented in the progress note is what counts when determining whether therapy has conformed to standard practices. In addition, case notes are critical when things get dicey; professionally kept progress notes are therapists' primary means of protecting against lawsuits and complaints.

However, if you take a walk down the halls of most community and public mental health agencies, you will hear grumbling about paperwork: "There's too much" and "It's a waste of time." This may be true, at least in part. However, if there is a clinical document therapists should not grumble about, it is progress notes. These are therapists' greatest sources of protection, and thanks to recent legislation, there is more clarity than ever about what should be in them.

Two Different Animals: Progress Notes versus Psychotherapy Notes

In 2003, the U.S. Department of Health and Human Services began enforcing a new set of medical documentation guidelines outlined in HIPAA (Health Insurance Portability and Accountability Act; USDHHS, 2003). Along with solving other health care issues such as portability of health care insurance coverage, HIPAA regulations included new privacy standards for medical documentation. Most significantly for therapists—and startling to those who had been practicing for years—was the new distinction between two sets of clinical documents: **progress notes** and **psychotherapy notes** (Halloway, 2003). Formerly, keeping two sets of notes was somewhere between unethical and illegal, depending on how you handled requests for information. However, to increase patient privacy, the new HIPAA legislation sanctioned the practice of keeping two different kinds of documents:

PROGRESS NOTES AND PSYCHOTHERAPY NOTES

- **Progress notes:** These make up the "official" medical file—the formal medical record that is shared with other medical professionals, clients (upon written request), and/or in response to subpoenas. Third-party payers generally have detailed requirements for the content of these notes.

- **Psychotherapy notes:** These are the property of the therapist (or person who created them) and remain separate from the formal medical file *if they are kept separately* (in a separate physical file). These records may include personal impressions, analyses of the client, hypotheses, and so forth. They have much greater protection under HIPAA legislation (if kept separately) and are rarely, if ever, disclosed to an outside third party. There are no standards for what information should be placed in these records because their purpose is to help therapists think through, plan, and reflect on client progress.

Progress Notes

Because psychotherapy notes are kept separate and private and have few guidelines, therapists' primary concern is with progress notes, which constitute the formal medical file. **HIPAA regulations** encourage psychotherapists to keep potentially damaging information in progress notes to a minimum because they are likely to be shared with other professionals, courts, and other parties. The goal is to *maximize client privacy* while simultaneously *documenting competent treatment that conforms to professional standards of care*. Rather than names, conversation topics, or the personal content of a client's life or the therapeutic conversation, third-party payers prefer detailed information about: (a) the frequency and duration of symptoms and (b) the specific interventions used to treat these symptoms. Such notes increase client privacy by *not* including potentially damaging information, such as fantasies of an affair, details about family interactions, and names of colleagues and friends.

Crisis situations are the most notable exception to this general principle of including minimal private information. When stabilizing a suicidal, self-harming, abused, or homicidal client, therapists must include detailed information about the assessment of safety, the safety plan (including the names and roles of people who are part of the plan), and specific actions taken to ensure safety and conform with legal requirements. When stabilizing a crisis situation, a therapist gains additional "insurance" by documenting prudent, professional care in this high-risk legal situation and also provides other health care professionals with the information they need to treat the client.

Progress Note Ingredients

HIPAA guidelines and third-party payers provide guidance on what to include in a progress note, thus increasing uniformity in the field. These common ingredients include the following:

- Client case number, not a name (to protect client confidentiality)
- Date, time, and length of session
- Who attended the session
- Provider's original signature (not initials) with professional license status or degree
- Client progress, including improvement or worsening of symptoms (with frequency and/or duration)
- Interventions used and client response
- Plan for future sessions; modification to treatment plan
- Assessment for crisis issues and description of how they are managed

Progress Note Options

The necessary ingredients for progress notes are generally agreed upon. However, just like any list of ingredients, there are many ways to combine them to serve up different dishes. Translated into the world of progress notes, this means that there is more than one right way to do a progress note. Many therapists choose to conform to HIPAA by adapting pre-HIPAA forms to the new standards; others use formats they create or that an agency has developed. Although one might assume that HIPAA regulations have unified the format of progress notes, my annual trips to agencies around town indicate that there are probably more types of progress notes than ice cream flavors at your local Baskin-Robbins. The most common are DAP and SOAP notes.

DAP Notes

Developed in response to early managed-care requirements, DAP (data, assessment, plan) notes are one of the more common formats for progress notes (Wiger, 2005). They include the following:

- Data: What happened in session, interventions, clinical observations, test results, symptom diagnosis, stressors
- Assessment: Assessment of symptoms, outcome of current session and overall course of therapy, treatment plan goals and objectives being met, areas needing more work, areas of progress
- Plan: Homework, interventions for next session, timing of next sessions, changes to treatment plan; some therapists use *P* for progress and emphasize any progress that was made

Although there is a general outline, DAP notes can be interpreted in numerous ways, and each practitioner or agency often develops a unique style, emphasizing different information in each section.

SOAP Notes

Another widespread format for progress notes is SOAP (subjective, objective, assessment, plan) notes (Wiger, 2005). Many medical professionals, including general practice doctors, chiropractors, and occupational therapists use them. Because SOAP notes were originally designed for documenting treatment of physical conditions, they are often awkward when applied to mental health. Therefore, as with DAP notes, the interpretation of each section can vary significantly across practitioners and agencies. SOAP notes include the following:

- Subjective observations: Description of client's narrative and/or reported symptoms; some mental health practitioners have adapted the *S* to mean "situation," referring to the concerns and problems brought by the client
- Objective observations: Therapists' observations, test results, findings from physical examination, vital signs
- Assessment: Summary of symptoms, assessment, and diagnosis; differential diagnosis considerations
- Plan: Plan to treat listed symptoms, including instructions and medications given to client

The All-Purpose HIPAA Form for Progress Notes

Unfortunately, neither DAP nor SOAP notes may be particularly helpful to new therapists. The following form was developed to address the most common requirements of private insurance and public agencies in a format that is easy to follow.

PROGRESS NOTE

Date: ____ **Time:** __:__ ☐ am/☐ pm   **Session Length:** ☐ 45 min ☐ 60 min ☐ Other: ___ minutes

Present: ☐ Adult Male ☐ Adult Female ☐ Child Male ☐ Child Female ☐ Other: _____

Billing Code: ☐ 90791 (eval) ☐ 90834 (45 min therapy) ☐ 90837 (60 min therapy) ☐ 90847 (family)
☐ Other: _____

Symptom(s)	Duration and Frequency Since Last Visit	Progress
1:		☐ Improved ☐ Progressing ☐ Maintained ☐ Regressed ☐ None ☐ Variable ☐ Not addressed
2:		☐ Improved ☐ Progressing ☐ Maintained ☐ Regressed ☐ None ☐ Variable ☐ Not addressed
3:		☐ Improved ☐ Progressing ☐ Maintained ☐ Regressed ☐ None ☐ Variable ☐ Not addressed

Explanatory Notes on Symptoms: _____

In-Session Interventions and Assigned Homework

Client Response/Feedback

> [blank box]

Plan

☐ Continue with treatment plan: plan for next session: _____

☐ Modify plan: _____

Next session: Date: _____   Time: ___:___   ☐ am/☐ pm

Crisis Issues: ☐ No indication of crisis/client denies ☐ Crisis assessed/addressed: describe below

> [blank box]

_____ ,   _____   _____
Clinician's Signature   License/Intern Status   Date

◇◇◇

Case Consultation/Supervision ☐ Not Applicable

Notes: _____

Collateral Contact ☐ Not Applicable

Name: _____   Date of Contact: _____   Time: ___:___   ☐ am/☐ pm

☐ Written release on file: ☐ Sent/☐ Received ☐ In court docs ☐ Other: _____

Notes: _____

_____ ,   _____   _____
Clinician's Signature   License/Intern Status   Date

_____ ,   _____   _____
Supervisor's Signature   License   Date

📝 You can download this form from www.cengagebrain.com or www.mastering competencies.com.

COMPLETING A PROGRESS NOTE FORM

Client Number

To protect confidentiality, client names should never be put on file labels or progress notes. If a note accidentally slips out of a binder at Starbucks (this has happened), it should be impossible to identify the client. Actually, notes should never leave the building, and therapists should never leave the building after seeing clients until they have completed their progress notes.

Date, Time, and Session Length

Each note should begin with the date of the session, the time the session started, and the length of the session.

Persons Present

Because more than one person may be in therapy, therapists should indicate who was there. I recommend the following notation system (previously cited in Chapter 11):

AF: Adult Female
AM: Adult Male
CF#: Child Female plus age (e.g., CF8 = eight-year-old girl)
CM#: Child Male plus age (e.g., CM8 = eight-year-old boy)

If these abbreviations are used throughout the note, supervisors who read the notes will know who's who without using names.

CPT Billing Codes

Insurance companies use CPT (Current Procedural Terminology) codes, which have been established and updated by the American Medical Association to identify what type of service was provided. New CPT codes for therapists were issued on January 1, 2013:

- 90791: Psychiatric diagnostic evaluation (generally used for the first session)
- 90832: Psychotherapy, 30 minutes with patient and/or family member
- 90834: Psychotherapy, 45 minutes with patient and/or family member (used for standard 45–50-minute session)
- 90837: Psychotherapy, 60 minutes with patient and/or family member
- 90845: Psychoanalysis
- 90846: Family psychotherapy, 45–50 minutes
- 90847: Family psychotherapy, conjoint psychotherapy with patient present, 45–50 minutes
- 90849: Multiple-family group psychotherapy
- 90853: Group therapy (other than multiple-family group)
- 90839: Psychotherapy for crisis, first 60 minutes; use **90840** for each additional 30 minutes
- 90785: Interactive complexity code used with evaluation and psychotherapy codes: 90791, 90832, 90834, 90837, and 90839

Most county mental health agencies have their own set of billing codes. Although they are often not standardized within the same state, they generally use categories similar to those of the CPT codes.

Symptoms and Progress

Each week, therapists document the *duration, frequency,* and *severity* of symptoms. Here are some examples:

- "Client reports mild depressed mood most days (or five out of seven days)."
- "Client reports one panic attack the past week, moderate severity."
- "Client reports decreased conflict with parents; two arguments past week."

The 1–10 scale can also be used to visually track progress and setbacks.

Interventions

Progress notes should clearly identify which interventions the therapist used to help the client address the problems identified in the treatment plan. Here it is best to use theory-specific language:

- "Used solution-focused scaling to identify steps to reduce depression over next week."
- "Used enactments to practice alternatives to conflict."
- "Created genogram to increase insight related to family drinking patterns."

Therapists should avoid statements such as:

- "Discussed work stress" (not a therapeutic intervention).
- "Talked about fears" (how does this distinguish you from a bartender or hairstylist?).

Client Response

Increasingly, therapists document how clients responded to treatment, that is, what did and did not work:

- "Client receptive to reframe related to work issues; less receptive to reframe of pattern related to relationship."
- "Client actively engaged in enactment; optimistic could work at home."
- "Client expressed enthusiasm about mindfulness exercises."

Plan

This section describes the agenda for the next session and/or thoughts about modifying the treatment plan; for example:

- "Will bring parents to next session."
- "Follow up on journal assignment."
- "Continue to assess for self-harm."

Crisis Issues

Therapists document any crisis issues that arose in session and any issues they followed up from prior sessions. If there have been crisis issues, such as cutting or suicidal ideation, therapists should continue noting *in writing* that they checked on these issues during subsequent sessions. If a crisis issue was detected, therapists must clearly detail: (a) the assessment process and the data used to support conclusions and (b) the specific actions taken to ensure the safety of the client and/or the public. Documenting crisis situations requires much more detailed and specific information than documenting general progress and interventions. Here are some examples:

- "Client reported suspected abuse of child in family; reported child hit with belt on more than one occasion; report called in to CPS at 7:15 pm; taken by Christine K.; full report placed in file."
- "Client reported passive suicidal ideation: 'wish I were dead'; denied plan or intent: 'I would never do it because of my kids'; developed safety plan of three names to call; went over emergency contact for therapist."
- "Client reported cutting twice this week; developed safety plan in which the client agreed to use scaling for safety to develop alternative action at level seven; client readily agreed to plan."
- "Client denies cutting this week; no new cuts on wrists evident."

Try It Yourself

Either based on a vignette, real situation, or video, write a case note using the form In this chapter, online, or at the end of Chapters 4 to 10.

Consultation and Supervision

When obtaining supervision, peer consultation, or legal consultation (from a lawyer), therapists should document recommendations and/or information, especially regarding ethical and legal issues.

Collateral Contacts

Whenever you contact another professional (teacher, physician, psychiatrist, social worker) or a family member regarding a client, the contact needs to be documented, noting that form permitting release of information is on file.

Signature

Finally, therapists must: (a) sign the progress notes by hand (no initials) and (b) indicate their license status. If a therapist is unlicensed, his or her supervisor typically also signs the progress notes.

A Time and Place for Progress Notes

The proper time for writing progress notes is simple: *immediately following the session.* Because therapists conduct 45- to 50-minute sessions, progress notes can be written in the 10 to 15 minutes between sessions. If this is not possible, therapists must complete progress notes before leaving at the end of the day. Anything less gets you into a gray ethical area because a session is hard to remember with the same level of detail a day or two later—no matter how good your memory is. Trust me, I've tried it once or twice, and it does not work; therefore, I recommend you put daily progress notes in your "religious practice" category: they get done every time on time for fear of eternal damnation, or worse, the wrath of an ethics review board.

In addition, there is only one place for progress notes: a locked file cabinet. Like all medical professionals, therapists are required to keep client files and progress notes securely locked when not in immediate use—in some cases, under two sets of locks (e.g., in a locked file cabinet in a locked room). Digital files require high levels of computer security, outlined in the HIPAA policy (USDHHS, 2003). Moreover, *any piece of paper that has identifying client information,* such as phone message pads or calendars, must also be locked when not in use. In most states, therapists must keep records for seven years past the age of majority (adulthood), after which time they may be destroyed (e.g., shredded). The up side of these security requirements is that they keep your desk clean, and, for many, the ritual act of shredding has the therapeutic benefit of releasing pent-up stress and frustration.

Electronic Record Keeping

The majority (78%) of mental health practitioners now complete their records electronically, either on a computer or online (Matthews, 2015). In a recent qualitative study of 33 clinicians about their experiences with electronic recording keeping, all participants reported preferring using digital record keeping to using traditional paper files (I have to agree with them). If you work in an agency, they will have record-keeping policies that you will need to follow and technology that you will need to use. Clinicians in private practice can choose from several companies that provide HIPAA-compliant medical records for mental health practitioners. If a clinician keeps confidential information on a computer, phone, or flash drive, numerous levels of protection should be in place in case the digital device is lost. I have listed some options for securing such information on www.masteringcompetencies.com.

Different ethical and legal issues are involved in keeping electronic records as compared with keeping paper records. Although it is hard to say which has more potential problems, it is fair to say digital ones are harder to predict and foresee. First, clinicians using digital records should inform clients of this and the potential to impact confidentiality. Second, mental health clinicians working in large agencies or integrated health settings in which numerous others have access to the electronic records need to carefully consider what information goes into the file, especially information about family members who may also be served at that facility (Nielsen, 2015). For example, a parent may give information about a child's biological parent that the child is unaware of and later this information is unintentionally revealed to the child by another medical professional. Similarly, one parent may give sensitive information about another parent for the purposes of treating the child, and this information is brought up later, to the surprise of the other parent.

Final Note on Notes

Progress notes are the heart of clinical documentation, and in many ways are the most important documents we produce because they provide the clearest record of what happens behind closed doors. They are the only place where we can document that we conducted ourselves as professionals, rendering appropriate and necessary medical services. Because they are the documents most likely to be viewed by outsiders should papers be released or subpoenaed, we must ensure that these notes protect us as well as our clients' privacy. The art of writing progress notes is one of the most important clinical skills to master. Thankfully, we get ample opportunity to practice.

QUESTIONS FOR PERSONAL REFLECTION AND CLASS DISCUSSION

1. What part of record keeping do you think will be the most challenging for you? How might you make it easier?
2. Some clinicians in large county agencies report that paperwork can take up to 50% of their work week. How would handle such a situation?
3. Has writing been a strength of yours? Have you ever done technical writing? How might you best approach learning how to efficiently write progress notes.

ONLINE RESOURCES

HIPAA Guidelines
www.hhs.gov/ocr/hipaa

CPT Codes from the AMA
www.ama-assn.org

Go to MindTap® for an eBook, videos of client sessions, activities, digital forms, practice quizzes, apps, and more—all in one place. If your instructor didn't assign MindTap, you can find out more information at CengageBrain.com.

REFERENCES

Halloway, J. D. (2003). More protections for patients and psychologists under HIPAA. *Monitor on Psychology, 34*(2), 22.

Jordan, K. (1999). Live supervision for being therapists in practicum: Crucial for quality counseling and avoiding litigation. *Family Therapy, 26*(2) 81–86.

Matthews, E. B. (2015). Integrating the electronic health record into behavioral health encounters: Strategies, barriers, and implications for practice. *Administration and Policy in Mental Health and Mental Health Services Research.* doi:10.1007/s10488-015-0676-3

Nielsen, B. A. (2015). Confidentiality and electronic health records: Keeping up with advances in technology and expectations for access. *Clinical Practice in Pediatric Psychology, 3*(2), 175–178. doi:10.1037/cpp0000096

U.S. Department of Health and Human Services (USDHHS). (2003). *Summary of HIPAA privacy rules.* Washington, DC: Author. Retrieved from www.hhs.gov/ocr/hipaa.

Wiger, D. E. (2005). *The psychotherapy documentation primer* (2nd ed.). New York: Wiley.

Afterword

Closing Thoughts: Where to Go from Here?

You have just finished a grand tour of the pragmatic and theoretical aspects of family therapy practice in the 21st century. You have been introduced to the clinical skills you will be expected to perform in field placements: case conceptualization, clinical assessment, treatment planning, progress assessments, and case notes. You have also been introduced to the most well-established therapeutic models in the field of family therapy, including the new evidence-based models. So, where do you go from here? The next step in mastering the competencies is to enter the real world of clinical practice, where you will learn to walk the talk.

Getting Started: Working with a Supervisor

If you have started field placement already, you already know that your supervisor is key to meaningfully mastering competencies. More so than your professors, your supervisor is the one who helps you translate book knowledge into action. Thus, it is important to learn how to "use" supervision well.

Realistic Expectations

Perhaps it is easiest to start with what *not* to do, which is *not* to expect your supervisor to be omniscient and omnipotent—or, in other words, don't confuse a supervisor with God. A common misunderstanding is that new trainees often expect their supervisors to have mastered all aspects of the profession: all theories, all techniques, all laws, all ethic codes, all diagnoses, all referral possibilities, all research methods—in short, everything. It's just not possible—or, at least, I have not met anyone who has. Instead, it is useful to approach each supervisor with the attitude that you have *something* to learn from them—it might be diagnosis, a specific theory, case notes, law and ethics, or group work. Every supervisor has something valuable to teach. Many of my trainees find that approaching their supervisors with more realistic expectations not only reduces their frustration with their supervisor, but it also makes them more realistic about their expectations of what they themselves should be mastering in the first few years of training.

Asking for What You Need

If for some reason you believe your supervisor is not helping you in a particular area—perhaps with treatment plans, diagnosis, or a specific theory—it often helps to *directly ask* for what you want. Most supervisors are more than happy to work such requests in the supervision process. If not, know that you will have many more supervisors who will provide further opportunities for learning.

Seeking Advanced Training

Another frequent misunderstanding that new trainees have is thinking that they are done with academic training once they receive a master's degree or a license. A master's degree is the *minimal* training you need to prepare you for licensure, and a license simply certifies that the state does not think you will hurt anybody without direct supervision. Those are pretty low standards. To become a competent therapist, you will need a minimum of 5 to 10 years of postdegree training in a specialty. Most importantly, it takes this level of training to provide the knowledge and skill foundations you will need to *prevent burnout*. Becoming a skilled therapist is a *long-term project*; a master's degree and a license are just the first step in the process.

The greatest barrier to advanced training is time and money. Once you graduate and have to start paying back student loans, it is hard to afford conferences and workshops—they are expensive, at least in the short term. However, they are an *investment*. Investing in advanced training is investing in your future, and it opens new opportunities to expand your practice. There are state and national conferences, special in-depth training offered by institutes specializing in particular approaches or populations, and an increasing number of quality online programs. You do not have to go broke, but you do need to put some time and money aside to ensure that you develop fully as an independent, creative professional. I have never met anyone who regretted investing in training. I recommend that you get as many training sessions as possible while you are in school and qualify for the "student" discount: those will look like bargain-basement prices once you graduate.

Belonging: Professional Organizations

Almost all professionals belong to professional organizations. But for therapists in the 21st century, membership is a matter of survival: namely, the ability to get hired and paid. Why? National professional organizations, such as the American Association for Marriage and Family Therapy (for LMFTs), the American Counseling Association (for LPCs), the National Association of Social Workers (for social workers), and the American Psychological Association (for psychologists) are the people who lobby in Congress, in state legislatures, and with third-party payers to ensure that their licensees have jobs and get reimbursed. Without these organizations working on behalf of their members, therapists would not be able to survive in today's marketplace. So, depending on which license you intend to pursue, it is important to join—and student membership is always cheapest.

Besides the not-so-minor issue of ensuring a paycheck, these organizations offer some of the best training and networking opportunities available. Attending national conventions and training keeps you on the cutting edge of the profession. Most also have state-level and regional meetings that keep you in the loop. The local meetings are often the source of great networking connections, whether you are just starting out and looking for a job or have been in the field for years and want to market yourself or hire someone else. All offer opportunities to join boards of directors and subcommittees, where you may shape the future direction of the profession. Professional organizations also provide free legal consultation—and if you have ever had to pay a lawyer, you know that one phone call pays for three years of membership. In the end, professional organizations are where it is all happening—so don't miss the party!

Self-Supervision

In addition to relying on your supervisor and knowledge from advanced training, it is still helpful to learn how to help yourself. Whether a veteran therapist or the new kid on the block, one of the most exciting parts of learning how to complete a case conceptualization (see Chapter 11) is that you can provide yourself with outstanding supervision at a moment's notice without paying a fee or waiting until next week's supervision session. You can use the case conceptualization form to walk yourself through the case and identify core issues and dynamics you can use to focus your treatment. This is most useful when you are feeling stuck, but it is also helpful with new clients or with clients who you have been seeing for a longtime who have undergone minor to moderate change. As simple as it may sound, this exercise has often helped my supervisees and me identify more effective ways to proceed—and all we did was answer questions we asked ourselves.

Last Words

I hope this introduction to family therapy has inspired you to work creatively and hopefully with individuals, couples, and families using family therapy theories, all of which view individuals and their problems as part of larger relational and social contexts. I trust you will find that they provide a remarkably rich foundation for helping people with all forms of suffering and life struggles. Most importantly, I hope the depth and humanity of these ideas are transferable from the pages of this book to your work with clients, so that with each interaction, you touch that ineffable part of their being that brings forth the best of who they are—and in doing so, also brings forth your best.

APPENDIX

A

The Family Therapy Core Competencies

The American Association for Marriage and Family Therapy (www.aamft.org) developed the following comprehensive set of core competencies with the input of practicing therapists as well as numerous third-party stakeholders. These competencies describe the knowledge and skills that practitioners should have to work independently (i.e., to be licensed) and are also used by universities and supervisors when training new therapists. Many of these competencies are addressed in the clinical forms covered in the text and are denoted by boldface text in the following tables.

HOW TO READ THE CORE COMPETENCIES

- **Number:** Each competency is identified with a three-part number.
  - *First number:* Domains 1–6
  - *Second number:* Subdomains 1–5
  - *Third number:* The specific competency in the subdomain
- **Subdomain:** The second column refers to the subdomain: conceptual, perceptual, executive, evaluative, or professional.
- **Competence:** The third column is the specific competence or skill.
- **Form:** The last column identifies the form or assignment where the competency is measured in *The Complete Marriage and Family Core Competencies Assessment System* (Gehart, 2007). A competency may be measured on one or more forms and may be measured more than once; *the number of measurements is indicated in parentheses, such as (2)*. Only four of the eight forms are included in this book. These are abbreviated as follows:

    CC = **Case Conceptualization** (see Chapter 11)

    CA = **Clinical Assessment** (see Chapter 12)

(continued)

HOW TO READ THE CORE COMPETENCIES (*CONTINUED*)

TP = Treatment Plan (see Chapter 13)

PN = Progress Notes (see Chapter 15)

- The remaining competencies (not included in this book) are measured in the following forms:

    PD = Professional Development Plan

    LI = Live Interview

    LE = Live Interview Evaluation

    RP = Research Proposal

- **Bold-Text Competencies:** Boldface indicates that this competency is taught and measured in a form included in this book.

DOMAIN 1: ADMISSION TO TREATMENT

NUMBER	SUBDOMAIN	COMPETENCE	FORM
1.1.1	Conceptual	**Understand systems concepts, theories, and techniques that are foundational to the practice of marriage and family therapy.**	CC (10)
1.1.2	Conceptual	**Understand theories and techniques of individual, marital, couple, family, and group psychotherapy.**	TP
1.1.3	Conceptual	**Understand the behavioral health care delivery system, its impact on the services provided, and the barriers and disparities in the system.**	TP
1.1.4	Conceptual	**Understand the risks and benefits of individual, marital, couple, family, and group psychotherapy.**	TP
1.2.1	Perceptual	**Recognize contextual and systemic dynamics (e.g., gender, age, socioeconomic status, culture/race/ ethnicity, sexual orientation, spirituality, religion, larger systems, social context).**	CC
1.2.2	Perceptual	**Consider health status, mental status, other therapy, and other systems involved in the clients' lives (e.g., courts, social services).**	CA
1.2.3	Perceptual	**Recognize issues that might suggest referral for specialized evaluation, assessment, or care.**	CA
1.3.1	Executive	**Gather and review intake information, giving balanced attention to individual, family, community, cultural, and contextual factors.**	CA
1.3.2	Executive	**Determine who should attend therapy and in what configuration (e.g., individual, couple, family, extrafamilial resources).**	CA (2) TP
1.3.3	Executive	**Facilitate therapeutic involvement of all necessary participants in treatment.**	TP LI
1.3.4	Executive	Explain practice-setting rules, fees, rights, and responsibilities of each party, including privacy, confidentiality policies, and duty to care to client or legal guardian.	LI
1.3.5	Executive	Obtain consent to treatment from all responsible persons.	LI

1.3.6	Executive	Establish and maintain appropriate and productive therapeutic alliances with the clients.	TP LI
1.3.7	Executive	Solicit and use client feedback throughout the therapeutic process.	PN LI
1.3.8	Executive	Develop and maintain collaborative working relationships with referral resources, other practitioners involved in the clients' care, and payers.	PN
1.3.9	Executive	Manage session interactions with individuals, couples, families, and groups.	LI
1.4.1	Evaluative	Evaluate case for appropriateness for treatment within professional scope of practice and competence.	TP
1.5.1	Professional	Understand the legal requirements and limitations for working with vulnerable populations (e.g., minors).	LI
1.5.2	Professional	Complete case documentation in a timely manner and in accordance with relevant laws and policies.	PN
1.5.3	Professional	Develop, establish, and maintain policies for fees, payment, record keeping, and confidentiality.	CA PN (2) LI

DOMAIN 2: CLINICAL ASSESSMENT AND DIAGNOSIS

Number	Subdomain	Competence	Form
2.1.1	Conceptual	Understand principles of human development; human sexuality; gender development; psychopathology; psychopharmacology; couples processes; and family development and processes (e.g., family, relational, and system dynamics).	CC CA
2.1.2	Conceptual	Understand the major behavioral health disorders, including the epidemiology, etiology, phenomenology, effective treatments, course, and prognosis.	CA (2)
2.1.3	Conceptual	Understand the clinical needs and implications of persons with comorbid disorders (e.g., substance abuse and mental health; heart disease and depression).	TP
2.1.4	Conceptual	Comprehend individual, marital, couple, and family assessment instruments appropriate to presenting problem, practice setting, and cultural context.	TP RP
2.1.5	Conceptual	Understand the current models for assessment and diagnosis of mental health disorders, substance use disorders, and relational functioning.	CA
2.1.6	Conceptual	Understand the strengths and limitations of the models of assessment and diagnosis, especially as they relate to different cultural, economic, and ethnic groups.	CA RP
2.1.7	Conceptual	Understand the concepts of reliability and validity, their relationship to assessment instruments, and how they influence therapeutic decision making.	RP
2.2.1	Perceptual	Assess each client's engagement in the change process.	LI
2.2.2	Perceptual	Systematically integrate client reports, observations of client behaviors, client relationship patterns, reports from other professionals, results from testing procedures, and interactions with client to guide the assessment process.	CC

(continued)

DOMAIN 2: CLINICAL ASSESSMENT AND DIAGNOSIS (*continued*)

NUMBER	SUBDOMAIN	COMPETENCE	FORM
2.2.3	Perceptual	Develop hypotheses regarding relationship patterns, their bearing on the presenting problem, and the influence of extratherapeutic factors on client systems.	CC (11)
2.2.4	Perceptual	Consider the influence of treatment on extratherapeutic relationships.	CA
2.2.5	Perceptual	Consider physical/organic problems that can cause or exacerbate emotional/interpersonal symptoms.	CA
2.3.1	Executive	Diagnose and assess client behavioral and relational health problems systemically and contextually.	CA
2.3.2	Executive	Provide assessments and deliver developmentally appropriate services to clients, such as children, adolescents, elders, and persons with special needs.	TP (2) LI
2.3.3	Executive	Apply effective and systemic interviewing techniques and strategies.	TP LI
2.3.4	Executive	Administer and interpret results of assessment instruments.	CA RP
2.3.5	Executive	Screen and develop adequate safety plans for substance abuse, child and elder maltreatment, domestic violence, physical violence, suicide potential, and dangerousness to self and others.	CA PN LI
2.3.6	Executive	Assess family history and dynamics using a genogram or other assessment instruments.	CC (2)
2.3.7	Executive	Elicit a relevant and accurate biopsychosocial history to understand the context of the clients' problems.	CC (3) LI
2.3.8	Executive	Identify clients' strengths, resilience, and resources.	CC (2)
2.3.9	Executive	Elucidate presenting problem from the perspective of each member of the therapeutic system.	CC (2) LI
2.4.1	Evaluative	Evaluate assessment methods for relevance to clients' needs.	CA LE
2.4.2	Evaluative	Assess ability to view issues and therapeutic processes systemically.	CA LE
2.4.3	Evaluative	Evaluate the accuracy and cultural relevance of behavioral health and relational diagnoses.	CA LE
2.4.4	Evaluative	Assess the therapist–client agreement of therapeutic goals and diagnosis.	CA LE
2.5.1	Professional	Utilize consultation and supervision effectively.	PN LI

DOMAIN 3: TREATMENT PLANNING AND CASE MANAGEMENT

NUMBER	SUBDOMAIN	COMPETENCE	FORM
3.1.1	Conceptual	Know which models, modalities, and/or techniques are most effective for presenting problems.	TP
3.1.2	Conceptual	Understand the liabilities incurred when billing third parties, the codes necessary for reimbursement, and how to use them correctly.	PN

3.1.3	Conceptual	Understand the effects that psychotropic and other medications have on clients and the treatment process.	CA
3.1.4	Conceptual	Understand recovery-oriented behavioral health services (e.g., self-help groups, 12-step programs, peer-to-peer services, supported employment).	TP LI
3.2.1	Perceptual	Integrate client feedback, assessment, contextual information, and diagnosis with treatment goals and plan.	TP PN LI
3.3.1	Executive	Develop, with client input, measurable outcomes, treatment goals, treatment plans, and aftercare plans with clients utilizing a systemic perspective.	TP
3.3.2	Executive	Prioritize treatment goals.	TP
3.3.3	Executive	Develop a clear plan of how sessions will be conducted.	TP (2)
3.3.4	Executive	Structure treatment to meet clients' needs and to facilitate systemic change.	TP
3.3.5	Executive	Manage progression of therapy toward treatment goals.	TP
3.3.6	Executive	Manage risks, crises, and emergencies.	TP CA LI
3.3.7	Executive	Work collaboratively with other stakeholders, including family members, other significant persons, and professionals not present.	PN
3.3.8	Executive	Assist clients in obtaining needed care while navigating complex systems of care.	TP LI
3.3.9	Executive	Develop termination and aftercare plans.	TP
3.4.1	Evaluative	Evaluate progress of sessions toward treatment goals.	PN
3.4.2	Evaluative	Recognize when treatment goals and plan require modification.	PN
3.4.3	Evaluative	Evaluate level of risks, management of risks, crises, and emergencies.	CA TP LI
3.4.4	Evaluative	Assess session process for compliance with policies and procedures of practice setting.	LE
3.4.5	Professional	Monitor personal reactions to clients and treatment process, especially in terms of therapeutic behavior, relationship with clients, process for explaining procedures, and outcomes.	LE
3.5.1	Professional	Advocate with clients in obtaining quality care, appropriate resources, and services in their community.	TP LI
3.5.2	Professional	Participate in case-related forensic and legal processes.	CA
3.5.3	Professional	Write plans and complete other case documentation in accordance with practice-setting policies, professional standards, and state/provincial laws.	TP PD (2) LE (2) RP (2)
3.5.4	Professional	Utilize time management skills in therapy sessions and other professional meetings.	LI

DOMAIN 4: THERAPEUTIC INTERVENTIONS

Number	Subdomain	Competence	Form
4.1.1	Conceptual	Comprehend a variety of individual and systemic therapeutic models and their application, including evidence-based therapies and culturally sensitive approaches.	TP LE
4.1.2	Conceptual	Recognize strengths, limitations, and contraindications of specific therapy models, including the risk of harm associated with models that incorporate assumptions of family dysfunction, pathogenesis, or cultural deficit.	TP LE
4.2.1	Perceptual	Recognize how different techniques may impact the treatment process.	TP (2)
4.2.2	Perceptual	Distinguish differences between content and process issues, their role in therapy, and their potential impact on therapeutic outcomes.	TP LI
4.3.1	Executive	Match treatment modalities and techniques to clients' needs, goals, and values.	TP LI
4.3.2	Executive	Deliver interventions in a way that is sensitive to special needs of clients (e.g., gender, age, socioeconomic status, culture/race/ethnicity, sexual orientation, disability, personal history, larger systems issues of the client).	PN LI
4.3.3	Executive	Reframe problems and recursive interaction patterns.	TP (2) LI
4.3.4	Executive	Generate relational questions and reflexive comments in the therapy room.	TP (2) LI
4.3.5	Executive	Engage each family member in the treatment process as appropriate.	TP (2) LI
4.3.6	Executive	Facilitate clients in developing and integrating solutions to problems.	TP (2) PN LI
4.3.7	Executive	Defuse intense and chaotic situations to enhance the safety of all participants.	LI
4.3.8	Executive	Empower clients and their relational systems to establish effective relationships with each other and larger systems.	TP (2) LI
4.3.9	Executive	Provide psychoeducation to families whose members have serious mental illness or other disorders.	TP (2) LI
4.3.10	Executive	Modify interventions that are not working to better fit treatment goals.	PN LI
4.3.11	Executive	Move to constructive termination when treatment goals have been accomplished.	TP
4.3.12	Executive	Integrate supervisor/team communications into treatment.	PN LI
4.4.1	Evaluative	Evaluate interventions for consistency, congruency with model of therapy and theory of change, cultural and contextual relevance, and goals of the treatment plan.	TP LE (2)
4.4.2	Evaluative	Evaluate ability to deliver interventions effectively.	PN LE
4.4.3	Evaluative	Evaluate treatment outcomes as treatment progresses.	PN LE
4.4.4	Evaluative	Evaluate clients' reactions or responses to interventions.	PN LI LE

4.4.5	Evaluative	Evaluate clients' outcomes for the need to continue, refer, or terminate therapy.	TP PN LE
4.4.6	Evaluative	Evaluate reactions to the treatment process (e.g., transference, family of origin, current stress level, current life situation, cultural context) and their impact on effective intervention and clinical outcomes.	LE
4.5.1	Professional	Respect multiple perspectives (e.g., clients, team, supervisor, practitioners from other disciplines who are involved in the case).	PN LI
4.5.2	Professional	Set appropriate boundaries, manage issues of triangulation, and develop collaborative working relationships.	LI
4.5.3	Professional	Articulate rationales for interventions related to treatment goals and plan, assessment information, and systemic understanding of clients' context and dynamics.	TP LE

DOMAIN 5: LEGAL ISSUES, ETHICS, AND STANDARDS

NUMBER	SUBDOMAIN	COMPETENCE	FORM
5.1.1	Conceptual	Know state, federal, and provincial laws and regulations that apply to the practice of marriage and family therapy.	CA LI
5.1.2	Conceptual	Know professional ethics and standards of practice that apply to the practice of marriage and family therapy.	CA LI
5.1.3	Conceptual	Know policies and procedures of the practice setting.	LI
5.1.4	Conceptual	Understand the process of making an ethical decision.	CA PN LE
5.2.1	Perceptual	Recognize situations in which ethics, laws, professional liability, and standards of practice apply.	CA PN LI
5.2.2	Perceptual	Recognize ethical dilemmas in practice setting.	PN LE
5.2.3	Perceptual	Recognize when a legal consultation is necessary.	PN LE
5.2.4	Perceptual	Recognize when clinical supervision or consultation is necessary.	PN LI
5.3.1	Executive	Monitor issues related to ethics, laws, regulations, and professional standards.	PN LI
5.3.2	Executive	Develop and assess policies, procedures, and forms for consistency with standards of practice to protect client confidentiality and to comply with relevant laws and regulations.	CA
5.3.3	Executive	Inform clients and legal guardian of limitations to confidentiality and parameters of mandatory reporting.	LI
5.3.4	Executive	Develop safety plans for clients who present with potential self-harm, suicide, abuse, or violence.	CA PN LI
5.3.5	Executive	Take appropriate action when ethical and legal dilemmas emerge.	CA PN LI
5.3.6	Executive	Report information to appropriate authorities as required by law.	CA PN LI
5.3.7	Executive	Practice within defined scope of practice and competence.	TP

(continued)

DOMAIN 5: LEGAL ISSUES, ETHICS, AND STANDARDS (*continued*)

NUMBER	SUBDOMAIN	COMPETENCE	FORM
5.3.8	Executive	Obtain knowledge of advances and theory regarding effective clinical practice.	PD
5.3.9	Executive	Obtain license(s) and specialty credentials.	PD (2)
5.3.10	Executive	Implement a personal program to maintain professional competence.	PD (3)
5.4.1	Evaluative	Evaluate activities related to ethics, legal issues, and practice standards.	LE
5.4.2	Evaluative	Monitor attitudes, personal well-being, personal issues, and personal problems to ensure they do not impact the therapy process adversely or create vulnerability for misconduct.	PD
5.5.1	**Professional**	**Maintain client records with timely and accurate notes.**	**PN**
5.5.2	**Professional**	**Consult with peers and/or supervisors if personal issues, attitudes, or beliefs threaten to adversely impact clinical work.**	**PN PD**
5.5.3	Professional	Pursue professional development through self-supervision, collegial consultation, professional reading, and continuing educational activities.	PD
5.5.4	**Professional**	**Bill clients and third-party payers in accordance with professional ethics, relevant laws, and policies, and seek reimbursement only for covered services.**	**PN**

DOMAIN 6: RESEARCH AND PROGRAM EVALUATION

NUMBER	SUBDOMAIN	COMPETENCE	FORM
6.1.1	**Conceptual**	**Know the extant marriage and family therapy (MFT) literature, research, and evidence-based practice.**	**TP RP**
6.1.2	Conceptual	Understand research and program evaluation methodologies, both quantitative and qualitative, relevant to MFT and mental health services.	RP
6.1.3	Conceptual	Understand the legal, ethical, and contextual issues involved in the conduct of clinical research and program evaluation.	RP
6.2.1	Perceptual	Recognize opportunities for therapists and clients to participate in clinical research.	RP
6.3.1	Executive	Read current MFT and other professional literature.	PD (2)
6.3.2	**Executive**	**Use current MFT and other research to inform clinical practice.**	**CC TP**
6.3.3	Executive	Critique professional research and assess the quality of research studies and program evaluation in the literature.	RP
6.3.4	Executive	Determine the effectiveness of clinical practice and techniques.	LE RP
6.4.1	Evaluative	Evaluate knowledge of current clinical literature and its application.	PD RP
6.5.1	Professional	Contribute to the development of new knowledge.	PD

Source: AAMFT. References: Gehart, D. (2007). The complete marriage and family therapy core competency assessment system: Eight outcome-based instruments for measuring student learning. Thousand Oaks, CA: Author. Available: www.mftcompetencies.com

A P P E N D I X

B

CACREP Competency-Based Standards

Below, you will find the new Council on the Accreditation of Counseling and Related Educational Programs (CACREP) competency-based standards for master students in marriage and family counseling. Students should be able to demonstrate these competencies prior to graduating. Faculty in CACREP programs can download scoring rubrics correlated to these and all other areas of CACREP specialization on the web page hosted by the publisher as well as masteringcompetencies.com.

Marriage, Couple, and Family Counseling

Students who are preparing to work as marriage, couple, and family counselors are expected to possess the knowledge, skills, and practices necessary to address a wide variety of issues in the context of relationships and families. In addition to the common core curricular experiences outlined in Section II.F of the CACREP 2016 Standards, programs must provide evidence that student learning has occurred in the following domains:

Foundations

F. Marriage, Couple, and Family Counseling

Students who are preparing to specialize as marriage, couple, and family counselors are expected to possess the knowledge and skills necessary to address a wide variety of issues in the context of relationships and families. Counselor education programs with a specialty area in marriage, couple, and family counseling must document where each of the lettered standards listed below is covered in the curriculum.

1. **Foundations**
   a. history and development of marriage, couple, and family counseling
   b. theories and models of family systems and dynamics
   c. theories and models of marriage, couple, and family counseling

    d. sociology of the family, family phenomenology, and family of origin theories

    e. principles and models of assessment and case conceptualization from a systems perspective

    f. assessments relevant to marriage, couple, and family counseling

2. Contextual Dimensions

    a. roles and settings of marriage, couple, and family counselors

    b. structures of marriages, couples, and families

    c. family assessments, including diagnostic interviews, genograms, family mapping, mental diagnostic status examinations, symptom inventories, and psychoeducational and personality assessments

    d. diagnostic process, including differential diagnosis and the use of current diagnostic classification systems, including the *Diagnostic and Statistical Manual of Mental Disorders* (DSM) and the *International Classification of Diseases* (ICD)

    e. human sexuality and its effect on couple and family functioning

    f. aging and intergenerational influences and related family concerns

    g. impact of crisis and trauma on marriages, couples, and families

    h. impact of addiction on marriages, couples, and families

    i. impact of interpersonal violence on marriages, couples, and families

    j. impact of unemployment, under-employment, and changes in socioeconomic standing on marriages, couples, and families

    k. interactions of career, life, and gender roles on marriages, couples, and families

    l. physical, mental health, and psychopharmacological factors affecting marriages, couples, and families

    m. cultural factors relevant to marriage, couple, and family functioning, including the impact of immigration

    n. professional organizations, preparation standards, and credentials relevant to the practice of marriage, couple, and family counseling

    o. ethical and legal considerations and family law issues unique to the practice of marriage, couple, and family counseling

    p. record keeping, third-party reimbursement, and other practice and management considerations in marriage, couple, and family counseling

3. Practice

    a. assessment, evaluation, and case management for working with individuals, couples, and families from a systems perspective

    b. fostering family wellness

    c. techniques and interventions of marriage, couple, and family counseling

    d. conceptualizing and implementing treatment, planning, and intervention strategies in marriage, couple, and family counseling

    e. strategies for interfacing with the legal system relevant to marriage, couple, and family counseling

Source: CACREP.

Psychology Benchmarks

Competency Benchmarks in Professional Psychology

I. Professionalism

1. Professional Values and Attitudes: As evidenced in behavior and comportment that reflect the values and attitudes of psychology.		
READINESS FOR PRACTICUM	**READINESS FOR INTERNSHIP**	**READINESS FOR ENTRY TO PRACTICE**
1A. Integrity—Honesty, personal responsibility, and adherence to professional values		
Understands professional values; honest, responsible	Adherence to professional values infuses work as psychologist-in-training; recognizes situations that challenge adherence to professional values	Monitors and independently resolves situations that challenge professional values and integrity
1B. Deportment		
Understands how to conduct oneself in a professional manner	Communication and physical conduct (including attire) is professionally appropriate, across different settings	Conducts self in a professional manner across settings and situations
1C. Accountability		
Accountable and reliable	Accepts responsibility for own actions	Independently accepts personal responsibility across settings and contexts
1D. Concern for the Welfare of Others		
Demonstrates awareness of the need to uphold and protect the welfare of others	Acts to understand and safeguard the welfare of others	Independently acts to safeguard the welfare of others

(continued)

1E. Professional Identity		
Demonstrates beginning understanding of self as professional: "thinking like a psychologist"	Displays emerging professional identity as psychologist; uses resources (e.g., supervision, literature) for professional development	Displays consolidation of professional identity as a psychologist; demonstrates knowledge about issues central to the field; integrates science and practice

2. Individual and Cultural Diversity: Awareness, sensitivity, and skills in working professionally with diverse individuals, groups, and communities who represent various cultural and personal background and characteristics defined broadly and consistent with APA policy.		
READINESS FOR PRACTICUM	READINESS FOR INTERNSHIP	READINESS FOR ENTRY TO PRACTICE
2A. Self as Shaped by Individual and Cultural Diversity (e.g., cultural, individual, and role differences, including those based on age, gender, gender identity, race, ethnicity, culture, national origin, religion, sexual orientation, disability, language, and socioeconomic status) **and Context**		
Demonstrates knowledge, awareness, and understanding of one's own dimensions of diversity and attitudes toward diverse others	Monitors and applies knowledge of self as a cultural being in assessment, treatment, and consultation	Independently monitors and applies knowledge of self as a cultural being in assessment, treatment, and consultation
2B. Others as Shaped by Individual and Cultural Diversity and Context		
Demonstrates knowledge, awareness, and understanding of other individuals as cultural beings	Applies knowledge of others as cultural beings in assessment, treatment, and consultation	Independently monitors and applies knowledge of others as cultural beings in assessment, treatment, and consultation
2C. Interaction of Self and Others as Shaped by Individual and Cultural Diversity and Context		
Demonstrates knowledge, awareness, and understanding of interactions between self and diverse others	Applies knowledge of the role of culture in interactions in assessment, treatment, and consultation of diverse others	Independently monitors and applies knowledge of diversity in others as cultural beings in assessment, treatment, and consultation
2D. Applications based on Individual and Cultural Context		
Demonstrates basic knowledge of and sensitivity to the scientific, theoretical, and contextual issues related to ICD (as defined by APA policy) as they apply to professional psychology. Understands the need to consider ICD issues in all aspects of professional psychology work (e.g., assessment, treatment, research, relationships with colleagues)	Applies knowledge, sensitivity, and understanding regarding ICD issues to work effectively with diverse others in assessment, treatment, and consultation	Applies knowledge, skills, and attitudes regarding dimensions of diversity to professional work

3. Ethical Legal Standards and Policy: Application of ethical concepts and awareness of legal issues regarding professional activities with individuals, groups, and organizations.

READINESS FOR PRACTICUM	READINESS FOR INTERNSHIP	READINESS FOR ENTRY TO PRACTICE
3A. Knowledge of Ethical, Legal and Professional Standards and Guidelines		
Demonstrates basic knowledge of the principles of the APA Ethical Principles and Code of Conduct [ethical practice and basic skills in ethical decision-making]; demonstrates beginning level knowledge of legal and regulatory issues in the practice of psychology that apply to practice while placed at practicum setting	Demonstrates intermediate level knowledge and understanding of the APA Ethical Principles and Code of Conduct and other relevant ethical/professional codes, standards and guidelines, laws, statutes, rules, and regulations	Demonstrates advanced knowledge and application of the APA Ethical Principles and Code of Conduct and other relevant ethical, legal, and professional standards and guidelines
3B. Awareness and Application of Ethical Decision-Making		
Demonstrates awareness of the importance of applying an ethical decision model to practice	Demonstrates knowledge and application of an ethical decision-making model; applies relevant elements of ethical decision-making to a dilemma	Independently utilizes an ethical decision-making model in professional work
3C. Ethical Conduct		
Displays ethical attitudes and values	Integrates own moral principles/ethical values in professional conduct	Independently integrates ethical and legal standards with all competencies

4. Reflective Practice/Self-Assessment/Self-Care: Practice conducted with personal and professional self-awareness and reflection; with awareness of competencies; with appropriate self-care.

READINESS FOR PRACTICUM	READINESS FOR INTERNSHIP	READINESS FOR ENTRY TO PRACTICE
4A. Reflective Practice		
Displays basic mindfulness and self-awareness; engages in reflection regarding professional practice	Displays broadened self-awareness; utilizes self-monitoring; engages in reflection regarding professional practice; uses resources to enhance reflectivity	Demonstrates reflectivity both during and after professional activity; acts upon reflection; uses self as a therapeutic tool
4B. Self-Assessment		
Demonstrates knowledge of core competencies; engages in initial self-assessment with regard to competencies	Demonstrates broad, accurate self-assessment of competence; consistently monitors and evaluates practice activities; works to recognize limits of knowledge/skills and to seek means to enhance knowledge/skills	Accurately self-assesses competence in all competency domains; integrates self-assessment in practice; recognizes limits of knowledge/skills and acts to address them; has extended plan to enhance knowledge/skills
4C. Self-Care (attention to personal health and well-being to assure effective professional functioning)		
Understands the importance of self-care in effective practice; demonstrates knowledge of self-care methods; attends to self-care	Monitors issues related to self-care with supervisor; understands the central role of self-care to effective practice	Self-monitors issues related to self-care and promptly intervenes when disruptions occur

(continued)

4D. Participation in Supervision Process		
Demonstrates straightforward, truthful, and respectful communication in supervisory relationship	Effectively participates in supervision	Independently seeks supervision when needed

II. Relational

5. Relationships: Relate effectively and meaningfully with individuals, groups, and/or communities.		
READINESS FOR PRACTICUM	READINESS FOR INTERNSHIP	READINESS FOR ENTRY TO PRACTICE
5A. Interpersonal Relationships		
Displays interpersonal skills	Forms and maintains productive and respectful relationships with clients, peers/colleagues, supervisors and professionals from other disciplines	Develops and maintains effective relationships with a wide range of clients, colleagues, organizations and communities
5B. Affective Skills		
Displays affective skills	Negotiates differences and handles conflict satisfactorily; provides effective feedback to others and receives feedback nondefensively	Manages difficult communication; possesses advanced interpersonal skills
5C. Expressive Skills		
Communicates ideas, feelings, and information clearly using verbal, nonverbal, and written skills	Communicates clearly using verbal, nonverbal, and written skills in a professional context; demonstrates clear understanding and use of professional language	Verbal, nonverbal, and written communications are informative, articulate, succinct, sophisticated, and well-integrated; demonstrate thorough grasp of professional language and concepts

III. Science

6. Scientific Knowledge and Methods: Understanding of research, research methodology, techniques of data collection and analysis, biological bases of behavior, cognitive–affective bases of behavior, and development across the lifespan. Respect for scientifically derived knowledge.		
READINESS FOR PRACTICUM	READINESS FOR INTERNSHIP	READINESS FOR ENTRY TO PRACTICE
6A. Scientific Mindedness		
Displays critical scientific thinking	Values and applies scientific methods to professional practice	Independently applies scientific methods to practice
6B. Scientific Foundation of Psychology		
Demonstrates understanding of psychology as a science	Demonstrates intermediate level knowledge of core science (i.e., scientific bases of behavior)	Demonstrates advanced level knowledge of core science (i.e., scientific bases of behavior)

6C. Scientific Foundation of Professional Practice

Understands the scientific foundation of professional practice	Demonstrates knowledge, understanding, and application of the concept of evidence-based practice	Independently applies knowledge and understanding of scientific foundations independently applied to practice

7. Research/Evaluation: Generating research that contributes to the professional knowledge base and/ or evaluates the effectiveness of various professional activities.

READINESS FOR PRACTICUM	READINESS FOR INTERNSHIP	READINESS FOR ENTRY TO PRACTICE

7A. Scientific Approach to Knowledge Generation

Participates effectively in scientific endeavors when available	Demonstrates development of skills and habits in seeking, applying, and evaluating theoretical and research knowledge relevant to the practice of psychology	Generates knowledge

7B. Application of Scientific Method to Practice

No expectation at this level	Demonstrates knowledge of application of scientific methods to evaluating practices, interventions, and programs	Applies scientific methods of evaluating practices, interventions, and programs

IV. Application

8. Evidence-Based Practice: Integration of research and clinical expertise in the context of patient factors.

READINESS FOR PRACTICUM	READINESS FOR INTERNSHIP	READINESS FOR ENTRY TO PRACTICE

8A. Knowledge and Application of Evidence-Based Practice

Demonstrates basic knowledge of scientific, theoretical, and contextual bases of assessment, intervention, and other psychological applications; demonstrates basic knowledge of the value of evidence-based practice and its role in scientific psychology	Applies knowledge of evidence-based practice, including empirical bases of assessment, intervention, and other psychological applications, clinical expertise, and client preferences	Independently applies knowledge of evidence-based practice, including empirical bases of assessment, intervention, and other psychological applications, clinical expertise, and client preferences

9. Assessment: Assessment and diagnosis of problems, capabilities and issues associated with individuals, groups, and/or organizations.

READINESS FOR PRACTICUM	READINESS FOR INTERNSHIP	READINESS FOR ENTRY TO PRACTICE

9A. Knowledge of Measurement and Psychometrics

Demonstrates basic knowledge of the scientific, theoretical, and contextual basis of test construction and interviewing	Selects assessment measures with attention to issues of reliability and validity	Independently selects and implements multiple methods and means of evaluation in ways that are responsive to and respectful of diverse individuals, couples, families, and groups and context

(continued)

9B. Knowledge of Assessment Methods

Demonstrates basic knowledge of administration and scoring of traditional assessment measures, models, and techniques, including clinical interviewing and mental status exam	Demonstrates awareness of the strengths and limitations of administration, scoring and interpretation of traditional assessment measures as well as related technological advances	Independently understands the strengths and limitations of diagnostic approaches and interpretation of results from multiple measures for diagnosis and treatment planning

9C. Application of Assessment Methods

Demonstrates knowledge of measurement across domains of functioning and practice settings	Selects appropriate assessment measures to answer diagnostic question	Independently selects and administers a variety of assessment tools and integrates results to accurately evaluate presenting question appropriate to the practice site and broad area of practice

9D. Diagnosis

Demonstrates basic knowledge regarding the range of normal and abnormal behavior in the context of stages of human development and diversity	Applies concepts of normal/abnormal behavior to case formulation and diagnosis in the context of stages of human development and diversity	Utilizes case formulation and diagnosis for intervention planning in the context of stages of human development and diversity

9E. Conceptualization and Recommendations

Demonstrates basic knowledge of formulating diagnosis and case conceptualization	Utilizes systematic approaches of gathering data to inform clinical decision-making	Independently and accurately conceptualizes the multiple dimensions of the case based on the results of assessment

9F. Communication of Assessment Findings

Demonstrates awareness of models of report writing and progress notes	Writes assessment reports and progress notes and communicates assessment findings verbally to client	Communicates results in written and verbal form clearly, constructively, and accurately in a conceptually appropriate manner

10. Intervention: Interventions designed to alleviate suffering and to promote health and well-being of individuals, groups, and/or organizations.

READINESS FOR PRACTICUM	READINESS FOR INTERNSHIP	READINESS FOR ENTRY TO PRACTICE

10A. Intervention Planning

Displays basic understanding of the relationship between assessment and intervention	Formulates and conceptualizes cases and plans interventions utilizing at least one consistent theoretical orientation	Independently plans interventions; case conceptualizations and intervention plans are specific to case and context

10B. Skills

Displays basic helping skills	Displays clinical skills	Displays clinical skills with a wide variety of clients and uses good judgment even in unexpected or difficult situations

10C. Intervention Implementation

Demonstrates basic knowledge of intervention strategies	Implements evidence-based interventions	Implements interventions with fidelity to empirical models and flexibility to adapt where appropriate

10D. Progress Evaluation

Demonstrates basic knowledge of the assessment of intervention progress and outcome	Evaluates treatment progress and modifies treatment planning as indicated, utilizing established outcome measures	Independently evaluates treatment progress and modifies planning as indicated, even in the absence of established outcome measures

11. Consultation: The ability to provide expert guidance or professional assistance in response to a client's needs or goals.

READINESS FOR PRACTICUM	READINESS FOR INTERNSHIP	READINESS FOR ENTRY TO PRACTICE

11A. Role of Consultant

No expectation at this level	Demonstrates knowledge of the consultant's role and its unique features as distinguished from other professional roles (such as therapist, supervisor, teacher)	Determines situations that require different role functions and shifts roles accordingly to meet referral needs

11B. Addressing Referral Question

No expectation at this level	Demonstrates knowledge of and ability to select appropriate means of assessment to answer referral questions	Demonstrates knowledge of and ability to select appropriate and contextually sensitive means of assessment/data gathering that answers consultation referral question

11C. Communication of Consultation Findings

No expectation at this level	Identifies literature and knowledge about process of informing consultee of assessment findings	Applies knowledge to provide effective assessment feedback and to articulate appropriate recommendations

11D. Application of Consultation Methods

No expectation at this level	Identifies literature relevant to consultation methods (assessment and intervention) within systems, clients, or settings	Applies literature to provide effective consultative services (assessment and intervention) in most routine and some complex cases

V. Education

12. **Teaching:** Providing instruction, disseminating knowledge, and evaluating acquisition of knowledge and skill in professional psychology.		
READINESS FOR PRACTICUM	**READINESS FOR INTERNSHIP**	**READINESS FOR ENTRY TO PRACTICE**
12A. Knowledge		
No expectation at this level	Demonstrates awareness of theories of learning and how they impact teaching	Demonstrates knowledge of didactic learning strategies and how to accommodate developmental and individual differences
12B. Skills		
No expectation at this level	Demonstrates knowledge of application of teaching methods	Applies teaching methods in multiple settings

13. **Supervision:** Supervision and training in the professional knowledge base of enhancing and monitoring the professional functioning of others.		
READINESS FOR PRACTICUM	**READINESS FOR INTERNSHIP**	**READINESS FOR ENTRY TO PRACTICE**
13A. Expectations and Roles		
Demonstrates basic knowledge of expectations for supervision	Demonstrates knowledge of, purpose for, and roles in supervision	Understands the ethical, legal, and contextual issues of the supervisor role
13B. Processes and Procedures		
No expectation at this level	Identifies and tracks progress achieving the goals and tasks of supervision; demonstrates basic knowledge of supervision models and practices	Demonstrates knowledge of supervision models and practices; demonstrates knowledge of and effectively addresses limits of competency to supervise
13C. Skills Development		
Displays interpersonal skills of communication and openness to feedback	Demonstrates knowledge of the supervision literature and how clinicians develop to be skilled professionals	Engages in professional reflection about one's clinical relationships with supervisees, as well as supervisees' relationships with their clients
13D. Supervisory Practices		
No expectation at this level	Provides helpful supervisory input in peer and group supervision	Provides effective supervised supervision to less advanced students, peers, or other service providers in typical cases appropriate to the service setting

VI. Systems

14. **Interdisciplinary Systems:** Knowledge of key issues and concepts in related disciplines. Identify and interact with professionals in multiple disciplines.		
READINESS FOR PRACTICUM	**READINESS FOR INTERNSHIP**	**READINESS FOR ENTRY TO PRACTICE**
14A. Knowledge of the Shared and Distinctive Contributions of Other Professions		
No expectation at this level	Demonstrates beginning, basic knowledge of the viewpoints and contributions of other professions/professionals	Demonstrates awareness of multiple and differing world-views, roles, professional standards, and contributions across contexts and systems; demonstrates intermediate level knowledge of common and distinctive roles of other professionals
14B. Functioning in Multidisciplinary and Interdisciplinary Contexts		
Cooperates with others	Demonstrates beginning knowledge of strategies that promote interdisciplinary collaboration vs. multidisciplinary functioning	Demonstrates beginning, basic knowledge of and ability to display the skills that support effective interdisciplinary team functioning
14C. Understands how Participation in Interdisciplinary Collaboration/Consultation Enhances Outcomes		
No expectation at this level	Demonstrates knowledge of how participating in interdisciplinary collaboration/consultation can be directed toward shared goals	Participates in and initiates interdisciplinary collaboration/consultation directed toward shared goals
14D. Respectful and Productive Relationships with Individuals from Other Professions		
Demonstrates awareness of the benefits of forming collaborative relationships with other professionals	Develops and maintains collaborative relationships and respect for other professionals	Develops and maintains collaborative relationships over time despite differences
15. **Management-Administration:** Manage the direct delivery of services (DDS) and/or the administration of organizations, programs, or agencies (OPA).		
READINESS FOR PRACTICUM	**READINESS FOR INTERNSHIP**	**READINESS FOR ENTRY TO PRACTICE**
15A. Appraisal of Management and Leadership		
No expectation at this level	Forms autonomous judgment of organization's management and leadership Examples: • Applies theories of effective management and leadership to form an evaluation of organization • Identifies specific behaviors by management and leadership that promote or detract from organizational effectiveness	Develops and offers constructive criticism and suggestions regarding management and leadership of organization Examples: • Identifies strengths and weaknesses of management and leadership or organization • Provides input appropriately; participates in organizational assessment

(continued)

15B. Management		
No expectation at this level	Demonstrates awareness of roles of management in organizations	Participates in management of direct delivery of professional services; responds appropriately in management hierarchy

15C. Administration		
Complies with regulations	Demonstrates knowledge of and ability to effectively function within professional settings and organizations, including compliance with policies and procedures	Demonstrates emerging ability to participate in administration of clinical programs

15D. Leadership		
No expectation at this level	No expectation at this level	Participates in system change and management structure

16. Advocacy: Actions targeting the impact of social, political, economic, or cultural factors to promote change at the individual (client), institutional, and/or systems level.

READINESS FOR PRACTICUM	READINESS FOR INTERNSHIP	READINESS FOR ENTRY TO PRACTICE
16A. Empowerment		
Demonstrates awareness of social, political, economic, and cultural factors that impact individuals, institutions, and systems, in addition to other factors that may lead them to seek intervention	Uses awareness of the social, political, economic, or cultural factors that may impact human development in the context of service provision	Intervenes with client to promote action on factors impacting development and functioning
16B. Systems Change		
Understands the differences between individual and institutional level interventions and system's level change	Promotes change to enhance the functioning of individuals	Promotes change at the level of institutions, community, or society

APPENDIX
D

Social Work 2015 Competencies

Competency 1: Demonstrate Ethical and Professional Behavior

Social workers understand the value base of the profession and its ethical standards, as well as relevant laws and regulations that may impact practice at the micro, mezzo, and macro levels. Social workers understand frameworks of ethical decision-making and how to apply principles of critical thinking to those frameworks in practice, research, and policy arenas. Social workers recognize personal values and the distinction between personal and professional values. They also understand how their personal experiences and affective reactions influence their professional judgment and behavior. Social workers understand the profession's history, its mission, and the roles and responsibilities of the profession. Social workers also understand the role of other professions when engaged in interprofessional teams. Social workers recognize the importance of life-long learning and are committed to continually updating their skills to ensure they are relevant and effective. Social workers also understand emerging forms of technology and the ethical use of technology in social work practice. Social workers:

- make ethical decisions by applying the standards of the NASW Code of Ethics, relevant laws and regulations, models for ethical decision-making, ethical conduct of research, and additional codes of ethics as appropriate to context;
- use reflection and self-regulation to manage personal values and maintain professionalism in practice situations;
- demonstrate professional demeanor in behavior; appearance; and oral, written, and electronic communication;
- use technology ethically and appropriately to facilitate practice outcomes; and
- use supervision and consultation to guide professional judgment and behavior.

Competency 2: Engage Diversity and Difference in Practice

Social workers understand how diversity and difference characterize and shape the human experience and are critical to the formation of identity. The dimensions of diversity are understood as the intersectionality of multiple factors including but not limited to age, class, color, culture, disability and ability, ethnicity, gender, gender identity and expression, immigration status, marital status, political ideology, race, religion/spirituality, sex, sexual orientation, and tribal sovereign status. Social workers understand that, as a consequence of difference, a person's life experiences may include oppression, poverty, marginalization, and alienation as well as privilege, power, and acclaim. Social workers also understand the forms and mechanisms of oppression and discrimination and recognize the extent to which a culture's structures and values, including social, economic, political, and cultural exclusions, may oppress, marginalize, alienate, or create privilege and power. Social workers:

- apply and communicate understanding of the importance of diversity and difference in shaping life experiences in practice at the micro, mezzo, and macro levels;
- present themselves as learners and engage clients and constituencies as experts of their own experiences; and
- apply self-awareness and self-regulation to manage the influence of personal biases and values in working with diverse clients and constituencies.

Competency 3: Advance Human Rights and Social, Economic, and Environmental Justice

Social workers understand that every person regardless of position in society has fundamental human rights such as freedom, safety, privacy, an adequate standard of living, health care, and education. Social workers understand the global interconnections of oppression and human rights violations, and are knowledgeable about theories of human need and social justice and strategies to promote social and economic justice and human rights. Social workers understand strategies designed to eliminate oppressive structural barriers to ensure that social goods, rights, and responsibilities are distributed equitably and that civil, political, environmental, economic, social, and cultural human rights are protected. Social workers:

- apply their understanding of social, economic, and environmental justice to advocate for human rights at the individual and system levels; and
- engage in practices that advance social, economic, and environmental justice.

Competency 4: Engage in Practice-informed Research and Research-informed Practice

Social workers understand quantitative and qualitative research methods and their respective roles in advancing a science of social work and in evaluating their practice. Social workers know the principles of logic, scientific inquiry, and culturally informed and ethical approaches to building knowledge. Social workers understand that evidence that informs practice derives from multidisciplinary sources and multiple ways of knowing.

They also understand the processes for translating research findings into effective practice. Social workers:

- use practice experience and theory to inform scientific inquiry and research;
- apply critical thinking to engage in analysis of quantitative and qualitative research methods and research findings; and
- use and translate research evidence to inform and improve practice, policy, and service delivery.

Competency 5: Engage in Policy Practice

Social workers understand that human rights and social justice, as well as social welfare and services, are mediated by policy and its implementation at the federal, state, and local levels. Social workers understand the history and current structures of social policies and services, the role of policy in service delivery, and the role of practice in policy development. Social workers understand their role in policy development and implementation within their practice settings at the micro, mezzo, and macro levels and they actively engage in policy practice to effect change within those settings. Social workers recognize and understand the historical, social, cultural, economic, organizational, environmental, and global influences that affect social policy. They are also knowledgeable about policy formulation, analysis, implementation, and evaluation. Social workers:

- identify social policy at the local, state, and federal level that impacts well-being, service delivery, and access to social services;
- assess how social welfare and economic policies impact the delivery of and access to social services;
- apply critical thinking to analyze, formulate, and advocate for policies that advance human rights and social, economic, and environmental justice.

Competency 6: Engage with Individuals, Families, Groups, Organizations, and Communities

Social workers understand that engagement is an ongoing component of the dynamic and interactive process of social work practice with, and on behalf of, diverse individuals, families, groups, organizations, and communities. Social workers value the importance of human relationships. Social workers understand theories of human behavior and the social environment, and critically evaluate and apply this knowledge to facilitate engagement with clients and constituencies, including individuals, families, groups, organizations, and communities. Social workers understand strategies to engage diverse clients and constituencies to advance practice effectiveness. Social workers understand how their personal experiences and affective reactions may impact their ability to effectively engage with diverse clients and constituencies. Social workers value principles of relationship-building and interprofessional collaboration to facilitate engagement with clients, constituencies, and other professionals as appropriate. Social workers:

- apply knowledge of human behavior and the social environment, person-in-environment, and other multidisciplinary theoretical frameworks to engage with clients and constituencies; and
- use empathy, reflection, and interpersonal skills to effectively engage diverse clients and constituencies.

Competency 7: Assess Individuals, Families, Groups, Organizations, and Communities

Social workers understand that assessment is an ongoing component of the dynamic and interactive process of social work practice with, and on behalf of, diverse individuals, families, groups, organizations, and communities. Social workers understand theories of human behavior and the social environment, and critically evaluate and apply this knowledge in the assessment of diverse clients and constituencies, including individuals, families, groups, organizations, and communities. Social workers understand methods of assessment with diverse clients and constituencies to advance practice effectiveness. Social workers recognize the implications of the larger practice context in the assessment process and value the importance of interprofessional collaboration in this process. Social workers understand how their personal experiences and affective reactions may affect their assessment and decision-making. Social workers:

- collect and organize data, and apply critical thinking to interpret information from clients and constituencies;
- apply knowledge of human behavior and the social environment, person-in-environment, and other multidisciplinary theoretical frameworks in the analysis of assessment data from clients and constituencies;
- develop mutually agreed-on intervention goals and objectives based on the critical assessment of strengths, needs, and challenges within clients and constituencies; and
- select appropriate intervention strategies based on the assessment, research knowledge, and values and preferences of clients and constituencies.

Competency 8: Intervene with Individuals, Families, Groups, Organizations, and Communities

Social workers understand that intervention is an ongoing component of the dynamic and interactive process of social work practice with, and on behalf of, diverse individuals, families, groups, organizations, and communities. Social workers are knowledgeable about evidence-informed interventions to achieve the goals of clients and constituencies, including individuals, families, groups, organizations, and communities. Social workers understand theories of human behavior and the social environment, and critically evaluate and apply this knowledge to effectively intervene with clients and constituencies. Social workers understand methods of identifying, analyzing, and implementing evidence-informed interventions to achieve client and constituency goals. Social workers value the importance of interprofessional teamwork and communication in interventions, recognizing that beneficial outcomes may require interdisciplinary, interprofessional, and interorganizational collaboration. Social workers:

- critically choose and implement interventions to achieve practice goals and enhance capacities of clients and constituencies;
- apply knowledge of human behavior and the social environment, person-in-environment, and other multidisciplinary theoretical frameworks in interventions with clients and constituencies;
- use interprofessional collaboration as appropriate to achieve beneficial practice outcomes;
- negotiate, mediate, and advocate with and on behalf of diverse clients and constituencies; and
- facilitate effective transitions and endings that advance mutually agreed-on goals.

Competency 9: Evaluate Practice with Individuals, Families, Groups, Organizations, and Communities

Social workers understand that evaluation is an ongoing component of the dynamic and interactive process of social work practice with, and on behalf of, diverse individuals, families, groups, organizations, and communities. Social workers recognize the importance of evaluating processes and outcomes to advance practice, policy, and service delivery effectiveness. Social workers understand theories of human behavior and the social environment, and critically evaluate and apply this knowledge in evaluating outcomes. Social workers understand qualitative and quantitative methods for evaluating outcomes and practice effectiveness. Social workers:

- select and use appropriate methods for evaluation of outcomes;
- apply knowledge of human behavior and the social environment, person-in-environment, and other multidisciplinary theoretical frameworks in the evaluation of outcomes;
- critically analyze, monitor, and evaluate intervention and program processes and outcomes; and
- apply evaluation findings to improve practice effectiveness at the micro, mezzo, and macro levels.

Index